The Fetus as a Patient

THE EVOLVING CHALLENGE

The Fetus as a Patient

THE EVOLVING CHALLENGE

Edited by

Frank A. Chervenak

New York Presbyterian Hospital – Cornell Medical Center,
New York, USA

Asim Kurjak

Department of Obstetrics and Gynecology,
University of Zagreb, Croatia

Zoltan Papp

1st Department of Obstetrics and Gynaecology,
Semmelweis University, Budapest, Hungary

The Parthenon Publishing Group
International Publishers in Medicine, Science & Technology

A CRC PRESS COMPANY

BOCA RATON   LONDON   NEW YORK   WASHINGTON, D.C.

Library of Congress Cataloging-in-Publication Data

Data available on request

British Library Cataloguing-in-Publication Data

The fetus as a patient: the evolving challenge
  1. Fetus – Diseases 2. Fetus – Abnormalities
  3. Fetus – Diseases – Diagnosis 4. Perinatology
  I. Chervenak, Frank A. II. Kurjak, Asim
  III. Papp, Z.
  618.3'2

ISBN 1-84214-157-0

Published in the USA by
The Parthenon Publishing Group
345 Park Avenue South
10th Floor
New York, NY 10010, USA

Published in the UK and Europe by
The Parthenon Publishing Group
23–25 Blades Court
Deodar Road
London SW15 2NU, UK

Copyright © 2002
The Parthenon Publishing Group

*No part of this book may be reproduced in any form
without permission from the publishers, except for the
quotation of brief passages for the purposes of review.*

Typeset by Speedlith Photo Litho Ltd, Manchester, UK
Printed and bound by Bookcraft (Bath) Ltd.,
Midsomer Norton, UK

Contents

Section 4   Current perspectives on clinical perinatology

List of principal contributors

A.J. Antsaklis
Division of Maternal Fetal Medicine
University of Athens
Athens
Greece

D. Blickstein
Institute of Hematology
Rabin Medical Center, Beilinson Campus
49100 Petach Tikva
Israel

I. Blickstein
Department of Obstetrics and Gynecology
Kaplan Medical Center
76100 Rehovot
Israel

S.T. Chasen
Department of Obstetrics and Gynecology
Weill Medical College of Cornell University
525 East 68th Street
New York
NY 10021
USA

F.A. Chervenak
Department of Obstetrics and Gynecology
New York Presbyterian Hospital
Weill Medical College of Cornell University
525 East 68th Street
New York
NY 10021
USA

L. Cornette
Division of Paediatrics and Child Health
Leeds General Infirmary
Leeds LS2 9NS
UK

E.V. Cosmi
2nd Institute of Obstetrics and Gynecology
University of Rome
'La Sapienza'
324-00161 Rome
Italy

V. D'Addario
4th Unit of Obstetrics and Gynecology
University Medical School of Bari
Policlinico
Piazza G. Cesare
70124 Bari
Italy

G.C. Di Renzo
Center of Perinatal and Reproductive Medicine
University Hospital Monteluce
06122 Perugia
Italy

M.Y. Divon
Department of Obstetrics and Gynecology
Lenox-Hill Hospital
100 East 77th Street
New York
NY 10021
USA

M.I. Evans
Department of Obstetrics and Gynecology
MCP Hahnemann University
245 North 15th Street
MS 495
Philadelphia, PA 19102
USA

S. Kupesic
Department of Obstetrics and Gynecology
Medical School, University of Zagreb
Sveti Duh Hospital
Sveti Duh 64
10000 Zagreb
Croatia

A. Kurjak
Department of Obstetrics and Gynecology
Medical School, University of Zagreb
Sveti Duh Hospital
Sveti Duh 64
10000 Zagreb
Croatia

J.J.A.M. Laudy
Department of Obstetrics and Gynecology
University Hospital Rotterdam
Dr. Molewaterplein 40
3015 GD Rotterdam
The Netherlands

K. Maeda
Department of Obstetrics and Gynecology
Seirei Mikatahara Hospital
Hamamatsu
Japan

G.P. Mandruzzato
Department of Obstetrics and Gynecology
Istituto per l'Infanzia
Via dell'Istria 65/1
34100 Trieste
Italy

M. Mahran
Department of Obstetrics and Gynecology
Ain Shams University
P.O.B. 1036
Cairo
Egypt

E. Mathieu
Service de Gynécologie Obstétrique et
    Médecine de la Reproduction
Hôpital Tenon
4 rue de la Chine
75020 Paris
France

A. Matias
Department of Obstetrics and Gynecology
Faculty of Medicine
University Hospital of S. João
4200 Porto
Portugal

P. Merviel
Department of Gynecology, Obstetrics and
    Reproductive Medicine
Hôpital Tenon
4 rue de la Chine
75020 Paris
France

G. Monni
Department of Obstetrics and Gynecology
Prenatal & Preimplantation Genetic Diagnosis
    – Fetal Therapy
Ospedale Regionale Microcitemie
Via Jenner s/n – 09121 Cagliari
Italy

J.P. Newnham
Department of Obstetrics and Gynecology
The University of Western Australia
King Edward Memorial Hospital
374 Bagot Road, Subiaco
Perth
Western Australia 608
Australia

Z. Papp
1st Department of Obstetrics and Gynecology
Faculty of Medicine
Semmelweis University
Barossa utca 27
1088 Budapest
Hungary

R.K. Pooh
Department of Perinatology
Taijukai-Keisei General Hospital
3-5-28 Muromachi
Sakaide City
Kagawa 762-0007
Japan

R.A. Quintero
Florida Institute for Fetal Diagnosis and
    Therapy
13601 Bruce B. Downs Boulevard, Suite 160
Tampa, FL 33613
USA

R. Romero
Perinatology Research Branch
National Institute of Child Health and
  Human Development
Department of Obstetrics – Gynecology
Hutzel Hospital
4707 St. Antoine Boulevard
Detroit, MI 48201
USA

J.G. Schenker
Department of Obstetrics and Gynecology
Hadassah Medical Center
PO Box 12000
The Hebrew University
91120 Jerusalem
Israel

T. Stefos
Department of Obstetrics – Gynecology
University of Ioannina
Greece

H. Takeuchi
Department of Obstetrics and Gynecology
Sanno Hospital
8-10-16 Akasaka
Minato-ku
Tokyo 107-0052
Japan

V. Váradi
St. Margaret Hospital
Bécsi u. 132
Budapest H-1032
Hungary

L.S. Voto
Fundacion Miguel Margulies
Juncal 2186
1125 Buenos Aires
Argentina

H.N. Winn
Division of Maternal–Fetal Medicine
St. Mary's Health Center
6420 Clayton Road
St. Louis, MO 63117
USA

C. Yabes-Almirante
Perinatal Center
Philippine Children's Medical Center
Quezon Avenue
Quezon City
The Philippines

J.H. Yang
Department of Obstetrics and Gynecology
Yonsei University College of Medicine
Seoul
South Korea

I.E. Zador
Department of Obstetrics and Gynecology
Wayne State University
Hutzel Hospital
4707 St. Antoine Boulevard
Detroit, MI 48201
USA

Color plates

Color Plate A Power Doppler reveals the onset of heart activity

Color Plate B Vascular anatomy of 8-week-old embryo. Note the abdominal aorta with the umbilical artery branching at the caudal pole. The umbilical vein can be followed from the abdominal umbilical insertion through the fetal liver, and ending below the heart

Color Plate C A normal embryo at 9 weeks' gestation. Three-dimensional power Doppler reveals the entire embryonic circulation obtained from different angles

Color Plate D Surface view of the fetus at 10 weeks' gestation. Three-dimensional ultrasound allows simultaneous visualization of the fetal anatomy and corresponding circulation. The entire fetal circulation is presented from different angles. The aorta and umbilical vessels are prominent. Vessels responsible for perfusion of the brain can be seen at the base of the skull. Because of the development of the central nervous system, body movements are very rich and complex

Color Plate E A fetus at 12 weeks of gestation. Note the two major vascular supplies to the brain: the internal carotid artery and the vertebral artery. Three-dimensional power Doppler sonography precisely depicts the spatial relationship of the vessels and bones of the skull

Color Plate F The blood supply to the choroid plexus has some particular characteristics. Detected by pulsed spectral Doppler, arterial blood flow velocity waveforms show pandiastolic flow earlier than any other embryonic artery. This is evidence that, at this gestational age, a great portion of cerebral perfusion is directed to the choroid plexus

Color Plate G Transvaginal color Doppler scan of an 8-week gestation complicated by retrochorionic hematoma. Spiral arteries and embryonic heart activity are clearly displayed

Color Plate H Transvaginal color Doppler sonogram of uterine vessels in a case of retrochorionic hematoma. Blood flow signals extracted from radial arteries demonstrate the absence of diastolic flow ($RI = 1.0$)

Color Plate I Transvaginal color Doppler scan of missed abortion at 8 weeks' gestation. Color Doppler reveals blood flow within the maternal vessels and absence of flow in the fetal vessels. Note the hydropic degeneration of the yolk sac demonstrated by the increased diameter and altered echogenicity

Color Plate J Transvaginal color Doppler scan of a richly vascularized blighted ovum. Color Doppler facilitates the visualization of dilated spiral arteries in close proximity to the empty gestational sac

Color Plate K Transvaginal color Doppler scan of another case of anembryonic pregnancy. Note the irregular shape of the empty gestational sac and discrete blood flow signals at its periphery

Color Plate L Transvaginal color Doppler scan of blood flow signals obtained from the intervillous space. Note the low vascular resistance of artery-like signals ($RI = 0.39$) characteristic of this pathology

Color Plate M Transvaginal color Doppler scan of missed abortion. Note the prominent blood flow signals obtained from maternal vessels and the absence of fetal heart activity

Color Plate N Increased resistance index ($RI = 0.51$) of the artery-like signal within the intervillous space obtained in a patient with missed abortion

Color Plate O Transvaginal color Doppler scan of retained products of conception

Color Plate P The fetal pulmonary circulation visualized with color Doppler from a cross-section of the fetal chest at the level of the cardiac four-chamber view. Sp, fetal spine; H, fetal heart. (Reprinted with permission from Laudy JJAM, *et al*. The fetal lung 2: Pulmonary hypoplasia. *Ultrasound Obstet Gynecol* 2000;16: 482–90)

Color Plate Q Metaphase images obtained following hybridization of the degenerate oligonucleotide primed polymerase chain reaction (DOP-PCR) product from a single female fetus cell labelled with Spectrum Green together with the DOP-PCR product from normal female DNA labelled with Spectrum Red. The fluorescence ratios for all chromosomes are within the cut-off threshold of 0.8–1.2

Color Plate R Comparative genomic hybridization fluorescent ratio profiles obtained following hybridization of the degenerate oligonucleotide primed polymerase chain reaction (DOP-PCR) product from a single female fetus cell labelled with Spectrum Green together with the DOP-PCR product from normal female DNA labelled with Spectrum Red. The fluorescence ratios for all chromosomes are within the cut-off threshold of 0.8–1.2

Color Plate S Metaphase images obtained following hybridization of the degenerate

oligonucleotide primed polymerase chain reaction (DOP-PCR) product from a single trisomy 21 male fetus cell labelled with Spectrum Green together with the DOP-PCR product from normal female DNA labelled with Spectrum Red. The fluorescence ratios for all chromosomes except 21 and X are within the cut-off threshold of 0.8–1.2. The profile for the X chromosome shows a deviation to the left and the profile for chromosome 21 shows a deviation to the right, indicating increased copy number for 21 in the test cell

Color Plate T Comparative genomic hybridization fluorescent ratio profiles obtained following hybridization of the degenerate oligonucleotide primed polymerase chain reaction (DOP-PCR) product from a single female fetus cell labelled with Spectrum Green together with the DOP-PCR product from normal female DNA labelled with Spectrum Red. The fluorescence ratios for all chromosomes are within the cut-off threshold of 0.8–1.2. The profile for the X chromosome shows a deviation to the left and the profile for chromosome 21 shows a deviation to the right, indicating increased copy number for 21 in the test cell

Color Plate U Three-dimensional reconstruction of trophoblastic erosion of endometrial capillaries at 6 weeks' gestation

Color Plate V Angio four-dimensional reconstruction of trophoblastic erosion of endometrial capillaries

Color Plate W Three-dimensional color Doppler right uterine artery coupled with protodiastolic notch in a pregnant woman at 9 weeks' gestation, age 38 years, gravida 1, para 0. Note the high resistance index (RI) (0.99).

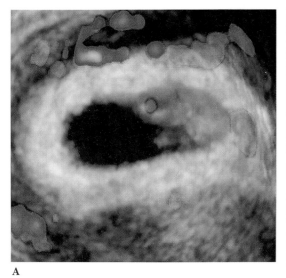

A

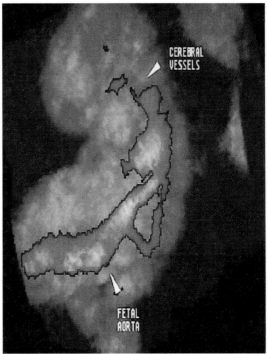

B

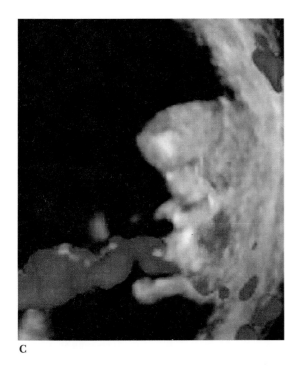

C

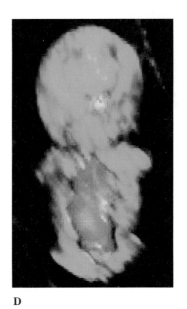

D

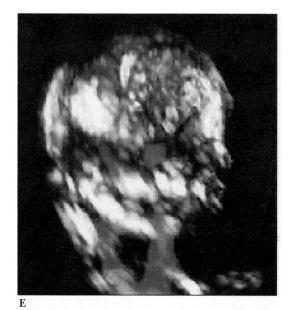

E

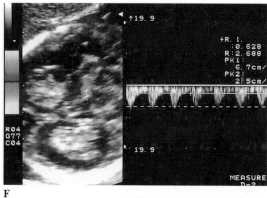

F

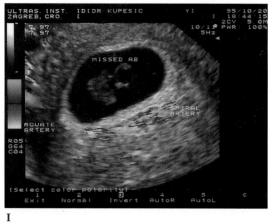

G

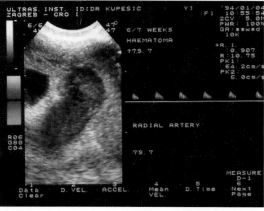

H

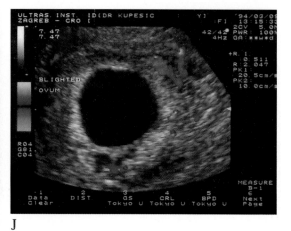

I

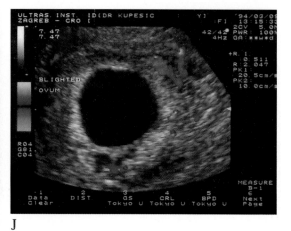

J

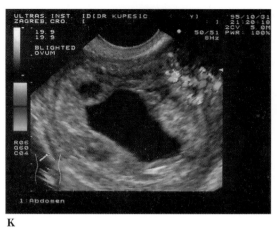

K

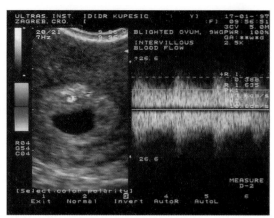

L

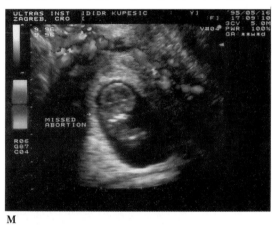

M

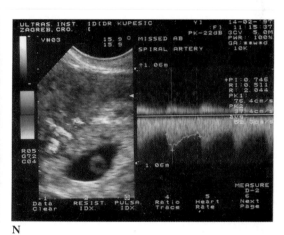

N

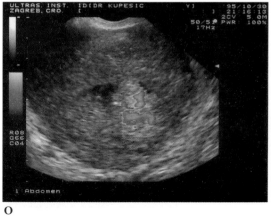

O

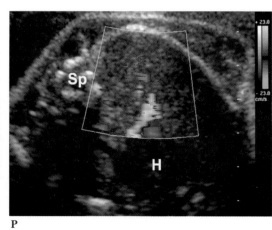

P

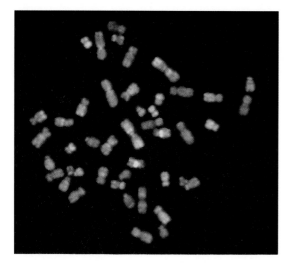

Q

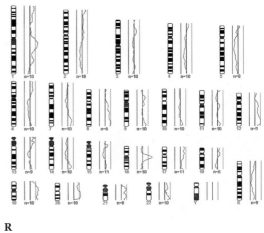

R

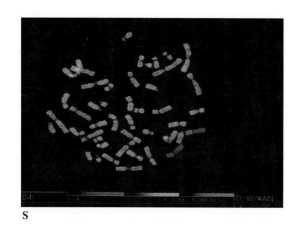

S

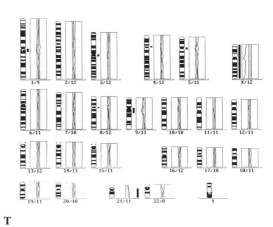

T

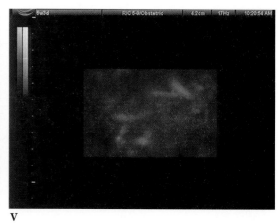

U

V

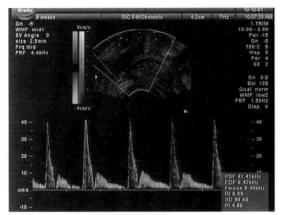

W

Foreword

The International Society of the Fetus as a Patient is dedicated to improving all dimensions of fetal diagnosis and therapy. This book, *The Fetus as a Patient: The Evolving Challenge*, bears testament to the current work of the Board of Directors and invited speakers of our Society.

The introductory chapter addresses the moral foundations of leadership in fetal medicine and defines both the virtues that leaders should strive for as well as the vices that they should avoid.

More than any other modality, ultrasound permits visualization of the fetus and fetal diagnosis. New developments in three-dimensional and color Doppler ultrasound permit new insights into early embryonic structure and function. These insights enhance the physician's ability to address such clinical topics as threatened abortion and ectopic pregnancy, and diagnosis of fetal anomalies, especially brain abnormalities. This section closes with a quintessential example of the application of ultrasound technology to a clinical challenge, the sonographic examination of the uterine cervix and its application to clinical medicine.

Section 2 highlights the state of the art of prenatal diagnosis and therapy. Counselling regarding the important topics of pre-embryonic research, genetic counselling and prenatal informed consent for sonogram are addressed. The prenatal diagnosis of hemoglobinopathies and the evaluation of fetal blood in the maternal circulation are reviewed, as well as the important invasive procedures of amniocentesis and selective reduction.

Section 3 tackles the continuing challenge of fetal assessment. Cardiotocography, ultrasound imaging, Doppler ultrasound and the analysis of nucleated red blood cells are used to address the important topics of intrauterine growth restriction, macrosomia and multiple gestations, including the especially problematic twin-to-twin transfusion syndrome. Hydrops in both its immune and non-immune forms is analyzed as well as the continuing challenge of the diagnosis of intrapartum asphyxia.

Current perspectives on clinical perinatology are presented in the last section on a wide variety of clinical topics, including the Internet, low-molecular-weight heparin, breast cancer, substance abuse, toxoplasmosis, the use of antenatal steroids, pre-eclampsia and neonatal intensive care.

The editors are grateful to the Board of Directors and invited speakers of the International Society of the Fetus as a Patient. They have each made a special effort to present their best current work in a concise and clinically valuable fashion. Each contribution, while unique, blends together with the others to reflect the scope of the evolving challenge of the fetus as a patient.

Frank A. Chervenak
Asim Kurjak
Zoltan Papp

The moral foundations of leadership in fetal medicine

1

F. A. Chervenak, L. B. McCullough, A. Kurjak and Z. Papp

Leadership in fetal medicine requires both managerial and moral excellence[1]. In ancient Greece, Plato argued in *The Republic* that the ideal leader is someone who commits himself to and is trained for a life of service and devotion to fellow citizens[2]. The power of the philosopher–king should be directed to the good of others in order for that power to have moral authority. When directed primarily to self-interest, Plato also taught, such power and authority corrupts its holders and becomes dangerous. In other words, leadership requires competence and the direction of that competence toward the good of others.

Plato would recognize and endorse the following description of leadership from the Drucker Foundation[3]. This foundation was established by Peter F. Drucker, internationally recognized as one of the leading scholars of business management.

> Leadership without direction is useless. Uninformed by ideas about what is good and bad, right and wrong, worthy and unworthy, it is not only inconsistent, but dangerous. As the pace of change in our world continues to accelerate, strong basic values become increasingly necessary to guide leadership behavior.

This view is echoed in current texts on leadership and management[4–6]. Physicians are familiar with the far-reaching changes in the structure and financing of medical care. Physician–leaders must provide the right direction for this change. We cannot, and therefore should not, look to insurance companies or the government to provide this needed direction.

The first component of leadership, which is essential, is managerial: mastery of the management knowledge and skills necessary to protect the organization's economic interests and organize its human and material resources[3–6]. In years past in the USA, when there were seemingly unlimited sources of funding from indemnity insurers and the government, the level of management knowledge and skill required of medical leaders was low. With the advent of managed care in its many forms and the changes in Medicare and Medicaid reimbursements, the level of management skills required of physician–leaders has risen enormously. Management styles that had been successful in the past, in an era of economic abundance in health care, are at risk for becoming prescriptions for failure today in an era of quality and cost control. It should be obvious that mastery of the complex knowledge and skills required to manage the contemporary health-care organization in conditions of economic scarcity is essential for medical leadership. A crucial antidote to disillusionment with some physician–leaders is that they become competent managers. In the absence of such competence, creating and sustaining a culture of professionalism in fetal medicine becomes impossible.

In our view, competent management skills are a necessary, but not sufficient, condition for leadership in fetal medicine. As Plato and The Drucker Foundation would teach us, management skills can be used, on the one hand, in the pursuit of the goal of excellence in patient care, medical education, and clinical and basic science research, with the protection of the organization's economic interest an important means for achieving this goal[6]. On the other hand, the protection of the organization's economic interest can become the end or overriding goal of management decisions[7]. We should not lead our institutions toward this latter goal. Instead, we should lead on the basis of a core concept in the history of medical ethics, the physician as the moral fiduciary of the patient. The purpose of this paper is to argue for this core concept of medical ethics as the moral foundation of medical leadership in fetal medicine and to argue for the role of physician–leaders in creating and sustaining a moral culture of professionalism in fetal medicine.

PHYSICIAN AS FIDUCIARY

The concept of the physician as the fiduciary of the patient was introduced into the English-language literature of medical ethics by Dr John Gregory (1724–73)[8], and into the ethics of health-care organizations by Dr Thomas Percival (1740–1803)[9]. Their ideas crossed the Atlantic and influenced American medical ethics, starting in the 18th century with Benjamin Rush, continuing in the 19th century with the American Medical Association's *Code of Ethics* of 1847, and defining the professional nature of the doctor–patient relationship to this day[10–12]. Their work in medical ethics was also widely influential in Europe. Pelligrino and Thomasma have emphasized the central role of the virtues of this relationship[13].

Gregory and Percival described fiduciary physicians and organizations in a way that Plato would recognize and that anticipates contemporary literature on leadership and management. Physicians and health-care institutions should act primarily to protect and promote the interests of patients, keep self-interest in a systematically secondary position, and have confidence that a commitment to scientific and moral excellence in patient care will result in the long run in sufficient remuneration and deserved prestige[14]. Making the pursuit and protection of economic interests the primary goal of patient care in fetal medicine is unethical, because doing so undermines the physician's ability to maintain his or her professionalism.

Gregory took the maintenance of professionalism to be the task and responsibility of individual physicians. Physicians should form their character and conduct themselves in practice by accepting the requirements of the concept of the physician as fiduciary of the patient. Percival was one of the first in the history of medical ethics to understand that, in the setting of the hospital and other health-care organizations, successful maintenance of professionalism also vitally depended on the moral culture of the organization, especially the decisions of those responsible for leading and managing it. In the era of managed care in the USA and limited resources in other countries, and the consequent need to improve quality and control costs, maintenance of professionalism depends even more on the decisions of managers and the moral culture that their decisions create in a health-care organization. Physicians can no longer maintain their professionalism alone. Creating and sustaining a moral culture of profession-alism in health-care organizations therefore requires moral leadership. Moral leadership means that physician–leaders should make the concept of the physician as fiduciary the moral foundation of their management decisions about patient care[7,15], medical education[7,16] and clinical research[7].

FOUR PROFESSIONAL VIRTUES

From Gregory and Percival came four professional virtues that form the moral basis of the professional, fiduciary relationship of physician to patient[14]. These virtues are self-effacement, self-sacrifice, compassion and integrity[17]. In the clinical setting, self-effacement means that clinical judgement should not be affected by differences between doctors and patients, such as class, gender and race, that can introduce irrelevant and destructive bias into clinical judgement and practice[18,19]. Similarly, self-effacement requires physician–leaders to be unbiased by such factors as their own specialty or subspecialty, friends and colleagues, gender or ethnicity, and other factors that could result in arbitrary and unfair treatment of subordinates.

In the clinical setting, self-sacrifice means that the physician should be willing to take reasonable risks to himself or herself regarding such forms of self-interest as health, income and job security when required to do so to meet the needs of patients[13,17]. Similarly, the physician–leader should be willing to restrain self-interest, including organizational self-interest, as required for subordinates to sustain their primary focus on their fiduciary responsibilities to patients, trainees, or research subjects. The physician–leader should also be willing to take risks to job security, as required to create a moral culture of the organization defined by professionalism, grounded in the fiduciary obligations of physicians and health-care organizations to their patients.

In the clinical setting, compassion means that the physician should always be aware of the patient's pain, suffering and distress, and promptly seek to ameliorate them[13,17]. The main obligation in compassion of the physician–leader is to the physician–patient relationship and its fiduciary character. For physician–leaders, compassion requires recognition of two kinds of suffering and distress on the part of their colleagues. The first kind occurs when the physician's ability to meet fiduciary obligations to patients is adversely affected by decisions to ration resources that do not take those fiduciary obligations into account, and from serious threats to legitimate self-interests of subordinates for adequate income and job security as institutions cut services and downsize. The second kind of stress occurs when the physician experiences reductions in resources that can be shown to be consistent with fulfilling fiduciary obligations to patients. The physician–leader, out of compassion, may be obliged to commiserate with colleagues experiencing this second kind of stress in response to change, but to actively review and, if necessary, change his or her management decisions in response to the first kind of stress. In this respect, the physician–leader should routinely ask subordinates, 'What can I do to help?'.

In the clinical setting, integrity requires the physician to practice fetal medicine according to standards of intellectual and moral excellence[13,17]. This does *not* mean doing the most for patients, but what will benefit them clinically according to evidence and rigorous clinical judgement. Integrity requires the physician–leader to make management decisions based on scientific evidence, well-documented outcomes, reliable, well-formed clinical judgements and sound, balanced economic judgements, especially at the interface between professional colleagues and organizational resources[6]. Essential to integrity is open and honest communication with subordinates and accountability for the bases of management decisions. In this way the physician–leader creates and sustains a moral culture of professionalism in fetal medicine, i.e. a stable, transparent pattern of management decisions that sustains doctor–patient relationships in the organization as moral fiduciary relationships. Part of open communication is accessibility, e.g. not using subordinate administrators or staff to buffer or block access.

FOUR VICES

Corresponding to these four professional virtues are vices, which physician–leaders in fetal medicine should rigorously avoid. In the clinical setting unwarranted bias, the antithesis of self-effacement, harms patients. An example is the psychological harm done to women who have experienced romantic or sexual overtures or contact from their doctors[20]. For the physician–leader, negative bias based on race or gender can lead to unethical and even illegal forms of discrimination in hiring or promotion. The more insidious version of this vice takes the form of positive bias in hiring or promotion or the allocation of resources based on gender, personal relationship, or shared specialty or subspecialty. When institutions merge, this vice can take the form of favoring departments or individuals in one's home institution when those departments or individuals are not objectively better than their counterparts in the merger partner. Physician–leaders in managed care who preferentially contract work to friends or former associates show similar unwarranted bias. Self-effacement requires the physician–leader to be rigorously impartial in all decisions about employment, promotion, contracting for services and allocation of resources.

In the clinical setting, self-sacrifice is violated when physicians put self-interest above the health-related interests of patients, e.g. referring less frequently than warranted to maximize their year-end payment under a withhold-compensation plan. The clinical investigator violates self-sacrifice when he or she uses the 'thumb screw of persuasion'[21] in order to put undue pressure on their own patients to enroll in their own clinical trials, or when he or she advertises for subjects in a potentially misleading way, problems from which fetal medicine is not free. The academic physician–leader violates self-sacrifice when, as a chairman or division chief, he or she insists on being senior author on every paper coming from the department or division, a form of self-aggrandizement and arrogance that threatens the intellectual and moral integrity of the academic enterprise. The managed-care physician–leader who inappropriately denies appeals for expensive medical care in order to maximize his or her year-end bonus acts on greed, which at best threatens and at worst undermines the culture of professionalism and therefore the fiduciary relationships of colleagues, contributing to a morally corrupt organizational culture. The physician–leader who claims attention, especially in the electronic media, for the clinical work or innovation of subordinates compromises the virtue of self-sacrifice. Self-sacrifice requires the physician–leader to be other-directed, not self-directed, and to display humility by focusing on the professional interests of subordinates, not on his or her own money, prestige or power[3].

In clinical practice, physicians violate compassion when they are indifferent to the pain, suffering and distress of their patients. When physicians confront unavoidable pain and suffering, or must cause it themselves in order to help patients, compassion requires them to do so reluctantly, so that they will not overlook less painful or stressful alternatives, e.g. considering a trial of vaginal delivery after a Cesarean section. The physician–leader who

utilizes salary freezes, salary reductions, or terminations, in order to control costs for justifiable reasons of overall organizational well-being, but who does not also take serious account of the impact of such decisions on the lives of employees and their families lacks compassion. For example, rather than taking the expeditious course of termination, compassion for an employee who might still be of value to the organization argues for working with that individual to be productive and contribute to the organization's goals. When physicians lack compassion they become hard-hearted, against which Gregory warned us[8]. Hard-heartedness damages the moral sensibilities of the physician, therefore threatening the fiduciary relationship. The physician–leader who seeks productivity improvement by demanding that everyone do more with less, but without seriously considering the professional and personal impact on subordinates, lacks compassion and risks creating a work environment that is exploitative and even inhumane. Such an environment is antithetical to the moral culture of a fiduciary health-care organization. The physician–leader who never sees patients risks diminution of the moral sensibilities required of physicians and thus risks indifference to or an invidious distance from the professional life of colleagues. Such a physician–leader would be of little help, for example, to their colleagues who experience a catastrophic loss of unexpected mortality from an unexpected pulmonary embolism after a normal vaginal delivery. Compassion requires the physician–leader consistently to evaluate each physician's behavior and contributions to the organization from the perspective of the clinician on the front line.

The physician in practice violates integrity when he or she tells a hospitalized patient that the payor requires the physician to order early discharge when the real reason is that the physician is trying to avoid becoming an outlier regarding length-of-stay after Cesarean delivery. This is deception in the form of a lie. Deception can take more subtle forms, such as providing incomplete information to the patient or using terms that are deliberately ambiguous, e.g.

quoting success rates for assisted reproduction and level of risk for Cesarean delivery from the literature only, but leaving out one's own experience, or implying that medical students are doctors by introducing them as 'my associates'. In addition, the physician who refuses, despite overwhelming evidence, to take responsibility for a bad outcome violates integrity. Lofty mission statements, promulgated by 'leaders' whose own behavior contradicts and even undermines the values expressed in those mission statements, create a Kafkaesque organizational culture that corrupts everyone in it.

When physician–leaders try to avoid accountability for both action and inaction by saying different things to different subordinates, thus creating obfuscation and stress, they lack integrity. Frank deception may be less of a problem than such strategic ambiguity. A medical director of a managed-care plan who makes allocation decisions about medical necessity or appropriateness about non-excluded clinical intervention that results in harm to patients, and subsequently hides behind the language of the law or claims that he or she is simply making a business – not a clinical – decision, lacks integrity[7]. Similarly, physician–leaders who blame others for poor administrative decisions as a way to avoid accountability lack integrity. When a physician–leader creates or exploits levels of organizational bureaucracy to diffuse and therefore avoid accountability for decisions that he or she has made, he or she lacks integrity. In summary, such physician–leaders corrupt themselves and their organizations, by putting self-interest – in power, authority, income, or job security – ahead of their obligation to sustain a moral organizational culture of fiduciary service to patients. Integrity requires the physician–leader to be open and honest in all communications with subordinates and to be accountable to subordinates for management decisions. Fulfilling this obligation requires the physician–leader to prevent obfuscation in bureaucratic structures and not to exploit it when it emanates from such structures.

As we have noted already in several places, whether the physician–leader makes virtues or vices the basis of his or her management decisions and organizational policy matters vitally to the moral life of health-care organizations, because virtues are the right direction and vices the wrong direction. The tools of medical management, such as finance, communication and strategic planning, are indifferent to whether the physician–leader uses them with virtuous or vicious foundations. When a physician–leader consistently uses institutional power and authority as an advocate for the professional virtues of the physician as a moral fiduciary of the patient and physician–patient relationships based on these virtues, he or she will create and sustain a moral culture of professionalism in his or her organization. This will be preventive ethics at its best, in the service of professionalism.

When physician–leaders follow the vices described here, they create an organizational culture of unbridled self-interest, which undermines fiduciary responsibility and therefore professionalism. Such an organizational culture is antithetical to the moral life of service that defines the physician as the fiduciary of the patient. This would be an organizational culture devoid of moral worth, occupied by physicians who would, in T.S. Eliott's words, be 'hollow men' and 'stuffed men'[22], working in the 'dead land'. This is indeed the world we will find ourselves in, if too many physician–leaders lead fetal medicine in the wrong direction.

CONCLUSION

Ancient thinkers of both the West, such as Plato[2], and the East, such as Confucius[23], argued, correctly, that living according to the virtues we have described here sustains leaders and their subordinates in ways that money, prestige and power cannot. Gregory echoes this thinking when he tells his readers that the trust of patients, which is earned by living according to these virtues, cannot be 'purchased by the wealth of India'[8]. In our view, a physician–leader today is defined as the fiduciary of the professionalism of the doctor–patient relationship in clinical practice, medical education and medical research[7,15]. The professional virtues of self-effacement, self-sacrifice, compassion and integrity – rather than the vices of unwarranted bias, the primacy of self-interest, hard-heartedness and corruption – should provide the moral foundation of the physician–leader's motivations, decisions and actions. The physician–leader who acts on these virtues will lead fetal medicine in the right direction, toward a moral culture of professionalism.

This is crucial, because institutions play a central role in fetal medicine. Patients are 'covered lives', the responsibility of large organizations such as managed-care organizations, physician–hospital alliances and academic practice plans. Because individual physicians specializing in fetal medicine discharge their fiduciary obligations in and through institutions, the moral culture of health-care organizations has become a vital element in sustaining their professionalism. Physician–leaders, along with individual physicians in practice, bear the responsibility for shaping organizations' cultures that support the fiduciary professionalism of physicians with daily responsibility for patient care, medical education and research. All three are vital to the ongoing development and success of fetal medicine. Fiduciary professionalism provides the moral foundation for directing that development to the good of the patients, both maternal and fetal.

References

1. Chervenak FA, McCullough LB. The moral foundation of medical leadership: the professional virtues of the physician as fiduciary of the patient. *Am J Obstet Gynecol* 2001;184:875–80
2. Plato. *Republic*. In Cooper JM, Hutchinson DS, eds. *Complete Works*. Indianapolis: Hackett Publishing Company, 1997
3. Hesslebein F, Goldsmith M, Beckhard R, eds. *The Drucker Foundation. The Leader of the Future.* San Francisco: Jossey-Bass Publishers, 1996
4. Bradford DL, Cohen AR. *Managing for Excellence*. New York: John Wiley & Sons, 1997
5. Kotter JP. *Leading Change*. Boston: Harvard Business School Press, 1996
6. Curry W, ed. *New Leadership in Health Care Management: The Physician Executive*, 2nd edn. Tampa: American College of Physician Executives, 1994
7. McCullough LB, Chervenak FA. Ethical challenges in the managed practice of obstetrics and gynecology. *Obstet Gynecol* 1999;93:304–7
8. Gregory J. *Lectures on the Duties and Qualifications of a Physician*. London: W. Strahan and T. Cadell, 1772. In McCullough LB, ed. *John Gregory's Writings on Medical Ethics and Philosophy of Medicine*. Dordrecht: Kluwer Academic Publishers, 1998
9. Percival T. *Medical Ethics, or a Code of Institutes and Precepts, Adopted to the Professional Conduct of Physicians and Surgeons*. London: Johnson and Bickerstaff, 1803. In Pelligrino E, ed. *The Classics of Medicine Library*. Birmingham: Gryphon Editions, 1985
10. Baker R, Porter D, Porter R. *The Codification of Medical Morality: Historical and Philosophical Studies of the Formalization of Western Medical Morality in the Eighteenth and Nineteenth Centuries*, vol 1. *Medical Ethics and Etiquette in the Eighteenth Century*. Dordrecht: Kluwer Academic Publishers, 1993
11. Baker R. *The Codification of Medical Morality: Historical and Philosophical Studies of the Formalization of Western Medical Morality in the Eighteenth and Nineteenth Centuries*, vol 2. *Anglo American Medical Ethics and Medical Jurisprudence in the Nineteenth Century*. Dordrecht: Kluwer Academic Publishers, 1995
12. Baker RB, Latham SR, Caplan AL, Emanuel LL. *The American Medical Ethics Revolution: How the AMA's Code of Ethics Has Transformed Physicians' Relationships to Patients, Professionals and Society*. Baltimore: The Johns Hopkins University Press, 1999
13. Pelligrino ED, Thomasma DC. *The Virtues in Medical Practice*. New York: Oxford University Press, 1993
14. McCullough LB. *John Gregory and the Invention of Professional Medical Ethics and the Profession of Medicine*. Dordrecht: Kluwer Academic Publishers, 1998
15. Chervenak FA, McCullough LB, Chez R. Responding to the ethical challenges of managed

care in the practice of obstetrics and gynecology. *Am J Obstet Gynecol* 1996;175:523–7

16. Fries MH. Professionalism in obstetrics–gynecology residency education: the view of program directors. *Obstet Gynecol* 2000;95:314–16

17. McCullough LB, Chervenak FA. *Ethics in Obstetrics and Gynecology*. New York: Oxford University Press, 1994

18. Kopelman LM, Lannin DR, Kopelman AE. Preventing and managing unwarranted biases against patients. In McCullough LB, Jones JW, Brody BA, eds. *Surgical Ethics*. New York: Oxford University Press, 1998:242–54

19. Kopelman L. Help from Hume reconciling professionalism and managed care. *J Med Philos* 1999;24:396–410

20. McCullough LB, Chervenak FA, Coverdale JH. Ethically justified guidelines for defining sexual boundaries between obstetrician–gynecologists and their patients. *Am J Obstet Gynecol* 1996;175: 496–500

21. Ingelfinger FJ. Informed (but uneducated) consent. *N Engl J Med* 1972;287:465–6

22. Eliott TS. The hollow men. In Untermeyer L, ed. *Modern American Poetry*. New York: Harcourt Brace & World, 1962:395–6

23. Leys S (translator and notes). *The Analects of Confucius*. New York: WW Norton, 1997

The assessment of morphological and vascular development of the early embryo

2

A. Kurjak, T. Hafner and I. Bekavac

EVOLUTION OF ULTRASOUND MODALITIES IN IMAGING EARLY HUMAN DEVELOPMENT

Our expanding capability for ultrasound imaging in normal pregnancies has focused attention on the early weeks of gestation. The embryonic period extending from conception until 9 weeks of gestation is extremely important. Most major anatomic structures and organ systems are formed and developed during this period. It is during this period that most major developmental anomalies originate.

A prerequisite for embryo imaging is a high-frequency ultrasound probe. Subtle details of the developing embryo can be depicted by the use of the higher frequency of ultrasound. This, however, has necessitated the ultrasound transducer to be positioned in close proximity to the embryo. By the use of the standard two-dimensional transvaginal probe it was possible *in vivo* to depict and analyze many details previously known only from embryological textbooks[1-4]. Sonoembryology, a new sonographic discipline, was established. However, because of anatomic constraints, manipulation with the transvaginal probe was quite limited, causing difficulty for sonographers in their efforts to obtain the proper scanning plane. Examinations were often prolonged, producing increased discomfort to the patients, and substantially increasing the cumulative ultrasound energy transmitted to the vulnerable embryo.

Three-dimensional sonography greatly improved the quality of visualization of the fetus[5-12]. It particularly improved the first-trimester scan[13-18]. The most significant contribution to the study of early brain development has been done by the Oslo team (Blaas *et al.*)[19]. The limited manipulative capacity of the transvaginal probe has no impact on the quality of the scans. The acquired volume containing data of the embryonic morphology can be rotated and transected in an unlimited number of planes. Additionally, specific details of importance can be emphasized by different modalities of image rendering. Hidden details of inner embryonic structures can be depicted and clearly presented by the use of 'electronic scalpel'. Measurements have been brought to a higher level. Besides the standard one-dimensional measurements of length, three-dimensional sonography measures the precise volume of complex, irregular biological structures in a way that is simple and fast. The time of embryo exposure to ultrasound energy is reduced to a minimum. Volume acquisition takes only a few seconds. Data are stored in digital form and can be used for analysis at any time, without any loss of quality. In the same form, data are ready for telemedical application.

Multicenter studies have shown some limitations of three-dimensional ultrasound scanning[20]. Fetal and maternal movements during the scanning process lead to motion artifacts that can degrade the quality of an image. Fetal surface rendering primarily depends on sufficient amniotic fluid volume in front of the region of interest. In some cases, oligohydramnios and superimposed structures make surface rendering impossible. Finally, three-dimensional examination of stored volumes is a time-consuming operation. Beginners will need plenty of time and assisted education to become adept at data acquisition, orientation and manipulation; this is mandatory for three-dimensional ultrasound imaging.

VISUALIZATION OF EARLY VASCULAR DEVELOPMENT

With structures as minute as newly formed vascular channels, visualization presents a problem. The first technique used to analyze the developing embryo was light microscopy. By slicing paraffin blocks containing the embryo, it was possible to visualize the arrangement and development of tissues. However, the obvious problem was that these were all non-viable specimens. The anatomy could be studied, but not the physiological changes within the tissue. New possibilities were opened with immune staining. The basic principle is to bind antibodies to the cells that need to be visualized. When attached to the antigen, a part of this antibody molecule gives off light. The cells can then be studied by fluorescence microscopy. Drake and colleagues used this method to depict all vessels and angioblasts within embryos[21].

The embryology in classical textbooks is also based on non-viable specimens. The first imaging technique to depict an active, viable vascular system was color Doppler. This kind of ultrasound is specially designed to detect movement, the movement of erythrocytes within blood vessels in particular. The latest, most sophisticated kind of color Doppler is three-dimensional power Doppler ultrasound.

Kurjak and colleagues[13] used combined B-mode and power Doppler imaging in order to evaluate fetal growth and the development of the fetal circulation. Their study included 270 normally developing pregnancies. They used a fully digital three-dimensional device with complete storage of three-dimensional power Doppler data (Kretz, 530 D, Kretz-Medison, Zipf, Austria and Seoul, Korea). Different rendering modes were used in color-coded data processing and presentation. A minimum-intensity projection was used for a surface-rendered vascular image. The former was superior in assessment of the spatial inter-relationships of vascular structures, and the latter was useful in the assessment of the morphology and outer surface of a confined vascular structure.

TYPICAL MORPHOLOGICAL AND VASCULAR DEVELOPMENTAL FEATURES OF THE EARLY EMBRYO

Five weeks

The gestational sac can be visualized from the middle of the 5th week of amenorrhea as a small, spherical anechoic structure placed inside one of the endometrial leaves. Planar mode tomograms are helpful in distinguishing an early intraendometrial gestational sac from a collection of free fluid between the endo-metrial layers (pseudogestational sac). Three-dimensional sonography enables precise measurement of the exponentially expanding gestational sac volume during the first trimester (Table 1). The amniotic cavity volume can be obtained in correlation with crown–rump length (CRL) measurements. At the beginning of the 5th week, the small secondary yolk sac is visible as the earliest sign of the developing embryo. Planar mode tomograms are useful for detecting the embryonic pole inside the gestational sac. Adjacent to the yolk sac, the

Table 1 *Gestational sac volume (mean ± SD) determined by three-dimensional ultrasound between 5 and 12 weeks' gestation*

Gestational age (weeks)	n	Gestational sac volume (cm³)
5	18	1.62 ± 0.58
6	27	2.15 ± 1.15
7	42	8.05 ± 1.85
8	55	18.90 ± 2.50
9	48	40.02 ± 3.84
10	31	72.20 ± 7.90
11	28	120.50 ± 12.00
12	21	205.55 ± 22.05
Total	270	58.62 ± 6.48

embryo can be seen as a small straight line when it reaches 2–3 mm in length at the end of the 5th week.

Blood flow in the spiral arteries can be observed by transvaginal color Doppler as early as the end of 4 weeks from the last menstrual period. A color signal from the spiral arteries is seen within a hyperechoic area in close proximity to the gestational sac. The blood flow velocities in systole and diastole are very low. Sometimes it is possible to obtain a color Doppler signal from the endometrium where a gestational sac will develop. At this time, the observed color signal is the only sign of early pregnancy. The color flow signal is probably obtained from the spiral arteries, which are altered, owing to the activity of the tropho-blast[22].

Three-dimensional power Doppler reveals intense vascular activity from the first sonographic evidence of the developing pregnancy during the 5th week of gestation. A hyperechoic chorionic ring is interrupted by color-coded sprouts that penetrate its border. Future development of the three-dimensional power Doppler program should include three-dimensional gray-scale (anatomic) information

and simultaneous power Doppler and shift spectrum information.

Six weeks

The three-dimensional image of an embryo during the 6th week of pregnancy is characterized by a rounded, bulky head and a thin body. The head is prominent, owing to the developing forebrain. Limb buds are rarely visible at this stage of pregnancy. However, the umbilical cord and vitelline duct are always clearly visible.

Transvaginal sonography is able to detect embryonic heartbeats as early as 5 weeks and 4 days of menstrual age, at the embryo CRL of 3–4 mm. The color Doppler signal accurately indicates the position of the embryonic heart pulsations. At this very early stage, this finding may help clinicians to differentiate between a living and a non-living embryo in cases of missed abortion (Figure 1).

Three-dimensional power Doppler allows clear depiction of aortic and umbilical blood flow within the embryo's trunk. The initial branches of the umbilical vessels are visible at the placental umbilical insertion. Pulsed

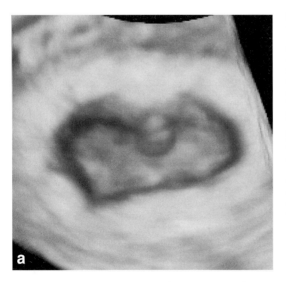 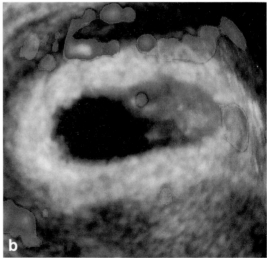

Figure 1 *(a) During the 6th week of pregnancy, the embryo can be seen, adjacent to the yolk sac, as a small straight line when it reaches 2–3 mm in length. There are no specific ultrasound features that can be distinguished. (b) Power Doppler reveals the onset of heart activity (see Color Plate A)*

Doppler signals from the aorta and umbilical artery obtained by conventional color Doppler demonstrate absent end-diastolic flow, while the umbilical vein blood flow is pulsatile.

Seven weeks

During the 7th week of pregnancy the head is strongly flexed anteriorly, being in contact with the chest. Limb buds are often visible laterally to the body (Figure 2). The amnion that can be seen as a spherical hyperechoic membrane is still close to the embryo. The chorion frondosum can be distinguished from the chorion laeve.

The intracranial circulation becomes visible as early as the 7th week of gestation. At this time, discrete pulsations of the internal carotid arteries are detectable at the base of the skull. Three-dimensional power Doppler depicts features of early vascular anatomy at the base of the skull, with branches evolving laterally to the mesencephalon and cephalic flexure. Pulsed Doppler analysis reveals absent end-diastolic velocities in the arteries.

Eight weeks

The arms and feet are clearly visible. The insertion of the umbilical cord is visible on the anterior abdominal wall. During the 8th and 9th weeks, the developing intestine is being herniated into the proximal umbilical cord.

The visualization rate of the fetal aorta and umbilical artery is now higher (Figure 3). Blood flow in the fetal heart and aorta as well as in the umbilical artery and spiral arteries is clearly visualized. Three-dimensional power Doppler imaging allows visualization of the entire fetal circulation. There are no significant hemodynamic changes in these blood vessels in comparison to the earlier period of pregnancy in the uteroplacental or fetal circulation.

Nine to ten weeks

Herniation of the midgut is present. The dorsal column, the early spine, can be examined in its whole length. The arms with elbow, and legs

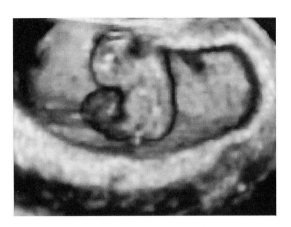

Figure 2 *Normal embryo at 7 weeks' gestation. Note the anterior flexion of the head, in contact with the chest. Adjacent to the embryo, the yolk sac can be seen*

with knee, are clearly visible. The feet can be seen approaching the midline (Figures 4 and 5).

The common and internal carotid arteries may be visualized at the end of the 8th gestational week and the beginning of the 9th week. A cerebral circulation can be documented at 8 weeks in the form of discrete pulsations of the intracerebral part of the internal carotid artery. From the 9th gestational week, arterial pulsations can be detected on transverse section, lateral to the mesencephalon and cephalic flexure. The circle of Willis and its major branches can be depicted by three-dimensional power Doppler.

A characteristic waveform profile, i.e. a systolic component with absent end-diastolic frequencies, is visible from the 7th to the 10th gestational week, suggesting a high vascular resistance at the embryonic (aorta) and umbilical placental level as compared with that of late pregnancy[23].

Eleven to twelve weeks

In the 11th week of pregnancy, development of the head and neck continues. The herniated midgut returns into the abdominal cavity. Planar mode enables detailed analysis of the embryonic body with visualization of the stomach and urinary bladder. The kidneys are also often visible. The arms and legs continue

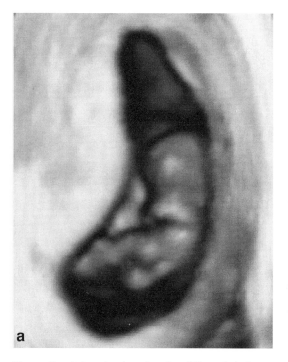

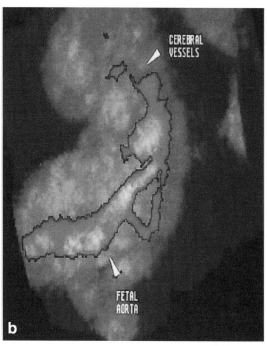

Figure 3 *At 8 weeks, the embryo has different body features to be observed (a). The head has less flexion, and the limbs are elongated. The careful observer can distinguish segments of the arms and legs. The umbilical cord is a prominent structure. Proportionally, it is thick and rather stiff. Vascular anatomy can be seen in increasing detail (b). Note the abdominal aorta with the umbilical artery branching at the caudal pole. The umbilical vein can be followed from the abdominal umbilical insertion through the fetal liver, and ending below the heart (see Color Plate B)*

with their development. The long bones can be visualized as hyperechoic elongated structures inside the upper and lower extremities. Fingers and toes are visible (Figure 6). Facial details such as the nose, orbits, maxilla and mandible are often visible. Detailed three-dimensional analysis of the fetal spine, chest and limbs is obtainable by using the transparent, X-ray-like mode.

At this stage, the pulsations of the middle cerebral artery can easily identify it as a separate vessel. However, until the end of the 10th gestational week, the ultrasonically detected vascular network should be called the 'intracranial circulation'. Until the end of the first trimester, the absence of end-diastolic blood flow in fetal and placental components of the circulation is a normal physiological finding. Establishment of the end-diastolic component of blood flow is in direct correlation with an increase in all maternal arteries.

Between the 10th and 14th weeks, diastolic velocities in fetal blood vessels begin to emerge, but are incomplete and inconsistently present. The umbilical artery and fetal aorta are still the most prominent vessels for color Doppler assessment. A significant decrease of the pulsatility index (PI) is observed in the intracranial vessels with advancing gestational age, and it is present 2 weeks earlier than it is noted in other parts of the fetal circulation. End-diastolic velocities are also present earlier in the cerebral vessels than in the fetal aorta and umbilical artery. These data suggest low vascular impedance in the fetal brain, independent of changes in the vascular resistance of the fetal trunk or uteroplacental circulation. This apparently independent and autoregulatory mechanism provides an adequate blood supply

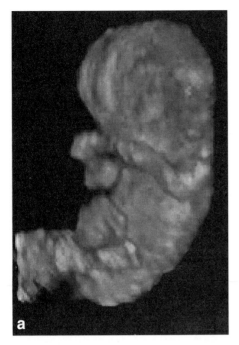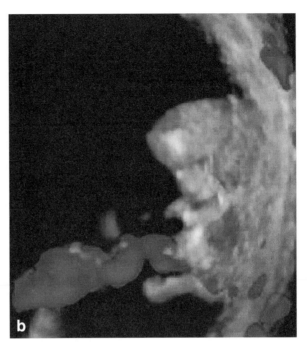

Figure 4 *A normal embryo at 9 weeks' gestation (a). The size of the lateral ventricles has increased rapidly. The third ventricle is still relatively wide at the beginning of this week, owing to the growth of the thalami. In the fetuses of ≥ 25 mm in crown–rump length, there is a clear gap between the rhombencephalic and the mesencephalic cavity, owing to the growing cerebellum. Three-dimensional power Doppler (b) reveals the entire embryonic circulation obtained from different angles (see Color Plate C)*

to the growing fetal brain. This physiological response is similar to the brain-sparing effect that has been described in hypoxic fetuses in the late second and third trimesters. Some scientists suggest that the full establishment of intervillous flow leads to increased oxygen transport and decreased resistance in the peripheral embryonic circulation.

With the use of three-dimensional power Doppler it is possible to depict the major branches of the aorta: the common iliac and renal arteries. The circle of Willis and its branches are easily visible (Figure 7).

Determining chorionicity and amnionicity during the end of the first trimester may be much easier by three-dimensional surface rendering (Figure 8). All of the relevant criteria can be used. These include: counting the number of placentas; determining whether each embryo is within its own amniotic sac; describing the appearance of the dividing membrane; and looking for the presence of a triangular projection of placental tissue beyond the chorionic surfaces (lambda or twin peak sign)[24,25].

Owing to the superb quality of the images, three-dimensional sonography enables detection of developmental anomalies[26–31]. Three-dimensional sonography will certainly improve early detection of fetal anomalies, and possibly become the screening method for them. Three-dimensional sonography can improve the accuracy and success rate of nuchal translucency measurement in pregnancy between 10 and 14 weeks' gestation (Figure 9). In a series of 120 pregnancies Kurjak and Kupesic[32] were able to obtain the mid-sagittal section and measure nuchal translucency in 100% of cases using three-dimensional transvaginal sonography (Table 2). By the use of standard two-dimensional sonography this was possible in only 85% of cases. In addition, three-dimensional sonography produced better intraobserver reproducibility of results. Three-dimensional sonography with the potential of complex and sophisticated post-processing of images has

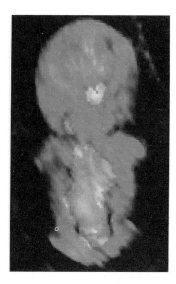

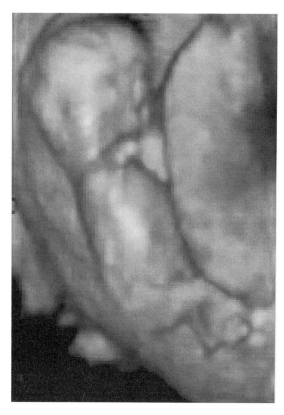

Figure 5 *Surface view of the fetus at 10 weeks' gestation. Three-dimensional ultrasound allows simultaneous visualization of the fetal anatomy and corresponding circulation. The entire fetal circulation is presented from different angles. The aorta and umbilical vessels are prominent. Vessels responsible for perfusion of the brain can be seen at the base of the skull. Because of the development of the central nervous system, body movements are very rich and complex (see Color Plate D)*

Figure 6 *Three-dimensional surface image of a fetus at 12 weeks' gestation. Note the regular morphology of the fetal head, body and extremities*

proved to be a useful tool in experimental embryology. Using a special off-line imaging computer device, Blaas and co-workers[33] produced a series of *ex vivo* obtained images of human embryos emphasizing development of the brain cavities during the first trimester. This new technology moved embryology from post-mortem studies to the *in vivo* environment.

NEUROSONOGRAPHY IN THE FIRST TRIMESTER OF PREGNANCY

The central nervous system (CNS) of the embryo mainly occupies the head, which is the most prominent anatomical structure. In the embryo or the fetus, the ratio of the size of the head to that of the whole body is one-half to one-third. Accordingly, the CNS occupies the main part of the morphological assessment of fetal development.

Gestational age 5 and 6 weeks

The first ultrasound appearance of the embryo begins in the 5th week of pregnancy. The embryonic pole is depicted as a hyperechoic line close to the yolk sac. During the 5th and 6th weeks, the embryonic pole grows, reaching the size of 5–6 mm, with visible heart action. At this stage neural structures cannot be depicted by ultrasound. However, soon, at the end of the 6th week and during the 7th week (CRL 8–14 mm) the embryonic cephalic pole is clearly distinguishable from the embryonic torso[13].

Gestational age 7 weeks

The main feature of the cephalic pole is the rhombencephalon (hindbrain) seen as a hypoechoic vesicle below the calvarial roof. Anteriorly, the narrow mesencephalon and prosencephalon

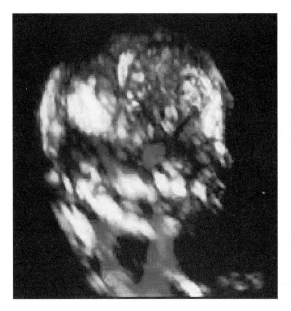

Figure 7 *A fetus at 12 weeks of gestation. Note the two major vascular supplies to the brain: the internal carotid artery and the vertebral artery. Three-dimensional power Doppler sonography precisely depicts the spatial relationship of the vessels and bones of the skull (see Color Plate E)*

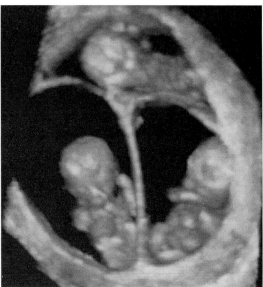

Figure 8 *Triplets visualized by three-dimensional sonography*

can occasionally be identified. Owing to the pronounced anterior flexion of the embryonic head, the anterior parts of the embryonic brain lie very close to the heart bulge. Between the 6th and 8th week from the last menstruation a secondary canalization takes place. The prosencephalon (forebrain) differentiates into the telencephalon and diencephalon. The rhombencephalon divides into the metencephalon and myelencephalon. Including the mesencephalon (midbrain) that does not change significantly, the brain consists of five secondary brain vesicles[34–36]. Three-dimensional multiplanar imaging is superb for ultrasonic visualization of these processes.

Gestational age 8 weeks

At 8 weeks (CRL 15 mm) the most prominent structure is the posteriorly positioned rhombencephalon[37]. The anterior mesencephalic cavity is connected to the rhombencephalic cavity by the narrow isthmus rhombencephali. A few days later (CRL 19 mm) in a sagittal section it is

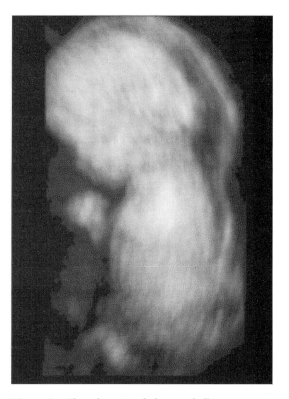

Figure 9 *Three-dimensional ultrasound allows assessment of the mid-sagittal section in all fetuses between 12 and 14 weeks' gestation; this is mandatory for accurate measurement of nuchal translucency*

Table 2 *Data on nuchal translucency (NT) visualization rates between 10 and 14 weeks of gestation by two- and three-dimensional (2D and 3D) transvaginal ultrasound (TVS)*

Gestational age (weeks)	Cases (n)	NT visualization rates			
		2D TVS		3D TVS	
		n	%	n	%
10–11	9	8	88.9	9	100
11–12	21	18	85.7	21	100
12–13	48	42	87.5	48	100
13–14	33	25	75.8	33	100
14–14^{+5}	9	9	100.0	9	100
Total	120	102	85.0	120	100

clear that the mesencephalon and diencephalon are developing faster than the rhombencephalon. The size of the rhombencephalon is less prominent in comparison to the size of other cavities. Owing to the initial size and prominence of the rhombencephalon, this can be misinterpreted as an abnormal cystic structure[6]. With further development of the brain, the rhombencephalon reduces the proportion of its size. The rhombencephalon accounts for 54% of the embryonic brain at the 7th gestational week, reducing its relative size to 36% at the 9th gestational week[38]. By selecting the appropriate oblique axial section on the three-dimensional multiplanar analysis, it is possible to depict the spatial relationship between different parts of the developing brain. The youngest part of the brain, the telencephalon, can also be depicted at this gestational age (8.5 weeks). Telecephalic cavities are visualized laterally to the diencephalic cavity. The diencephalon, which gives rise to the future third ventricle, appears as a large central cavity. It is interposed between the two precursors of the lateral ventricles and brain hemispheres (telencephalon)[35]. The growth of the prosencephalon is much faster than that of the other parts of the brain. The telencephalon forms the cerebral hemispheres and the lateral ventricles with the choroid plexi. The diencephalon is the origin of the thalamus and third ventricle.

Gestational age 9 weeks

The cerebral hemispheres contain hyperechoic choroid plexi. The cavity of the mesencephalon, the future aqueduct of Sylvius, is still a large cavity. During the 9th week the head begins to assume its round shape, and the biparietal diameter (BPD) measures between 9 and 12 mm[34,39]. At this time a part of the rhomben-cephalon, the metencephalon, starts its thickening, forming the future cerebellum and the fourth ventricle.

Gestational age 10 weeks

At 10 weeks of pregnancy, the embryonic period is over. The fetus gains its human resemblance. At the transverse section through the fetal head the most prominent structures are the cerebral hemispheres with the lateral ventricles. The lateral ventricles are almost completely filled with the hyperechoic choroid plexus. The size of the third ventricle has been reduced in favor of the development of the thalamus. The third ventricle is visualized as a thin gap between hypoechoic thalamic bodies. At the end of the 10th week of gestation the caudal brain structure, the metencephalon, differentiates into the posterior cerebellum and anterior pons.

Gestational age 11 weeks

In the 11th week of pregnancy a butterfly-like choroid plexus is clearly visible in the transverse section through the head (Figure 10). The BPD at this time measures 18–19 mm[34]. In the oblique axial section, the cerebellum and cysterna magna can be analyzed. The thalamus is connected with the cerebellum through the hypoechoic cerebellar peduncles. Besides the brain structures there are some other structures that can be analyzed at this gestational age. Three-dimensional sonography can exactly depict the formation of the bones of the head. This can ascertain the normal development of the calvaria, and help in early detection of major brain and head abnormalities. Depiction of the fetal face can be obtained by the use of three-dimensional multiplanar analysis.

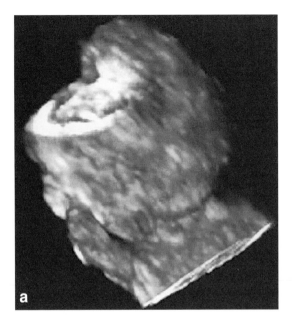

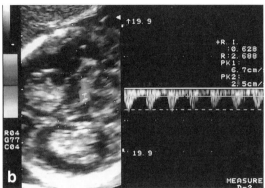

Figure 10 *Butterfly-like hyperechoic choroid plexus is the most prominent feature of the fetal brain after the 10th week of pregnancy. Normally, it fills the lateral ventricles, and it is responsible for production of the cerebrospinal fluid. Three-dimensional sonography accurately depicts the anatomy of the developing central nervous system (a). The blood supply to the choroid plexus has some particular characteristics. Detected by pulsed spectral Doppler (b), arterial blood flow velocity waveforms show pandiastolic flow earlier than any other embryonic artery. This is evidence that, at this gestational age, a great portion of cerebral perfusion is directed to the choroid plexus (see Color Plate F)*

Examination of the fetal face is important and must be performed as a part of the CNS examination. Some severe CNS anomalies have substantial impact on the development of the fetal face[34].

THREE-DIMENSIONAL SONOGRAPHY OF EXTRAEMBRYONIC STRUCTURES: THE YOLK SAC

Three-dimensional ultrasound imaging may give additional data to functional Doppler studies for research into developmental anatomy and embryology. This method allows a detailed morphological and volumetric analysis of static extraembryonic structures. Conventional methods for measuring volumes of fluid-filled spaces include modelling of shapes (e.g. using an ellipsoidal approximation). Using the three-dimensional planar mode, the position of the yolk-sac wall is accurately spatially assessed. Measurement of the volume, rather than estimation from a simple geometric model, increases the accuracy of the measurement. The growth and appearance of the yolk sac

have been correlated with the outcome of pregnancy[40]. Kupesic and co-workers[23] measured gestational sac volume and yolk sac volume and vascularity in 80 women with an uncomplicated pregnancy between 5 and 12 weeks of gestation. Regression analysis revealed exponential growth of the gestational volume throughout the first trimester of pregnancy. Gestational sac volume measurements can be used for the estimation of gestational age in early pregnancy. An abnormal gestational sac volume measurement could potentially be used as a prognostic marker for pregnancy outcome. The yolk sac volume was found to increase from 5 to 10 weeks of gestation (Table 3). However, when the yolk sac reaches its maximum volume at around 10 weeks it has already started to degenerate, which can be indirectly proved by a significant reduction in visualization rates of the yolk sac vascularity. Therefore, the disappearance of the yolk sac in normal pregnancies is probably the result of yolk sac degeneration rather than of a mechanical compression of the expanding cavity. These events suggest that the evaluation of the biological function of the yolk

Table 3 *Yolk sac volume (mean ± SD) and vascularity determined by three-dimensional ultrasound and color Doppler between 5 and 12 weeks of gestation*

Gestational age (weeks)	n	Yolk sac volume (mm^3)	Yolk sac vascularity visualization rates (%)
5	18	7.30 ± 1.40	0
6	27	14.20 ± 2.10	37.04
7	42	38.90 ± 4.85	83.33
8	55	51.55 ± 5.14	90.91
9	48	56.00 ± 5.35	81.25
10	31	61.60 ± 6.15	64.52
11	28	57.75 ± 5.80	25.00
12	21	52.28 ± 5.15	14.28
Total	270	42.45 ± 4.49	49.54

sac by measuring the diameter and/or the volume is limited. Therefore, a combination of functional and volumetric studies is necessary to identify some of the more important moments during early pregnancy.

FOUR-DIMENSIONAL SONOGRAPHY

A superb tool that enables depiction of the whole complexity of developmental stages in early human development is four-dimensional sonography. We can investigate embryonic movements and behavior that are a product of developing morphological, hemodynamic and metabolic functions of the embryo. Developmental stages of embryonic behavior are backed up by typical features of morphological and hemodynamic sonographic findings.

At 5–6 weeks of gestation, the embryonic pole is positioned adjacent to the yolk sac. There are no specific ultrasound features that can be distinguished. Apart from the present fetal heart action, there are no embryonic movements. At 7 weeks of gestation, embryonic movements are observed. They are not frequent and consist mainly of changing the position of the head towards the rest of the body. Limb movements are absent.

At 8 weeks, embryonic movements can be divided into two main groups: gross body movements that consist of changing of the position of the head towards the body; and movements of the extremities. The arms and legs are moved vigorously. However, no flexion or extension in the elbow or knee can be seen.

At 10 weeks of gestation, fetal movements are rich. The fetus has gained total human resemblance. Many details are visible. The careful observer should visualize the face with both eyes, nose and mouth. All three segments of the upper and lower extremities are visible. Movements of the body are complex. They are a product of advanced development of the central nervous system.

CONCLUSION

Many details involved in this process are still obscure to our knowledge. We believe that studies including a combination of *in vivo* three-dimensional data with post-mortem histology specimens can yield new and interesting facts about this period of human development, full of incomparable intensity. Undoubtedly, rapid technological development will allow real-time three-dimensional ultrasound to provide improved patient care on the one hand, and increased knowledge of developmental anatomy on the other.

References

1. Kossoff G, Griffith KA, Dixon CE. Is the quality of transvaginal images superior to transabdominal ones under matched conditions? *Ultrasound Obstet Gynecol* 1991;1:29–35

2. Timor-Tritsch IE, Farine D, Rosen MG. A close look at early embryonic development with the high-frequency transvaginal transducer. *Am J Obstet Gynecol* 1988;159:676–81

3. Achiron R, Achiron A. Transvaginal ultrasonic assessment of the early fetal brain. *Ultrasound Obstet Gynecol* 1991;1:336

4. Kushnir U, Shalev J, Bronshtein M, *et al*. Fetal intracranial anatomy in the first trimester of pregnancy: transvaginal ultrasonographic evaluation. *Neuroradiology* 1989;32:222–5

5. Baba K, Satch K, Sakamoto S, *et al*. Development of an ultrasonic system for three-dimensional reconstruction of the fetus. *J Perinat Med* 1989;17:19–24

6. Fredfelt KE, Holm HH, Pedersen JF. Three-dimensional ultrasonic scanning. *Acta Radiol Diagn* 1984;25:237–9

7. Merz E, Bahlaman F, Weber G, *et al*. Three-dimensional ultrasonography in prenatal diagnosis. *J Perinat Med* 1995;23:213–22

8. Merz A, Macchiela D, Bahlamann F, *et al*. Three-dimensional ultrasound for the diagnosis of fetal malformations. *Ultrasound Obstet Gynecol* 1992;2:137–9

9. Miric-Tesanic D, Kurjak A. Trodimenzionalni ultrazvuk u ginekologiji i porodništvu. *Gynaecol Perinatol* 1997;6:43–6

10. Merz E, Bahlmann F, Weber G, *et al*. Volume 3D scanning – a new dimension in the evaluation of fetal malformations. *Ultrasound Obstet Gynecol* 1993;3:131–4

11. Bonilla-Musoles F, Raga F, Osborne N, Blanes J. The use of three-dimensional (3D) ultrasound for study of normal pathologic morphology of the human embryo and fetus: preliminary report. *J Ultrasound Med* 1995;14:757–65

12. Kurjak A, Hafner T, Kos M, Kupesic S, Stanojevic M. Three-dimensional sonography in prenatal diagnosis: a necessity or a luxury? *J Perinat Med* 2000;28:194–209

13. Kurjak A, Kupesic S, Banovic I, Hafner T, Kos M. The study of morphology and circulation of early embryo by three-dimensional ultrasound and power Doppler. *J Perinat Med* 1999;27:145–57

14. Bonilla-Musoles F. Three-dimensional visualization of the human embryo: a potential revolution in prenatal diagnosis [Editorial]. *Ultrasound Obstet Gynecol* 1996;7:393–7

15. Maymon J, Halperin Z, Weinraub A, Herman A, Schneider D. Three-dimensional sonography of conjoined twins at 10 weeks: a case report. *Ultrasound Obstet Gynecol* 1998;11:292–4

16. Kurjak A, Kupesic S. Three dimensional transvaginal ultrasound improves measurement of nuchal translucency. *J Perinat Med* 1999;27:97–102

17. Kupesic S, Kurjak A. Volume and vascularity of the yolk sac studied by three-dimensional ultrasound and color Doppler. *J Perinat Med* 1999;27:91–6

18. Blaas HG, Eik-Nes SH, Kiserund T, Berg S, Angelsen B, Olstad B. Three-dimensional imaging of the brain cavities in human embryos. *Ultrasound Obstet Gynecol* 1995;5:228–32

19. Blaas HG, Eik-Nes SH, Kiserud TW, Berg S, Angelsen B, Olstad B. Three-dimensional imaging of the brain cavities in human embryos. *Ultrasound Obstet Gynecol* 1995;5:228–32

20. Pretorius DH, Nelson TR. Three-dimensional ultrasound [Opinion]. *Ultrasound Obstet Gynecol* 1995;5:219–21

21. Drake CJ, Cheresh DA, Little CD. An antagonist of integrin alpha v beta 3 for angiogenesis. *J Cell Sci* 1995;108:2655–7

22. Kurjak A, Laurini R, Kupesic S, Kos M, Latin V, Bulic K. A combined Doppler and morphopathological study of intervillous circulation. *Ultrasound Obstet Gynecol* 1995;6(Suppl 2):116

23. Kupesic S, Kurjak A, Ivancic-Kosuta M. Volume and vascularity of the yolk sac studied by three-dimensional ultrasound and color Doppler. *J Perinat Med* 1999;27:91–6

24. Benoit B. Three-dimensional surface mode for demonstration of normal fetal anatomy in the second and third trimester. In Merz E, ed. *3D Ultrasound in Obstetrics and Gynecology*. Philadelphia: Lippincot Williams and Wilkins, 1998:95–100

25. Kurjak A, Kos M. Three dimensional ultrasonography in prenatal diagnosis. In Chervenak FA, Kurjak A, eds. *Fetal Medicine*. Carnforth, UK: Parthenon Publishing, 1999:102–8

26. Pretorius DH, Nelson TR. Three-dimensional ultrasound of fetal surface features. *Ultrasound Obstet Gynecol* 1992;2:166–8

27. Lee A, Deutinger J, Bernaschek G. Three-dimensional ultrasound: abnormalities of the fetal face in surface and volume rendering mode. *Br J Obstet Gynaecol* 1995;102:40–3

28. Lee A, Deutinger J, Bernaschek G. Voluvision: three-dimensional ultrasonography of fetal malformations. *Am J Obstet Gynecol* 1994;170:1312–14

29. Lee A, Kratochwil A, Deutinger J, *et al.* Three-dimensional ultrasound in diagnosing phocomelia. *Ultrasound Obstet Gynecol* 1995;5:238–40

30. Bonilla-Musoles F, Raga F, Osborne N, Blanes J. The use of three-dimensional (3D) ultrasound for study of normal pathologic morphology of the human embryo and fetus: preliminary report. *J Ultrasound Med* 1995;14:757–65

31. Bonilla-Musoles F. Three-dimensional visualization of the human embryo: a potential revolution in prenatal diagnosis [Editorial]. *Ultrasound Obstet Gynecol* 1996;7:393–7

32. Kurjak A, Kupesic S. Three-dimensional trans-vaginal ultrasound improves measurement of nuchal translucency. *J Perinat Med* 1999;27:91–6

33. Blaas HG, Eik-Nes SH, Berg S, Torp H. *In-vivo* three-dimensional ultrasound reconstructions of embryos and early fetuses. *Lancet* 1998;352:1182–6

34. Achiron R, Achiron A. Transvaginal fetal neurosonography: the first trimester of pregnancy. In Chervenak FA, Kurjak A, Comstock CH, eds. *Ultrasound and the Fetal Brain*. Carnforth, UK: Parthenon Publishing, 1995:95–108

35. Blaas HG, Eik-Nes SH, Kiserud T, *et al.* Early development of the forebrain and midbrain: a longitudinal study from 7 to 12 postmenstrual weeks of gestation. *Ultrasound Obstet Gynecol* 1994;4:183–92

36. Blaas HG, Eik-Nes SH, Kiserud T, *et al.* Early development of the hindbrain: a longitudinal study from 7 to 12 weeks of gestation. *Ultrasound Obstet Gynecol* 1995;5:151–60

37. Cyr DR, Mack LA, Nyberg DA, Sheppard TH, Shuman WP. Fetal rhombencephalon: normal ultrasound findings. *Radiology* 1988;166:691–2

38. Jenkins GB. Relative weight and volume of the component parts of the brain of the human embryo at different stages of development. *Contr Embryol Carneg Instn* 1921;13:41–60

39. Blaas HG, Eik-Nes SH. Ultrasound assessment of early brain development. In Jurkovic D, Jauniaux E, eds. *Ultrasound and Early Pregnancy*. Carnforth, UK: Parthenon Publishing, 1996:3–18

40. Lindsay DJ, Lyons EA, Levi CS, Zheng XH. Endovaginal appearance of the yolk sac in early pregnancy: normal growth and usefulness as a predictor of abnormal pregnancy outcome. *Radiology* 1988;166:109–12

Threatened abortion: new insights by color Doppler, three- and four-dimensional ultrasound

3

S. Kupesic, A. Kurjak and A. Aksamija

INTRODUCTION

Early pregnancy failure is the spontaneous ending of a pregnancy before the fetus has reached a viable gestational age[1]. The most common pathological symptom is vaginal bleeding. Threatened abortion is a clinical term to describe this symptom during the first 20 weeks of pregnancy in women who, on the basis of clinical evaluation, are considered to have a potentially living embryo[2].

Threatened and spontaneous abortions are the most common complications of early pregnancy. Sometimes we are not even aware that a woman has been pregnant and that she aborted. If we take into consideration these cases also, the incidence of spontaneous abortions is estimated as up to 70%[3]. Only one out of three embryos continues further development, and 50% of abortions occur before the time of expected menstruation[3,4]. These types of abortion usually cause the symptoms of sterility rather than infertility, because it seems as if the woman is not able to conceive. Thirty to forty per cent of pregnancies fail after implantation, and only 10–15% manifest with clinical symptoms[4–6]. Of all clinically recognized pregnancies, 15–20% end in miscarriage; 25% of women will have at least one miscarriage in their reproductive life[7]. Patients with a spontaneous abortion usually present during the 8–10 weeks from their last menstrual period with symptoms of vaginal bleeding and abdominal pain, with or without the expulsion of products of conception[8]. As a definition, incomplete abortion is the passage of some but not all fetal or placental tissue through the cervical canal. In complete abortion, all products of conception are expelled through the cervix[9]. The uterine debris may consist of a combination of products of conception, blood and decidua[10].

Recent studies have demonstrated that the risk for a repeated spontaneous abortion depends exclusively on the number of previous spontaneous abortions and their cause. Even though many different risk factors have been thoroughly researched, the cause of around 60% of unsuccessful pregnancies remains unknown[11]. The diagnostic and therapeutic response to a couple with pregnancy loss is not decided by the number of miscarriages. The response is significantly influenced by the woman's age, the couple's level of anxiety, and factors readily identified in the family and medical history. The degree of response will range from an educational discussion to a full diagnostic evaluation with appropriate treatment. It is helpful to consider pregnancy losses according to the following criteria[12].

Normal statistics

It is useful to keep in mind that the risk of spontaneous miscarriage is higher in older women. Spontaneous miscarriage occurs in 29% of women of 40 or more years, undergoing *in vitro* fertilization, after the demonstration of fetal heart motion by ultrasonography[13].

Genetic factors

It is worth trying to uncover causes for repetitive first-trimester miscarriages, because one recognized cause of the problem is a genetic abnormality. Karyotyping of couples will reveal that 3–8% have some abnormality, most frequently balanced chromosomal rearrangement, a translocation. Other abnormalities include sex chromosome mosaicism, chromosome inversions and ring chromosomes. Besides spontaneous miscarriages, these abnormalities are associated with high risk of malformations and mental retardation. Karyotyping is especially vital if the couple has had a malformed infant or fetus in addition to miscarriages. It is important to emphasize that karyotyping uncovers only a percentage of those pregnancies lost because of genetic abnormalities. There may be single gene defects that are not manifested by chromosomal abnormalities, and it is highly likely that a percentage of those patients, considered to have unexplained repetitive pregnancy loss, have this type of genetic defect. In addition, karyotyping of blood cells misses abnormalities of meiosis, which can be found in sperm cell lines. The karyotyping is expensive, but very helpful in making decisions if there is a positive family history[12].

Environmental factors

Smoking, alcohol and heavy coffee consumption have been reported to be associated with an increased risk of recurrent pregnancy losses[14]. In women who smoke, the increase of risk is proportional to the number of cigarettes smoked. In these cases, the fetal chromosomes are normal. More recently, the link with caffeine intake was not supported[15]. The use of electric blankets and heated water beds is also not associated with increased risk of spontaneous miscarriage[16].

Endocrine factors

Mild or subclinical endocrine diseases are not causes of recurrent miscarriages. Patients who have significant thyroid disease or uncontrolled diabetes mellitus may suffer spontaneous miscarriages, but it is unlikely that laboratory assessments of thyroid function and carbohydrate metabolism are worthwhile in relatively healthy women.

Anatomic causes

Uterine abnormalities can result in impaired vascularization of a pregnancy and limited space for a fetus, owing to distortion of the uterine cavity. Approximately 12–15% of women with recurrent miscarriages have a uterine malformation, and this can be best diagnosed by vaginal ultrasonography (especially with saline instillation and three-dimensional ultrasound)[12]. Hysterosalpingography (HSG) is relatively inaccurate and decisions should not be based upon HSG alone.

Infectious causes

Looking at the first-trimester miscarriage, Donders and colleagues found a firm correlation with bacterial vaginosis-associated microorganisms[17].

Thrombophilia

The major cause of thrombosis in pregnancy is an inherited predisposition for clotting, especially the factor V Leiden mutation. Deficiencies of antithrombin III, protein C and protein S are inherited in an autosomal dominant pattern, accounting for 10–15% of familial thrombosis. Mutation in the prothrombin gene and factor V Leiden mutation are the most common inherited causes of venous thromboembolism[18]. The factor V Leiden mutation is found in approximately 30% of individuals who develop venous thromboembolism[19]. The highest prevalence (3–4% of the general population) of the factor V Leiden mutation is found in Europeans, and its occurrence in populations not of European descent is very rare, perhaps explaining the low frequency of thromboembolic disease in Africa, Asia, and in native Americans[20]. The mutation is believed to have arisen in a single ancestor approximately 21 000 to 34 000 years ago[21]. The next most common inherited disorder is a guanine to adenine change in the gene encoding prothrombin[18,22]. The prevalence of this abnormality in the White population is estimated to range from 0.7 to 4%[23].

Immunological problems

Immunological problems can be classified into two groups: autoimmunity (self antigens), and alloimmunity (foreign antigens). In auto-immunity, a humoral or cellular response is directed against a specific component of the host. The lupus anticoagulant and anticardio-lipin antibodies are antiphospholipid antibodies, which arise as the result of an autoimmune disease. Several series have demonstrated that 10–16% of women with recurrent miscarriages have had antiphospholipid antibodies[2,3]. These antibodies are also associated with growth restriction and fetal death in addition to recurrent miscarriages. The anticardiolipin antibody and lupus anticoagulant can be identified and titered by specific immunoassays. Other individual antiphospholipid antibodies have not been associated with recurrent miscarriages[24]. The preferred treatment for significant titers of antiphospholipid antibodies consists of the combination of low-dose aspirin (80 mg daily) and low-dose heparin as soon as pregnancy is diagnosed[25,26].

Unfortunately, treatment is not always successful. Because of the risks associated with anticoagulation, aspirin and heparin treatment should be confined to women with recurrent pregnancy losses who have antiphospholipid antibodies and who have experienced first-trimester and/or second-trimester losses[27]. Alloimmunity refers to all causes of pregnancy loss related to an abnormal maternal immune response to antigens on placental or fetal tissues. Normally, the maintenance of pregnancy requires the formation of blocking factors (probably complexes of antibody and antigen) that prevent maternal rejection of fetal antigens. It has been argued that couples with repetitive miscarriages have increased sharing of human leukocyte antigens (HLA), a condition that would not allow the mother to make blocking antibodies. However, many investigators have failed to confirm that sharing of HLA antigens is found to a greater degree in couples with recurrent miscarriages[28], and at least five randomized placebo-controlled studies have failed to demonstrate a beneficial effect of immunotherapy in these cases[29].

Finally, the outcome of assisted reproductive technologies is not certain in women with a large number of recurrent miscarriages. In one series of 12 women with a history of recurrent abortions, eight women delivered at term after *in vitro* fertilization[30]. In addition, *in vitro* fertilization outcome seems to be reduced in women with positive antiphospholipid antibodies[31]. However, in another study, although the pregnancy rates were good, a high rate of spontaneous miscarriages (>50%) occurred in women with three or more consecutive losses[32]. Good results have been reported with oocyte donation in women with recurrent pregnancy loss[33]. However, decisions for undergoing oocyte donation are individual and heavily influenced by psychological, ethical and financial resources.

It should be emphasized that continued attempts at conception are rewarded with success in the majority of women (70–75%) labelled as recurrent aborters without identifiable cause[34].

From all these statements arises the constant need for further improvement of diagnostic methods in order to be able, as early as possible, to recognize symptoms of spontaneous abortion, and especially signs of threatened abortion at the stage when further complications could be prevented. The main problems in management of such patients lie in early diagnosis. When vaginal bleeding occurs the clinician should ask several questions that can radically alter the management:

(1) Is the patient pregnant?
(2) What is the gestational age?
(3) Is the fetus alive or dead?
(4) Is there any evidence to suggest that the pregnancy is extrauterine?
(5) In the event of an abortion, is it complete or incomplete?
(6) Is there any associated pelvic mass?

It is only after such differentiation that control and possibly therapeutic measures can be applied to cases where a normal outcome of the pregnancy can be expected. After an accurate diagnosis has been made, the selection of possible therapeutic measures is easier.

Ultrasound has become an irreplaceable diagnostic tool in the follow-up of the development and complications of early pregnancy. With the introduction of transvaginal sonography (TVS) the possibility for early morphological and biometric ultrasound examinations has been improved. The application of color Doppler has enabled functional hemodynamic examinations to be performed virtually after implantation. Threatened and spontaneous abortions are not usually of vital importance to a patient, but they play an important role in further reproductive functioning. Basic ultrasound markers for normal pregnancy are an intrauterine gestational sac, a normal embryo and its heart action. A fundamental aim of early ultrasound examination, besides the actual diagnosis of pregnancy, is to distinguish between an abnormal and a normal, vital pregnancy. A normal embryonic echo in 90% of cases suggests a normal pregnancy outcome[35]. If the crown–rump length (CRL) is <5 mm, the possibility of pregnancy loss is around 8%; if the CRL measures 6–10 mm, the possibility of pregnancy loss is around 3–4%; and if the CRL is >10 mm, the possibility of pregnancy loss is below 1%.

At present, ultrasonography is considered to be the best diagnostic method for detecting early pregnancy complications. The skill of the ultrasonographer is put to the test, since a verdict of pregnancy failure will often result in surgical intervention. With a normal intrauterine pregnancy, the chorion frondosum is undoubtedly the most common source of vaginal bleeding in the first trimester. Sonographic evidence of such bleeding can be identified as perigestational hemorrhage in 5–22% of women with symptoms of threatened abortion[1,2]. However, some precautions must be taken, because a perigestational hemorrhage is occasionally difficult to distinguish from a blighted twin. The prognostic significance of identifying perigestational hemorrhage during the first trimester remains uncertain. Most of the small hemorrhages resolve without clinical sequelae, but in some cases spontaneous abortion may occur[36].

INTRAUTERINE HEMATOMAS

Intrauterine hematomas have become a subject of morphological and hemodynamic research all over the world. They are defined as sonolucent crescent- or wedge-shaped structures between chorionic tissue and the uterine wall or fetal membranes[37] (Figure 1). By localization we can divide them into:

(1)   Retroplacental;
(2)   Subchorionic;
(3)   Marginal;
(4)   Supracervical.

Mantoni and Pedersen[38] were the first to describe the ultrasound image of an intrauterine hematoma, which has been clearly defined later by other authors[37,39,40]. The most severe are large, central, retroplacental hematomas in which there is separation of chorionic tissue from the basal decidua by a mechanism similar to that of abruption. The most common causes are:

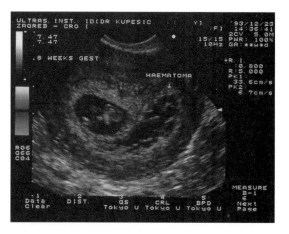

Figure 1 *Transvaginal color Doppler scan of an 8-week gestation complicated by retrochorionic hematoma. Spiral arteries and embryonic heart activity are clearly displayed (see Color Plate G)*

(1) Disturbed trophoblast invasion and a defect in spiral artery transformation;
(2) Infection;
(3) Mechanical factors;
(4) Autoimmune factors;
(5) Hematological factors.

There are two main explanations for the mechanism of early separation of chorionic tissue and hematoma formation[41]. The first suggests marginal bleeding at the edge of the trophoblast tissue, where disturbance in the local venous circulation occurs, mainly owing to inflammatory events. The second interpretation deals with formation of a retroplacental (central) hematoma where, pathohistologically, decidual arterial vasculopathy caused by disturbed primary and secondary trophoblast invasion has been discovered.

The finding of an intrauterine hematoma does not immediately indicate spontaneous abortion, but rather classifies this pregnancy into a high-risk group, with additional necessity for further intensive monitoring. Table 1 demonstrates the frequency of spontaneous abortions and preterm deliveries in patients with an intrauterine hematoma[37]. Prognostically, there are two main elements that determine the pregnancy outcome: localization and size.

Localization

According to Mantoni and Pedersen[38] and Kurjak and associates, this is a more predictive sign than the volume of the hematoma[37,40]. Much emphasis has been put on the volume of the hematoma, but not on the location of the hemorrhage. It is likely that, if the bleeding occurs at the level of the definitive placenta (under the cord insertion), it may result in placental separation and subsequent abortion[39]. Conversely, a subchorionic hematoma detaching only a membrane opposite to the cord insertion could probably reach a significant volume before it affects normal pregnancy development[36]. A supracervical hematoma has a much better prognosis, because of its easier drainage into the vagina and its location, which does not cause mechanical compression

of the uteroplacental circulation. A higher incidence of spontaneous abortions has been reported in cases where the hematoma has been localized in the fundal or corporal region, which could be attributed to placental location in that area[37]. Retroplacental or central hematomas have the worst prognosis, because they cause the largest effect on the uteroplacental circulation and placental tissue[41]. Table 2 presents data of Kurjak et al.[37] on hematoma site and pregnancy outcome[37].

Kurjak and co-workers reported on an increase in resistance to blood flow and a decrease in velocity through spiral arteries on the side of the subchorionic hematoma, a consequence of mechanical compression of the hematoma itself[37,38] (Figure 2). With the progression of pregnancy and growth of trophoblast tissue, gradual disappearance of the disturbance and normalization of the

Table 1 *Frequency of spontaneous abortions and preterm deliveries in patients with a subchorionic hematoma and controls. From reference 37, with permission*

	Patients	Spontaneous abortions		Preterm deliveries	
		n	%	n	%
Control	135	8	6.0	9	7.0
Subchorionic hematoma	59	10	16.9*	3	5.0
Total	194	18	9.2	12	6.2

*Fisher exact test vs. controls: one-tailed, $p = 0.006$, two-tailed, $p = 0.02$

Table 2 *Hematoma site and pregnancy outcome. From reference 37, with permission*

Site	Patients	Spontaneous abortion		Preterm delivery	
		n	%	n	%
Supracervical	30	2	6.7	2	6.7
Fundus–corpus	29	8	27.5*	1	3.4
Total	59	10	16.9	3	5.0

*Fisher exact test: one-tailed, $p = 0.01$, two-tailed, $p = 0.03$

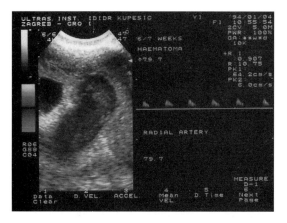

Figure 2 *Transvaginal color Doppler sonogram of uterine vessels in a case of retrochorionic hematoma. Blood flow signals extracted from radial arteries demonstrate the absence of diastolic flow (RI = 1.0) (see Color Plate H)*

circulation occur, but the pregnancy still remains in the high-risk group, with necessity for intensive monitoring. However, Alcazar reported that early fetal circulation does not seem to be affected by the presence of a retrochorionic hematoma[42]. His results were confirmed by Kurjak and associates[43] and Rizzo and colleagues[44]. In Alcazar's series, a possible explanation of these findings could be the fact that most of the hematomas were small and located marginally. Thus, they did not substantially affect the chorion frondosum and the delivery of nutrients and oxygen to the fetus, and therefore did not cause hemodynamic alterations or disturbances in the fetal circulation[42]. Most pregnancies that ended in spontaneous abortion had a centrally located hematoma (70%), but even in these cases they did not find any alteration in fetal hemodynamics as compared with the control group. On the other hand, hematoma volume was not associated with pregnancy outcome, which is in agreement with the results reported by Kurjak and co-workers[43].

Size

Modern ultrasonographic machines and the transvaginal approach enables us to measure the size of a hematoma accurately in relation to the trophoblast tissue, and its distance from the internal os[45]. Furthermore, software of the newest machines makes possible the spatial three-dimensional imaging of hematomas and surrounding structures, as well as measurement of their volume and dynamic follow-up of biometric changes. At the same time, Doppler measurements can evaluate the already mentioned compression effect on the adjacent uteroplacental circulation[37,40].

Threatened abortion is a common clinical situation in which vaginal bleeding occurs during the first half of pregnancy and the presence of a living embryo is suspected. The advent of TVS has allowed the improved assessment of threatened abortion, clarifying the differential diagnosis of missed abortion, ectopic pregnancy, blighted ovum and threatened abortion with a living embryo. Embryo vitality can be established reliably by documenting cardiac activity on real-time, B-mode ultrasonography.

In patients with normal pregnancies, when embryo vitality is confirmed, the rate of pregnancy loss is low (3.2%)[3]. However, in patients with threatened abortion with a living embryo, the rate of loss has been reported to be five-fold higher[45]. The ultimate cause of threatened abortion cannot be determined in most cases. When bleeding occurs, it could be speculated that vascular injury might be the primary or secondary cause. Indeed, histological studies have shown that insufficient invasion of spiral arteries may result in spontaneous abortion of live fetuses[46]. Therefore, an assessment of early placentation could be useful for predicting pregnancy outcome in cases of threatened abortion with a living embryo.

With the introduction of transvaginal color Doppler ultrasound, assessment of the early uteroplacental circulation has become feasible. Several studies have evaluated the uteroplacental circulation in patients with abnormal early pregnancies. These studies are interesting from a pathophysiological point of view, but may not be relevant for clinical practice, because diagnosis can be made with B-mode ultrasound, and assessment of the uteroplacental circulation does not add clinical or prognostic information.

However, the situation is different in patients with threatened abortion and a living embryo. In such cases, information regarding the uteroplacental circulation obtained with the use of color Doppler ultrasound could provide prognostic information. Based on our knowledge, only a few studies have addressed this issue. Stabile and co-workers[47] evaluated the uteroplacental circulation in a series of 48 women with first-trimester threatened abortion. After the exclusion of five women with missed abortion and three with ectopic pregnancy, only two of 40 women had spontaneous abortion. The investigators found no differences in the resistance index (RI) from the uterine arteries between patients with spontaneous abortion and those with normal pregnancy outcome. However, the number of cases that ended in spontaneous abortion was too low to allow any definitive conclusions to be drawn. More recently, Kurjak and associates[43] evaluated the uteroplacental circulation in 60 patients with threatened abortion. Eight of 50 patients with a living embryo had a spontaneous abortion. These investigators found no differences in Doppler parameters of the uterine vessels between these patients and controls[43]. Results of Alcazar and Ruiz-Perez[48] are also in agreement with those of the previous studies, and suggest that there is no alteration in the uteroplacental circulation in patients with first-trimester threatened abortion with a living embryo. They speculated that this fact could be explained by a minimal vascular injury that could not be detected by Doppler ultrasound.

GESTATIONAL SAC AND EMBRYONIC ECHO

Biometric and morphological characteristics of the gestational sac and an embryonic echo can be used as a predictive factor in the diagnosis of threatened abortion. Decreased values of gestational sac diameter and/or its irregular shape can suggest an impending incident and can be used as a marker for chromosomopathies. Early spontaneous abortion is usually connected with triploidy and trisomy[49,50]. Early growth restriction, identified on the basis of decreased CRL values in relation to the gestational age and proportional dimensions of the gestational sac, could indicate early hemodynamic disturbances or chromosomal aberrations. Several studies have demonstrated that sonographic findings, particularly CRL measurements, have prognostic value[45,49,51]. On the basis of CRL measurements it is possible to predict spontaneous miscarriage and possible birth weight[45]. Diabetes mellitus and aneuploidy are already recognized causes of reduced embryonic cell division during the first trimester[50]. In maternal diabetes mellitus a small CRL for gestational age is associated with subsequent delivery of a small-for-gestational-age infant. Findings showing that the embryo grows so that the values of CRL measurements always move within certain centile limits also point to a possible connection between embryo size in early pregnancy and birth weight. The reliability of CRL measurements depends on embryo size and on the fact that the measurements are precise only when the greatest long axis reaches 18–22 mm. In smaller embryos, an error of merely a few millimeters results in a large deviation. In embryos over 18 mm, when the CRL is measured and the anatomic structures are visible, the possibility of an error is smaller. Apart from the necessity of a precise measurement, the risk of adverse pregnancy outcome depends on the gestational age and embryo size. However, some results suggest that the measurement of fetal CRL may be a useful predictor of spontaneous miscarriage and a small-for-gestational age fetus in pregnancies with threatened miscarriage[51].

The embryonic heart rate demonstrates physiological variability within its normal range of frequencies, which is 150–190 beats/min for an embryo larger than 10 mm at 8–12 weeks of gestation. Bradycardia or arrhythmia could be considered as predictors of heart action cessation. In such cases, early hemodynamic heart failure was noted with consequential gestational sac enlargement, yolk sac enlargement (more than 6 mm) and initial generalized hydrops. This type of hemodynamic disturbance can occur in patients presenting with massive intrauterine hematomas prior to fetal demise[52]. Reduced body movements of the embryo during the first and second trimesters are also included in possible predictors of early pregnancy complications[52].

YOLK SAC

The yolk sac is the first recognizable structure inside the gestational sac in early pregnancy. The earliest TVS visualization demonstrates a regularly rounded extra-amniotic structure when the gestational sac is 8–10 mm[53]. Normal biometric values of the inner diameter of the yolk sac during the first trimester are 3–6 mm.

The following changes are related to the prediction of spontaneous abortion[53]:

(1) Too large – more than 6 mm (over 2 SD, sensitivity 16%, specificity 97%, positive predictive value (PPV) 60%);
(2) Too small – less than 3 mm (below 2 SD, sensitivity 15%, specificity 95%, PPV 44%);
(3) Irregular shape – mainly wrinkled with indented walls;
(4) Degenerative changes – abundant calcifications with decreased translucency of the yolk sac;
(5) Number of yolk sacs – has to be equal to the number of embryos.

It is currently supposed that yolk sac abnormalities are rather the consequence than the cause of altered embryonic development[54,55] (Figure 3). Table 3 shows the yolk sac diameter and vascularity between 6 and 12 weeks of gestation in normal pregnancies[54]. Table 4 presents data on yolk sac diameter and vascularity between 6 and 12 weeks of gestation in patients with missed abortion[55].

ANEMBRYONIC PREGNANCY

A blighted ovum is a gestational sac in which the embryo either failed to develop or died at a stage too early to visualize. The diagnosis of anembryonic pregnancy is based on the absence of embryonic echoes within a gestational sac large enough for the structures to be visible, independently of the clinical data or the menstrual cycle[36]. The gestational sac, in these patients, represents only an empty chorionic cavity (Figure 4). In an anembryonic pregnancy, a fertilized ovum develops into a blastocyst, but the inner cell mass and resultant fetal pole never develop. The gestational sac invades the endometrium and acts partially like a normally developing pregnancy. The syncytiotrophoblast invades the endometrium and produces human chorionic gonadotropin, which produces a positive pregnancy test, tender breasts and other clinical signs of pregnancy. The normal appearances, however, are short-lived. The gestational sac fails to grow and develop normally, and the uterus fails to develop as expected[36]. Anembryonic pregnancy is associated with chromosomopathies in 60% of cases[5]. The trophoblastic tissue continues its hormonal activity, which enables these pregnancies to exist for a long time before the start of necrotic changes. It also shows hydropic changes, so the size of the gestational sac can

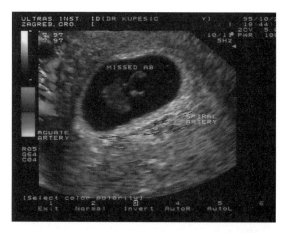

Figure 3 *Transvaginal color Doppler scan of missed abortion at 8 weeks' gestation. Color Doppler reveals blood flow within the maternal vessels and absence of flow in the fetal vessels. Note the hydropic degeneration of the yolk sac demonstrated by the increased diameter and altered echogenicity (see Color Plate I)*

Table 3 *Yolk sac diameter and vascularity between 6 and 10 weeks of gestation in normal pregnancies. From reference 54, with permission*

Gestational age (weeks)	*Yolk sac diameter*				*Yolk sac vascularity*		
	n	*Mean* (mm)	*Range*	*Significance*	*n*	*%*	*Significance*
6	9	3.1	2.5–3.8		3	33.33	
7	15	3.6	2.9–4.4	$p < 0.05$	12	80.00	$p < 0.005$
8	19	4.1	3.6–5.1	$p < 0.05$	17	89.47	$p < 0.05$
9	18	4.5	4.1–5.9	$p < 0.05$	15	83.33	$p < 0.05$
10	14	5.3	4.3–6.0	$p < 0.001$	8	57.14	$p < 0.001$
11	12	5.0	4.1–5.9	$p < 0.05$	3	25.00	$p < 0.005$
12	10	4.3	3.4–4.9	$p < 0.001$	0	0	$p < 0.001$
Total	87	4.2	2.5–6.0		58	66.67	

Table 4 *Yolk sac diameter and vascularity between 6 and 12 weeks of gestation in patients with missed abortion. From reference 55, with permission*

Gestational age (weeks)	*Yolk sac diameter*				*Yolk sac vascularity*	
	n	≥ 6.1 mm	2.5–6.0 mm	≤ 2.4 mm	*n*	*%*
6	4	2	1	1	0	0
7	9	4	3	2	2	22.22
8	11	5	4	2	3	27.27
9	7	3	2	2	2	28.57
10	6	2	2	2	1	16.67
11	6	2	2	2	1	16.67
12	5	3	1	1	0	0
Total	48	21	15	12	9	18.54

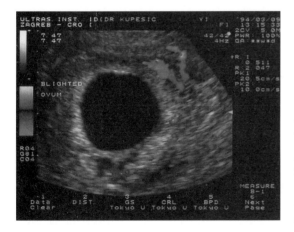

Figure 4 *Transvaginal color Doppler scan of a richly vascularized blighted ovum. Color Doppler facilitates the visualization of dilated spiral arteries in close proximity to the empty gestational sac (see Color Plate J)*

sometimes demonstrate a much larger diameter than would be expected for gestational age.

Advances in TVS allow us to detect this kind of abnormality at a mean sac diameter of 15 mm[56]. If the volume of the sac is less than 2.5 ml, in a pregnancy that fails to increase in size by at least 75% over the period of 1 week, this pregnancy could also be diagnosed as a blighted ovum. When a large empty sac measuring 12–18 mm in mean diameter is found, the absence of a living embryo is suspicious for non-viability, but this finding should be correlated with other clinical and sonographic data, including the presence of a yolk sac. According to Tongsong and co-workers[57], a gestational sac with a diameter of 17 mm or larger without a detectable embryonic echo is a confident marker for anembryonic pregnancy, even on the basis of only one transvaginal ultrasound examination (specificity 100%, PPV 100%). The same can be applied to the gestational sac larger than 13 mm without a visible yolk sac.

Large empty gestational sacs are usually related to chromosomopathies and a 'real' blighted ovum that is paternal in origin (Figure 4). The expression 'real' blighted ovum is used deliberately, because the ultrasonographic finding of an anembryonic pregnancy in differential diagnosis includes retained missed abortion, where a complete resorption of an embryo may occur (Figure 5). In those cases the gestational sac is usually smaller than expected for gestational age.

With falling levels of human chorionic gonadotropin, progesterone and estrogen, the feeling of being pregnant and the associated pelvic fullness and breast tenderness are also lost. The diagnosis of blighted ovum can be made in 100% of cases by two real-time ultrasonography examinations performed a week apart[56]. The fact that a fetus is never observed in spite of very careful study is of primary importance[57]. Some Doppler studies have shown that there was no significant difference in RI values of the spiral arteries between pregnancy failures and normal pregnancies[58–60]. Studies of the intervillous circulation demonstrated lower pulsatility index (PI) values (0.54 ± 0.04) of the artery-like signals in patients with a blighted ovum when compared to those with a normal pregnancy (0.80 ± 0.04) and a missed abortion (0.75 ± 0.04)[61,62]. A lower PI from the intervillous space of the anembryonic pregnancy group may reflect changes in the placental stroma, where the individual villi are prone to edema (Figure 6). One could speculate that lower velocities of the venous flow obtained from the intervillous space in women with an anembryonic pregnancy may result from reduced drainage[61]. Furthermore, the lower impedance to blood flow observed in the spiral arteries indicates that a massive and continuous infiltration of the maternal blood without effective drainage causes further disruption of the maternal–embryonic

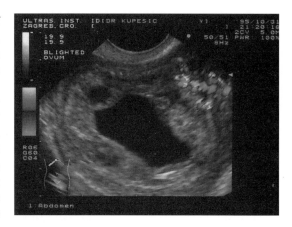

Figure 5 *Transvaginal color Doppler scan of another case of anembryonic pregnancy. Note the irregular shape of the empty gestational sac and discrete blood flow signals at its periphery (see Color Plate K)*

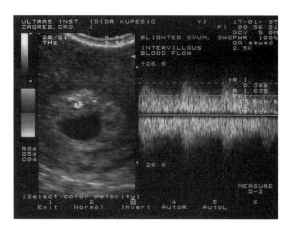

Figure 6 *Transvaginal color Doppler scan of blood flow signals obtained from the intervillous space. Note the low vascular resistance of artery-like signals (RI = 0.39) characteristic of this pathology (see Color Plate L)*

interface, resulting in abortion. Therefore, it seems that the impedance to blood flow in the intervillous space is lower when embryonic death takes place early and when mesenchymal tissue turgor is low[63]. In cases with a short retention period and normal internal tissue turgor and no villous edema, Doppler results are similar to those obtained in normal pregnancy. Combined studies from cytogenetics, pathology, ultrasound and Doppler flow are needed for a better understanding of the pathophysiology of early pregnancy failure.

MISSED ABORTION

The diagnosis of missed abortion is characterized by the identification of a fetus that does not demonstrate any heart activity[58] (Figure 7). It is also determined as a type of spontaneous abortion where, after fetal demise, spontaneous expulsion of the conceptus out of the uterus does not occur[11].

Ultrasound findings can be differentiated according to the time that has passed from the incident that caused the fetal demise and the break in circulation[11,56]:

(1) *Gestational sac image* recent – normal shape, later – collapsed, changed in shape and size;

(2) *Embryo without heart action and dynamics* recent – morphology preserved, later – smaller with altered morphology, completely amorphous or fragmented;

(3) *Changes of trophoblast tissue* heterogeneous, degeneratively changed (hydropic or calcified), intrauterine hematomas, separation of membranes.

It is relatively easy to make this diagnosis by means of the transvaginal color Doppler facilities. The main parameter is the absence of heart activity and the lack of a color flow signal at its expected position after the 6th gestational week[63]. However, one should be aware that the length of time elapsing between arrest of embryonic development and clinical presentation will determine the sonographic image and should be considered in the interpretation. If ultrasound facilities are available, the diagnosis of embryonic demise is not improved by the measurement of any placental hormone or protein.

Histological studies of material obtained after spontaneous abortions have shown insufficient trophoblastic invasion into the spiral arteries. Such findings suggest defective transformation of spiral arteries as a possible cause of spontaneous abortion[63]. Recent Doppler studies did not show any difference

in terms of RI and PI for the intervillous arterial flow and spiral arteries between women with missed abortion and those with normal pregnancy[64,65] (Figure 8). In long-standing demise, the cessation of the embryonic portion of the placental circulation leaves the fluid-pumping action of the trophoblast unaffected, as it remains nourished by maternal intervillous blood[61]. As a consequence, the trophoblast-conveyed fluid in the villous stroma is no longer drained by the embryonic circulation. Progressive accumulation of the

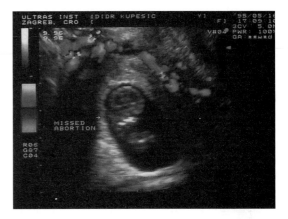

Figure 7 *Transvaginal color Doppler scan of missed abortion. Note the prominent blood flow signals obtained from maternal vessels and the absence of fetal heart activity (see Color Plate M)*

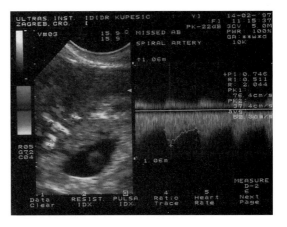

Figure 8 *Increased resistance index (RI = 0.51) of the artery-like signal within the intervillous space obtained in a patient with missed abortion (see Color Plate N)*

fluid may result in significant reduction of the intervillous blood flow[61,62]. As chromosomal abnormalities are one of the most important factors for spontaneous abortion, occurring in more than 50%, it is not surprising that Doppler studies have not demonstrated any significant difference in terms of vascular resistance between normal pregnancies and those with missed abortions. However, further investigation is needed to clarify the link between chromosomal abnormalities and impaired hemochorial placentation[66].

TRANSVAGINAL SONOGRAPHY AS AN AID IN THERAPY

For years surgical uterine evacuation has remained the universally accepted method for management of early pregnancy loss, but recent studies have provided evidence supporting the role of expectant and medical management in early pregnancy[67-69]. Nielsen and Hahlin[70], in a small randomized study of expectant and surgical management of early pregnancy loss, demonstrated that there was a spontaneous resolution in 80% of cases managed expectantly. Even though expectant management of early pregnancy loss is used sporadically by clinicians, little is known about the natural history of this process. Hence, information regarding the likelihood of success, the spectrum and duration of symptoms, is not available to clinicians and patients in planning management.

Some studies have been performed to compare the sonographic evaluation of the endometrial echogenicity and thickness with the histopathological findings after dilatation and curettage (D&C), to determine whether TVS could identify those patients who might avoid surgical procedures[71,72].

It is well known that the surgical procedure of D&C has several risks, such as hemorrhage, infection, formation of uterine adhesions, cervical trauma, secondary infertility, chronic pelvic pain, dyspareunia and psychological problems[7,73,74]. The correct use of TVS can significantly reduce these risks and maintain a woman's future fertility[73]. Many authors have

researched the ability of TVS to distinguish the cases with complete evacuation of the endometrial cavity, consequently avoiding D&C. Ballagh and colleagues[7] in their recent study doubted the necessity for D&C in all cases of abortion during the first trimester and proposed that the more accurate ultrasound diagnosis in these cases would reduce unnecessary surgical procedures.

Sariam and co-workers[75] performed the largest clinical study to outline the natural history of spontaneous early pregnancy loss. The findings of this study have established that expectant management of miscarriage is feasible and effective, especially in the group of women with an ultrasound diagnosis of incomplete miscarriage. The fact that none of 305 women managed expectantly required blood transfusion or developed infective morbidity confirms that expectant management of miscarriage is safe. The success rate in women with incomplete miscarriage was 96%, significantly higher than in those with missed miscarriage (62%). Other studies have also proposed the use of hormone assays or ultrasound facilities to predict the likelihood of successful expectant management, with a success rate in the group with the missed miscarriage of 62%[76,77]. In the study performed by Schwarzler and associates[77] the success rate at the end of 2 weeks of assessment was 62%, which improved significantly to 84% after 28 days of expectant management of missed miscarriage. This is significantly higher than that quoted by Jurkovic and colleagues[78], who reported that only 20% of women with missed miscarriages underwent a compete miscarriage at the end of a 2-week assessment. Waiting for a further 2 weeks in the current study might well have improved the success rate. Additionally, inclusion of asymptomatic women with missed miscarriages may also have contributed to the lower success rate, as they might be less likely to miscarry in the specified follow-up period[74,75].

Haines and co-workers[79] used sonographically derived measurements (transverse and sagittal cavity area of the uterus) to select cases suitable for conservative treatment. In this study, 64% of the cases fulfilled the criteria for non-surgical treatment. Cetin and Cetin[8] evaluated the maximum anteroposterior diameter of the uterine cavity on the long-axis view and the echo pattern of the retained products of conception. They found that conservative management could be a choice in patients with a uterine cavity containing fluid mixed with solid components, or containing only solid components, if the maximum anteroposterior diameter of the uterine cavity on the long-axis view was less than 10 mm and 8 mm, respectively. TVS findings can be used as a decision factor in the management of patients with first-trimester spontaneous abortion to reduce the need for an elective curettage by approximately 58%[8].

Kurtz and Shlansky-Goldberg[9] showed that a thick endometrium (> 5 mm in maximum anteroposterior diameter) was always associated with retained products of conception. Conversely, a thin endometrium of < 2 mm was almost always indicative of no products of conception. More work is needed to substantiate this finding and to determine the thickness of the endometrium that can be used to predict when all products of conception have been spontaneously passed. The results of the study performed by Chung and colleagues[74] suggest that the use of misoprostol may be justified as a preliminary treatment in the management of spontaneous abortion. The proportion of women requiring curettage may become smaller with further experience of misoprostol, when optimal dosage, frequency and duration of the treatment become more clear. These authors concluded that further experience with TVS may also reduce the number of women subjected to unnecessary treatment[74]. Rulin and associates[80] found that ultrasonography was highly reliable in the management of presumed complete spontaneous abortion in the first trimester. Histopathological examination performed in that study showed that in 69% of patients with retained uterine products the endometrial thickness was >10 mm. The results of Botsis and co-workers[81] were in accordance with those of Rulin and colleagues[80] regarding endometrial thickness, although the most reliable parameter in their study seemed to be the endometrial echogenicity.

Color Doppler may provide additional help for decision making in the therapeutic approach. Although the diagnostic capacity of color Doppler ultrasound and its value as a predictor of pregnancy outcome are still unclear, it has markedly reduced uncertainties in the diagnosis of early pregnancy failure[47,82]. Incomplete abortion varies with the stage of embryological development at the time of demise and the amount of gestational tissue passed. Variable amounts of disorganized echogenic debris, fluid, or both are often present in the endometrial cavity. A mixed endometrial pattern characterized by the presence of both hyperechoic and hypoechoic areas remains the mainstay in the diagnosis of incomplete abortion. Transvaginal color Doppler demonstrates rich perfusion of the unexpelled gestational tissue (Figure 9). Abundant color flow is caused by dilated spiral arteries and the venous system, probably in response to the active trophoblastic tissue. Low vascular impedance (RI = 0.41 ± 0.01) can be detected at the endometrial level even without clear viability of the products of conception[82].

TVS is a simple and reliable method for the evaluation of the endometrial stripe and echogenicity, in order to reduce the number of unnecessary curettage procedures in those

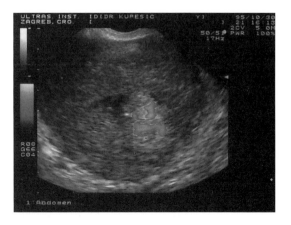

Figure 9 *Transvaginal power Doppler scan of retained products of conception (see Color Plate O)*

patients presenting with clinical symptoms of spontaneous abortion during the first trimester of pregnancy. The expectant management of spontaneous early miscarriages is known to provide an outcome (both medical and psychological morbidity) equivalent to that from surgical evacuation of the uterus, with no adverse effect on future fertility[83]. For appropriate patients, this approach with effective support can be easier and less distressing.

The patient with early miscarriage usually presents as an anxious, frustrated individual on the verge of despair[84]. Evaluation should be spaced over several visits, allowing the clinician to establish communication and rapport with the patient. Frequent communication between the clinician and the patient during the first trimester of the next pregnancy is essential. The emotional support that the clinician can bring to this interaction will be most useful and in some cases may even be therapeutic. Some studies have demonstrated that the availability and desirability of routine follow-up care is associated with reduced psychological morbidity following pregnancy loss[84,85].

ROLE OF THREE- AND FOUR-DIMENSIONAL ULTRASOUND IN THE ASSESSMENT OF THREATENED ABORTION

Three-dimensional (3D) ultrasound is an exciting new technology that provides valuable information in the investigation and management of patients with early pregnancy pathology. In the not too distant future, this examination may become the method of choice for assessing morphology of the uterus and its cavity[86].

With conventional 2D ultrasonography, the assessment of the overall structures relevant for differentiating a normal from an abnormal early pregnancy is often difficult and time consuming. Three-dimensional ultrasonography allows visualization of the intrauterine content in all three dimensions at the same time, providing an improved overview and a more clearly defined demonstration of different anatomical planes[87]. With the advent of 3D

ultrasound, we are now able to review the sections in all three mutually perpendicular (orthogonal) planes. We can also scrutinize all features in surface-rendered and transparent views. Already, a number of investigators have effectively demonstrated that 3D ultrasound offers various advantages over conventional 2D imaging[88,89].

Although the development of this diagnostic modality started a decade ago, it was only in the 1990s that we obtained the high quality of reconstruction based on the development of advanced computer systems. This opened unexpected avenues in diagnosis in obstetrics and gynecology[90–92]. The use of 3D imaging can now be extended to follow pregnancy from conception to term.

The expanded capability for 3D imaging in normal pregnancies has focused attention on the early weeks of gestation. The embryonic period, extending from conception until 9 weeks of gestation, is extremely important. Most of the major anatomic structures and organ systems are formed and developed during this period. The sequential appearance of embryonic and fetal structures can be visualized by TVS as much as 3 weeks earlier than with the use of transabdominal ultrasound[89]. Endoscopic uterine sonography and embryoscopy[93] have also been able to delineate embryonic structures much earlier than TVS and with a more clearly outlined configuration. However, these two techniques are invasive procedures and neither their safety nor guidelines for their use have yet been established. Three-dimensional ultrasound is a valuable, non-invasive tool for the study of embryonic and fetal development, which can replace invasive methods of investigation.

This method allows a detailed morphological and volumetric analysis of the embryo and static extraembryonic structures. Using the 3D planar mode the position of the yolk sac is accurately spatially assessed. Three-dimensional sonography produces better intraobserver reproducibility of the obtained results in comparison to conventional 2D sonography. Kupesic and co-workers[94] measured gestational sac volume and yolk sac volume and vascularity in 80 women with an uncomplicated pregnancy between 5 and 12 weeks of gestation. Regression analysis revealed exponential growth of gestational sac volume throughout the first trimester of pregnancy. Gestational sac volume measurements could be used for the estimation of gestational age in early pregnancy. An abnormal gestational sac volume measurement could potentially be used as a prognostic marker for pregnancy outcome. The yolk sac was found to increase from 5 to 10 weeks of gestation. However, when the yolk sac reaches its maximum volume at around 10 weeks it has already started to degenerate, which can be indirectly confirmed by a significant reduction in visualization rates of the yolk sac vascularity. These events suggest that the evaluation of the biological function of the yolk sac by measuring the diameter and/or the volume is limited. Therefore, a combination of functional and volumetric studies is necessary to identify some of the more important moments during early pregnancy.

Kurjak and colleagues[54] reported on the vascularization of the yolk sac in normal pregnancies between 6 and 10 weeks of gestation. Pulsed Doppler signals characterized by low velocity and high pulsatility were obtained in 85.71% of the yolk sacs during the 7th and 8th gestational weeks. Although the reports on the yolk sac and vitelline circulation are very exciting, it should be noted that such studies are not ethically feasible in ongoing human pregnancies, since the secondary yolk sac is the source of primary germ cell and blood stem cells[95]. Kurjak and Kupesic[62] performed a study analyzing the vascularization of the yolk sac in 48 patients with missed abortions. In 18.5% of these patients three types of abnormal vascular signals were derived from the yolk sac:

(1) Irregular blood flow;
(2) Permanent diastolic flow;
(3) Venous blood flow.

The prognostic significance of analyzing the secondary yolk sac circulation is not clearly established, since these vessels persist inside the wall of the yolk sac up to 1 month after the cellular death of the other components[96]. Therefore, changes in vascular pattern as well as changes in yolk sac appearance (size, shape and echogenicity) seem to be a consequence of poor embryonic development or even embryonic death, rather than a primary cause of early pregnancy failure. Three-dimensional ultrasound may significantly contribute to *in vivo* observations of the yolk sac, enabling scanning time to be reduced and the yolk sac's honeycomb surface pattern to be observed. Automatic volume calculation will allow us to estimate the precise relationship between the yolk sac and gestational sac volumes, as well as to obtain the correlation between yolk sac and CRL measurements. Furthermore, 3D ultrasound and power Doppler will allow study of turgescent blood vessels rising above the surface of the yolk sac. The same technique can be used to study the evolution from the embryo–vitelline towards the embryo–placental circulation. Alterations in the yolk sac circulatory system may also have prognostic value for predicting pregnancy outcome.

In the light of these considerations it is of great importance to stress that, by adding colored blood flow signals to the gray-scale image, or extracting only color-coded signals, it is possible to depict a three-dimensional image of the vascular features of an early pregnancy. This enables elucidation of the longitudinal changes in the embryonic and early uteroplacental circulation.

Three-dimensional power Doppler enables clear visualization of the entire embryonic circulation starting from the 7th week of gestation, and visualization of the intensive blood circulation under the early placenta. The number of areas in which blood penetrates the intervillous space increases gradually with gestation. The number of areas with an established intervillous circulation increases with embryonic and placental growth, in order to maintain a state of metabolic balance. It is expected that three-dimensional power Doppler and spectral pulsed Doppler data with post-mortem histology specimens will yield new and important facts about this period of human development.

The straightforward development of three-dimensional ultrasound has acquired the possibility of performing 3D imaging in real-time mode. This technique is called four-dimensional (4D) ultrasound, because time becomes a parameter within the three-dimensional imaging sequence. The display of such a sequence of 3D images can give information about movements[97].

Recently, a few ultrasound machines have become commercially available that can provide a 4D mode. These systems rely on specially designed probes and fast rendering devices. They can reach up to 20 images per second, depending on the volume size, resolution and mechanics of the probe. Problems arising from this technology have led to the incorporation of a special design of probes and require fast computer rendering. Learning the skills needed for three-dimensional and four-dimensional ultrasound requires new training, but good experience in 2D ultrasound is essential[97].

Clinical research about the possible applications of 4D ultrasound is still missing. Four-dimensional ultrasound is especially helpful in increasing the quantity of image information, because the acquisition of the right moment is easier when there are sequential volumes from which to choose. In the case of threatened abortion, possible advantages are the improvement of image quality, better anatomic orientation and demonstration of eventual uterine contractions. Another benefit may result from the improvement of the response interval between the investigator and the machine. High-speed rendering decreases the calculation time between re-adjustments and three-dimensional image output. This allows fast adjustment of imaging parameters and fast post-processing with a reduction in volume data.

CONCLUSION

With the advent of TVS, the assessment of early pregnancy has greatly improved. Ultrasound examination of the pelvis by a transvaginal probe combined with color and pulsed Doppler assessment may increase the reliability of ultrasound diagnosis in early pregnancy. This technique has enabled us to measure, in detail and with accuracy, blood flow through the vessels of the embryo, uterus and ovaries, which have previously not been measurable by any existing diagnostic method in the 6th week of pregnancy. Embryonic and fetal vessels can be easily visualized by this method, and the pulsed Doppler beam can thus be easily guided to the vessels of interest. If only pulsed Doppler is used, the localization of blood flow is a time-consuming and relatively difficult procedure. The guidance of the pulsed Doppler beam by color helps to locate areas of most abundant flow and thus makes the examination much faster and more accurate.

Just when it appeared that diagnostic ultrasound has reached the limits of its technical development and that further refinements would be of a minor nature, three-dimensional imaging has come on the scene. This technology has reached a stage where structures of only a few millimeters can be imaged *in vivo* in three dimensions. This significantly contributes to research into the developing embryo.

Three-dimensional power Doppler allows more precise and earlier evaluation of the embryonic, fetal and intervillous circulatory systems in normal and abnormal pregnancies. We believe that recent developments in ultrasound technology will contribute to better understanding of the pathology of early pregnancy and threatened abortion.

References

1. Barnea E. Epidemiology and etiology of early pregnancy disorders. In Barnea E, Hustin J, Jauniaux E, eds. *The First Twelve Weeks of Gestation.* Heidelberg: Springer-Verlag, 1992: 263–79

2. Kupesic S, Kurjak A, Chervenak F. Doppler studies of subchorionic hematomas in early pregnancy. In Chervenak F, Kurjak A, eds. *Current Perspectives on the Fetus as a Patient.* Carnforth, UK: Parthenon Publishing, 1996: 33–9

3. Edmonds DK, Lindsky KS, Miller JF. Early embryonic mortality in women. *Fertil Steril* 1982; 38:447–53

4. Hakim RB, Gray RH, Zacur H. Infertility and early pregnancy loss. *Am J Obstet Gynecol* 1995; 172:1510–17

5. Wilcox AJ, Weinbert C, O'Connor JF. Incidence of early loss in pregnancy. *N Engl J Med* 1988; 319:159–64

6. Alberman E. The epidemiology of repeated abortion. In Beard RW, Bishop F, eds. *Early Pregnancy Loss: Mechanism and Treatment.* New York: Springer-Verlag, 1988:9–17

7. Ballagh SA, Harris HA, Demasio K. Is curettage needed for uncomplicated incomplete spontaneous abortion? *Am J Obstet Gynecol* 1998;179: 1279–82

8. Cetin A, Cetin M. Diagnostic and therapeutical decision-making with transvaginal sonography for first trimester spontaneous abortion, clinically thought to be complete or incomplete. *Contraception* 1998;57:393–7

9. Kurtz AB, Shlansky-Goldberg BB. Detection of retained products of conception following spontaneous abortion in the first trimester. *J Ultrasound Med* 1991;10:387–95

10. Chung TKH, Cheung LP, Sahota DS, Haines CJ, Chang AMZ. Evaluation of the accuracy of transvaginal sonography for the assessment of retained products of conception after spontaneous abortion. *Gynecol Obstet Invest* 1998;45: 190–3

11. Kos M, Kupesic S, Latin V. Diagnostics of spontaneous abortion. In Kurjak A, eds. *Ultrasound in Gynecology and Obstetrics.* Zagreb: Art Studio Azinovic, 2000:314–21

12. Speroff L, Glass RH, Kase NG, eds. Recurrent early pregnancy loss. *Clinical Gynecologic Endocrinology and Infertility.* London: Williams and Wilkins, 1999:1043–55

13. Deaton JL, Honoré GM, Huffman CS, Bauguess P. Early transvaginal ultrasound following an accurately dated pregnancy: importance of finding a yolk sac or fetal heart motion. *Hum Reprod* 1997;12:2820–3

14. Windham GC, Voin Behren J, Fenster L, Schaefer C, Swan SH. Moderate maternal alcohol consumption and risk of spontaneous abortion. *Epidemiology* 1997;8:509–14

15. Fenster L, Hubbard AE, Swan SH, *et al.* Caffeinated beverages, decaffeinated coffee, and spontaneous abortion. *Epidemiology* 1997;8: 515–23

16. Belanger K, Leaderer B, Hellenbrand K, *et al.* Spontaneous abortion and exposure to electric blankets and heated water beds. *Epidemiology* 1998;9:36–42

17. Donders GGG, Odds A, Veercken A, *et al.* Abnormal vaginal flora in the first trimester, but not full blown bacterial vaginosis, is associated with preterm birth. *Prenat Neonat Med* 1998;3: 558–93

18. Martinelli I, Sacchi E, Landi G, Taioli E, Duca F, Mannucci PM. High risk of cerebral-vein thrombosis in carriers of prothrombin-gene mutation and in users of oral contraceptives. *N Engl J Med* 1998;338:1793–7

19. Zoller B, Hillarp A, Berntorp E, Dahlback B. Activated protein C resistance due to common factor V gene mutation is a major risk factor for venous thrombosis. *Ann Rev Med* 1997;48: 45–58

20. Rees DC, Cox M, Clegg JB. World distribution of factor V Leiden. *Lancet* 1995;346:1133–4

21. Zivelin A, Griffin JH, Xu X, *et al.* A single genetic origin for a common Caucasian risk factor for venous thrombosis. *Blood* 1997;89:397–402

22. Poort SR, Rosendaal FR, Reitsma PH, Bertina RM. A common genetic variation in the 3'-untranslated region of the prothrombin gene is associated with elevated plasma prothrombin levels and an increase in venous thrombosis. *Blood* 1996;88:3698–703

23. Rosendaal FR, Doggen CJM, Zivelin A, *et al.* Geographic distribution of the 20210 G to A prothrombin variant. *Thromb Heamost* 1998;79: 706–8

24. Branch DW, Silver R, Pierangeli S, van Leeuwen I, Harris EN. Antiphospholipid antibodies other than lupus anticoagulant and anticardiolipin antibodies in women with recurrent pregnancy loss, fertile controls, and antiphospholipid syndrome. *Obstet Gynecol* 1997;89:549–55

25. Cowchock FS, Reece EA, Balaban D, Branch DW, Plouffe L. Repeated fetal losses associated with antiphospholipid antibodies: a collaborative randomized trial comparing prednizone with

low-dose heparin treatment. *Am J Obstet Gynecol* 1992;166:1318–23

26. Rai R, Cohen H, Dave M, Regan L. Randomized controlled trial of aspirin and aspirin plus heparin in pregnant women with recurrent miscarriage associated with phospholipid antibodies. *Br Med J* 1997;314:253–7

27. Simpson JL, Carson SA, Chesney C, *et al.* Lack of association between antiphospholipid antibodies and first-trimester spontaneous abortion: prospective study of pregnancies detected within 21 days of conception. *Fertil Steril* 1998;69:814–20

28. Karhukorpi J, Laitinen T, Tiilikainen AS. HLA-G polymorphism in Finnish couples with recurrent spontaneous miscarriages. *Br J Obstet Gynaecol* 1997;104:1212–14

29. Perino A, Vassilaides A, Vucetich A. Short term therapy for recurrent abortion using short-term intravenous immunoglobulins: results of double blind placebo-controlled Italian study. *Hum Reprod* 1997;12:2388–92

30. Balasch J, Creus M, Fabregues F, *et al.* In vitro fertilization treatment for unexplained recurrent abortion: a pilot study. *Hum Reprod* 1996;11:1579–82

31. Denis AL, Guido M, Adler RD, Bergh PA, Brenner C, Scott RT Jr. Antiphospholipid antibodies and pregnancy rates and outcome in *in vitro* patients. *Fertil Steril* 1997;67:1084–90

32. Raziel A, Herman A, Strassburger D, Soffer Y, Bukovsky I, Ron-El R. The outcome in *in vitro* fertilization in unexplained habitual aborters concurrent with secondary infertility. *Fertil Steril* 1997;67:88–92

33. Remohi J, Gallardo E, Levy M, *et al.* Oocyte donation in women with recurrent pregnancy loss. *Hum Reprod* 1996;11:2048–51

34. Clifford K, Rai R, Regan L. Future pregnancy outcome in unexplained recurrent first-trimester miscarriage. *Hum Reprod* 1997;12:387–9

35. Goldstein SR. Embryonic death in early pregnancy: a new look at the first trimester. *Obstet Gynecol* 1994;84:294–7

36. Kurjak A, Kupesic S. Blood flow studies in normal and abnormal pregnancy. In Kurjak A, Kupesic S, eds. *An Atlas of Transvaginal Color Doppler*. Carnforth, UK: Parthenon Publishing, 2000:41–51

37. Kurjak A, Schulman H, Kupesic S, Zudenigo D, Kos M, Goldenberg M. Subchorionic hematomas in early pregnancy: clinical outcome and blood flow patterns. *J Matern Fetal Med* 1996;5:41–4

38. Mantoni M, Pedersen JF. Intrauterine hematoma: an ultrasound study of threatened abortion. *Br J Obstet Gynaecol* 1981;88:47–50

39. Jauniaux E, Gavril P, Nicolaides KH. Ultrasonographic assessment of early pregnancy complication. In Jurkovic D, Jauniaux E, eds. *Ultrasound and Early Pregnancy*. Carnforth, UK: Parthenon Publishing, 1995:53–64

40. Kurjak A, Chervenak F, Zudenigo D, Kupesic S. Early pregnancy hemodynamics assessed by transvaginal color Doppler. In Chervenak F, Kurjak A, eds. *The Fetus as a Patient*. Carnforth, UK: Parthenon Publishing, 1994:435–55

41. Laurini RN. Abruptio placentae: from early pregnancy to term. In Chervenak F, Kurjak A, eds. *The Fetus as a Patient*. Carnforth, UK: Parthenon Publishing, 1996:433–44

42. Alcazar JL. Assessment of fetal circulation in patients with retrochorionic hematoma during the first trimester of pregnancy. *Prenat Neonat Med* 1998;3:458–63

43. Kurjak A, Zudenigo D, Predanic M, Kupesic S, Funduk B. Assessment of the fetomaternal circulation in threatened abortion by transvaginal color Doppler. *Fetal Diagn Ther* 1994;9:341–7

44. Rizzo G, Capponi A, Soregaroli M, Arduini D, Romani C. Early fetal circulation in pregnancies complicated by retroplacental hematoma. *J Clin Ultrasound* 1995;23:525–9

45. Falco P, Milano V, Pilu G, *et al.* Sonography of pregnancies with first-trimester bleeding and viable embryo: a study of prognostic indicators by logistic regression analysis. *Ultrasound Obstet Gynecol* 1996;7:65–9

46. Khong TY, Liddell HS, Robertson WG. Defective hemochorial placentation as a cause of miscarriage: a preliminary study. *Br J Obstet Gynaecol* 1987;94:649–55

47. Stabile I, Grudzinkas J, Campbell S. Doppler ultrasonographic evaluation of abnormal pregnancies in the first trimester. *J Clin Ultrasound* 1990;18:497–501

48. Alcazar JL, Ruiz-Perez ML. Uteroplacental circulation in patients with first-trimester threatened abortion. *Fertil Steril* 2000;73:130–5

49. Bromley B, Harlow BL, Laboda LA, Benacerraf BR. Small sac size in the first trimester: a predictor of poor fetal outcome. *Radiology* 1991;178:375–7

50. Dickey RP, Gasser R, Oltar TT, Taylor SN. Relationship of initial chorionic sac diameter to abortion and abortus karyotype based in new growth curves for the 16th to 49th postovulation day. *Hum Reprod* 1994;9:559–65

51. Reljic M. The significance of crown–rump length measurement for predicting adverse pregnancy outcome of threatened abortion. *Ultrasound Obstet Gynecol* 2001;17:510–12

52. Birnholz JC, Kent FB. The embryo as a patient: early pregnancy loss. In Chervenak F, Kurjak A, eds. *The Fetus as a Patient*. Carnforth, UK: Parthenon Publishing, 1996:345–7

53. Lindsay DJ, Lovett IS, Lyons EA. Endovaginal appearance of the yolk sac in pregnancy: normal growth and usefulness as a predictor of abnormal pregnancy. *Radiology* 1992;183:115–18

54. Kurjak A, Kupesic S, Kostovic Lj. Vascularization of yolk sac and vitelline duct in normal pregnancy studied by transvaginal color *Doppler J Perinat Med* 1994;22:433–40

55. Kurjak A, Kupesic S, Kos M, Latin V, Kos MA. Ultrasonic and Doppler studies of human yolk sac. In Chervenak F, Kurjak A, eds. *The Fetus as a Patient*. Carnforth, UK: Parthenon Publishing, 1996:21–32

56. De Crespigni LC. Early diagnosis pregnancy failure with transvaginal ultrasound. *Am J Obstet Gynecol* 1988;159:408–9

57. Tongsong T, Wanapirak C, Srisomboon J, *et al.* Transvaginal ultrasound in threatened abortion with empty gestational sac. *Int Gynecol Obstet* 1994;46:297–301

58. Jaffe R, Warsof SL. Color Doppler imaging in the assessment of uteroplacental blood flow in abnormal first trimester intrauterine pregnancies: an attempt to define an etiologic mechanism. *J Ultrasound Med* 1992;11:41–4

59. Kurjak A, Kupesic S, Di Renzo GC, Pooh R, Kos, M, Hafner T. Recent advances in prenatal sonography. *Prenat Neonat Med*, 1998;3:194–207

60. Kurjak A, Kupesic S, Banovic I, Hafner T, Kos M. The study of morphology and circulation of the early embryo by three-dimensional ultrasound and power Doppler. *J Perinat Med* 1999; 27:145–57

61. Kurjak A, Kupesic S. Doppler assessment of intervillous blood flow in normal and abnormal early pregnancy. *Obstet Gynecol* 1997;89:252–6

62. Kurjak A, Kupesic S. Parallel Doppler assessment of yolk sac and intervillous circulation in normal pregnancy and missed abortion. *Placenta* 1998;19:619–23

63. Szulman AE. The natural history of early human spontaneous abortion. In Barnea ER, Check JH, Grudzinkas JG, Marvo T, eds. *Implantation and Early Pregnancy in Humans*. Carnforth, UK: Parthenon Publishing, 1993:309–21

64. Jaffe R. Investigation of abnormal first trimester gestations by color Doppler imaging. *J Clin Ultrasound* 1993;21:521–6

65. Kurjak A, Zudenigo D, Predanic M, Kupesic S. Recent advances in Doppler study of early feto-maternal circulation. *J Perinat Med* 1994;22:419–39

66. Jauniaux E, Zaidi J, Jurkovic D, Campbell S, Hustin J. Comparison of color Doppler features and pathological findings in complicated early pregnancy. *Hum Reprod* 1994;9:2432–7

67. Kaplan B, Pardo J, Rabinerson D. Future fertility following conservative management of complete abortion. *Hum Reprod* 1996;11:92–4

68. Chipchase J, James D. Randomization trial of expectant versus surgical management of spontaneous miscarriage. *Br J Obstet Gynaecol* 1997;104:840–1

69. Hurd WW, Whitfield RR, Randolph JF, Kercher ML. Expectant management versus elective curettage for the treatment of spontaneous abortion. *Fertil Steril* 1997;68:601–6

70. Nielsen S, Hahlin M. Expectant management of the first trimester spontaneous abortion. *Lancet* 1995;365:84–6

71. Nielsen S, Hahlin M. Expectant management of first trimester miscarriage. *Lancet* 1995;345:84–6

72. Alcazar JL, Baldonado C, Laparte C. The reliability of transvaginal ultrasonography to detect retained tissue after first trimester spontaneous abortion, clinically thought to be complete. *Ultrasound Obstet Gynecol* 1995;6:126–9

73. Kaplan B, Pardo J, Rabinerson D, Fisch B, Neri A. Future fertility following conservative management of complete abortion. *Hum Reprod* 1996;11:92–4

74. Chung TKH, Cheung LP, Leung TY, Heines CJ, Chang AMZ. Misoprostol in the management of spontaneous abortion. *Br J Obstet Gynaecol* 1995; 102:832–5

75. Sariam S, Khare M, Michailidis S, Thilaganathan B. The role of ultrasound in the expectant management of early pregnancy loss. *Ultrasound Obstet Gynecol* 2001;17:506–9

76. Nielsen S, Hahlin M, Oden A. Using a logistic model to identify women with first trimester abortion suitable for expectant management. *Br J Obstet Gynaecol* 1996;103:1230–5

77. Schwarzler P, Holden D, Nielsen S, Hahlin M, Sladkevicius P, Bourne TH. The conservative management of the first trimester miscarriages and the use of color Doppler sonography for patient selection. *Hum Reprod* 1999;14:1341–5

78. Jurkovic D, Ross JA, Nicolaides KH. Expectant management of missed miscarriage. *Br J Obstet Gynaecol* 1998;105:670–1

79. Haines CJ, Chung T, Leung DYL. Transvaginal ultrasonography and conservative management of spontaneous abortion. *Gynecol Obstet Invest* 1994;37:14–17

80. Rulin MC, Bornstein SG, Campbell JD. The reliability of ultrasonography in the management of the spontaneous abortion clinically thought to be complete: a prospective study. *Am J Obstet Gynecol* 1993;168:12–16

81. Botsis D, Panagopoulos P, Kondorvadis A, *et al.* The accuracy of transvaginal sonography in detecting retained products of conception after first-trimester spontaneous abortion. *Prenat Neonat Med* 2001;6:112–15

82. Jauniaux E, Jurkovic D, Campbell S. *In vivo* investigation of the anatomy and the physiology

of early human placental circulation. *Ultrasound Obstet Gynecol* 1991;1:435–45

83. Blohm F, Hahlin M, Nielsen S, Milsom I. Fertility under randomized trial of spontaneous abortions managed by surgical evacuation or expectant management. *Lancet* 1997;349:995

84. Lee C, Slade P, Vygo VEN. The influence of psychological debriefing on emotional adaptation in women following early miscarriage: a preliminary study. *Br J Med Psychol* 1996;69: 47–58

85. Nikcevic AV, Tunkel SA, Nicolaides KH. Psychological outcomes following missed abortions and provision of follow-up care. *Ultrasound Obstet Gynecol* 1998;11:123–8

86. Bonilla-Musolles F. Three-dimensional visualization of the human embryo: a potential revolution in prenatal diagnosis. *Ultrasound Obstet Gynecol* 1996;7:393–7

87. Merz E, Bahlmann F, Weber G, Macchiella D. Three-dimensional ultrasonography in prenatal diagnosis. *Am J Obstet Gynecol* 1995;23:213–22

88. Pretorius DH, House M, Nelson TR. Fetal face visualization using three-dimensional ultrasonography. *J Ultrasound Med* 1995;14:349–56

89. Kurjak A, Hafner T, Kos M, Kupesic S, Stanojevic M. Three-dimensional sonography in prenatal diagnosis: a luxury or a necessity? *J Perinat Med* 2000;28:194–209

90. Sohn C, Bastert G. The technical requirements of stereoscopic three-dimensional ultrasound imaging. *Sonoace Int* 1996;3:16–25

91. Kurjak A, Kupesic S. Three dimensional ultrasound improves measurement of nuchal translucency. *J Perinat Med* 1999;27:97–102

92. Kurjak A, Sparac V, Kupesic S, Bekavac I. Three-dimensional ultrasound and three-dimensional power Doppler in the assessment of adnexal masses. *Ultrasound Rev Obstet Gynecol* 2001;2: 167–84

93. Fujiwaki R, Hata T, Hata K, Kitao M. Intra-uterine sonographic assessment of embryonic development. *Am J Obstet Gynecol* 1995;173: 1770–4

94. Kupesic S, Kurjak A, Ivancic-Kosuta M. Volume and vascularity of the yolk sac studied by three-dimensional ultrasound and color Doppler. *J Perinat Med* 1999;27:91–6

95. Kurjak A, Zodan T, Kupesic S. Three-dimensional sonoembryology of the first trimester. In Kurjak A, Kupesic S, eds. *Clinical Application of 3D Sonography*. Carnforth, UK: Parthenon Publishing, 2000:109–20

96. Hustin J, Jauniaux E. Implantation of the yolk sac. In Kurjak A, eds. *Textbook of Perinatal Medicine*. Carnforth, UK: Parthenon Publishing, 1998:960–8

97. Lee A. Four-dimensional ultrasound in prenatal diagnosis: leading edge in imaging technology. *Ultrasound Rev Obstet Gynecol* 2001;1:144–8

Venous return evaluation in monochorionic twin pregnancies in the late first trimester

4

A. Matias and N. Montenegro

> '...Two nations are in thy womb,
> and two manners of people shall be separated;
> and the one people shall be stronger than
> the other people;
> and the elder shall serve the younger...'
>
> *Genesis, XXXVI 25*

Twin-to-twin transfusion syndrome (TTTS) is a frightening complication in about 15% of monochorionic twin pregnancies still far from being effectively anticipated and treated. Strong evidence suggests that increased fetal nuchal translucency thickness (NT) in one of the monochorionic twins can be predictive of TTTS. One of the most plausible mechanisms for increased NT is heart failure, which can be indirectly manifested by abnormal blood flow in the ductus venosus. In the present chapter we specify the contribution of ductus venosus Doppler flowmetry in the evaluation of monochorionic twins and in the anticipation of occasional hemodynamic imbalance.

CHORIONICITY VERSUS ZYGOSITY

Over the past decade, perinatal mortality in singleton pregnancies has fallen, owing to advances in fetal medicine and improvement in perinatal care. A similar reduction has not been observed in multiple pregnancies, in which perinatal loss still remains six times higher than in singleton pregnancies. Even more striking is the perinatal mortality of monochorionic twins (260‰) which remains three- to five-fold higher than in dichorionic pregnancies (90‰). The rate of perinatal loss before 24 weeks in monochorionic compared with dichorionic pregnancies is 12.2% versus 1.8%[1].

Clearly it is chorionicity rather than zygosity that determines several aspects of antenatal management and perinatal outcome. Zygosity reflects the type of conception whereas chorionicity denotes the type of placentation. The type of placentation, according to Corner's theoretical model[2], depends on the time of splitting of the fertilized ovum.

Monozygotic twinning occurs in one-third of twin pregnancies. In about one-third, placentas will be dichorionic, if splitting occurs within 3 days of fertilization. However, splitting occurs most commonly (75%) between 3 and 8 days after fertilization when a monochorionic diamniotic placenta is formed (single placenta with two amniotic cavities). In less than 1% of monozygotic conceptions twinning occurs 8 days after fertilization: a single placental mass is formed with no dividing membrane (monochorionic monoamniotic placentation). Conjoined twins are a rare variant of monochorionic monoamniotic placentation when splitting occurs more than 14 days following fertilization.

An example of a complication almost unique to monozygotic twinning is TTTS. The first historical reference to this syndrome appears in the Bible telling about two pairs of twins: the first – Jacob and Esau (who was also called 'the red') and the second – Jacob's grandsons Pharez and Zerah ('Sunrise', wearer of the red thread). This syndrome was always recognized as a devastating complication of identical twins. Its severity is responsible for 15–17% of overall perinatal loss in monochorionic twins[3]. By way of intertwin vascular connections, blood is transfused from the donor, who becomes growth-restricted and develops high-output cardiac insufficiency and oligohydramnios, to the recipient, who develops circulatory overload with congestive heart failure and polyhydramnios. Therefore, this entity reflects primarily a circulatory imbalance.

Could this situation in any way display indirect signs of hemodynamic compromise as early as the first trimester of pregnancy? Data gathered from the literature show that increased NT at 10–14 weeks of gestation was found twice as often in monochorionic as in singleton pregnancies, and the likelihood ratio of developing TTTS in those twins with increased NT was 3.5[4]. Considering that monochorionic pregnancies do not show a higher prevalence of chromosomal abnormalities, the higher prevalence of increased NT in those twins could be ascribed to cardiac dysfunction.

Recently our group provided evidence on early heart failure in fetuses with increased NT and chromosomopathies[5–7] and/or cardiac defects[7,8] by showing alterations in the ductus venosus (DV) blood flow. More incipiently abnormal flow in the DV found in monochorionic twins with discrepant NT between 11 and 14 weeks was also implicated in the subsequent development of TTTS[9].

In this review we present data on the contribution of the combined evaluation of NT and DV blood flow at 11–14 weeks of gestation for the screening of those monochorionic pregnancies at risk of developing TTTS later in pregnancy.

During a 3-year period, 20 monochorionic diamniotic pregnancies were identified in our ultrasound unit during routine ultrasonographic assessment at 11–14 weeks of gestation. NT and Doppler blood flow waveforms in the DV were recorded in both twins at 11–14 weeks of gestation. A right ventral mid-sagittal plane of the fetal trunk was obtained during fetal quiescence and the pulsed Doppler gate was placed intermittently in the distal portion of the umbilical sinus[10]. An average of five consecutive high-quality waveforms was used to measure the peak velocity during ventricular systole (S-wave) and diastole (D-wave), the lowest forward velocity during atrial contraction in late diastole (A-wave) and the pulsatility index

(PI). Doppler blood flow waveforms were also recorded from the umbilical vein (UV) and umbilical artery (UA).

A second scan was performed at about 17–18 weeks of gestation to look for signs of TTTS. Severe TTTS was defined ultrasonographically by the presence of anhydramnios and a non-visible bladder in the donor in combination with polyhydramnios and a dilated bladder in the recipient. Doppler blood flow waveforms were obtained in the DV, UV and UA at the time of TTTS identification and every 2 weeks after selective laser photocoagulation of communicating vessels.

In Table 1 the characteristics of the 20 cases are shown, with emphasis on NT measurement, characteristics of ductal A-wave and eventual development of TTTS.

In cases 1 and 3 increased NT was found in at least one fetus in combination with discordant patterns of DV waveform: reversed A-wave in the fetus with increased NT and slightly reduced velocity during atrial contraction in the other fetus (Figures 1 and 2). Pulsatile flow in the UV was recorded in the first fetus. End-diastolic blood flow was present in the UA of both fetuses.

At 17 weeks of gestation, ultrasonographic signs of TTTS appeared in both cases. The larger fetus (presumed recipient) had a distended bladder and presented polyhydramnios. The smaller twin (presumed donor) showed oligohydramnios and the bladder was not visible. Major fetal anomalies were discarded. In the 'recipient' the A-wave velocity in the DV was nearly zero and the umbilical artery PI was within the normal range[11]. In the 'donor' the umbilical artery PI was increased and the A-wave velocity in the DV was diminished (Figures 3 and 4).

Both patients were referred to the Harris Birthright Research Centre for Fetal Medicine (London, UK) for fetoscopic laser separation of the vascular anastomosis at 17 weeks of gestation. One week later, the amniotic fluid around the 'donor' had recovered and the bladder became visible in both cases. Both twins subsequently showed normalization of Doppler blood flow parameters (Figures 5 and 6).

Table 1 *Parameters of the 20 monochorionic twin pregnancies evaluated, including maternal age, gestational age at the time of the first examination, nuchal translucency thickness (NT), difference in NT (ΔNT) and A-wave velocity in the ductus venosus (DV). The ultimate occurrence of twin–twin transfusion syndrome (TTTS) and the type of treatment are shown*

Case no.	Maternal age (years)	Gestational age (weeks)	NT	ΔNT	DV (A wave)	TTTS	Treatment
1	28	12	3.3/3.7	0.4	N/rev	yes	laser
2	33	12	1.6/1.7	0.1	N/N	no	–
3	27	12	1.0/3.7	2.7	N/rev	yes	laser
4	41	12	1.5/1.0	0.5	N/N	no	–
5	28	12	1.5/1.3	0.2	N/N	no	–
6	31	12	0.7/0.8	0.1	N/N	no	–
7	40	12	1.7/1.7	0	N/N	no	–
8	36	13	2.7/1.4	1.3	N/N	no	–
9	33	11	1.6/1.7	0.1	N/N	no	–
10	44	12	1.5/1.5	0	N/N	no	–
11	36	12	0.9/0.9	0	N/N	no	–
12	33	11	1.0/1.0	0	N/N	no	–
13	33	12	1.1/1.6	0.5	N/N	no	–
14	32	11	1.0/1.1	0.1	N/N	no	–
15	15	11	2.0/2.6	0.6	N/N	no	–
16	31	12	1.3/1.4	0.1	N/N	no	–
17	35	13	2.1/2.3	0.2	N/N	no	–
18	31	13	1.1/1.3	0.2	N/N	no	–
19	33	13	1.3/1.1	0.2	N/N	no	–
20	27	13	1.9/1.7	0.2	N/N	no	–

N, normal flow; rev, reverse flow during atrial contraction in the DV

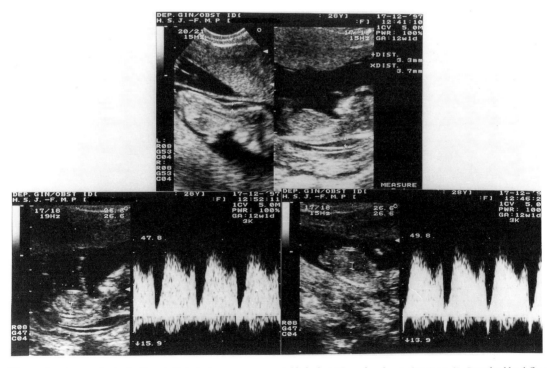

Figure 1 *A monochorionic diamniotic twin pregnancy was established at 12 weeks of gestation (case 1). Doppler blood flow waveforms in both fetuses were obtained in the ductus venosus (DV). A nuchal translucency (NT) discrepancy was noted (NT = 3.3/3.7 mm). The fetus with the highest NT shows an inverted A-wave in the DV. (Reprinted with permission from Twin Research)*

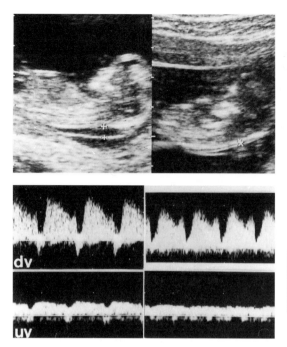

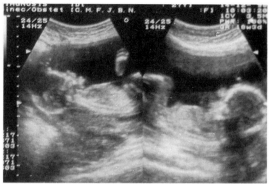

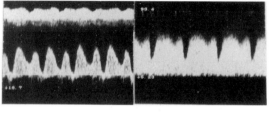

Figure 3 *Doppler blood flow waveforms in the ductus venosus (DV) obtained in case 1 at 18 weeks of gestation, when twin–twin transfusion was detected. Abnormal flow in the DV (absent flow during atrial contraction) and umbilical vein (pulsatile flow) was recorded in the recipient*

Figure 2 *A monochorionic diamniotic twin pregnancy was established at 12 weeks of gestation (case 3). Doppler blood flow waveforms in both fetuses were obtained in the umbilical vein (UV) and ductus venosus (DV) in the same scan. A nuchal translucency (NT) discrepancy was noted (NT = 3.7/1.0 mm). The fetus with increased NT shows an inverted A-wave in the DV and dicrote pulsatility in the UV. (Reprinted with permission from Twin Research)*

In cases 4, 8, 13 and 15, although discrepant NT was detected between the two fetuses at 12–13 weeks of gestation, the Doppler blood flow pattern in the DV was normal for both twins. None of these fetuses developed signs of TTTS later in pregnancy.

In the remaining cases NT measurements were similar for both twins (difference in NT < 0.5 mm). Doppler blood flow waveforms recorded in the DV at 12–13 weeks were normal in both twins and no signs of TTTS were observed later in gestation.

In one case of dichorionic diamniotic twin pregnancy a discrepancy of NT measurements was found: 1.1 mm and 5.7 mm. Doppler blood flow evaluation of the DV showed a normal waveform pattern in the former fetus and retrograde flow during atrial contraction in the latter (Figure 7). Amniocentesis performed in both sacs revealed a normal female

fetus and a trisomy 21 fetus, respectively, suggesting a different cause for the discrepant NT.

DUCTAL FLOW AT 11–14 WEEKS: AN ANTICIPATORY SIGN OF HEMODYNAMIC IMBALANCE IN MONOCHORIONIC TWINS

Twin pregnancies exhibit significantly increased morbidity and mortality rates in comparison with singleton pregnancies. While accounting for only 2.5% of the population, twins are responsible for 12.6% of the perinatal mortality. In the particular case of monochorionic twinning the fetal loss rate is even more pronounced and there is an increased risk of adverse perinatal outcome. Therefore, targeted surveillance of monochorionic twins at earlier stages of gestation could anticipate and provide timely management of the pregnancies at risk of one of the most devastating type-specific complications – TTTS.

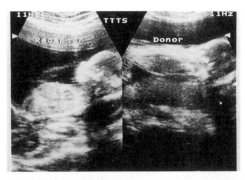

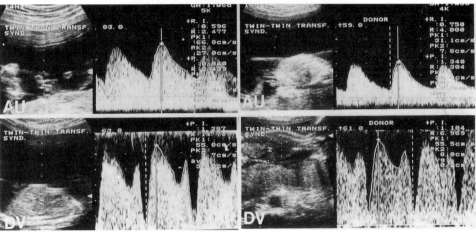

Figure 4 *Doppler blood flow waveforms in the umbilical artery (AU) and ductus venosus (DV) obtained in case 3 at 17 weeks of gestation, when twin–twin transfusion was detected. In both fetuses, abnormal flow in the DV (decreased velocity during atrial contraction) was recorded. The umbilical artery showed normal blood flow waveforms. Note the 'stuck-twin' with oligohydramnios (donor) and the polyhydramnios around the recipient. (Reprinted with permission from Twin Research)*

This syndrome is estimated to affect 15% (4–35%) of all monochorionic multiple pregnancies as a consequence of intertwin vascular anastomoses. It accounts for 17% of perinatal mortality[12], nearly 12% of neonatal deaths and 8.4% of infant deaths in twins. This is 3–10 times higher than in singletons. Neurodevelopment abnormalities are 6–8 times more frequent in twins than in singletons[13,14]. Cardiac abnormalities are frequently reported in the larger twin, ranging from mild to critical pulmonary stenosis or lethal cardiomyopathy[15].

The progressive nature of TTTS *in utero* is thought to be due to one twin (the donor) slowly pumping blood to the other (the recipient) through these anastomoses. Monochorionic monoamniotic placentas and most monochorionic diamniotic placentas are believed to display such anastomoses[16]. It is believed that, if these vascular anastomoses are scarce and with unidirectional flow, the risk for developing TTTS is increased, owing to uncompensated arteriovenous flow from recipient to donor[17]. In addition to more frequent vascular patterns in monochorionic twins developing TTTS, other factors such as discordant/asymmetrical chorion development and more prevalent velamentous insertion should also be considered. Consequently, in about one-third of cases, this circulatory imbalance will eventually result in the development of the acute polyhydramnios/oligohydramnios sequence in the second trimester of pregnancy[3,18].

The pathophysiology of TTTS is poorly understood, and, although transfusion has been confirmed *in vivo*[19], the pathophysiology

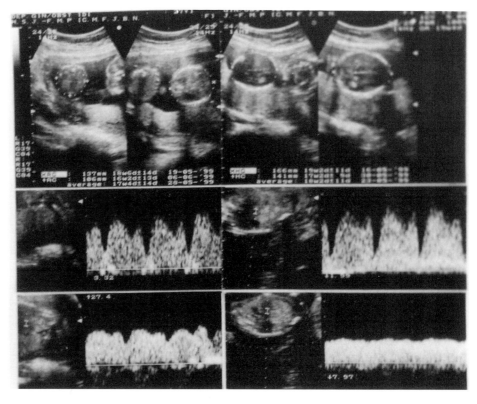

Figure 5 *Improvement of ductus venosus waveforms in the recipient (case 1) 1 week after fetoscopic laser coagulation*

of TTTS includes more than shunting of blood from donor to recipient. A vicious cycle of hypervolemia–polyuria–hyperosmolality is established, leading to polyhydramnios and congestive heart failure in the recipient. Cardiac overload and dilatation could promote high atriopeptin secretion by the dilated atria. This could occur very early in gestation as a consequence of early cardiac overload, and trigger TTTS. Knowing more about how and when the vascular problems occur could help improve the management and outcome of the twins.

Alterations in cardiac hemodynamics are indirectly demonstrated by alterations in venous blood flow waveforms. The abnormal pulsatile pattern consists of increased velocity of blood flow away from the heart during atrial contraction and has been reported in the fetus with a failing heart[20,21]. The most striking feature is the reduced or reversed flow during atrial contraction in the DV commonly found in fetuses with congenital heart defects[8,20], growth restriction[21] and TTTS[9,22]. In all these clinical situations this particular hemodynamic alteration seems to reflect impaired cardiac performance and is a sign of dismal prognosis.

Hecher and co-workers[22] found highly pulsatile venous waveforms in the recipient with fully established TTTS. Umbilical vein pulsations and absent or reversed flow during atrial contraction in the DV are signs of congestive heart failure due to hypervolemia and increased preload from placental vascular anastomotic transfusion. Zosmer and colleagues[23] showed that some surviving twins of TTTS had a persistent right ventricular hypertrophic cardiomyopathy and proposed that cardiac dysfunction could be induced *in utero* by sustained strain upon the heart by TTTS, predominantly affecting the right ventricle. The right ventricle is stiffer and more

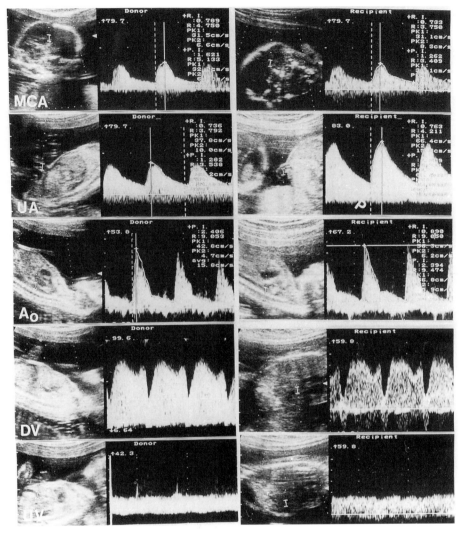

Figure 6 *Normal Doppler blood flow profiles (arterial and venous) obtained in both fetuses (case 3) 1 week after fetoscopic laser coagulation. MCA, middle cerebral artery; UA, umbilical artery; Ao, descending aorta; DV, ductus venosus; UV, umbilical vein*

afterload-sensitive than the left ventricle, mostly owing to the redistribution of blood in the cerebral arteries which decreases the left ventricular afterload. In contrast, the significant reduction of blood flow velocity in the UA recorded in the 'donor' is consistent with hypovolemia and increased placental resistance, increasing cardiac afterload and decreasing umbilical venous return.

Can this circulatory imbalance, fully expressed later in pregnancy, disclose indirect signs of cardiac dysfunction in earlier stages of gestation? Sebire and co-workers[1,4] recently demonstrated a higher prevalence of increased NT among monochorionic twins at 10–14 weeks of gestation and a four-fold increase in the risk of developing TTTS in this subgroup. In more recent studies of vascular hemodynamics in fetuses with increased NT at 10–14 weeks, the abnormal flow in the DV more frequently recorded in fetuses with chromosomopathies, with or without cardiac

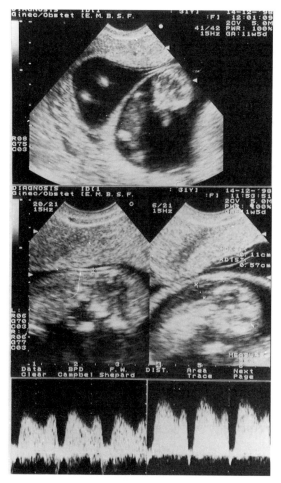

Figure 7 *A dichorionic diamniotic twin pregnancy identified at 11 weeks (note the twin-peak sign). Nuchal translucency (NT) was measured in both fetuses (NT = 1.1/5.7 mm). Doppler blood flow waveforms were obtained in the ductus venosus (DV) of each fetus: the fetus with the highest nuchal translucency (right) showed an inverted A-wave in the DV (amniocentesis showed trisomy 21) while the fetus with a measurement within the normal range (left) presented a normal waveform pattern (normal female karyotype). (Reprinted with permission from Twin Research)*

defects, was related to heart strain[5-9]. These findings are in good agreement with the overt hemodynamic alterations found in TTTS later in pregnancy[22]. Therefore, strong evidence suggests that increased NT along with abnormal flow in the DV, even in the presence of a normal karyotype, may be early signs of cardiac impairment or defect[5-9]. Following the same rationale, hemodynamic changes associated with TTTS may manifest between 10 and 14 weeks of gestation as increased NT in the recipient[1,4], owing to congestive heart failure. With advancing gestation, this transient heart failure eventually resolves, with increased diuresis and ventricular compliance.

DV appreciation as a regulatory shunt of oxygenated blood can add valuable information to fetal venous hemodynamic evaluation. Blood flow in the DV is characterized by forward flow throughout the cardiac cycle with high velocity during ventricular systole (S-wave) and diastole (D-wave). Only in cardiac failure, when end-diastolic pressure becomes elevated, does atrial systole produce large atrial pressure waves and cause reversal in the atrial waveform of the DV[5-8,20,21].

Concerning the safety of ultrasound bioeffects in such a vulnerable period as the first trimester of pregnancy, it is accepted that the combination of intermittent pulsed Doppler with much lower energy output techniques, such as color Doppler and power Doppler, makes the identification of vascular structures easier and shortens the time of fetal exposure to the ultrasound beam[24]. Finally, bone ossification is incipient at this stage of pregnancy, reducing the danger of aggressive thermal effects.

Until now, we could diagnose TTTS in monochorionic pregnancies only between 17 and 26 weeks, when it was fully established, by identifying the disparity in fetal size and amniotic fluid volume between donor and recipient. However, perinatal morbidity and mortality rates could be dramatically decreased if TTTS could be identified at earlier stages of pregnancy. It may well be that the combination of discrepant NT and abnormal flow in the DV at 11–14 weeks of gestation in monochorionic twins represents the alarm sign predictive of the subsequent development of TTTS. Both first-trimester clues could anticipate the early development of heart dysfunction and should motivate the ultrasonographer to undertake a closer monitoring of these twins more prone to develop TTTS. Therefore, positive screening could provide timely therapeutic strategies and thus improve the outcome of these threatened pregnancies.

References

1. Sebire NJ, D'Ercole, C, Hughes K, Carvalho M, Nicolaides KH. Increased nuchal translucency thickness at 10–14 weeks of gestation as a predictor of severe twin-to-twin transfusion syndrome. *Ultrasound Obstet Gynecol* 1997;10:86–9

2. Corner GW. The observed embryology of human single-ovum twins and other multiple births. *Am J Obstet Gynecol* 1995;70:933–51

3. Cincotta RB, Fisk N. Current thoughts on twin–twin transfusion syndrome. *Clin Obstet Gynecol* 1997;40:290–302

4. Sebire NJ, Souka A, Skentou H, Geerts L, Nicolaides KH. Early prediction of severe twin-to-twin transfusion syndrome. *Hum Reprod* 2000;15: 2008–10

5. Montenegro N, Matias A, Areias JC, Castedo S, Barros H. Increased nuchal translucency: possible involvement of early cardiac failure. *Ultrasound Obstet Gynecol* 1997;10:265–8

6. Matias A, Montenegro N, Areias JC, Brandão O. Anomalous venous return associated with major chromosomopathies in the late first trimester of pregnancy. *Ultrasound Obstet Gynecol* 1998;11: 209–13

7. Matias A, Gomes C, Flack N, Montenegro N, Nicolaides KH. Screening for chromosomal defects at 11–14 weeks: the role of ductus venosus blood flow. *Ultrasound Obstet Gynecol* 1998;12:380–4

8. Matias A, Huggon I, Areias JC, Montenegro N, Nicolaides KH. Cardiac defects in chromosomally normal fetuses with abnormal ductus venosus blood flow at 10–14 weeks. *Ultrasound Obstet Gynecol* 1999;14:307–10

9. Matias A, Montenegro N, Areias JC. Anticipating twin–twin transfusion syndrome in monochorionic twin pregnancy. Is there a role for nuchal translucency and ductus venosus blood flow evaluation at 11–14 weeks? *Twin Res* 2000;3:65–70

10. Montenegro N, Matias A, Areias JC, Barros H. Ductus venosus revisited: a Doppler blood flow evaluation in the first trimester of pregnancy. *Ultrasound Med Biol* 1997;23:171–6

11. Montenegro N, Beires J, Pereira Leite L. Reverse end-diastolic umbilical artery blood flow at 11 weeks' pregnancy. *Ultrasound Obstet Gynecol* 1995;5:141–2

12. Powers WF, Kiely JL. The risks confronting twins: a national perspective. *Am J Obstet Gynecol* 1994; 170:456–61

13. Williams K, Hennessy E, Alberman E. Cerebral palsy: effects of twinning, birthweight and gestational age. *Arch Dis Child* 1996;75:F178–82

14. Denbow ML, Battin MR, Cowan F, Azzopardi D, Edwards AD, Fisk N. Neonatal cranial ultrasonographic findings in preterm twins complicated by severe fetofetal transfusion syndrome. *Am J Obstet Gynecol* 1998;178:479–83

15. Zosmer N, Bajoria R, Weiner E, Rigby M, Vaughan J, Fisk N. Clinical and echographic features of *in utero* cardiac dysfunction in the recipient twin-to-twin transfusion syndrome. *Br Heart J* 1994;72:74–9

16. Benirschke K, Kim CK. Multiple pregnancy. *N Engl J Med* 1973;288:1276–84

17. Bajoria R, Wigglesworth J, Fisk NM. Angioarchitecture of monochorionic placentas in relation to twin–twin transfusion syndrome. *Am J Obstet Gynecol* 1995;172:856–63

18. Bebbington MW, Wittman BK. Fetal transfusion syndrome: antenatal factors affecting outcome. *Am J Obstet Gynecol* 1989;160:913–15

19. Tanaka M, Natori M, Ishimoto H, Kohno H, Kobayashi T, Nosawa S. Intravascular pancuronium bromide infusion for prenatal diagnosis of twin-to-twin transfusion syndrome. *Fetal Diagn Ther* 1992;7:36–40

20. Kiserud T, Eik-Nes SH, Hellevik LR, Blas HG. Ductus venosus blood velocity changes in fetal cardiac diseases. *J Matern Fetal Invest* 1993;3:15–20

21. Kiserud T, Eik-Nes SH, Blaas HG, Hellevik LR, Simensen B. Ductus venosus blood velocity and the umbilical circulation in the seriously growth retarded fetus. *Ultrasound Obstet Gynecol* 1994;4: 109–14

22. Hecher K, Ville Y, Snijders R, Nicolaides KH. Doppler studies of the fetal circulation in twin-to-twin transfusion syndrome. *Ultrasound Obstet Gynecol* 1995;5:318–24

23. Zosmer N, Bajoria R, Weiner E, Rigby M, Vaughan J, Fisk N. Clinical and echographic features of *in utero* cardiac dysfunction in the recipient twin-to-twin transfusion syndrome. *Br Heart J* 1994;72:74–9

24. European Committee for Ultrasound Radiation Safety. Clinical Safety Statement. *Eur J Ultrasound* 1996;4:145

First-trimester diagnosis of fetal abnormalities by two- and three-dimensional sonoembryology

5

H. Takeuchi

With the advent of the concept of sonoembryology by two-dimensional (2D) transvaginal ultrasound about 10 years ago, the scientific observation and description of fetal morphology in early pregnancy has become feasible. Consequently, fetal anomalies are able to be diagnosed at an earlier stage with more precise observation.

It was also about 10 years ago that the 3D ultrasound machine appeared on the market. However, the feasibility of 3D sonoembryological observation for diagnosing fetal anomalies at an early stage of pregnancy was first reported only about 5 years ago. Since then, anomaly cases successfully diagnosed by 3D transvaginal ultrasound in the first trimester of pregnancy have gradually increased.

Several kinds of technique for 3D ultrasound examination have been developed. Among them, the orthogonal multiplanar display method that uses conventional 2D imaging, and the surface rendering method that can demonstrate fetal appearance, both provide new and useful diagnostic information in the evaluation of fetal morphology by conventional 2D sonoembryology.

It is considered that the supplemental use of 3D multiplanar and surface image information to the conventional 2D sonoembryology contributes to the diagnosis of fetal anomalies in the first trimester of pregnancy.

This article reviews the early diagnosis of fetal abnormalities by sonoembryology at 8–14 weeks of pregnancy, with particular consideration of the contribution of 3D ultrasound, showing our own cases.

NON-IMMUNE HYDROPS FETALIS

Non-immune hydrops fetalis is thought to be a common symptom of fetal disease at any stage, even in the first trimester of pregnancy. Although Hernadi and Torocsik[1] did not find hydrops fetalis among their 3991 unselected population at 12 weeks pregnancy, Iskalos and associates[2] presented 45 cases of fetal hydrops between 11 and 17 weeks. Generalized skin edema is believed to be the first feature of fetal hydrops, and when increased nuchal thickness is included in its signs, abnormality of the fetal neck was reported to be diagnosed as early as 9 weeks of gestation[3,4]. In their early detected hydrops, Iskalos and co-workers[2] described that, in addition to generalized edema, ascites and pleural effusion were observed in 8.9% and 2.2% of the cases, respectively.

Cases of non-immune hydrops presenting at an early gestation will be missed, because hydrops developing during the first half of pregnancy is more likely to resolve or to lead to fetal demise, depending on the severity of the underlying anomaly[5]. Non-immune hydrops cases diagnosed at an early gestational age have a higher incidence of abnormal karyotype and a higher perinatal mortality rate[2,6].

Fetal hydrops can be diagnosed from generalized formation of a demonstrable separation of the skin from the body wall, which is most clearly observed at the level of the fetal head and in particular at the back of the neck. Iskalos and colleagues[2] found that placental edema was the most commonly associated feature with generalized skin edema. Ascites is considered to be commonly found in early hydrops, but pleural effusions are believed to be rarely observed before 15 weeks, except in cases of Turner syndrome.

In our first case, a coronal section of a fetus at the end of 8 weeks or the beginning of 9 weeks was obtained by conventional 2D ultrasound as shown in Figure 1. The fetal shape as a whole is depicted quite clearly. Fluid retention in thoracic and abdominal cavities, namely pleural effusions and ascites with generalized subcutaneous edema, is clearly delineated. A two-dimensional sectional image at the appropriate cross-section is indispensable to delineate fluid retention in the body cavity. For obtaining the appropriate cross-sectional view, multiplanar display by 3D ultrasound is extremely useful.

The second case at 9 weeks of pregnancy shows hydrops with noticeable subcutaneous edema by surface display of 3D ultrasound (Figure 2). The characteristic appearance of hydrops can be shown more clearly by surface display than by conventional 2D imaging. No fluid accumulation in the thoracic and abdominal cavities was found by multiplanar display of 3D ultrasound.

CYSTIC HYGROMA

Cystic hygroma is defined as fluid-filled sacculations of the lateral neck and nuchal region that result from lymphatic dysplasia. However, the differential diagnosis by ultrasound between cystic hygroma and increased nuchal thickness is often ambiguous. In many cases it is difficult to distinguish simple nuchal edema from uniloculated hygroma. Cystic hygromas are often associated with generalized skin edema. Cullen and colleagues[7] reported that cystic hygromas were the most common anomaly in the first trimester.

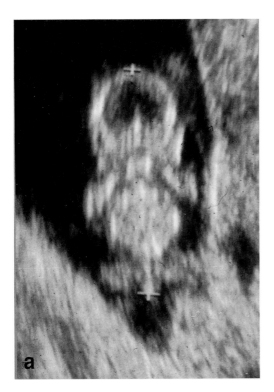 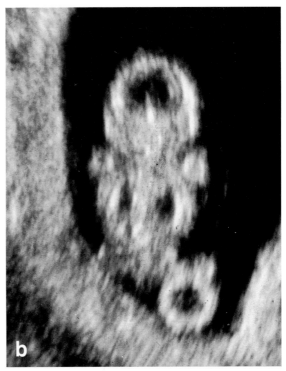

Figure 1 *Coronal scans of fetuses at 8 weeks of gestation. The echogram (a) was obtained from a normal fetus with crown–rump length (CRL) of 18 mm. A large echo-free space in the head shows the fourth ventricle. Echogram (b) delineates almost the same size of a fetus (CRL 20 mm) with apparent echo-free spaces in the thoracic region as well as swollen and double-layered thoracic wall. Pleural effusion with edematous skin was the most likely condition*

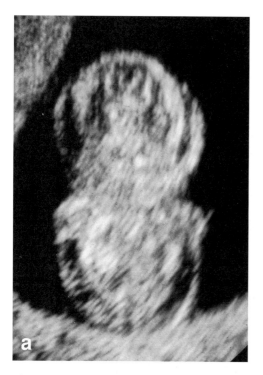 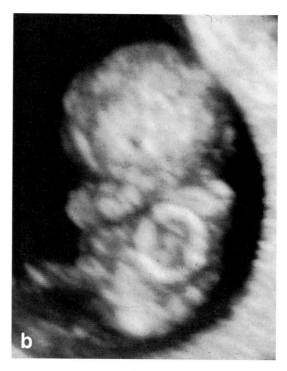

Figure 2 *A fetus with hydrops fetalis at 9 weeks of gestation shown two-dimensionally (a) and three-dimensionally (b). The two-dimensional echogram depicts generalized edema on the head and trunk. The round, swollen appearance is well shown by surface rendering of transvaginal 3D ultrasound. A ring-like structure on the thorax is the yolk sac*

Recently, Rosati and Guariglia[8] included in the group of cystic hygroma those cases with a large and collar-like structure with internal septations around the lateral and posterior neck in the axial plane, and cystic dilatations larger than 3 mm in diameter in the antero-lateral aspects of the cervical region. Nuchal translucency was defined as a cystic swelling dorsal to the spine and extending from the occiput to the upper posterior part of the spine, presenting in the mid-sagittal plane of the cervical region.

It is considered that, for delineating cystic hygroma with septations (Figure 3), 2D multi-planar display of 3D ultrasound is more useful than conventional 2D ultrasound. Evaluation of the region of the cyst at the anterolateral aspect of the cervix can be carried out more easily by 3D surface rendering than by the 2D cross-sectional view, as shown in Figure 4.

CONJOINED TWINS

Conjoined twins are a very rare entity of abnormality in monozygotic twins and occur in every 50 000 to 100 000 births. Although separation of conjoined twins can be success-fully accomplished in selected cases, the feasibility and subsequent morbidity are dependent upon the degree of organ and vascular communication. Therefore, meticulous and detailed visualization of the fetuses is required as early as possible[9].

However, early and accurate diagnosis of conjoined twins is still a challenge, owing to difficulties in visualizing a complete separation of the twins, observing two fetal spines in unusual proximity, presenting unusual embry-onic or fetal shapes and presenting more than three vessels in the umbilical cord as well as a single cardiac motion[10]. An accurate prenatal

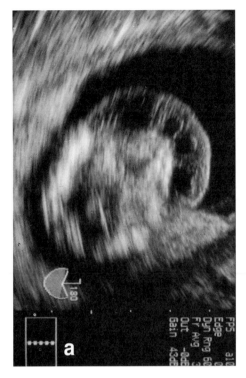
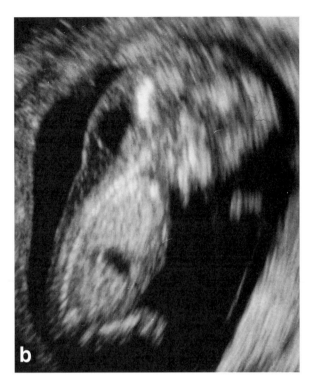

Figure 3 *Two fetuses with cystic hygroma at 14 weeks of gestation. A two-dimensional transverse section at the neck (a) shows severe edema with multiple cystic fluid retention at the dorsal area. A similar edema with fluid retention, particularly at the nuchal region, is seen in a sagittal sectional view (b)*

diagnosis of conjoined twins can be made by 2D ultrasound as early as the first trimester of pregnancy. One should suspect conjoined twins when there is inability to observe a clear separation between fetal anatomic segments (Figure 5). The diagnosis, however, should only be made after careful and extensive scanning, combining the ultrasound examination with transducer-induced fetal movements. A careful anatomic and vascular mapping to determine the extent of organ sharing is of vital importance to determine prognosis.

Detailed evaluation at this stage would be beneficial, owing to the high frequency of associated anomalies related to fusion, which include neural tube defect, orofacial cleft, imperforate anus and diaphragmatic hernia. In this respect, transvaginal 3D ultrasound seems to be an improvement over routinely applied 2D ultrasound. It provides accurate

data regarding fetal structures and biometry, using multiplanar imaging, as well as spatial surface animation, which may enhance the diagnosis of fetal malformations, especially during the first trimester of pregnancy. Bega and co-workers[9] reported that, using a combination of multiplanar display and surface rendering, they were able to confirm the diagnosis of conjoined twins at 10 weeks' gestation and ascertain the level and extent of organ connection. The importance of 3D ultrasound for early accurate diagnosis of cephalopagus twins was reported by Kuroda and colleagues[11]. It is not suggested that 3D ultrasound is critical for the diagnosis of conjoined twins. However, it might be suggested that 3D ultrasound could help to classify more accurately the type of conjoined twins detected.

Several authors have reported that conjoined twins were able to be diagnosed more easily

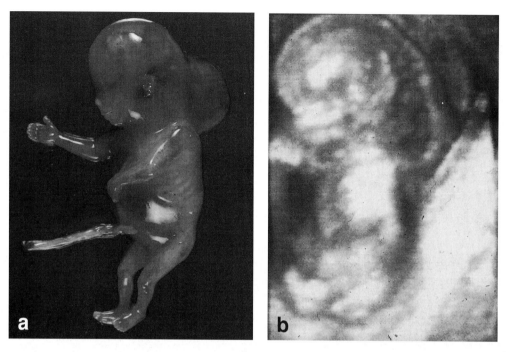

Figure 4 *A fetus with cystic hygroma after termination of pregnancy (a) and a 3D echogram (b) of the same fetus in utero at 15 weeks of gestation. The cystic part of the nuchal region is clearly delineated by surface mode of 3D ultrasound*

and in more detail by using 3D ultrasound[9-13]. As Bonilla-Musoles and co-workers[13] stated, color Doppler in combination with 3D ultrasound can be a useful complement to 2D ultrasound in confirming early diagnosis and in determining the extent of organ sharing and definitive classification of conjoined twins.

HYDROCEPHALUS AND HOLOPROSENCEPHALY

The initial main object of sonoembryology was examination of the central nervous system (CNS)[14], because the developing stage of the brain ventricles from 7 weeks onward can be confirmed by a conventional 2D image. For example, in the mid-sagittal sectional image of the fetus at the end of 8 weeks of pregnancy, from the rostaral portion, each of the lateral ventricles, the third ventricle, mid-ventricle and the forth ventricle, are clearly delineated as curved and connected tubular structures. Blaas and associates[15,16], by using a method

obtaining an optimal 2D image by their own 3D machine with the computerized reconstruction technique, successfully showed the growing process of the diencephalon, mesencephalon and rhombencephalon quantitatively from these lengths, widths and heights, and from the calculated volumes.

As for diagnosis of ventricular abnormalities in early pregnancy, it should be known from which gestational age a particular structural abnormality can be depicted. For instance, in the case of hydrocephalus, ventriculomegaly develops after the 14th week of gestation. Hernadi and Torocsik[1] reported that they could delineate ventriculomegaly in only two cases at the 11–14-week scan among eight cases of hydrocephaly.

On the other hand, earlier diagnosis is possible in a case of severe anomaly such as holoprosencephaly. Gonzalez-Gomez and colleagues[17] reported successful diagnosis of alobar holoprosencephaly at 10 weeks of gestation with its single ventricular cavity.

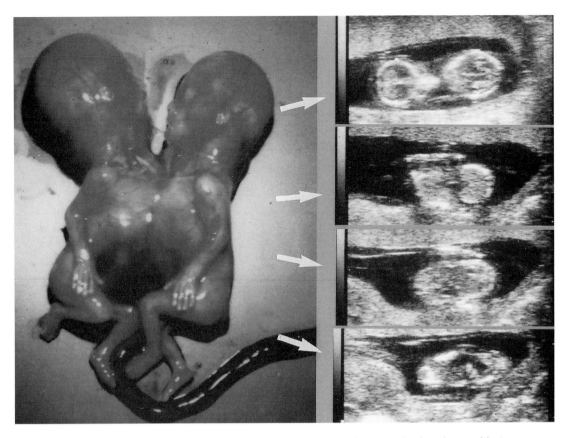

Figure 5 *Conjoined twins at 13 weeks of gestation. Top row: two completely separate heads with normal brain structures are seen. Second row: almost the same size of thoraces fused anteriorly. Only one heart exists at the center of the fused thoraces. Third row: transverse section at the level of the stomach visualized complete anterior fusion of the upper abdominal region with two separate stomachs. Bottom row: two pelves with lower extremities are independently shown in opposite positions*

However, for the earliest diagnosis of this anomaly, detailed observation of ventricular structures is required, because the degree of the abnormality depends on the degree of forebrain cleavage. Blaas and colleagues[18] reported that, when they diagnosed alobar holoprosencephaly at 9 weeks, the use of 3D ultrasound made additional diagnostic ultrasound tomograms possible, and the volume reconstructions improved the imaging and the understanding of the condition.

We had a case of semi-lobar holoprosencephaly at 12 weeks of gestation. A 2D image in an appropriate cross-section of the head is essential for observing abnormalities of the ventricles. In this case, the semi-coronal view of the head, which showed symmetrical ventricu-lomegaly without a cortex, partially interrupted falx cerebri and fused thalami, was most diagnostic (Figure 6). For delineating the partial segmentation of the ventricle, the 3D multiplanar display for obtaining the exact sectional view is very useful.

In a case of hydranencephaly, the relatively small head and sloping forehead without normal lateral ventricle structures in an 11-week fetus was noted by Lam and Tan[19]. A large fluid-filled intracranial cavity with small cerebral hemispheres, which is characteristic of hydranencephaly, was readily shown in a case of 12 weeks' pregnancy by Lin and co-workers[20]. For detecting this kind of abnormality in early pregnancy, multiplanar presentation of the head by 3D ultrasound is very useful.

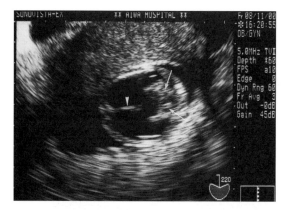

Figure 6 *Coronal section of the head obtained by conventional 2D ultrasound in a case of holoprosencephaly at 12 weeks of gestation. Enlarged ventricles without cortex, interrupted falx cerebri (arrowhead) and fused thalami (arrows) are characteristically visualized*

ACRANIA AND EXENCEPHALY/ANENCEPHALY

As a result of a screening study carried out in the UK in unselected women with live fetuses at 10–14 weeks of gestation, a prevalence of one case of anencephaly in 1175 fetuses was reported[21]. Now it is considered that acrania and exencephaly are precursors of anencephaly that develop as a result of a defective closure of the rostral neuropore during 5 weeks of gestation. Its morphological abnormality, namely an absent skull and disorganized brain tissue extruded from the skull, is relatively easily delineated. In the case of a lack of a skull echo and some volume of disorganized irregular brain echo, the diagnosis of acrania and exencephaly should be suspected. Van Zalen-Sprock and co-workers[22] reported that, in their series of diagnosis of CNS anomalies at 6–16 weeks of pregnancy, they did not find any case of anencephaly, whereas 12 cases of exencephaly were successfully diagnosed. A screening system for acrania and exencephaly by 2D ultrasound has already been established. Johnson and co-workers[21] reported that, when sonographers were instructed specifically to look for and record the presence or absence of acrania at the 10–14-week screening scan, all cases of anencephaly could be successfully diagnosed.

In our experience, acrania and exencephaly could be diagnosed as early as 7 weeks of gestation by depicting absence of the skull and deformed brain tissue without showing brain ventricle structures two-dimensionally (Figure 7). However, even by the 9–10-week scan, the condition can be overlooked when depicting the optimal section is difficult. To prevent this, observation by 3D ultrasound is useful. By the multiplanar display, depicting the correct sagittal section and coronal section, acrania and exencephaly are rather easily diagnosed. Also, by the surface mode, the abnormality of the head is shown more clearly (Figure 8).

SPINA BIFIDA

Spina bifida is a failure of closure of the neural tube, which normally occurs by the 6th week of gestation. The neural tube itself can be delineated as two parallel lines in the coronal section of an embryo as early as 7 weeks of gestation[14]. The closure of the neural canal should be confirmed by visualization of three ossification centers presented from the 10th week of gestation. Braithwaite and associates[23] reported successful depiction of the vertebrae and overlying skin in both the transverse and the coronal sections in all fetuses at 12–13 weeks of gestation. However, it is noted that, even in early diagnosis of spina bifida, the cranial and cerebellar signs should be observed[24].

Recently, Blaas and colleagues[25] reported successful detection of three cases of lumbosacral myelomeningocele by using their high-frequency transvaginal machine. In targeted ultrasound examination at 9 weeks of gestation in all cases, the 2D coronal section revealed the irregularities of the spine. Repeated examinations at 10 and 12 weeks confirmed the diagnosis of spina bifida. These authors reported that 3D evaluation at 9 weeks in case 1 confirmed the irregularity of the spine by any plane slicing through the defect, but did not add new information. They also stated that, in case 3, 3D imaging at 9 weeks visualized the defect from different angles, but this did not improve the diagnosis.

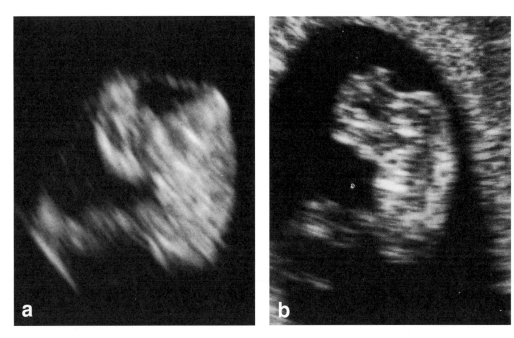

Figure 7 *Sagittal sectional views of almost the same size of a normal embryo with 15-mm crown–rump length (CRL) (a) and a 14.5-mm-CRL embryo with acrania and exencephaly (b). In the normal embryo a distinct fourth ventricle at the region of the rhrombencephalon and the smooth shape of the head can be seen. However, in embryo (b), the bizarre irregular shape of the head indicates acrania and, without ventricular structure in the brain, this is an important sonoembryological sign of exencephaly*

However, it is my opinion that 3D surface imaging makes a significant contribution to accurate diagnosis of myelomeningocele, because this can demonstrate the spinal area very clearly (Figure 9). By using commercial 3D equipment, Bonilla-Musoles successfully showed a surface image of spina bifida and myelomeningocele at 9.5 weeks' gestation[26].

OMPHALOCELE

Although a birth prevalence of omphalocele was described as about one in 3000, a result of a screening study at 10–14 weeks of gestation showed one omphalocele in 874 unselected pregnancies[27]. All fetuses at 8–10 weeks demonstrate herniation of the midgut that is visualized as a hyperechogenic mass at the base of the umbilical cord. Retraction of the midgut into the abdominal cavity is completed by the end of 11 weeks. Blaas and co-workers[28] stated that, as long as the herniation is physiological, its size does not exceed 6.5 mm. Accordingly,

even before 12 weeks of gestation, pathological herniation can be diagnosed by the shape and size of the herniated mass (Figure 10). Brown and colleagues[29] and Pagliano and colleagues[30] diagnosed omphalocele as early as 10 weeks of gestation by 2D ultrasound.

For accurate measurements of the size of an omphalocele, 3D multiplanar display was thought to be more effective than single use of 2D ultrasound. In my opinion, the surface rendering method, when it is adequately applied, is effective in the differential diagnosis between physiological and pathological herniation (Figure 11). Chang and associates[31] reported a case of omphalocele at 14 weeks of gestation successfully visualized by the surface rendering method of transabdominal 3D ultrasound.

GASTROSCHISIS

In gastroschisis, herniation of the intestine occurs through an abdominal wall defect

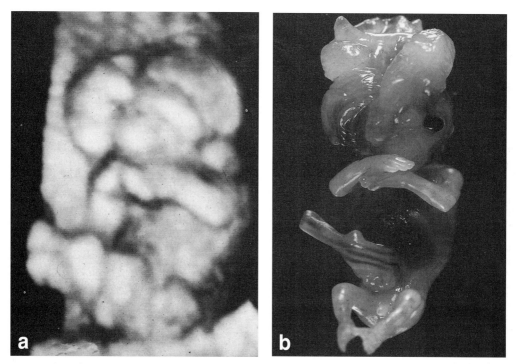

Figure 8 *Three-dimensional surface image of a fetus with acrania and exencephaly* in utero *at 10 weeks of gestation (a) and a photograph of the same fetus after termination of pregnancy (b). Characteristic irregularity of the fetal head was sufficiently delineated by the 3D surface image*

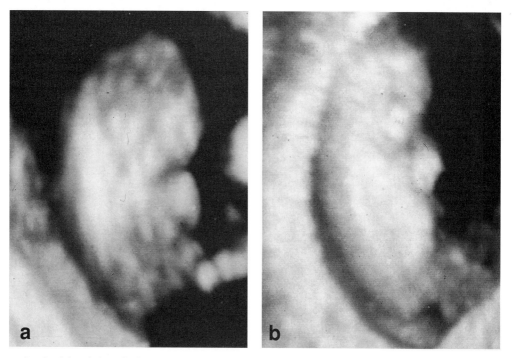

Figure 9 *Semi-dorsal view of a fetus at 8 weeks (a) and 9 weeks of gestation (b) visualized by 3D surface image. The spinal region is more clearly delineated in a fetus at 9 weeks and, when there is an abnormality such as myelomeningocele in the spinal region, this might be easily delineated*

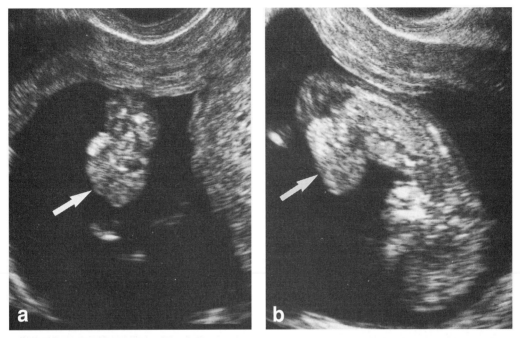

Figure 10 *2D images of omphalocele at 12 weeks of gestation. Exomphalos (arrow) is depicted in transverse (a) and sagittal sections (b). In the transverse section of this large herniation, it is possible to observe that the herniation contains stomach and liver*

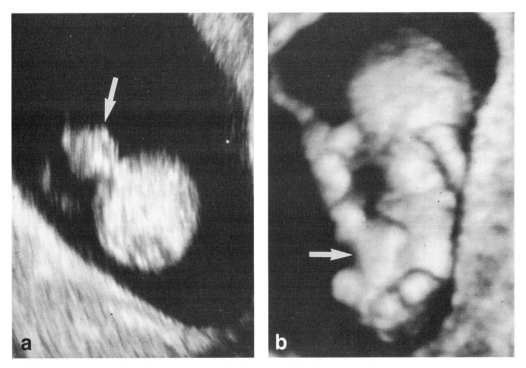

Figure 11 *Physiological midgut herniation into the cord visualized by a conventional 2D image (a) and 3D surface image (b). The size of the mass of herniation (arrow) does not exceed the diameter of 8 mm. The image (a) was obtained from a fetus at 11 weeks of gestation. By using 3D imaging, the small mass of midgut herniation (arrow) can be identified even at 9 weeks of gestation*

located just lateral and usually to the right of an intact umbilical cord. Ultrasound diagnosis of gastroschisis is based on the demonstration of the normal location of the umbilicus and the herniated loops of intestine, which are free-floating (Figure 12). Although the incidence of gastroschisis by ultrasound examinations in the second trimester of pregnancy was reported to be similar to that of omphalocele, scarcity of reports on the first-trimester diagnosis is noted[32]. Guzman[33] reported successful diagnosis of gastroschisis at 12 weeks of pregnancy. Cullen and colleagues[7] visualized bowel herniation from a lateral anterior wall defect remote from the cord insertion in an 11-week fetus. Earlier diagnosis might be made by using 3D ultrasound in the future.

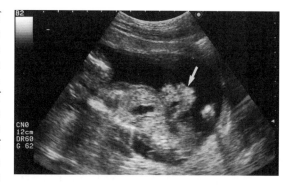

Figure 12 *Gastroschisis at 18 weeks of gestation, visualized by conventional 2D imaging. Eviscerated bowel (arrow) was floating in the amniotic cavity. 3D ultrasound is thought to be a useful technique to delineate this kind of abnormality in earlier stages of gestation*

SKELETAL DYSPLASIA

It has already been described that, sono-embryologically, limb buds are first seen at about 8 weeks, the femur and humerus are seen from 9 weeks, the tibia/fibula and radius/ulna from 10 weeks and the digits of the hands and feet from 11 weeks; all long bones are consistently seen from 11 weeks. Zorzoli and co-workers[34] presented a reference range of fetal limb bone lengths with gestation from 10 weeks, showing similar linear growth of the humerus, radius/ulna, femur and tibia/fibula from about 6 mm at 11 weeks to 13 mm at 14 weeks. Reports on ultrasound diagnosis of a wide range of skeletal defects in the first trimester are seen in the literature. Souka and Nikolaides[32] collected the cases, which contain achondrogenesis type II at 11 weeks[35], thanatophoric dwarfism at 13 weeks[36], osteogenesis imperfecta at 13 weeks[37], asphyxiating thoracic dystrophy at 14 weeks[38], Roberts syndrome at 10 weeks[39], Jarcho–Levin syndrome at 12 weeks[40], ectodactyly, ectodermal dysplasia and cleft palate (EEC) syndrome at 14 weeks[41] and akinesia deformation sequence at 13 weeks[42]. After this review[32], we had reports on ultrasound diagnosis of cleidocranial dysplasia at 14 weeks[43], congenital hypophosphatasia at 14 weeks[44], hemoglobin Bart's disease at 10 weeks[45] and chondroectodermal dysplasia at 12 weeks[46].

The 2D ultrasound findings of these skeletal dysplasias in the first trimester are mainly short limbs, and in some cases deformed or fractured bones with or without hypomineralization. It is interesting that, in these 18 cases, five cases had increased nuchal translucency.

By using 3D sonoembryology, it is feasible to visualize the entire length of extremities from 8 weeks of gestation[47]. The elbow and hand, knee and foot can be recognized from 9 weeks. Accordingly 3D sonography is superior to 2D sonography in delineation of the whole length of the extremities. Although there is no report on early diagnosis of skeletal dysplasia by 3D ultrasound to date, it is considered that there is room for its application in the future.

This case showed a large nuchal translucency, hypomineralization of vertebral bodies and short limbs at 12 weeks. Normal mineralization of the skull was seen, and therefore skeletal dysplasia and dwarfism were diagnosed. Based on these ultrasound findings, achondrogenesis type II was the most likely condition. In a 14-week scan, short and wide upper extremities, and short femurs and tibiae/fibulae in a crossed position were noted by conventional trans-abdominal sonography (Figure 13). As shown in Figure 14, these abnormalities were better visualized with the surface mode of 3D ultra-sound. The prenatal counselling to mother and family was facilitated by this 3D image of the fetus.

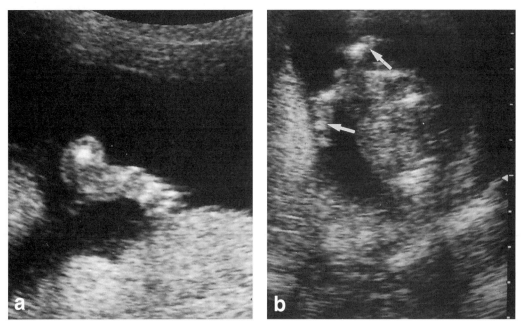

Figure 13 *Extremities of a case of dwarfism at 14 weeks of gestation, shown by conventional 2D imaging. A short and wide arm is successfully visualized (a). A short femur and tibia/fibula (arrows) are in an unusual crossing position (b)*

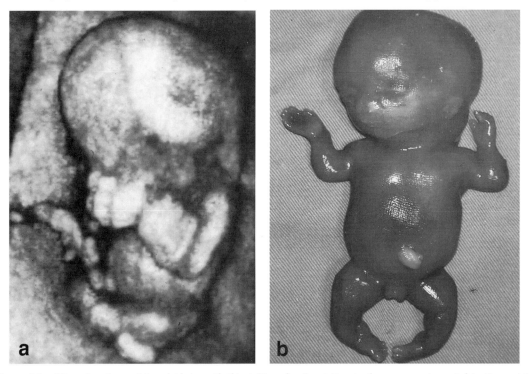

Figure 14 *3D surface image (a) and photograph (b) at 16 weeks of gestation in the same case presented in Figure 13. Characteristics of dwarfism such as large head and short trunk and short and wide extremities are well visualized in the 3D image. Crossed lower extremities are successfully visualized*

References

1. Hernadi L, Torocsik M. Screening for fetal anomalies in the 12th week of pregnancy by transvaginal sonography in an unselected population. *Prenat Diagn* 1997;17:753–9

2. Iskalos J, Jauniaux E, Rodeck C. Outcome of non-immune hydrops fetalis diagnosed during the first half of pregnancy. *Obstet Gynecol* 1997;90;321–5

3. Shulman LP, Emerson DS, Grevengood C, *et al*. Clinical course and outcome of fetuses with isolated cystic nuchal lesions and normal karyotypes detected in the first trimester. *Am J Obstet Gynecol* 1994;171:1278–81

4. Trauffer PML, Anderson CE, Johnson A, *et al*. The natural history of euploid pregnancies with first-trimester cystic hygromas. *Am J Obstet Gynecol* 1994;170:1279–84

5. Jauniaux E. Diagnosis and management of early non-immune hydrops fetalis. *Prenat Diagn* 1997; 17:1261–8

6. Santolaya J, Alley D, Jaffe R, *et al*. Antenatal classification of hydrops fetalis. *Obstet Gynecol* 1992;79:256–9

7. Cullen MT, Green J, Whetham J, *et al*. Transvaginal ultrasonographic detection of congenital anomalies in the first trimester. *Am J Obstet Gynecol* 1990;163:466–76

8. Rosati P, Guariglia L. Prognostic value of ultrasound findings of fetal cystic hygroma detected in early pregnancy by transvaginal sonography. *Ultrasound Obstet Gynecol* 2000;16:245–50

9. Bega G, Wapner R, Lev-Toaff A, *et al*. Diagnosis of conjoined twins at 10 weeks using three-dimensional ultrasound: a case report. *Ultrasound Obstet Gynecol* 2000;16:388–90

10. Maymon R, Halperin R, Weinraub Z, *et al*. Three-dimensional transvaginal sonography of conjoined twins at 10 weeks: a case report. *Ultrasound Obstet Gynecol* 1998;11:292–4

11. Kuroda K, Kamei Y, Kozuma S, *et al*. Prenatal evaluation of cephalopagus conjoined twins by means of three-dimensional ultrasound at 13 weeks of pregnancy. *Ultrasound Obstet Gynecol* 2000;16:264–6

12. Jonson D, Pretorius E, Budorick N. Three dimensional ultrasound of conjoined twins. *Obstet Gynecol* 1997;90:701–2

13. Bonilla-Musoles F, Raga F, Bonilla F Jr, *et al*. Early diagnosis of conjoined twins using two-dimensional color Doppler and three-dimensional ultrasound. *J Natl Med Assoc* 1998;90:552–6

14. Takeuchi H. Sonoembryology in the central nervous system. In Kurjak A, Chervenak A, eds. *The Fetus as a Patient*. Carnforth, UK: Parthenon Publishing, 1994:141–50

15. Blaas H-G, Eik-Nes SH, Kiserud T, *et al*. Early development of the forebrain and midbrain: a longitudinal ultrasound study from 7 to 12 weeks of gestation. *Ultrasound Obstet Gynecol* 1994;4: 183–92

16. Blaas H-G, Eik-Nes SH, Kiserud T, *et al*. Early development of the hindbrain and midbrain: a longitudinal ultrasound study from 7 to 12 weeks of gestation. *Ultrasound Obstet Gynecol* 1995;5: 151–60

17. Gonzalez-Gomez F, Salamanca A, Padilla M, *et al*. Alobar holoprosencephalic embryo detected via transvaginal sonography. *Eur J Obstet Gynecol Reprod Biol* 1992;47:266–70

18. Blaas H-G, Eik-Nes SH, Vainio T, *et al*. Alobar holoprosencephaly at 9 weeks gestational age visualized by two- and three-dimensional ultra-sound. *Ultrasound Obstet Gynecol* 2000;15:62–5

19. Lam YH, Tan MHY. Serial sonographic features of a fetus with hydranencephaly from 11 weeks to term. *Ultrasound Obstet Gynecol* 2000;16:77–9

20. Lin YS, Chang FM, Liu CH. Antenatal detection of hydranencephaly at 12 weeks menstrual age. *J Clin Ultrasound* 1992;20:62–4

21. Johnson SP, Sebire NJ, Snijders RJM, *et al*. Ultrasound screening for anencephaly at 10–14 weeks of gestation. *Ultrasound Obstet Gynecol* 1997;9:14–16

22. Van Zalen-Sprock RM, van Vugt JM, van Geijn HP. First and early second trimester diagnosis of anomalies of the central nervous system. *J Ultrasound Med* 1995;14:603–10

23. Braithwaite JM, Armstrong MA, Economides DL. Assessment of fetal anatomy at 12 to 13 weeks of gestation by transabdominal and transvaginal sonography. *Br J Obstet Gynaecol* 1996;103:82–5

24. Blumenfeld Z, Siegler E, Bronshtein M. The early diagnosis of neural tube defects. *Prenat Diagn* 1993;13:863–71

25. Blaas H-G, Eik-Nes SH, Isaksen CV. The detection of spina bifida before 10 gestational weeks using two- and three-dimensional ultra-sound. *Ultrasound Obstet Gynecol* 2000;16:25–9

26. Bonilla-Musoles F. Three-dimensional visualization of the human embryo: a potential revolution in prenatal diagnosis. *Ultrasound Obstet Gynecol* 1996;7:393–7

27. Snijders RJM, Sebire NJ, Souka A, *et al*. Fetal exomphalos and chromosomal defects: relationship to maternal age and gestation. *Ultrasound Obstet Gynecol* 1995;6:250–5

28. Blaas H-G, Eik-Nes SH, Kiserud T, *et al*. Early development of the abdominal wall, stomach and heart from 7 to 12 weeks of gestation: a

longitudinal ultrasound study. *Ultrasound Obstet Gynecol* 1995;6:240–9

29. Brown DL, Emerson DS, Shulman LP, *et al.* Sonographic diagnosis of omphalocele during 10th week of gestation. *Am J Roentgenol* 1989; 153:825–6

30. Pagliano M, Mosseti M, Ragno P. Echographic diagnosis of omphalocele in the first trimester of pregnancy. *J Clin Ultrasound* 1990;18:658–60

31. Chang L, Chang C-H, Yu C-H, *et al.* Three-dimensional sonographic visualization of a fetal omphalocele at 14 weeks of gestation. *Prenat Diagn* 2000;20:523–4

32. Souka AP, Nikolaides KH. Diagnosis of fetal abnormalities at the 10–14-week scan. *Ultrasound Obstet Gynecol* 1997;10:429–42

33. Guzman EP. Early prenatal diagnosis of gastroschisis with transvaginal sonography. *Am J Obstet Gynecol* 1990;162:1253–4

34. Zorzoli A, Kustermann A, Caravelli FE, *et al.* Measurements of fetal limb bones in early pregnancy. *Ultrasound Obstet Gynecol* 1994;4:29–33

35. Fisk NM, Vaughan J, Smidt M, *et al.* Transvaginal recognition of nuchal oedema in the first trimester diagnosis of achondrogenesis. *J Clin Ultrasound* 1991;9:588–90

36. Benacerraf B, Lister J, Du Ponte BL. First trimester diagnosis of fetal abnormalities. *J Reprod Med* 1988;9:777–80

37. Dimaio MS, Barth R, Koprivnikar KE, *et al.* Prenatal diagnosis of osteogenesis imperfecta type 2 by DNA analysis and sonography. *Prenat Diagn* 1993;13:589–96

38. Ben Ami M, Perlitzz Y, Haddad S, *et al.* Increased nuchal translucency is associated with asphyxiating thoracic dysplasia. *Ultrasound Obstet Gynecol* 1997;10:297–8

39. Otano L, Matayoshi T, Lippold S. Roberts syndrome: first trimester prenatal diagnosis by cytogenetics and ultrasound in affected and non-affected pregnancies. *Am J Hum Genet* 1993;53: 1445

40. Eliyahu S, Weiner E, Lahav D, *et al.* Early sono-graphic diagnosis of Jarcho–Levin syndrome: a prospective screening program in one family. *Ultrasound Obstet Gynecol* 1997;9:314–18

41. Bronshtein M, Gershoni-Baruch R. Prenatal transvaginal diagnosis of ectodactyly, ectodermal dysplasia, cleft palate (EEC) syndrome. *Prenat Diagn* 1993;13:519–22

42. Hyett JA, Noble P, Sebire NJ, *et al.* Lethal con-genital arthrogryposis presents with increased nuchal translucency at 10–14 weeks of gestation. *Ultrasound Obstet Gynecol* 1997;9:310–13

43. Wallerstein AR, Moran E, Lee M-J. Early prenatal ultrasound diagnosis of cleidocranial dysplasia. *Ultrasound Obstet Gynecol* 2000;15:154–6

44. Tongsong T, Pongsatha S. Early prenatal sono-graphic diagnosis of congenital hypophosphatasia. *Ultrasound Obstet Gynecol* 2000;15:252–5

45. Lam YH, Tang MHY. Limb reduction defects as the sonographic manifestation of hemoglobin Bart's disease at 10 weeks of gestation. *Ultrasound Obstet Gynecol* 2000;16:587–9

46. Dygoff L, Thieme G, Hobbins JC. First trimester prenatal diagnosis of chondroectodermal dysplasia (Ellis–van Creveld syndrome) with ultrasound. *Ultrasound Obstet Gynecol* 2001;17:86–8

47. Takeuchi H. Advanced sonoembryology by transvaginal three-dimensional ultrasound. In Chervenak FA, Kurjak A, eds. *Fetal Medicine.* Carnforth, UK: Parthenon Publishing, 1999: 16–23

Chiari II malformation in the fetus   6

V. D'Addario, V. Pinto and L. Di Cagno

INTRODUCTION

Hydrocephaly is one of the most commonly diagnosed malformations encountered during prenatal ultrasonographic screening. It is a dilatation of the cerebral ventricles as a result of an increased amount of cerebrospinal fluid (CSF), with an accompanying increase in intraventricular pressure and, subsequently, an increase in fetal head size[1]. Hydrocephaly may be an isolated finding (0.4–0.9/1000 live births), but it is more frequently associated with other brainstem, cerebellar and/or spinal defects (0.5–3/1000 live births)[1]. According to the communication between the ventricles and the subarachnoid space, hydrocephaly may be classified as non-communicating or communicating. In the former there is obstruction to the flow of CSF occurring within the intraventricular system, and the CSF cannot freely flow to the subarachnoid space. In communicating hydrocephaly the CSF can flow freely from the ventricles to the subarachnoid space, because the obstruction to the flow of CSF is extraventricular at the level of the subarachnoid space[1].

Although the diagnosis of fetal hydrocephaly may be easily accomplished by well-established biometric and morphological criteria[2], the diagnosis of the cause of the ventriculomegaly still represents a difficult task. Ventricular dilatation may be caused by different congenital abnormalities carrying different prognoses, such as Chiari II malformation, aqueductal stenosis, Dandy–Walker malformation, intracranial masses, schizencephaly, dysgenesis of the corpus callosum, encephalocele, leptomeningeal inflammation, lissencephaly, or absence of arachnoid granulations. Chiari II malformation is, together with aqueductal stenosis, the most common cause of congenital hydrocephaly. Chiari malformation is a complex abnormality, consisting of various combinations of brainstem and cerebellar malformations, usually associated with ventriculomegaly and spinal defects[3]. Four types were classically defined in the 1890s, each representing a different and unrelated anomaly of the hindbrain. Today some authors do not include types III and IV in the modern grouping of Chiari malformations.

Type I is ectopia of the cerebellar tonsils; the anomaly is usually an isolated feature encountered in adults.

Type II, also known as Arnold–Chiari malformation, is a complex entity appearing in the early developmental stages, characterized by spinal myelomeningocele associated with cerebellar hypoplasia and displacement of the tonsils and of the elongated distal brainstem through the enlarged foramen magnum. The posterior fossa is small and shallow with low position of the venous sinuses, low-lying and hypoplastic tentorium with large incisura, shortening of the clivus along the basisphenoid, loss of the pontine flexure, aqueductal stenosis or forking, caudal displacement of the pons, medulla and basilar artery, descent and elongation of the cerebellar vermis through the foramen magnum, descent and chinking of the brainstem and upward herniation of the superior cerebellum through the incisura. Polygyria, cortical heterotopia and dysgenesis of the corpus callosum may be associated. Hydrocephaly is almost constantly associated.

Type III is herniation of the cerebellum through cervical spina bifida with a defect of the basal occipital bone.

Type IV is cerebellar hypoplasia.

PATHOGENESIS

The pathogenesis of the Chiari II malformation, the most important type in the prenatal diagnosis, is still a cause for debate[4]. Several theories have been proposed:

(1) The cord remains attached at the myelomeningocele level, preventing its ascent during development and causing a downward displacement of the brainstem and cerebellum[5].

(2) Hydrocephaly is the initial event, pushing the brainstem and cerebellum downward[6].

(3) The pontine flexure fails to form, leading to an elongated brainstem with subsequent bending of the medulla over the spinal cord[7].

(4) The deformity belongs to the group of dysraphic disorders with primary mesoderm and posterior fossa abnormality[8].

The last is the most recent and accredited theory, based on cellular research by McLone and Knepper[8] with the delayed Splotch (Spd/Spd) mouse embryo, which has genetically abnormal neurulation resulting in a sacral neural tube defect. According to this theory, Chiari II malformation is the final result of a cascade of effects on the developing brain, starting from the primitive spinal defect. Normally, in the developing central nervous system there is a transient occlusion of the spinal neurocele (the cavity of the primitive neural tube), which seems to be necessary to retain CSF within the developing brain and to expand the primitive ventricular system. This expansion is required to provide the mechanical support for outward migration of neuroblasts and for expansion of the surrounding mesenchyme, permitting it to condense into cartilage or into bone of a size appropriate to future growth. A defective occlusion of the spinal neurocele or a leakage of CSF through a spinal defect causes a decompression and collapse of the ventricular cavities. Failure of the rhombencephalic cavity to distend causes the development of a small

and abnormal posterior fossa; in the absence of adequate distension the pliable basal cranial mesoderm develops and condenses around a partially collapsed rhombencephalic vesicle, giving origin to a small fossa that is inadequate to house the developing cerebellum. Simultaneously, lack of the distension of the third and lateral ventricles causes abnormalities of the thalami (large massa intermedia), gray matter heterotopia, disorganization of the cerebral gyri and dysgenesis of the corpus callosum. Finally, hydrocephaly is the consequence of the obstruction of the outlets of the fourth ventricle, the stretching and narrowing of the cerebral aqueduct, the obliteration of the subarachnoid space at the level of the foramen magnum and the obstruction at the level of the dysplastic tentorium. In conclusion, hydrocephaly is the result of the Chiari II hindbrain malformation and not the cause.

ANATOMIC DERANGEMENTS OF HINDBRAIN AND SPINAL CORD

Necroscopic, as well as CT and MRI observations[3,9,10], have provided useful signs in the detection of hindbrain defects in the Chiari II malformation.

In Chiari II patients, the bony posterior fossa is extremely small. The foramen magnum is symmetrically enlarged, and frequently exhibits a small notch at the opisthion. The upper cervical spinal canal is usually enlarged and the bony posterior arch of C1 is incomplete in 70% of cases. The lower vertebral column nearly always shows posterior spina bifida with myelocele or myelomeningocele. The cervical cord is displaced caudally for a variable distance and is also compacted along its long axis by herniation of the hindbrain above it. The medulla and even the pons may also be displaced downward into the cervical spinal canal. The medulla may descend purely vertically, so it remains in line above the displaced spinal cord. More commonly, however, the medulla buckles backward and downward as it descends, forming a cervicomedullary spur behind and below the upper cervical cord. This spur typically lies somewhere between C2 and C4, but may be found as low as the upper thoracic level. The Chiari II cerebellum is smaller than normal; the vermis and adjacent medial cerebellar hemispheres are often poorly differentiated from each other. The tongue-like projection of the cerebellum extends into the spinal canal and overlies the upper part of the spinal cord, the medulla and the fourth ventricle. The Chiari II fourth ventricle is elongated craniocaudally and narrowed transversally. It may be twice the normal length and has nearly parallel side walls with no definable angles. The greatest sagittal dimension of the fourth ventricle typically lies at or below the foramen magnum within the upper cervical spinal canal. The downward protrusion of spinal cord, medulla, fourth ventricle and vermis forms an overlapping series of hernias, each of which causes anterior displacement and compression of the structures in front. Thus, cervical cord segments C3–C6 are typically flattened sagittally and broadened transversely as compared with normal segments. Also, the medulla is flattened sagittally. The compression on the inferior vermis produces both acute and chronic change and the tongue-like elongation of the cerebellum shows cortical atrophy. Finally, the cervical spinal cord is abnormal in 96% of all Chiari II patients. Hydromyelia is frequent and is most marked in the lower cervical segments[9].

CLINICAL FINDINGS

The complex hindbrain malformation is the principal cause of death in children with myelomeningocele, despite surgical intervention and aggressive medical management. The majority of clinical manifestations of Chiari II malformation occur in infancy, usually before the age of 3 months. They are related to the dysplasia of the brainstem in the newborn, to the progressive hydrocephaly, the hindbrain compression and the spinal defects in the infant or older child. Approximately 20% of children with myelomeningocele develop symptoms of hindbrain, cranial nerve and spinal cord compression. The site and

extent of the spinal lesion correlate with the neurological outcome. The higher and larger the lesion, the more severe the neurological dysfunction of the neonate[1]. Further clinical signs are related to the frequently associated cerebral anomalies (polygyria, cortical heterotopia, dysgenesis of the corpus callosum, large massa intermedia).

PRENATAL DIAGNOSIS

The prenatal detection of the Chiari II malformation as the cause of the ventriculomegaly is of help in offering the parents an accurate prognosis on the perspectives of life of the future newborn. In Chiari II malformation with associated spinal defect, the evaluation of the posterior fossa is a crucial part of the ultrasonic examination, since a small posterior fossa is one of its typical signs. The radiographic evaluation of the brain in adults shows a variety of linear, angular, surface area and volume measurements of the posterior fossa, both in normal and pathological cases[11-13]. To correctly evaluate the shape and accurately measure the size of the posterior fossa, Vega et al.[11] suggest making the following measurements on a lateral conventional skull X-ray: length of the clivus (from the basion to the base of the posterior clinoid process), length of the Chamberlain's line (from the opisthion to the posterior aspect of the palate), length of the Twining's line (from the internal occipital protuberance to the tuberculum sellae), length of the Twining–opisthion line (perpendicular line from the opisthion to Twining's line), basal angle (nasion–center of sella turcica–basion) and Boogard's angle (opisthion–basion–tuberculum sellae). They define the posterior fossa area as the area below the Twining's line. They found a significant difference between adult patients with Chiari I malformation and a control group, mainly regarding the surface area and the clivus length. Milhorat et al.[13] performed similar measurements on sagittal MRI scans of the brain in adults: they measured the length of the supraocciput along a line drawn from the center of the internal occipital protuberance to the opisthion, the length of the clivus, the slope of the tentorium (calculated by the angle formed by the tentorium and the supra-occiput) and the distance between the tip of the cerebellar tonsils and the line drawn from the basion to the episthion. They also calculated the volume of the posterior fossa using the Cavalieri stereological method, which is simpler and quicker than computer-based programs[14]. They found a significant difference between adult patients with Chiari I malformation and a control group, in both the linear and the volumetric measurements.

A small posterior fossa is also reported as a typical radiological, CT and MRI sign of Chiari II malformation. However, authors reporting on this anomaly in adults refer mainly to the morphological features of the malformation, rather than to the biometric ones. Naidich[15], who published an accurate study on the correlation between surgical, pathological and CT findings in infants with Chiari II malformation, reported the following typical CT signs: lacunar skull, petrous scalloping, hypoplastic tentorium, small posterior fossa, enlarged foramen magnum and upper cervical canal, incomplete fusion of the posterior arches of C1 and lower cervical vertebrae, cascading protrusions of the vermis, fourth ventricle, medulla and cervical cord into the spinal canal, and cervico-medullary kinking. Similarly, as regards the MRI signs of the malformation, the morphological features are preferred to the biometric features. MRI accurately reveals the relationship of the soft tissues and osseous structures and provides, non-invasively and with the proper delineation of brainstem, cerebellum and spinal canal, the best imaging method in the evaluation of borderline cases and in differentiation of Chiari I and II malformations[16].

The detailed findings and the complex measurements achievable on X-ray films or MRI scans in the adult cannot be completely transferred to the fetal sonograms. The small size of the fetal skull leads to poor-quality sonographic images as compared to X-ray and MRI, which precisely show the bones and

brain tissues, respectively. For this reason the prenatal sonographic findings of Chiari II malformation described so far are all indirect signs of the typically funnelling shape of the posterior fossa. They can be found on an axial scan of the posterior fossa and range from the 'effacement of the cisterna magna'[17], to the so-called 'banana sign'[18], to the 'absent cerebellum'[19], according to the severity of the posterior fossa dysmorphism. In the less severe forms the cerebellum still looks normal but its transverse diameter is smaller than normal and the cisterna magna is effaced or absent. The smaller the posterior fossa, the higher the cerebellar dysmorphism, and the fetal cerebellum assumes the typical banana shape. In the most severe cases little or no cerebellar tissue can be identified. The posterior fossa findings described so far are almost constantly associated with ventriculomegaly of varying degrees, and to a spinal defect with myelomeningocele, most frequently located at the lumbosacral level. Owing to the constant association with the spinal defect, the posterior fossa findings, particularly the 'banana sign', as well as a typical bossing of the frontal bones, known as the 'lemon sign', are commonly used as indirect signs of spina bifida and are successfully used to screen this defect with high sensitivity. Moreover, according to Naidich's CT observations[9] and to the dysraphic unified pathogenetic theory of McLone and Knepper[8] a correlation should be expected between the severity of the posterior fossa abnormality and the severity of ventriculomegaly. Such a correlation has been demonstrated in fetuses with myelomeningocele by Babcook et al.[20]. They subjectively graded the severity of the posterior fossa abnormality as mild (smaller than normal cisterna magna with cerebellum easily identifiable and not misshapen), moderate (small posterior fossa, effaced cisterna magna and misshapen cerebellum), or severe (very small posterior fossa, effaced cisterna magna and little or no identifiable cerebellar tissue) and found a correlation between the severity of the posterior fossa abnormality and the severity of the ventriculomegaly.

In no paper regarding the prenatal diagnosis of Chiari II malformation was a direct measurement of the posterior fossa reported. For this reason we have recently focused our attention on the shape and size of the posterior fossa, since a small posterior fossa is universally recognized as a specific sign of Chiari (both I and II) malformation[21]. To obtain this goal, we moved our attention from the traditionally used axial scan to the sagittal scan of the posterior fossa, showing the clivus anteriorly and the supraocciput posteriorly. In order to avoid complicated calculations, we suggested only the measurement of the angle defined by two lines drawn on the clivus and the supraocciput as a direct and objective sign of the shape of the posterior fossa[21] (Figure 1). This measurement is easily achieved in almost all cases. It becomes difficult and time-consuming before 16 and after 34 weeks of gestation; in early pregnancy the size of the bones (particularly the clivus) is too small to correctly draw a line on; in late gestation the visualization of the head in the sagittal view is severely limited in fetuses lying in the cephalic position. Despite this limitation the clivus–supraocciput angle is the easiest measurement that objectively represents the shape of the posterior fossa and, indirectly, its volume. Unlike the transverse cerebellar diameter, which is traditionally used as an indirect sign of the posterior fossa size, it has the advantage of being independent of gestational age. The normal value through gestation is 79.3 ± 6°. In our experience all cases of Chiari II malformation showed a value below the 5th centile (mean value 65.1°; range 61–71°) (Figure 2). Therefore, the cut-off value below which a Chiari malformation can be suspected is 72°. This measurement has also proved to be useful in differentiating fetal ventriculomegaly due to Chiari II malformation from that caused by other abnormalities. In fact, the values found in cases of ventriculomegaly due to other causes (aqueductal stenosis, Dandy–Walker malformation, dysgenesis of the corpus callosum, isolated borderline ventriculomegaly, schizencephaly) fell within the normal range, excluding six (two aqueductal

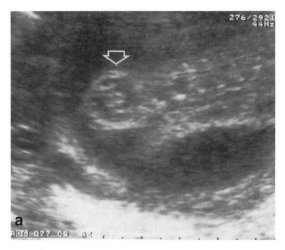

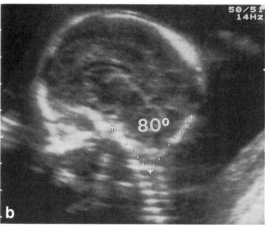

Figure 1 *Measurement of the clivus–supraocciput angle in a normal 21-week-old fetus. Two lines are electronically drawn on the clivus and the supraocciput; the angle defined by their intersection is measured (80°)*

stenosis, two dysgenesis of the corpus callosum, one borderline ventriculomegaly, one ventriculomegaly due to porencephaly) that showed values above the 90th centile; only two cases (both dysgenesis of the corpus callosum) showed values (74°) between the 10th and the 5th centiles (Figure 3).

The measurement of the clivus–supraocciput angle is particularly useful in cases of late diagnosis or referral of fetal ventriculomegaly, when the visualization of the classic indirect signs of Chiari II

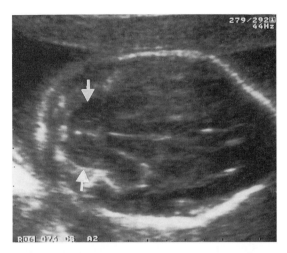

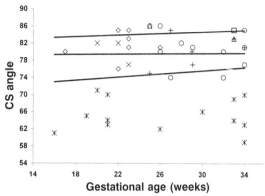

Figure 3 *The relationship between the clivus–supraocciput (CS) angle and gestational age; lines represent the 10th, 50th and 90th centiles. The values found in 44 cases of fetal ventriculomegaly are reported. ✳ Chiari II malformation; ◇ aqueductal stenosis; ✕ Dandy–Walker malformation; ○ dysgenesis of the corpus callosum; + borderline ventriculomegaly; △ porencephaly*

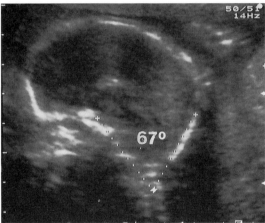

Figure 2 *Measurement of the clivus–supraocciput angle in a 21-week-old fetus affected by Chiari II malformation. The angle (67°) is lower than normal*

malformation may be limited. The 'lemon' sign is present in virtually all cases between 16 and 24 postmenstrual weeks, but after 24 weeks of gestation it is a less reliable marker and is present in only 13–50% of fetuses with a spinal defect[1,19,22]. The recognition of the 'banana sign' or small cerebellum and the effaced cisterna magna is possible in 95–100% of the cases[1,19,22], although, after 24 weeks, cerebellar absence is the most commonly seen 'cerebellar' sign[19]. The visualization of all of these signs may be limited in late gestation by the increased skull calcification, which obscures the intracranial structures. Finally, the examination of the spine may be limited by the fetal position and by the relative reduction of the amount of amniotic fluid, as compared to the fetal body volume.

References

1. Monteagudo A, Timor-Tritsch IE. Fetal neurosonography of congenital brain anomalies. In Timor-Tritsch, Monteagudo, Cohen. *Ultrasonography of the Prenatal and Neonatal Brain.* New York: McGraw Hill, 2001

2. Cardoza JD, Goldstein RB, Filly RA. Exclusion of fetal ventriculomegaly with a single measurement: the width of the lateral ventricular atrium. *Radiology* 1988;169:711–14

3. Gilbert-Barness E, ed. *Potter's Pathology of the Fetus and Infant,* vol 2. St Louis: Mosby Year Book, 1997

4. McLone DG, Naidich TP. Development morphology of the subarachnoid space, brain

vasculature, and contiguous structures, and the cause of the Chiari II malformation. *Am J Nucl Radiol* 1992;13:463–82

5. Penfield W, Coburn DF. Arnold–Chiari malformation and its operative treatment. *Arch Neurol Psychiatry* 1938;40:328–33

6. Padget DH. Neuroschisis on human embryonic maldevelopment: new evidence on anencephaly, spina bifida, and diverse mammalian defects. *J Neuropathol Exp Neurol* 1970;29:192–5

7. Daniel PM, Strich SJ. Some observations on the congenital deformity of central nervous system known as the Arnold–Chiari malformation. *J Neuropathol Exp Neurol* 1958;17:255–60

8. McLone DG, Knepper PA. The cause of Chiari II malformation: a unified theory. *Pediatr Neurosci* 1989;15:1–12

9. Naidich TP, McLone DG, Fulling KH. The Chiari II malformation: part IV. The hindbrain deformity. *Neuroradiology* 1983;25:179–97

10. Naidich TP, Pudlowski RM, Naidich JB, Gornish M, Rodriguez FJ. Computed tomographic signs of the Chiari II malformation. Part I: skull and dural partitions. *Radiology* 1980;134:65–71

11. Vega A, Quintana F, Berciano J. Basichondrocranium anomalies in adult Chiari type I malformation: a morphometric study. *J Neurol Sci* 1990;99:137–45

12. Nishikawa M, Sakamoto H, Hakuba A, Nakanishi N, Inoue Y. Pathogenesis of Chiari malformation: a morphometric study of the posterior cranial fossa. *J Neurosurg* 1997;86:40–7

13. Milhorat TH, Chou MW, Trinidad EM, *et al.* Chiari I malformation redefined: clinical and radiographic findings for 364 symptomatic patients. *Neurosurgery* 1999;40:1005–17

14. Clatterbuck RE, Sipos EP. The efficient calculation of neurosurgically relevant volumes from computed tomographic scans using Cavalieri's direct estimator. *Neurosurgery* 1997;40:339–43

15. Naidich TP. Cranial CT signs of the Chiari II malformation. *J Neuroradiol* 1981;8:207–27

16. Gammal TE, Mark EK, Brooks BS. MR imaging of Chiari II malformation. *Am J Nucl Radiol* 1987;35:1037–44

17. Goldstein RB, Podrasky AE, Filly RA, Callen PW. Effacement of the fetal cisterna magna in association with myelomeningocele. *Radiology* 1989;172:409–13

18. Nicolaides KH, Campbell S, Gabbe SG, Guidetti R. Ultrasound screening for spina bifida: cranial and cerebellar signs. *Lancet* 1986;2:72–4

19. Van den Hof MC, Nicolaides KH, Campbell J, Campbell S. Evaluation of the lemon and banana signs in one hundred thirty fetuses with open spina bifida. *Am J Obstet Gynecol* 1990;162:322–7

20. Babcook CJ, Goldstein RB, Barth RA, Damato NM, Callen PW, Filly RA. Prevalence of ventriculomegaly in association with myelomeningocele: correlation with gestational age and severity of posterior fossa deformity. *Radiology* 1994;190,703–7

21. D'Addario V, Pinto V, Del Bianco A *et al.* The clivus–supraocciput angle: a useful measurement to evaluate the shape and size of the fetal posterior fossa and to diagnose Chiari II malformation. *Ultrasound Obstet Gynecol* 2001;18: 146–9

22. Thiagarajah S, Henke J, Hogge WA, Abbitt PL, Breeden N, Ferguson JE. Early diagnosis of spina bifida: the value of cranial ultrasound markers. *Obstet Gynecol* 1990;76:54–7

Transvaginal three-dimensional volume assessment of the fetal brain structure

7

R. K. Pooh and K. H. Pooh

INTRODUCTION

Three-dimensional (3D) sonography, recently introduced into the field of prenatal diagnosis[1,2], has several abilities, such as surface imaging, multiplanar two-dimensional detection of inside of the organ, volume calculation and circulatory demonstration. Transvaginal sonography using cranial sutures and fontanelles as ultrasound windows[3-6] produces high-resolution images of the brain structure in the sagittal and coronal sections and has established a new field of 'neurosonography'[7]. Volume acquisition of the fetal brain by transvaginal 3D ultrasound enables intracranial multiplanar image assessment[8-12]. 3D volume imaging of fetal brain cavities in early pregnancy was reported by Blaas *et al.*[13,14]. We use transvaginal 3D sonography in mid- and late pregnancy for objective brain assessment.

PATIENTS AND METHODS

A total of 48 normal singleton fetuses with cephalic position between 12 and 38 weeks of gestation were studied. VOLUSON 530D (Medison Co., Seoul, Korea) with transvaginal 3D transducer was used. Whole volume data of the fetal brain were obtained on magneto-optical disks. Volume analyses were performed by the use of PC 3D-View, version 3.2 (Kretztechnik AG, Zipf, Austria). The lateral ventricle, choroid plexus and the intracranial cavity were manually traced on the image with repeating 15° or 30° rotation (Figure 1). Volume changes of the intracranial structures during normal pregnancy were analyzed.

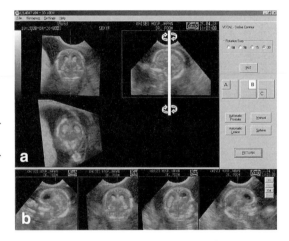

Figure 1 *3D volumetry of normal fetal brain. After 2–6 s of fan-scan of the fetal brain, three orthogonal views can be obtained (a) and parallel slicing of each view is possible. Volume image of target organ of the intracranial cavity can be rotated by 15–30° manually traced (b). When finishing image rotation and manual tracing, extracted images of target organ and estimated volume were automatically demonstrated*

In eight cases with mild or moderate ventriculomegaly, volume changes of the lateral ventricle and choroid plexus were studied and in two cases with glioependymal cyst with unilateral ventriculomegaly, cystic volume was calculated.

RESULTS

Volume analysis was successful in all normal brain cavities. During normal pregnancy, the volume of the intracranial cavity (Figure 2),

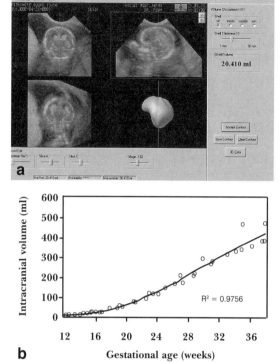

Figure 2 *Intracranial cavity volume imaging (a) and its volume change during pregnancy (b)*

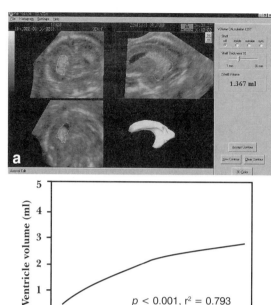

Figure 3 *Lateral ventricle volume imaging (a) and its volume change during pregnancy (b)*

ventricle (Figure 3) and choroid plexus (Figure 4) significantly increased. Changing appearance of the lateral ventricle and choroid plexus during pregnancy is shown in Figure 5. In all eight cases with mild or moderate ventriculomegaly, volumes of not only lateral ventricle, but also choroid plexus were larger than those found in normal fetuses (Figures 6 and 7). In two cases with glioependymal cyst, the cyst occupying lesions were calculated at 8% and 35% (Figure 8).

DISCUSSION

Volumetry of the fetal organ is one of the most interesting fields in prenatal fetal imaging. Magnetic resonance imaging (MRI) is one possible modality which can calculate organ volume and recent reports have shown its possibility to demonstrate fetal organ volumetry[15-17]. Kinoshita *et al.*[18] measured the volume changes of the lateral ventricle and germinal matrix in

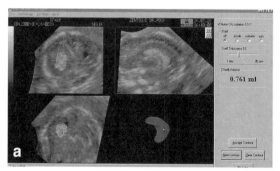

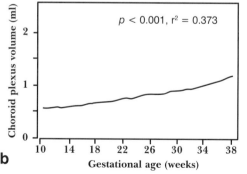

Figure 4 *Choroid plexus volume imaging (a) and its volume change during pregnancy (b)*

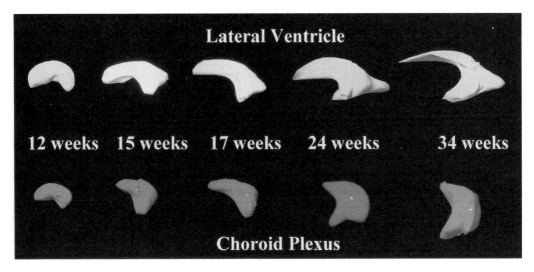

Figure 5 *Changing appearance of lateral ventricle and choroid plexus during pregnancy*

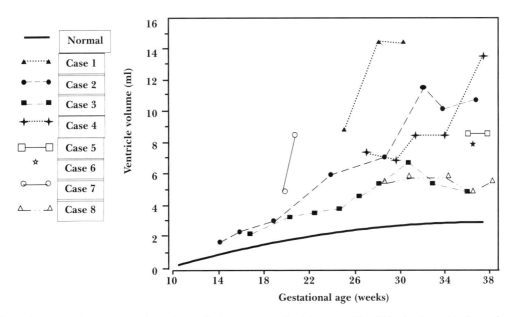

Figure 6 *Lateral ventricular volume change during pregnancy in eight cases with mild/moderate ventriculomegaly*

post-mortem fetuses using an experimental 4.7 tesla MRI system. Transvaginal 3D neuroscan has enabled clear demonstration of the intracranial structures in the sagittal, coronal and axial sections. Scanning duration is short[8,9] and off-line volume evaluation is quite helpful for *in vitro* assessment of fetal intracranial condition[12]. Our results showed that volume analysis could produce comprehensive volume imaging of the brain cavity, and provide us with longitudinal evaluation of the intracranial morphological change.

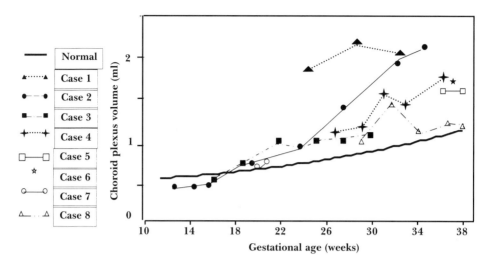

Figure 7 *Choroid plexus volume change during pregnancy in eight cases with mild/moderate ventriculomegaly*

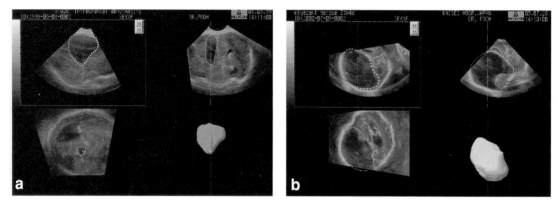

Figure 8 *Volume imaging of glioependymal cyst in two cases. (a) Intrahemispheric cyst occupying 8% (shell volume 15.6 ml) of intracranial cavity and (b) supra-to-infra-tentorial cyst occupying 35% (shell volume 184.7 ml) of intracranial cavity*

CONCLUSION

Intracranial volumetric study of fetuses may have a great potential in the fields of fetal development and fetal neurology.

ACKNOWLEDGEMENTS

This study was done with co-operation of Medison Co. (Seoul, Korea) and Kretztechnik AG (Zipf, Austria).

References

1. Kurjak A, Hafner T, Kos M, Kupesic S, Stanojevic M. Three-dimensional sonography in prenatal diagnosis: a luxury or a necessity? *J Perinat Med* 2000;28:194–9

2. Merz E. Three-dimensional ultrasound – a requirement for prenatal diagnosis. *Ultrasound Obstet Gynecol* 1998;12:225–6

3. Monteagudo A, Reuss ML, Timor-Tritsch IE. Imaging the fetal brain in the second and third trimesters using transvaginal sonography. *Obstet Gynecol* 1991;77:27–32

4. Monteagudo A, Timor-Tritsch IE, Moomjy M. *In utero* detection of ventriculomegaly during the second and third trimesters by transvaginal sonography. *Ultrasound Obstet Gynecol* 1994;4:193–8

5. Pooh RK, Maeda K, Pooh KH, Kurjak A. Sonographic assessment of the fetal brain morphology. *Prenat Neonat Med* 1999;4:18–38

6. Pooh RK, Nakagawa Y, Nagamachi N, Pooh KH, Nakagawa Y, Maeda K, *et al.* Transvaginal sonography of the fetal brain: detection of abnormal morphology and circulation. *Croat Med J* 1998;39:147–57

7. Timor-Tritsch IE, Monteagudo A. Transvaginal fetal neurosonography: standardization of the planes and sections by anatomic landmarks. *Ultrasound Obstet Gynecol* 1996;8:42–7

8. Pooh RK. Fetal brain assessment by three-dimensional ultrasound. In Kurjak A, Kupesic S, eds. *Clinical Application of 3D Sonography*. Carnforth, UK: Parthenon Publishing, 2000:171–9

9. Pooh RK, Pooh K, Nakagawa Y, Nishida S, Ohno Y. Clinical application of three-dimensional ultrasound in fetal brain assessment. *Croat Med J* 2000;41:245–51

10. Monteagudo A, Timor-Tritsch IE, Mayberry P. Three-dimensional transvaginal neurosonography of the fetal brain: 'navigating' in the volume scan. *Ultrasound Obstet Gynecol* 2000;16:307–13

11. Timor-Tritsch IE, Monteagudo A, Mayberry P. Three-dimensional ultrasound evaluation of the fetal brain: the three horn view. *Ultrasound Obstet Gynecol* 2000;16:302–6

12. Pooh RK, Pooh KH. Transvaginal 3D and Doppler ultrasonography of the fetal brain. *Semin Perinatol* 2001;25:38–43

13. Blaas HG, Eik-Nes SH, Kiserud T, Berg S, Angelsen B, Olstad B. Three-dimensional imaging of the brain cavities in human embryos. *Ultrasound Obstet Gynecol* 1995;5:228–32

14. Blaas HG, Eik-Nes SH, Berg S, Torp H. *In-vivo* three-dimensional ultrasound reconstructions of embryos and early fetuses. *Lancet* 1998;352: 1182–6

15. Baker PN, Johnson IR, Gowland PA, Hykin J, Adams V, Mansfield P, Worthington BS. Measurement of fetal liver, brain and placental volumes with echo-planar magnetic resonance imaging. *Br J Obstet Gynaecol* 1995;102:35–9

16. Garden AS, Roberts N. Fetal and fetal organ volume estimations with magnetic resonance imaging. *Am J Obstet Gynecol* 1996;175:442–8

17. Gong QY, Roberts N, Garden AS, Whitehouse GH. Fetal and fetal brain volume estimation in the third trimester of human pregnancy using gradient echo MR imaging. *Magn Reson Imaging* 1998;16:235–40

18. Kinoshita Y, Okudera T, Tsuru E, Yokota A. Volumetric analysis of the germinal matrix and lateral ventricles performed using MR images of postmortem fetuses. *Am J Neuroradiol* 2001;22: 382–8

Human fetal pulmonary arterial blood flow

8

J. J. A. M. Laudy and J. W. Wladimiroff

INTRODUCTION

Color-coded Doppler techniques allow study of the normal lung circulation during fetal development. Post-mortem examination of lethal lung hypoplasia has demonstrated well-defined changes in arterial pulmonary vascular morphology. It would, therefore, be worthwhile to explore the fetal arterial pulmonary circulation during the second half of pregnancy. It should be realized that only a descriptive analysis of Doppler velocity waveforms can be obtained.

NORMAL FETAL LUNG GROWTH

Fetal lung growth and lung maturation are related, but appear to be separately controlled. Normal lung growth refers to an increase in cell number and seems to be influenced primarily by physical factors such as intrauterine and intrathoracic space, lung liquid volume and pressure and breathing movements. Lung maturation refers to the distensibility or compliance of the lung and is divided into two components, structural and biochemical (surfactant).

An important physical factor that may influence lung growth is the intrauterine space, which depends on the amniotic fluid volume. A normal amount of amniotic fluid seems to be important for fetal lung growth[1,2]. Next to fetal urine, which is the primary component of amniotic fluid, actively secreted fetal lung fluid also constitutes a significant portion (about one-third) of amniotic fluid[3]. Fetal swallowing is the principal means of amniotic fluid resorption (Figure 1). Bilateral renal agenesis, obstructive lesions of the urinary tract and early preterm rupture of membranes are the most common conditions that cause oligohydramnios[4].

Several mechanisms have been put forward to explain the association between oligohydramnios and pulmonary hypoplasia. First, is decreased space for lung growth due to compression of the uterine wall upon the fetal chest and abdomen. Second, is restriction of fetal breathing movements by prolonged thoracic compression. Fetal breathing movements may stimulate lung growth by intermittently distending the lungs with fluid aspirated into the trachea[2]. However, as shown in some animal experiments, it seems unlikely

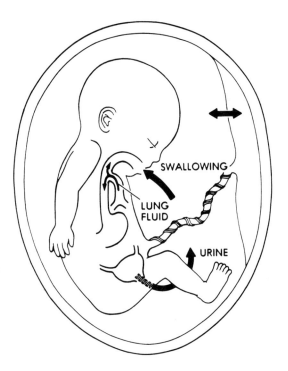

Figure 1 *A schematic illustration of the dynamic process of amniotic fluid formation and resorption. (Reprinted with permission from reference 3)*

that inhibition of fetal breathing is the predominant etiology of oligohydramnios-related pulmonary hypoplasia. Third, is increased efflux of lung liquid from the intrapulmonary space to the amniotic space, resulting in a decrease of intrapulmonary pressure[1,2]. This highlights the importance of the presence of intrapulmonary fluid and of a normal balance of volume and pressure on the developing fetal lung. Fetal lung liquid is formed by active transport across the pulmonary epithelium into the tracheobronchial lumen, where it establishes a positive pressure within the developing fetal lung[4,5]. The presence of a positive pressure in the trachea relative to amniotic pressure shows that there is resistance to outflow[5]. When breathing movements are absent, the pressure in the fetal trachea is even higher, which may be important in regulating the volume of fluid within the lungs. There is evidence that lung fluid acts as an internal stent for the lung, distending potential airways and stimulating growth and differentiation[4]. Oligohydramnios may increase lung fluid loss by compression of the lungs, with consequent decreased lung volume within the potential airways, thus leading to pulmonary hypoplasia. Based on several experimental animal studies it may be concluded that positive intratracheal pressure, amplitude of pressure changes as well as tidal volume changes during fetal breathing movements may influence fetal lung growth[2,4,5].

Another important physical factor that can interfere with fetal lung growth is the intrathoracic cavity. A smaller than normal intrathoracic space may be responsible for the development of fetal pulmonary hypoplasia[1,2,5]. Conditions that can be named in this respect are congenital diaphragmatic hernia, fetal hydrops, tumors of the thorax including adenomatoid malformations and skeletal anomalies deforming the thoracic cage[2,6–8]. Paralysis of the diaphragm may, apart from limiting the intrathoracic space, interfere with fetal breathing movements and this may have an additional negative effect on fetal lung growth[2,5].

Finally, normal pulmonary arterial flow during the canalicular and alveolar stages of fetal lung development appears to be essential for normal lung growth[9]. Ligation of the left pulmonary artery during the late canalicular stage of lung development in the fetal sheep creates pulmonary hypoplasia with significantly reduced lung weight and lung volume of the future gas exchange portion of the lung (future air spaces, parenchymal tissue and capillary content).

PHYSIOLOGY OF THE FETAL PULMONARY CIRCULATION

In the fetus, normal gas exchange is placental in origin and the pulmonary vascular circuit is a high-resistance, high-pressure, low-flow system[10]. In human fetuses blood supply to the lungs is 13% of total cardiac output at 20 weeks, increasing to 25% at 30 weeks. It remains constant during the last trimester[11]. This implies that pulmonary blood flow increases and pulmonary vascular resistance decreases with advancing gestation.

Fetal pulmonary blood flow is low despite the dominance of the right ventricle, which ejects about two-thirds of total cardiac output. Most of the right ventricular output is diverted away from the lungs through the widely patent ductus arteriosus to the thoracic aorta, then reaching the placenta through the umbilical circulation for oxygenation[12]. Since the ductus arteriosus is patent during intrauterine life, pulmonary arterial pressure is considered to be maintained at least equal to systemic arterial pressure[13]. Maintenance of a low-flow pulmonary vascular circuit depends on the high resistance of the pulmonary vasculature.

ABNORMAL LUNG DEVELOPMENT: PULMONARY HYPOPLASIA

Definition and morphological features

Pulmonary hypoplasia, either unilateral or bilateral, is a poorly defined condition of incomplete development of the lung, so that it fails to reach adult size[8]. This defective development is due to a decrease in the number of lung cells, airways and alveoli, with a resulting decrease in organ size and weight[7,14–17]. It has been postulated that impairment of pulmonary development during the pseudoglandular stage (before 16 weeks' gestation) causes reduced bronchiolar branching, cartilage development, acinar complexity and maturation, and retarded vascularization and thinning of the air–blood barrier[15]. Insults occurring after the pseudoglandular stage (after 16 weeks' gestation) impair acinar complexity and maturation[15].

Since growth of the pulmonary blood vessels parallels development of the airways (pre-acinar blood vessels with the conducting airways and intra-acinar blood vessels with alveolar development), it is not surprising that disturbance of the pulmonary vascular bed coincides with pulmonary hypoplasia. A decrease in total size of the pulmonary vascular bed, a decrease in the number of vessels per unit of lung tissue and increased pulmonary arterial smooth muscle have been described[18]. The last has been expressed in an increased medial wall thickness as a percentage of the external thickness[19]. Peripheral extension of muscle into arteries smaller than normal have been observed[16,19] and the intrapulmonary arteries are smaller than normal but appropriate for the reduced volume of the lung[16]. These features form the morphological basis for the increased pulmonary vascular resistance.

Epidemiology and etiology

The reported incidence of pulmonary hypoplasia in the general population ranges from 9 to 11 per 10 000 live births and is 14 per 10 000 of all births[20,21]. This must be an underestimate of the true incidence, since infants with lesser degrees of hypoplasia undoubtedly survive the neonatal period. The reported incidence of this condition in autopsies ranges from 7.8 to 22%[8,17,20,21] and more than 85% of those cases will display significant associated anomalies[8]. Perinatal mortality is high, approximately 70% in most series (55–100%)[22–26].

Pulmonary hypoplasia may be a primary or secondary phenomenon. Bilateral pulmonary hypoplasia occurring as an isolated anomaly has been considered as extremely rare[27]. It has been suggested that infants with primary pulmonary hypoplasia represent a group subject to decreased respiratory activity *in utero*, although the amount of amniotic fluid at delivery was not described in these instances[27]. Most cases of pulmonary hypoplasia are secondary to congenital anomalies or pregnancy complications that inhibit lung development. Factors important in lung growth are discussed in the previous sections. An exhaustive list of the numerous conditions reportedly associated with pulmonary hypoplasia was compiled by Sherer *et al.*[6]. Based on this adjusted list the categories can be grouped (Table 1).

Most cases, such as renal anomalies, congenital diaphragmatic hernia and hydrops fetalis, indicate interference with lung growth during the early developmental stage mainly before 16 weeks of gestation, whereas oligohydramnios due to prolonged rupture of membranes possibly impairs pulmonary development after 16 weeks[15]. Wigglesworth *et al.*[7] could detect no difference between the structural appearance of the lungs after rupture of the membranes dating from before 20 weeks' gestation in the presence of normal kidneys and that seen in cases of bilateral renal agenesis.

Renal and non-renal prolonged oligohydramnios are one of the major causes of pulmonary hypoplasia. The occurrence of bilateral renal agenesis and pulmonary hypoplasia was first recognized by Potter in 1946[28]. Later it became apparent that lethal pulmonary hypoplasia was also a consistent feature in babies with no renal function at birth, because of bilateral renal dysplasia with or without cyst formation. The common features associated with these anomalies are known as the Potter's syndrome: profound oligohydramnios, characteristic facial and limb deformities and pulmonary hypoplasia[29–31]. Growth deficiency, if delivered after 34 weeks, is also reported to be a common, although not a major feature in association with Potter's syndrome[31]. There is no evidence that pulmonary hypoplasia is genetically or teratologically related to the various urinary tract anomalies[29,32]. One hypothesis for the development of Potter's syndrome is that it is the consequence of multiple early mesodermal defects[30], although the widely accepted view is that the structural abnormalities of the face, lungs and limbs are secondary to oligohydramnios[29]. Also, other non-renal causes of prolonged oligohydramnios such as chronic amniotic fluid leakage may lead to the described non-renal features of Potter's syndrome[33]. Therefore, these secondary features are also known as the oligohydramnios sequence or oligohydramnios tetrad[33] (Figure 2).

It has been reported that oligohydramnios due to prolonged premature rupture of membranes (PROM) may be associated with pulmonary hypoplasia[22–25,33–35] even in the absence of the full complex of malformations connected with the oligohydramnios tetrad[23,24,36]. PROM, mostly defined as rupture

Table 1 *Etiological categories and examples of related anomalies associated with pulmonary hypoplasia*

Categories	Anomalies
Intrathoracic masses	congenital diaphragmatic hernia, congenital cystic adenomatoid malformation, bronchogenic cyst, etc.
Oligohydramnios based on renal or urinary tract anomalies	bilateral renal agenesis or dysplasia, bladder outlet obstruction, etc.
Non-renal oligohydramnios	prolonged preterm rupture of membranes
Skeletal malformations	osteogenesis imperfecta, thanatophoric dwarfism, etc.
Neuromuscular and central nervous system anomalies	fetal akinesia, anencephaly, etc.
Pleural effusions	rhesus and non-rhesus hydrops, etc.
Cardiac lesions	hypoplastic right or left heart, pulmonary stenosis, etc.
Abdominal wall defects	omphalocele, gastroschisis, etc.
Syndromes associated with pulmonary hypoplasia	trisomy 13, 18, 21, Robert syndrome, etc.

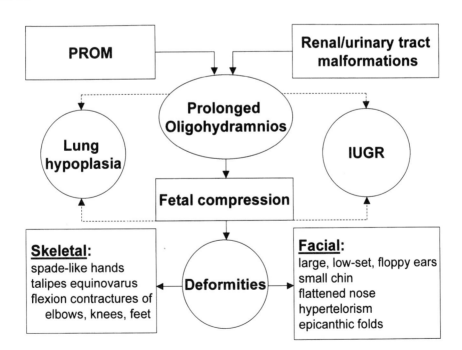

Figure 2 *Features of the Potter syndrome or oligohydramnios tetrad. PROM, premature rupture of membranes; IUGR, intrauterine growth restriction. (Reprinted with permission from Laudy JAM, et al. The fetal lung 2: Pulmonary hypoplasia.* Ultrasound Obstet Gynecol *2000;16:482–90)*

of the fetal membranes prior to the onset of labor, is a common obstetric problem that occurs in approximately 10% of all pregnancies, with worldwide reports varying between 5% and 45%[37]. Ninety per cent of the patients who present with this problem have a latent phase of less than 1 week[38]. The other 10%, who are largely preterm patients, present a dilemma in management[22,37,39]. Prolonged PROM is associated with an increased chance of infection in both the mother and the fetus, perinatal death as a result of prematurity, and fetal distress during labor because of cord compression[24,39]. The risks of early delivery and hyaline membrane disease must be weighed against those of expectant management, such as pulmonary hypoplasia, sepsis and fetal deformities. The incidence of neonatal infection following preterm membrane rupture has been reported to be between 0.5% and 25%[37]. It was demonstrated by McIntosh et al.[25] that pulmonary hypoplasia is a much more serious problem following preterm prolonged membrane rupture than is infection. This was confirmed by Tibboel et al.[34], who emphasized that, in case of prolonged PROM, prenatal care should not merely focus on the occurrence and prevention of infections, but rather on the occurrence of oligohydramnios, because of the risk of pulmonary hypoplasia increasing with its duration.

Even a period of oligohydramnios as short as 6 days may interfere with fetal lung development and cause pulmonary hypoplasia[23]. The reported incidence of pulmonary hypoplasia due to oligohydramnios based on chronic amniotic leakage varies between 8 and 26%, of which 55–100% was lethal[22–25]. The overall mortality rate after prolonged preterm PROM in these studies was 17–41% with a mortality rate due to pulmonary hypoplasia of 29–58%.

DOPPLER RECORDING TECHNIQUE

The introduction of more sensitive color-coded Doppler systems has led to identification of the human fetal pulmonary circulation[10,40]. (Figure 3, see Color Plate P). Consequently, Doppler velocimetry has recently been used to study the arterial pulmonary circulation in normal human fetuses[10,41–49]. Pulsed Doppler measurements of the right or left pulmonary arterial branches can be attempted from a transverse cross-section of the fetal chest at the level of the four-chamber view after visualization with color Doppler and during fetal apnea. Technically acceptable and reproducible arterial flow velocity waveforms across the left and right fetal lung, including the most distal vascular branches close to the inner thoracic wall, can be obtained in at least three-quarters of all recordings[43,49]. Recording failures are determined by fetal (breathing) movements, unfavorable fetal position or maternal obesity.

Most Doppler studies of the human fetal pulmonary circulation have been performed in the *proximal* arterial pulmonary branches and demonstrated a unique Doppler waveform pattern[41–46] (Figure 4a). Agreement exists regarding the nature of the systolic component of the proximal arterial pulmonary waveform, which is characterized by a rapid initial flow acceleration phase followed by an equally rapid deceleration phase. However, opinions differ about the end-diastolic component, ranging from forward flow being absent[10], present[43,44] or a combination of present and absent flow[42]. Further, discrepancies appear to

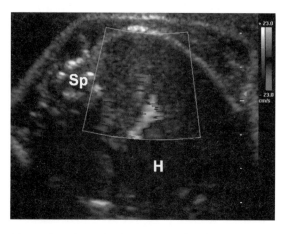

Figure 3 *The fetal pulmonary circulation visualized with color Doppler from a cross-section of the fetal chest at the level of the cardiac four-chamber view. Sp, fetal spine; H, fetal heart. (Reprinted with permission from Laudy JAM, et al. The fetal lung 2: Pulmonary hypoplasia. Ultrasound Obstet Gynecol 2000;16:482–90). (See Color Plate P)*

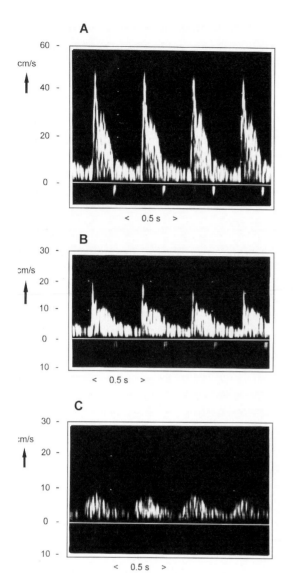

Figure 4 *Doppler ultrasound recording of blood flow velocity waveforms from the (a) proximal, (b) middle and (c) distal branch of the pulmonary artery from the same fetal lung at 25 weeks of gestation. (Reprinted with permission from reference 49)*

exist regarding reported peak systolic velocities in the proximal arterial pulmonary branches, which vary from a significant increase[10,42,44,46] to lack of gestational age dependency[41,43]. Finally, in the same vessel, the pulsatility index (PI) as well as the resistance index (RI)[45] have been described as remaining constant[10,43,45] or demonstrating a gestational age-related decrease[42,44–46]. Probably, sample-site differences and equipment-related differences (high-pass filter setting) play a role in the occurrence of these discrepancies. Based on knowledge mainly derived from fetal lamb studies of the pulmonary arterial circulation, high downstream impedance and the presence of a patent ductus arteriosus may be responsible for the nature of this particular profile[12,14].

Several studies have reported on Doppler velocimetry of fetal *peripheral* arterial pulmonary branches in uncomplicated pregnancies[42,45,47–49]. Also here, methodological differences such as defining the Doppler sample site for distal pulmonary arteries have made a comparison difficult. Laudy *et al.* showed that flow velocity waveforms, obtained from the middle part of the lung at equal distance from the outer border of the fetal heart and the inner thoracic wall, were similar to the waveforms from the proximal arterial branches, although with lower maximum peak systolic velocities in the middle arterial branches[43,49] (Figure 4b). The most distal arterial pulmonary branches as close as possible to the inner thoracic wall are characterized by a monophasic flow velocity profile with low forward flow velocities throughout the cardiac cycle[49] (Figure 4c).

None of all the reported Doppler flow velocity studies could detect significant differences between right and left arterial proximal or peripheral pulmonary branches.

PREDICTION OF PULMONARY HYPOPLASIA

An accurate prenatal test for detecting pulmonary hypoplasia is highly desirable from the obstetrician's point of view, because of the high perinatal mortality rate. Since the prediction of the non-lethal forms of pulmonary hypoplasia will not drastically change obstetric management, the reliable prenatal prediction of the lethal form might alter obstetric management. Therefore, we need an accurate and patient-friendly method of separating lethal from non-lethal pulmonary hypoplasia. One should realize that, in clinical practice dealing with an individual patient, such a particular test should display a positive predictive value of 100%.

We discuss clinical, biometric and hemodynamic features that have been proposed in this respect. For this purpose we focus on oligohydramnios-related pulmonary hypoplasia.

Clinical features

The relationship between PROM, persistent oligohydramnios and pulmonary hypoplasia was the subject of study for several authors. Table 2 presents four major papers on this subject with their conclusions. Although these reports vary more or less in their final statements, one may conclude that the onset of PROM plays an important role in the prediction of pulmonary hypoplasia – that is the earlier the onset, the higher the risk. The presence of persistent severe oligohydramnios will increase this risk even further. However, these clinical features are not predictive enough for clinicians dealing with an individual patient.

Biometric features

One of the most commonly used parameters in the prenatal prediction of pulmonary hypoplasia is the thoracic circumference, which can be obtained in a transverse cross-section through the fetal chest at the level of the cardiac four-chamber view with the atrioventricular valves in diastole. In most series the bony thoracic circumference has been used; this displays a linear correlation with gestational age.

Although the first reports on the application of fetal thoracic circumference in the prediction of lung hypoplasia were quite promising, other and some more recent studies revealed that this measurement has a lower sensitivity and accuracy compared with other biometric methods (shown in Table 3). It should be emphasized that most of these studies represent very heterogeneous patient cohorts and use different definitions of thoracic and lung dimensions and of pulmonary hypoplasia. Owing to these various findings, it is difficult to compare and consequently select a prenatal predicting test reliable enough for changing clinical management.

Until now, there are no studies available on the applicability of three-dimensional ultrasonography for fetal lung volume measurement in the prediction of lung hypoplasia.

Hemodynamic features

The underlying theory that Doppler velocimetry of the arterial pulmonary circulation could help us further in the prenatal prediction of pulmonary hypoplasia is based on observations in post-mortem studies that pulmonary hypoplasia is associated with

Table 2 *List of reports on the relation between clinical features and pulmonary hypoplasia*

Authors	Source	Conclusions
Nimrod *et al.*	*Am J Obstet Gynecol* 1984[22]	greatest impact: PROM < 26 wk and duration of rupture > 5 wk
Rotschild *et al.*	*Am J Obstet Gynecol* 1990[24]	onset of PROM best predictor with no case of PH > 26 wk no correlation of duration and degree of oligohydramnios with PH 50% estimated probability of PH when PROM at 19 wk
Vergani *et al.*	*Am J Obstet Gynecol* 1994[50]	onset of PROM + oligohydramnios independent predictors 50% estimated probability of PH when PROM at 25 wk
Kilbride *et al.*	*Am J Obstet Gynecol* 1996[26]	severe oligohydramnios > 2 wk after PROM < 25 wk: predicted neonatal mortality > 90% (87% due to PH)

PROM, premature rupture of membranes; PH, pulmonary hypoplasia

Table 3 *List of reports on the relation between biometric indices other than the thoracic circumference and pulmonary hypoplasia*

Authors	Source	Study group	Best prediction
Vintzileos *et al.*	*Am J Obstet Gynecol* 1989[51]	$n = 13$ 4 renal 4 PROM < 26 wk, > 5 wk 5 idiopathic oligohydramnios > 5 wk	(thoracic–heart area) × 100/thoracic area
Roberts and Mitchell	*Am J Obstet Gynecol* 1990[52]	$n = 20$ 20 PROM < 24 wk, > 1 wk	lung length
Yoshimura *et al.*	*Am J Obstet Gynecol* 1996[53]	$n = 21$ 13 renal 6 skeletal 2 PROM < 26 wk, > 5 wk	lung area TC/AC ratio
Merz *et al.*	*Prenat Diagn* 1999[54]	$n = 32$ 11 renal 7 CDH 7 skeletal 2 hydrops 5 miscellaneous	lung diameter

PROM, premature rupture of membranes; CDH, congenital diaphragmatic hernia; TC, thoracic circumference; AC, abdominal circumference

underdevelopment and structural changes of the pulmonary vascular bed such as a decrease in total size of the pulmonary vascular bed, a decrease in the number of vessels per unit of lung tissue and an increase of pulmonary arterial smooth muscle thickness. These changes may lead to increased pulmonary vascular resistance and decreased pulmonary arterial compliance. This may consequently affect pulmonary blood flow which may result in changes of both systolic and diastolic components of the pulmonary artery flow velocity waveform.

So far, only a few papers have dealt with this particular issue (Table 4). Unfortunately, these reports also present data from very small heterogeneous patient series and differ in Doppler sample site and examined Doppler parameters. Therefore, it is difficult to conclude from these results whether Doppler velocimetry is of any particular value in the prediction of pulmonary hypoplasia before birth. Nevertheless, nearly all studies agree that Doppler velocimetry may detect changes in blood velocity waveforms from the fetal arterial pulmonary circulation in the presence of pulmonary hypoplasia. However, whether this implies that Doppler assessment of the fetal arterial pulmonary circulation allows accurate differentiation between lethal and non-lethal pulmonary hypoplasia needs to be substantiated in larger prospective series.

This leads to a study, which was recently performed in our department, to determine the value of Doppler velocimetry of the arterial pulmonary circulation relative to fetal biometric indices and clinical correlates in the prenatal prediction of lethal lung hypoplasia associated with prolonged oligohydramnios due to PROM ($n = 31$) or bilateral renal pathology ($n = 11$)[57]. Despite marked oligohydramnios, recording of technically acceptable proximal and middle arterial pulmonary branch flow velocity waveforms was as successful as in normal pregnancies. However, in the presence of lethal lung hypoplasia, the percentage of technically acceptable distal waveforms was significantly reduced. It was hypothesized that unsuccessful distal arterial pulmonary flow velocity waveform recordings might be suspicious of lethal lung hypoplasia. When looking at the different components of the

Table 4 *List of reports on the relation between Doppler indices and pulmonary hypoplasia*

Authors	Source	Study group	Results
Mitchell *et al.*	*Ultrasound Obstet Gynecol* 1997[45]	*n* = 10 multicystic dysplastic kidney disease	in main pulmonary artery and proximal pulmonary branch: no significantly different Doppler waveforms in PH vs. controls in peripheral pulmonary artery: high resistant pattern in PH
Achiron *et al.*	*J Ultrasound Med* 1998[48]	*n* = 4 2 CDH 1 renal 1 skeletal	in right peripheral pulmonary artery: PI within 95% CI conclusion: PI poor indicator of PH
Yoshimura *et al.*	*Am J Obstet Gynecol* 1999[46]	*n* = 5 2 hydrops 2 skeletal 1 renal	in proximal branch pulmonary artery: PI significantly higher and PSV significantly lower in PH vs. controls
Chaoui *et al.*	*Eur J Obstet Gynecol Reprod Biol* 1999[55]	*n* = 9 (19–23 wk) 4 renal 2 CDH 3 miscellaneous including heart defects	in main stem of right/left pulmonary artery end systolic RV flow: normal values decreased PSV: 3/9 cases increased PI: 6/9 cases (all renal + CDH) conclusion: PI best parameter
Rizzo *et al.*	*Ultrasound Obstet Gynecol* 2000[56]	*n* = 20 20 PROM < 24 wk	in most peripheral pulmonary artery: PI sensitivity 63%, PPV 79%

CDH, congenital diaphragmatic hernia; PROM, premature rupture of membranes; PH, pulmonary hypoplasia; PI, pulsatility index; PSV, peak systolic velocity; RV, reversed flow; PPV, positive predictive value

arterial pulmonary waveforms, the most reliable parameters in the detection of lethal lung hypoplasia were peak systolic velocity in the proximal arterial pulmonary velocity waveform and time-averaged velocity and end-diastolic velocity in the middle arterial pulmonary velocity waveform with positive predictive values (PPV) of more than 70% and an accuracy of more than 75%. In the total group (*n* = 42), the lowest PPV for both the proximal and middle arterial pulmonary branches and overall accuracy was presented by the PI, which is in agreement with previous observations that the PI is not useful in the detection of changes in human fetal pulmonary vascular resistance[43]. Doppler velocimetry of the arterial pulmonary circulation displayed better PPVs and overall accuracy than the fetal chest and its cardiac and abdominal ratios. However, in the subset of PROM, the combination of onset of PROM at ≤ 20 weeks, duration of oligohydramnios for ≥ 8 weeks and degree of oligohydramnios of ≤ 1 cm was more predictive for lethal lung hypoplasia than Doppler velocimetry. Doppler velocimetry of the arterial pulmonary circulation, as a single test, failed to be reliable enough for clinical application.

Subsequently, it was questioned in this study, whether combining clinical (i.e. combination of onset of PROM at ≤ 20 weeks, duration of oligohydramnios for ≥ 8 weeks and degree of oligohydramnios of ≤ 1 cm), with biometric (thoracic/abdominal circumference ratio) and pulmonary Doppler parameters (peak systolic velocity from the proximal arterial branch) could improve the predictive value of lethal lung hypoplasia. In both the total study group and the subset of PROM, a PPV of 100% was achieved for the biometric and Doppler combination, but the sensitivity was low (≤ 50%). In the subset of PROM alone, a similar result was established for the combinations of combined clinical and biometric parameters; and combined clinical and Doppler parameters, which would limit its applicability in clinical management. However, in this particular subset, combination of all three clinical, biometric and Doppler parameters revealed not only a PPV of 100%, but also a considerable improvement in overall accuracy (93%) and sensitivity (71%), constituting the most favorable combination in the subset of PROM. Nevertheless, the clinical significance appears to be limited, owing to the restrictions in obtaining the necessary Doppler and biometric components of the combinations as well as the relatively low sensitivity. Whether these findings may be reliable enough to improve both obstetric management and parental counselling needs to be substantiated in further studies.

CONCLUSIONS

An accurate prenatal test for detecting pulmonary hypoplasia is highly desirable, since pulmonary hypoplasia is still associated with a high perinatal mortality rate. The various methods that have been proposed during the past two decades, based on clinical features and fetal two-dimensional thoracic and lung measurements, do not possess enough predictive value regarding the development of lethal lung hypoplasia, thus allowing reliable clinical decisions to be made. Doppler velocimetry has improved our knowledge of human fetal pulmonary hemodynamics under normal and abnormal conditions, and may detect changes in arterial intrapulmonary waveforms in cases of lung hypoplasia, but it seems clear that, currently, Doppler velocimetry alone is not accurate enough in predicting the lethal form of lung hypoplasia. Whether the addition of more recent techniques such as digital three-dimensional ultrasonography or fast MRI may contribute to a further improvement in the prenatal prediction of lethal lung hypoplasia should be elucidated in the not too distant future.

References

1. DiFiore JW, Wilson JM. Lung development. *Semin Pediatr Surg* 1994;3:221–32
2. Kitterman JA. Fetal lung development. *J Dev Physiol* 1984;6:67–82
3. Adzick NS, Harrison MR, Glick PL, Villa RL, Finkbeiner W. Experimental pulmonary hypoplasia and oligohydramnios: relative contributions of lung fluid and fetal breathing movements. *J Pediatr Surg* 1984;19:658–65
4. Shenker L, Reed KL, Anderson CF, Borjon NA. Significance of oligohydramnios complicating pregnancy. *Am J Obstet Gynecol* 1991;164:1597–600
5. Liggins GC. Growth of the fetal lung. *J Dev Physiol* 1984;6:237–48
6. Sherer DM, Davis JM, Woods JR. Pulmonary hypoplasia: a review. *Obstet Gynecol Surv* 1990; 45:792–803
7. Wigglesworth JS, Desai R, Guerrini P. Fetal lung hypoplasia: biochemical and structural variations and their possible significance. *Arch Dis Child* 1981;56:606–15
8. Page DV, Stocker JT. Anomalies associated with pulmonary hypoplasia. *Am Rev Respir Dis* 1982; 125:216–21
9. Pringle KC. Human fetal lung development and related animal models. *Clin Obstet Gynecol* 1986; 29:502–13
10. Emerson DS, Cartier MS. The fetal pulmonary circulation. In Copel JA, Reed KL, eds. *Doppler Ultrasound in Obstetrics and Gynecology*. New York: Raven Press, 1995:307–23
11. Rasanen J, Wood DC, Weiner S, Ludomirski A, Huhta JC. Role of the pulmonary circulation in the distribution of human fetal cardiac output during the second half of pregnancy. *Circulation* 1996;94:1068–73
12. Rudolph AM. Fetal and neonatal pulmonary circulation. *Ann Rev Physiol* 1979;41:383–95
13. Heymann MA, Rudolph AM. Control of the ductus arteriosus. *Physiol Rev* 1975;55:62–78
14. Thurlbeck WM. Prematurity and the developing lung. *Clin Perinatol* 1992;19:497–519
15. Nakamura Y, Harada K, Yamamoto I, *et al.* Human pulmonary hypoplasia. Statistical, morphological, morphometric and biochemical study. *Arch Pathol Lab Med* 1992;116:635–42
16. Kitagawa M, Hislop A, Boyden EA, Reid L. Lung hypoplasia in congenital diaphragmatic hernia. A

quantitative study of airway, artery, and alveolar development. *Br J Surg* 1971;58:342–6

17. Askenazi SS, Perlman M. Pulmonary hypoplasia: lung weight and radial alveolar count as criteria of diagnosis. *Arch Dis Child* 1979;54:614–18

18. Levin DL. Morphologic analysis of the pulmonary vascular bed in congenital left-sided diaphragmatic hernia. *J Pediatr* 1978;92:805–9

19. Barth PJ, Rüschoff J. Morphometric study on pulmonary arterial thickness in pulmonary hypoplasia. *Pediatr Pathol* 1992;12:653–63

20. Knox WF, Barson AJ. Pulmonary hypoplasia in a regional perinatal unit. *Early Hum Dev* 1986;114:33–42

21. Moessinger AC, Santiago A, Paneth NS, Rey HR, Blanc WA, Driscoll JM Jr. Time trends in necropsy prevalence and birth prevalence of lung hypoplasia. *Pediatr Perinat Epidemiol* 1989;3:421–31

22. Nimrod C, Varela-Gittings F, Machin G, Campbell D, Wesenberg R. The effect of very prolonged membrane rupture on fetal development. *Am J Obstet Gynecol* 1984;148:540–3

23. Thibeault DW, Beatty EC, Hall RT, Bowen SK, O'Neill DH. Neonatal pulmonary hypoplasia with premature rupture of fetal membranes and oligohydramnios. *J Pediatr* 1985;107:273–7

24. Rotschild A, Ling EW, Puterman ML, Farquharson D. Neonatal outcome after prolonged preterm rupture of the membranes. *Am J Obstet Gynecol* 1990;162:46–52

25. McIntosh N, Harrison A. Prolonged premature rupture of membranes in the preterm infant: a 7 year study. *Eur J Obstet Gynecol Reprod Biol* 1994;57:1–6

26. Kilbride HW, Yeast J, Thibeault DW. Defining limits of survival: lethal pulmonary hypoplasia after premature rupture of membranes. *Am J Obstet Gynecol* 1996;175:675–81

27. Swischuk LE, Richardson J, Nichols MM, Ingman MJ. Primary pulmonary hypoplasia in the neonate. *J Pediatr* 1979;95:573–7

28. Potter EL. Bilateral renal agenesis. *J Pediatr* 1946;29:68–76

29. Perlman M, Levin M. Fetal pulmonary hypoplasia, anuria and oligohydramnios. Clinicopathologic observations and review of literature. *Am J Obstet Gynecol* 1974;118:1119–23

30. Fitch N, Lachance RC. The pathogenesis of Potter's syndrome of renal agenesis. *Can Med Assoc J* 1972;107:653–6

31. Ratten G, Beischer N, Fortune D. Obstetric complications when the fetus has Potter's syndrome. *Am J Obstet Gynecol* 1973;115:890–5

32. Hack M, Jaffe J, Blankenstein R, Goodman M, Brish M. Familial aggregation in bilateral renal agenesis. *Clin Genet* 1974;5:173–7

33. Perlman M, Williams J, Hirsch M. Neonatal pulmonary hypoplasia after prolonged leakage of amniotic fluid. *Arch Dis Child* 1976;51:349–53

34. Tibboel D, Gaillard JLJ, Spritzer R, Wallenburg HCS. Pulmonary hypoplasia secondary to oligohydramnios with very premature rupture of fetal membranes. *Eur J Pediatr* 1990;149:496–9

35. Bhutani VK, Abbasi S, Weiner S. Neonatal pulmonary manifestations due to prolonged amniotic leak. *Am J Perinatol* 1986;3:225–30

36. Thibeault DW, Beatty EC, Hall RT, Bowen SK. Prolonged rupture of fetal membranes (PROM) and hypoplastic lungs without the oligohydramnios tetrad. *Pediatr Res* 1983;17:392A

37. Rudd EG. Premature rupture of the membranes. A review. *J Reprod Med* 1985;30:843–8

38. Garite TJ, Freeman RK, Linzey EM, Braly PS, Dorchester WL. Prospective randomized study of corticosteroids in the management of premature rupture of the membranes and the premature gestation. *Am J Obstet Gynecol* 1981;141:508–15

39. Morales WJ, Thomas T. Premature rupture of membranes at < 25 weeks: a management dilemma. *Am J Obstet Gynecol* 1993;168:503–7

40. DeVore GR. The use of color Doppler imaging to examine the fetal heart. Normal and pathologic anatomy. In Jaffe R, Warsof SI, eds. *Color Doppler Imaging in Obstetrics and Gynecology.* New York: McGraw-Hill, 1992:126–9

41. Stanley JR, Veille JC, Zaccaro D. Description of right pulmonary artery blood flow by Doppler echocardiography in the normal human fetus 17 to 40 weeks gestation. *J Matern Fetal Invest* 1994;4:S14

42. Rasanen J, Huhta JC, Weiner S, Wood DC, Ludomirski A. Fetal branch pulmonary arterial vascular impedance during the second half of pregnancy. *Am J Obstet Gynecol* 1996;174:1441–9

43. Laudy JAM, De Ridder MAJ, Wladimiroff JW. Doppler velocimetry in branch pulmonary arteries of normal human fetuses during the second half of gestation. *Pediatr Res* 1997;41:897–901

44. Chaoui R, Taddei F, Rizzo G, Bast C, Lenz F, Bollmann R. Doppler echocardiography of the main stems of the pulmonary arteries in the normal human fetus. *Ultrasound Obstet Gynecol* 1997;10:1–7

45. Mitchell JH, Roberts AB, Lee A. Doppler waveforms from the pulmonary arterial system in normal fetuses and those with pulmonary hypoplasia. *Ultrasound Obstet Gynecol* 1997;11:1–6

46. Yoshimura S, Masuzaki H, Miura K, Muta K, Gotoh H, Ishimaru T. Diagnosis of fetal pulmonary hypoplasia by measurement of blood flow velocity waveforms of pulmonary arteries with Doppler ultrasonography. *Am J Obstet Gynecol* 1999;180:441–6

47. Rizzo G, Capponi A, Chaoui R, Taddei F, Arduini D, Romanini C. Blood flow velocity waveforms from peripheral pulmonary arteries in normally grown and growth-retarded fetuses. *Ultrasound Obstet Gynecol* 1996;8:87–92

48. Achiron R, Heggesh J, Mashiach S, Lipitz S, Rotstein Z. Peripheral right pulmonary artery blood flow velocimetry: Doppler sonographic study of normal and abnormal fetuses. *J Ultrasound Med* 1998;17:687–92

49. Laudy JAM, de Ridder MAJ, Wladimiroff JW. Human fetal pulmonary artery velocimetry: repeatability and normal values with emphasis on middle and distal pulmonary vessels. *Ultrasound Obstet Gynecol* 2000;15:479–86

50. Vergani P, Ghidini A, Locatelli A, *et al.* Risk factors for pulmonary hypoplasia in second trimester premature rupture of membranes. *Am J Obstet Gynecol* 1994;170:1359–64

51. Vintzileos AM, Campbell WA, Rodis JF, Nochimson DJ, Pinette MG, Petrikovsky BM. Comparison of six different ultrasonographic methods for predicting lethal fetal pulmonary hypoplasia. *Am J Obstet Gynecol* 1989;161:606–12

52. Roberts AB, Mitchell JM. Direct ultrasonographic measurement of fetal lung length in normal pregnancies complicated by prolonged rupture of membranes. *Am J Obstet Gynecol* 1990;160: 1560–6

53. Yoshimura S, Masuzaki H, Gotoh H, Fukuda H, Ishimaru T. Ultrasonographic prediction of lethal pulmonary hypoplasia: comparison of eight different ultrasonographic parameters. *Am J Obstet Gynecol* 1996;175:477–83

54. Merz E, Miric-Tesanic D, Bahlmann F, Weber G, Halermann C. Prenatal sonographic chest and lung measurements for predicting severe pulmonary hypoplasia. *Prenat Diagn* 1999;19:614–19

55. Chaoui R, Kalache K, Tennstedt C, Lenz F, Vogel M. Pulmonary arterial Doppler velocimetry in fetuses with lung hypoplasia. *Eur J Obstet Gynecol Reprod Biol* 1999;84:179–85

56. Rizzo G, Capponi A, Angelini E, Mazzoleni A, Romanini C. Blood flow velocity waveforms from fetal perpheral pulmonary arteries in pregnancies with preterm rupture of the membranes: relationship with pulmonary hypoplasia. *Ultrasound Obstet Gynecol* 2000;15:98–103

57. Laudy JAM, Tibboel D, Robben SGF, de Krijger RR, de Ridder MAJ, Wladimiroff JW. Prenatal prediction of fetal pulmonary hypoplasia: clinical biometric and Doppler velocity correlates. *Pediatrics* 2002;109:259–61

Sonographic examination of the uterine cervix

9

T. Chaiworapongsa, J. Espinoza, K. Kalache, M.-T. Gervasi and R. Romero

INTRODUCTION

The uterine cervix plays a central role in the maintenance of normal pregnancy and in parturition. Mid-trimester cervical ripening, often referred to as 'cervical incompetence', is a major diagnostic and therapeutic challenge and a subject of intense debate among clinicians and researchers.

During normal pregnancy, most cervices remain firm and closed, despite a progressive increase in the size of the fetus and uterine distension. At the end of pregnancy and during labor, the cervix changes consistency (softens), shortens (effaces) and dilates to allow the expulsion of the conceptus. The term 'cervical ripening' refers to the anatomical, biophysical and biochemical processes which underlie the dramatic changes in cervical consistency, efface-ment and dilatation, that generally precede the onset of spontaneous labor.

Contrary to what was believed for many years, cervical ripening is an active metabolic process involving the extracellular matrix com-ponents of the cervix. These changes increase cervical compliance. Untimely cervical ripening could result in complications of pregnancy. For example, failure of the cervix to ripen before myometrial activation at term (i.e. onset of increased uterine contractility) may be the cause of a prolonged latent phase of labor; preterm premature cervical ripening may lead to mid-trimester spontaneous abortion or spontaneous preterm labor and delivery.

PHYSIOLOGY OF CERVICAL RIPENING

The uterine cervix is essentially a connective tissue organ, with smooth muscle cells accounting for less than 8% of the distal part of the cervix[1]. The ability of the cervix to retain the conceptus during pregnancy is unlikely to depend upon a traditional sphincteric mechanism. Indeed, perfusion of strips of human cervix with vasopressin, a hormone that stimulates smooth muscle contraction, induces a very modest contractile response in comparison to that induced by this hormone in strips from the uterine isthmus and the fundus, which contain more muscle[2].

It is now understood that the normal function of the cervix during pregnancy depends largely upon the regulation of connective tissue metabolism. This tissue is formed by abundant extracellular matrix that surrounds individual cells. The major macro-molecular components of the extracellular matrix are collagen, proteoaminoglycans, elastin and various glycoproteins, such as fibronectins. Collagen is considered the most important component of the extracellular matrix, determining the tensile strength of fibrous connective tissue. Changes in cervical characteristics during pregnancy have been attributed to changes in collagen content and metabolism[3]. Proteoaminoglycans have also been implicated in cervical physiology. The proteoaminoglycans decorin (PG-S$_2$) has a high affinity for collagen and can cover the surface of the collagen fibrils, stabilizing them and promoting the formation of thicker collagen bundles or fibers. In contrast, byglycan (PG-S$_1$) has no affinity for collagen and, therefore, can disorganize collagen fibrils. The predominant proteoglycan in the non-pregnant state is PG-S$_2$ and in the pregnant state is PG-S$_1$[4].

The biochemical events which have been implicated in cervical ripening are: decrease in total collagen content; increase in collagen solubility (probably indicating degradation or newly synthesized weaker collagen); and increase in collagenolytic activity (both collagenase and leukocyte elastase). Contrary to what is generally believed, extracellular matrix turnover in the cervix is very high[5]. Thus, mechanical properties of the cervix can change very quickly.

Uldbjerg et al.[4] have demonstrated the importance of collagen content in cervical dilatation. They reported a strong correlation between the collagen content (measured by hydroxyproline determination) of cervical biopsies obtained after delivery and the time required for the cervix to dilate from 2 to 10 cm[6]. Moreover, collagen concentration in the cervix of non-pregnant women is a function of parity: the higher the parity, the lower the collagen content[7]. This observation provides an explanation for why labor is shorter in parous women.

The changes in extracellular matrix components during cervical ripening have been likened to an inflammatory response[8]. Indeed, during cervical ripening there is an influx of inflammatory cells, including macrophages, neutrophils, mast cells and eosinophils into the cervical stroma. Considerable evidence supports a role for pro-inflammatory cytokines and chemokines in cervical ripening[9–13]. Interleukin-1 (IL-1), interleukin-8 (IL-8) and tumor necrosis factor-α can induce the morphological and biophysical changes associated with cervical ripening when locally applied to the cervix[14]. IL-8, a major chemokine capable of inducing chemotaxis, and thus infiltration of the cervix by inflammatory cells, has been considered as a central mediator of cervical ripening. Increased concentrations of this chemokine have been demonstrated in biopsies of the cervix. IL-8 concentrations increase six-fold in the cervix at term and show an additional 11-fold increase after cervical ripening associated with parturition[15]. Similar findings have been reported by Osmers et al. in biopsies obtained from the lower uterine segment[16]. Moreover, these investigators reported a strong correlation between the IL-8 concentrations and those of two metalloproteinases, matrix metalloproteinase (MMP)-8 and MMP-9.

Substantial evidence supports a role for matrix degrading enzymes in the process of cervical ripening. These enzymes are collectively known as MMPs. Cervical dilatation is associated with an increase in collagenolytic activity (MMP-1) in tissue and serum[17,18]. However, studies conducted by Osmers et al. have demonstrated that most of the cervical collagenase activity in the cervix/lower uterine segment during parturition is attributable to collagenase derived from neutrophils and specifically, MMP-8 (neutrophil collagenase)[16]. Uldbjerg et al. reported increases in leukocyte serine elastase associated with cervical ripening[6].

Several lines of evidence have been invoked to support the participation of sex steroid hormones in cervical ripening, a concept that has important clinical implications. This evidence includes: intravenous administration of 17β-estradiol induces cervical ripening[19]; estrogen stimulates collagen degradation in vitro[17]; progesterone blocks the estrogen-induced collagenolysis in vitro[17]; and administration of progesterone receptor antagonist induces cervical ripening in first-trimester pregnancy[20]. However, recent experimental evidence indicates that the role of sex steroid hormones in cervical ripening is far more complex. For example, cervical ripening in the rat begins long before a decrease in progesterone serum concentrations, suggesting that there must be a progesterone-independent mechanism capable of inducing cervical ripening in this species[21]. With regard to the role of estrogens, the administration of estrogen to pregnant women does not consistently result in cervical ripening. Moreover, the administration of neither estradiol nor its precursor (androstenedione) induces cervical ripening in the presence of high concentrations of progesterone in guinea pigs[22]. A puzzling observation is that the administration of estradiol to guinea pigs treated with onapristone (a progesterone receptor antagonist that induces cervical ripening) attenuates the cervical ripening normally induced by that compound[22]. Therefore, more work is required to elucidate the precise role of sex steroids in cervical ripening.

Prostaglandins (PGs) are used to induce cervical ripening prior to the induction of labor or abortion. Within hours of administration, PGE_2 can produce clinical and histological changes resembling physiological ripening which normally develop over several weeks of gestation. The mechanism of action of PGE_2 is thought to involve stimulation of collagenolytic activity and synthesis of $PG-S_1$ by cervical tissue[6]. However, the observation that neither indomethacin[23] nor the specific cyclooxygenase-II inhibitor, flosulide[20], inhibit the physiological and antiprogestin-induced cervical ripening raises questions about the central role attributed to prostaglandins in cervical ripening.

Nitric oxide (NO) has also been implicated in cervical ripening. The evidence for this is that the local application of NO donors can induce cervical ripening in guinea pigs and in humans[24,25], and that treatment of guinea pigs and rats with NO inhibitors (L-NAME) delays cervical ripening and results in prolonged delivery[25]. More studies are required to determine the precise role of this mediator in physiological and pathological cervical ripening.

Cervical modifications during pregnancy and parturition are not limited to physiological and biochemical changes (softening) but also involve anatomical changes (e.g. effacement and dilatation), which can be assessed with the use of ultrasound.

SONOGRAPHIC EVALUATION OF THE UTERINE CERVIX

Sonographic imaging of the cervix is a less invasive, more precise and objective method of assessing the cervical status than digital examination. Effacement (or cervical shortening), changes in the anatomy of the internal os (funnelling), endocervical canal dilatation, spontaneous modifications and changes following transfundal pressure can be determined by ultrasound scanning.

Technique and pitfalls

The cervix can be examined using a transabdominal, endovaginal and transperineal approach. We prefer the endovaginal technique for optimal assessment of the cervix. The close proximity of the probe to the cervix and the use of a high-frequency transducer improve image quality. Transabdominal sonography requires a full bladder for adequate visualization of the cervix. Over-distension of the bladder compresses and artificially lengthens the cervix[26]. Andersen[27] demonstrated that cervical length measurements obtained by transabdominal sonography were longer (5.2 mm on average) than those obtained using endovaginal sonography in a study of 186 pregnant women. Transabdominal measurements obtained with mild degrees of bladder filling were quite similar to those reported by transvaginal examination. The effect of an over-distended bladder is not detectable in non-pregnant women. The different behavior of the pregnant and non-pregnant cervix in response to the pressure exerted by the bladder is most likely due to the changes in extracellular matrix composition (collagen and glycosaminoglycans) during normal pregnancy[28]. In contrast, endovaginal scanning does not require a distended bladder.

The transperineal technique can be used when an endovaginal transducer is not available and does not require a full bladder[29,30]. The cervical length can be properly visualized and measured adequately by transperineal sonography in about 80% of patients. The presence of air in the vagina may render the examination non-informative. There is a high correlation between cervical length obtained by endovaginal and transperineal methods ($r = 0.93$; $p < 0.0001$). The degree of patient acceptability was similar[31].

Before conducting an endovaginal examination, patients are asked to empty their bladder. During the procedure, the patient lies in the supine position with flexed knees and hips. The probe is covered with either a glove or an appropriate sheath. Gel is placed between the transducer and the cover as well as on the surface sheath. The operator introduces the vaginal probe into the anterior fornix until a midline sagittal view of the cervix and lower uterine segment is seen. The internal os, external os, cervical canal and endocervical mucosa should be clearly identified (Figure 1). The endocervical mucosa is used to define the upper edge of the cervix. Otherwise, cervical length may erroneously include part of the lower uterine segment.

Excessive pressure with the probe may elongate the cervix. To avoid this pitfall, the probe is slowly withdrawn until the image blurs and is subsequently re-applied with an amount of pressure sufficient to restore the image. The cervical length is measured by freezing the screen three separate times. The reliability of measurements is increased if the variation between the measurements is not more than 2–3 mm; the optimal length of examination averages 5–10 min. For clinical purposes, the shortest cervical length is reported, provided that the image is adequate. The examination is recorded on videotape and the presence of a funnel or dynamic cervical changes is noted. A funnel is defined as dilatation of the upper portion of the cervical canal (Figure 2). This can only be recognized by being certain that the walls of

the funnel are formed by endocervical mucosa. Otherwise, the covering wall of the lower uterine segment can be erroneously considered as a funnel.

Several potential pitfalls should be avoided. When the cervical canal is curved, the cervical length can be determined by tracing along the canal or by adding the sum of two straight sections. To et al.[32] concluded in their prospective study conducted in 301 women at 23 weeks' gestation that the disparity of measurement, taken as a straight line or along the cervical canal, might not have any clinical significance because a short cervix (less than 16 mm) is always straight.

If the duration of the examination is too short and the patient has dynamic cervical changes during the examination, the cervical length may not represent the true baseline status of the cervix. This may account for some observations in which patients gain cervical length over time. The contours of the anterior and posterior lip of the ectocervix are usually clearly defined. However, in some instances the boundaries of the ectocervix cannot be discerned. In selected patients whose cervix cannot be adequately imaged, instillation of saline into the vagina allows precise recognition of the ectocervix[33]. Standardized measurements of a funnel are difficult as a funnel can be obliterated by pressure from the transducer, it is often transient, and a distended bladder can obscure it. Since the

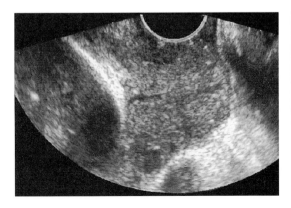

Figure 1 *Transvaginal sonographic appearance of a normal uterine cervix; the internal os, the external os and the endocervical canal can be easily visualized*

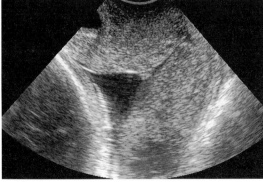

Figure 2 *Transvaginal sonographic appearance of a cervix with a V-shaped funnel*

longer the funnel, the shorter the remaining cervical length[34,35], it has been argued that the endocervical length contains most of the information required for the prediction of preterm delivery. Many favor cervical length measurement because it is far more reproducible than the assessment of funnelling. The value of detecting funnelling in the prediction of preterm delivery is reviewed later in this chapter. A rare pitfall in the examination of the cervix is that caused by the presence of a large endocervical polyp, which can make identification of the correct plane difficult to image[36]. Although cervical examination may appear simple to the experienced sonographer, certain patients may present significant challenges. For example, a cervix with an unusual orientation may be difficult to find. In a recent study, Yost *et al*. reported that 27% of the scans performed in 60 women presented some anatomical or technical difficulty[37].

THE COMMON TERMINAL PATHWAY OF PARTURITION

We have proposed that parturition has a common terminal pathway characterized by increased myometrial contractility, cervical ripening and membrane/decidual activation. These processes are required for both term and preterm parturition. Normal labor at term is characterized by co-ordinated activation of these three mechanisms and thus, patients will present with increased uterine contractility, cervical effacement and dilatation and eventually rupture their membranes. However, premature activation of different components can occur in a co-ordinated or unco-ordinated way. The premature co-ordinated activation of these mechanisms is observed in patients with classic preterm labor with progressive cervical dilatation leading to preterm delivery. Preferential activation of the cervical ripening component in the mid-trimester leads to the condition known as cervical incompetence. Later in pregnancy some patients will complain of vaginal pressure and will be recognized to have cervical dilatation and effacement out of proportion to the frequency and intensity of

myometrial contractility. Although these patients are traditionally considered to have preterm labor, clearly cervical ripening is the main component of the terminal pathway activated in these particular cases[38]. This model of preterm parturition is important because it suggests that premature cervical ripening may result in a spectrum of disease ranging from mid-trimester abortion to some forms of preterm labor and precipitous labor at term. Figures 3 and 4 describe the concepts outlined above. The hypothesis that there is a spectrum of cervical competence has been examined by several studies and will be reviewed in this chapter in the section entitled 'Cervical incompetence'.

Preterm birth and cervical sonography

Preterm birth is the leading cause of perinatal morbidity and mortality worldwide. Many interventions have been proposed to reduce the rate of prematurity, without success. Uterine activity monitoring has been used to identify activation of the myometrium, fetal fibronectin to detect decidual-membrane activation and cervical sonography to identify preterm cervical ripening. There is no evidence that home uterine monitoring can reduce the rate of prematurity[39,40] or that antibiotic administration to patients with a positive cervico/vaginal fibronectin is effective either[41].

Cervical sonography has been used in patients presenting with preterm labor, asymptomatic patients to assess the risk of preterm delivery and patients at high risk for preterm delivery and/or mid-trimester loss.

Cervical examination in patients presenting with preterm labor

Meta-analysis of randomized clinical trials in which patients with preterm labor are treated with either a placebo or β-adrenergic agents indicate that 47% of women treated with placebo deliver at term[42]. This has been interpreted as indicating that many patients are falsely diagnosed to have preterm labor. Assessment of the likelihood of preterm

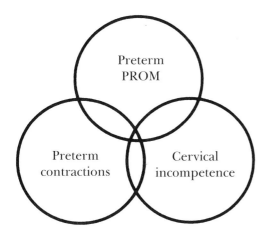

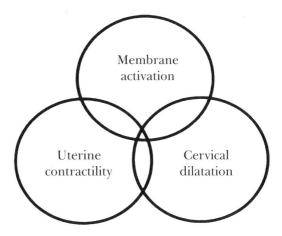

Figure 3 *The common terminal pathway of preterm and term parturition. PROM, premature rupture of membranes. From reference 38, with permission*

Figure 4 *Clinical manifestations of the premature activation of the common terminal pathway of human parturition. From reference 38, with permission*

delivery is of clinical interest because it may influence important clinical decisions such as administration of tocolysis and steroids, as well as transfer to a tertiary care center and/or discharge from the hospital.

There is now compelling evidence that examination of the cervix with ultrasound in patients presenting with preterm labor can assist in assessing the risk for preterm delivery. Table 1 summarizes the results of some of the studies published to date. In general, the shorter the cervix, the higher the risk for preterm delivery and vice versa.

Patients with preterm labor and a short cervix are at increased risk for intrauterine inflammation/infection. Gomez *et al.*[48] conducted a study in 187 patients presenting with preterm labor and cervical dilatation of less than 3 cm (as assessed by digital examination). All patients underwent amniocentesis. Intrauterine inflammation was defined as a positive amniotic fluid culture or Gram stain, or an amniotic fluid white blood cell count >100 cells/mm^3 or glucose <10 mg%. Patients with a short cervix (<20 mm) had a higher rate of intrauterine inflammation and preterm delivery at less than 35 weeks than those with a long cervix (intrauterine inflammation: short cervix, 19% (7/37) vs. long cervix, 3%

(5/150); $p < 0.05$ and for preterm delivery: short cervix, 59% (20/34) vs. long cervix, 16% (22/141); $p < 0.01$, respectively). Moreover, the shorter the cervix, the higher the frequency of intra-amniotic inflammation (χ^2 for trend; $p < 0.01$). A long cervix defined as 30 mm or more was associated with a 5% rate of preterm delivery (<35 weeks) while patients with a cervix of less than 20 mm delivered preterm in 77% of the cases.

An abnormal cervical index and the presence of funnelling also increases the risk of preterm delivery, as demonstrated by Gomez *et al.*[45] (Table 2). Timor Tritsch *et al.*[49] studied the clinical significance of funnelling for the prediction of preterm delivery in a population with symptoms of preterm labor. In 70 patients admitted to the hospital for threatened preterm labor, wedging of the internal os was associated with preterm delivery with a sensitivity of 100%, a specificity of 74%, a positive-predictive value of 59% and a negative-predictive value of 100%.

Another important observation of a study conducted in 60 singleton and twin pregnant women has been that all patients presenting with preterm labor and a cervix longer than 30 mm delivered at term[44]. The high negative-predictive value for preterm birth associated with a long cervix and with the absence of funnelling has important clinical implications in symptomatic patients.

In conclusion, cervical sonography is a powerful method to assess the risk of preterm delivery in patients presenting with preterm labor. In patients found to have long cervices, it would probably be beneficial to avoid aggressive intervention. The patients who had short cervices would have an increased risk of intrauterine inflammation/infection as well as a higher rate of preterm delivery and will probably be benefited with targeted interventions (i.e. steroid administration and transfer to a center with a newborn special care unit).

Cervical length in the prediction of preterm delivery in asymptomatic patients

Several studies have measured the cervical length of pregnant women using transabdominal, endovaginal and perineal scanning. In most cases, the cervical length is stable in

the first 30 weeks of pregnancy both in nulliparous and in multiparous women who delivered at term and a progressive, although not substantial, shortening of the cervix occurs in the third trimester of pregnancy[50–52]. Median or mean cervical lengths in low-risk populations in the mid-trimester are shown in Table 3.

A short cervix is a significant risk factor for preterm delivery. Andersen et al.[50] in a study of 113 women evaluated on one occasion before 30 weeks' gestation, reported that a cervical length of less than 39 mm is associated with a 25% risk of preterm delivery, while a long cervix (defined as a cervical length ≥ 39 mm) decreases the risk of preterm birth (4.7%). Furthermore, the risk of spontaneous preterm birth was inversely related to the cervical length. These findings have been confirmed by several other investigators, both in low-risk and high-risk asymptomatic populations[34,36,51,59–61].

Table 4 describes the details of some of the studies with adequate information to allow

Table 1 *Measurement of cervical length by transvaginal ultrasound in women with symptoms of preterm labor*

Authors	n	Gestational age (weeks)	Cut-off (mm)	Definition of PTD (weeks)	Prevalence of PTD (%)	Sensitivity (%)	Specificity (%)	PPV (%)	NPV (%)
Murakawa et al. (1993)[43]	32	18–37	<20	<37	34	27	100	100	72
			≥ 35			100	71	65	100
Iams et al. (1994)[44]	60	24–35	<30	<36	40	100	44	55	100
Gomez et al. (1994)[45]	59	20–35	≤ 18	<36	37	73	78	67	83
Rizzo et al. (1996)[46]	108	24–36	≤ 20	<37	43	68	79	71	76
Rozenberg et al. (1997)[47]	76	24–34	≤ 26	<37	26	75	73	50	89

PTD, preterm delivery; PPV, positive-predictive value; NPV, negative-predictive value

Table 2 *Diagnostic indexes and predictive values of different ultrasonographic cervical biometric findings in identification of preterm delivery in patients with acute preterm labor. Reproduced with permission from Gomez* et al.[45]

	Sensitivity	Specificity	PPV	NPV	Relative risk (95% CI)
Cervical index ≥ 0.52	76% (16/21)	94% (31/33)	89% (16/18)	86% (31/36)	6.4 (2.8–14.7)
Cervical length ≤ 18 mm	73% (16/22)	78% (29/37)	67% (16/24)	83% (29/35)	3.9 (1.8–8.5)
Funnel width ≥ 6mm	67% (14/21)	76% (25/33)	64% (14/22)	78% (25/32)	2.0 (1.4–6.0)
Funnel length ≥ 9mm	71% (15/21)	91% (30/33)	83% (15/18)	83% (30/36)	5.0 (2.3–10.7)
Funnelling present	77% (17/22)	54% (20/37)	50% (17/34)	80% (20/25)	2.5 (1.1–5.9)

PPV, positive-predictive value; NPV, negative-predictive value; CI, confidence interval calculation of diagnostic indices and predictive values. Our review will focus on the highlights of studies that significantly contribute to the understanding of the value of cervical sonography in screening for spontaneous preterm birth.

The Maternal–Fetal Medicine Units Network of the National Institute of Child Health and Human Development (NICHHD) conducted a prospective cohort study entitled the 'Preterm Prediction Study'. The value of clinical, demographic, microbiological, biochemical and sonographic parameters in the prediction of preterm birth were examined. Iams et al.[34] reported the cardinal observations of cervical sonography. A total of 2915 low-risk

asymptomatic patients were examined at 24 weeks' gestation and at 28 weeks by transvaginal sonography to evaluate the cervix and calculate the risk of delivering before 35 weeks. The shorter the cervix, the greater was the risk of spontaneous preterm birth (Figure 5). An exponential increase in the relative risk of delivering before 35 weeks was described (Figure 6). The diagnostic indices and predictive values for different cut-off values of cervical length, funnelling and Bishop score are displayed in Table 5. This large study confirmed the results of Andersen indicating that a short cervix increases the risk for preterm delivery while a long cervix decreases such risk and extended the observations by

Table 3 *Cervical length (mean or median) in low-risk populations in mid-trimester*

Authors	n	Cervical length (mm)
Ayers et al. (1988)[53]	150	52
Podobnik et al. (1988)[54]	80	48
Andersen et al. (1990)[50]	125	41
Kushnir et al. (1990)[51]	24	48
Andersen (1991)[27]	77	42
Murakawa et al. (1993)[43]	177	37
Zorzoli et al. (1994)[55]	154	42
Iams et al. (1995)[56]	106	37
Iams et al. (1996)[34]	2915	35
Cook et al. (1996)[57]	41	41
Tongsong et al. (1997)[58]	175	42
Heath et al. (1998)[59]	1252	38

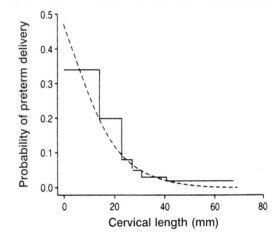

Figure 5 *Estimated probability of spontaneous preterm delivery before 35 weeks of gestation from the logistic-regression analysis (dashed line) and observed frequency of spontaneous preterm delivery (solid line) according to cervical length measured by transvaginal ultrasonography at 24 weeks. From reference 34, with permission*

Table 4 *Measurement of cervical length by ultrasound in low-risk asymptomatic pregnant women and preterm delivery (PTD) rate according to different cut-off values*

Authors	n	Gestational age (weeks)	Cut-off (mm)	Definition of PTD (weeks)	Prevalence of PTD (%)	Sensitivity (%)	Specificity (%)	PPV (%)	NPV (%)
Andersen et al. (1990)[50]	113	<30	<39	<37	15	76	59	25	93
Tongsong et al. (1995)[61]	730	28–30	≤ 35	<37	12	66	62	20	93
Iams et al. (1996)[34]	2915	24	<20	<35	4	23	97	26	97
Taipale et al. (1998)[62]	3694	18–22	≤ 25	<37	2	6	100	39	99
Heath et al. (1998)[63]	2702	23	≤ 15	≤ 32	1.5	58	99	52	99
Hassan et al. (1999)[64]	6877	14–24	≤ 15	≤ 32	3.6	8	99	47	97

PPV, positive-predictive value; NPV, negative-predictive value allowing discernment of the comparative value of cervical length with other predictors of preterm delivery (demographic, bio-chemical, microbiological and clinical).

An important series of studies reported by Heath et al.[59] and conducted at King's College Hospital in London examined the value of cervical sonography in the screening of preterm birth. Cervical length was measured by transvaginal sonography in a low-risk population of 2702 patients (for the distribution of cervical length at 23 weeks of gestation, Figure 7). Patients with a history of preterm birth, of Afro-Caribbean origin, of low

maternal age (<20 years) and thin (low body mass index) had a shorter cervix than those without such risk factors. However, when logistic regression analysis was used to examine the contribution of all these parameters to the prediction of preterm birth (<32 weeks), a short cervix was the only predictor of outcome[63]. These findings suggest that clinical and demographic risk factors associated with preterm birth operate through inducing cervical ripening. In this study, a cervix of 15 mm or less at 23 weeks of gestation in 1.7% of the population identified 60% of patients who subsequently had a

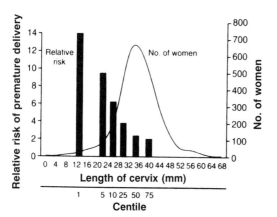

Figure 6 *Distribution of subjects among centiles for cervical length measured by transvaginal ultrasonography at 24 weeks of gestation (solid line) and relative risk of spontaneous preterm delivery before 35 weeks of gestation according to centiles for cervical length (bars). From reference 34, with permission*

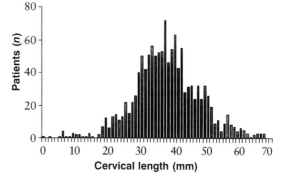

Figure 7 *Distribution of cervical length at 23 weeks of gestation in 2702 low-risk patients. From reference 59, with permission*

Table 5 *Sensitivity, specificity and predictive value of cervical length, funnelling and Bishop score for preterm delivery before 35 weeks of gestation. Reproduced with permission from Iams et al.[34]*

	Cervix at 24 weeks						Cervix at 28 weeks					
Variable	≤ 20 mm	≤ 25 mm	≤ 30 mm	Presence of funnel	Bishop score ≥ 6	Bishop score ≥ 4	≤ 20 mm	≤ 25 mm	≤ 30 mm	Presence of funnel	Bishop score ≥ 6	Bishop score ≥ 4
Sensitivity (%)	23.0	37.3	54.0	25.4	7.9	27.6	31.3	49.4	69.9	32.5	15.8	42.5
Specificity (%)	97.0	92.2	76.3	94.5	99.4	90.9	94.7	86.8	68.5	91.6	97.9	82.5
Positive-predictive value (%)	25.7	17.8	9.3	17.3	38.5	12.1	16.7	11.3	7.0	11.6	25.6	9.9
Negative-predictive value (%)	96.5	97.0	97.4	96.6	96.0	96.5	97.6	98.0	98.5	97.6	96.3	96.9

spontaneous preterm birth (<32 weeks) and 80% of those who had a spontaneous preterm birth at <28 weeks (Figure 8).

We conducted a retrospective cohort study[64] of 6877 women with cervical sonography performed between 14 and 24 weeks. Examinations were conducted transabdominally and, in cases of cervical length <30 mm or sub-optimal visualization, transvaginally. A cervical length of ≤ 15 mm had a positive-predictive value of 48%, a negative-predictive value of 97%, a sensitivity of 8% and a specificity of 99.7% for spontaneous preterm delivery at ≤ 32 weeks. A history of preterm delivery and African-American ethnic group were also associated with the occurrence of spontaneous preterm birth, although the odds ratio was considerably lower than that of a short cervix. The low sensitivity of a short cervix in this study is similar to that reported by Taipale and Hiilesmaa in a large study in Finland[62]. The apparent discrepancy among studies could be explained by the different gestational age at which ultrasound examination was conducted. We have evidence that the later scan is more predictive of preterm delivery than earlier scans. The study of Heath et al. includes exams conducted at 23 weeks, while the exams by Hassan et al. and Taipale et al. were performed at lower gestational ages.

In conclusion, a short cervix identifies a population at high risk for spontaneous preterm delivery. However, at least one-third and perhaps more patients who deliver preterm (<32 weeks) will not have a short cervix in the mid-trimester and, therefore, cervical length with ultrasound is not a screening tool but rather a method for risk assessment. The high positive-predictive value of a short cervix (nearly 50% for spontaneous preterm birth <32 weeks) justifies trials of intervention (see below).

Short cervix and the risk of preterm premature rupture of membranes and subsequent preterm delivery

An interesting study was conducted by the Maternal–Fetal Medicine Units Network to examine the relationship between a short

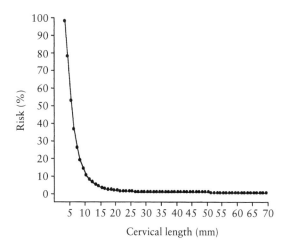

Figure 8 *Risk for spontaneous delivery at ≤ 32 weeks according to cervical length at 23 weeks. From reference 59, with permission*

cervix and preterm birth caused by preterm premature rupture of membranes (PROM)[65]. A total of 2929 were evaluated in ten centers between 23 and 24 weeks of gestation. The frequency of preterm birth at less than 37 weeks of gestation was 14.4% (422/2929). Preterm PROM occurred at less than 35 weeks' gestation and at less than 37 weeks' gestation in 2% and 4.5%, respectively, and this accounted for 32.6% of all preterm deliveries (<37 weeks). A short cervix, previous preterm birth caused by premature PROM and positive fetal fibronectin test were strong predictors for preterm birth caused by preterm PROM at both less than 35 and 37 weeks' gestation. Multivariate analysis indicated that a short cervical length at 23–24 weeks' gestation was consistently associated with preterm PROM among both nulliparous and multiparous women (at <35 weeks, nulliparous, odds ratio 9.9 (3.3–25.9) vs. multiparous, odds ratio 4.2 (2.0–8.90); and at less than 37 weeks, nulliparous, odds ratio 3.7 (1.8–7.7) vs. multiparous, odds ratio 2.5 (1.4–4.5)).

Longitudinal study of cervical ultrasound in asymptomatic patients

Zorzoli et al.[55] evaluated changes in cervical dimension of 154 pregnant women at a mean gestational age of 12, 16, 20, 25 and 31 weeks in a population with a prevalence of prematurity of 1.9% (defined as <35 weeks). They reported that cervical length did not change significantly ($p = 0.06$) with gestational age, whereas the anteroposterior diameter at mid-portion (cervical width) of the cervix shortened with advancing gestational age. Multiparous women had longer and thicker cervices than primigravidas or women with previous Cesarean sections or first-trimester abortions. Similarly, Cook et al. studied 41 patients longitudinally from 18 to 30 weeks' gestation[57]. The cervical length and cervical diameter were followed every 2 weeks. Cervical length and diameter were constant in both nulliparous ($n = 21$) and primiparous ($n = 20$) women throughout the studied period. The mean cervical length in primiparous was longer than that in nulliparous women (44 ± 5.1 mm vs. 41 ± 4.7 mm; $p < 0.001$).

Bergelin et al.[66] studied 19 healthy nulliparous women every 2 weeks from 22 weeks until delivery at term. In all but one woman, cervical length decreased and cervical width increased with advancing gestation. Three patterns of changes in cervical length were observed, a continuous decrease in 53% (10/19), an accelerated shortening rate after approximately 30 weeks in 26% (5/19) and a sudden shortening after 36 weeks in 16% (3/19) of patients.

Sonographic evaluation of cervical length in twin pregnancies

Twin gestations occur in 1% of all pregnancies and they are at increased risk of preterm birth. Several studies have examined the value of endovaginal sonography for the prediction of preterm delivery in twin pregnancies[67–74].

The preterm prediction study of the NICHHD Network of Maternal–Fetal Medicine Units examined risk factors for preterm delivery in twin gestations. Goldenberg et al.[68] reported that a short cervix, defined as a length of 25 mm or less, was more common in twin than in singleton gestations at 24 and 28 weeks. Moreover, at 24 weeks a short cervix was the only factor predictive of preterm birth. At 28 weeks, a positive fetal fibronectin was significantly associated with spontaneous preterm birth <32 weeks.

Souka et al.[72] studied ultrasound at 23 weeks' gestation in 215 twin pregnancies. The sensitivity of a short cervix defined as a length of ≤ 25 mm in the prediction of spontaneous preterm delivery at 28, 30, 32 and 34 weeks was 100%, 80%, 47% and 35%, respectively (Table 6). The rate of spontaneous delivery at or before 32 weeks increased exponentially with decreasing cervical length measured at 23 weeks (Figure 9). An interesting observation was that the risk of preterm delivery for patients with a cervical length of ≤ 25 mm in twin pregnancies was similar to the risk in singleton pregnancies with a cervical length of 15 mm or less (52%). This has been interpreted as indicating that the cervical length required in twin gestations to confer protection against preterm delivery is greater than that of singleton gestations.

Guzman et al.[73] reported a prospective longitudinal study of 131 twin pregnancies between 15 and 28 weeks of gestation. A short cervix (≤ 20 mm), regardless of gestational age, was equally good in predicting preterm delivery as funnel width, funnel length, percentage of funnelling and cervical index.

Yang et al.[74] studied 65 twin pregnancies between 18 and 26 weeks' gestation. Transvaginal or translabial cervical sonography was used to evaluate cervical length and the presence of a funnel. The prevalence of preterm delivery (defined as <35 weeks of gestation) was 23% (15/65). Cervical length of 25 mm or less and 30 mm or less was associated with sensitivities of 27% and 53% in predicting preterm delivery. The positive-predictive value was 67% and 62%, respectively, for each cut-off (relative risk (RR) = 4.6 (2.0–10.3) and RR = 3.6 (1.6–7.8), respectively).

A long cervix in twin gestations is reassuring. Imseis et al.[71] reported that 97% of twin gestations with a cervical length of 35 mm or more delivered after 34 weeks of gestation.

Table 6 *Rate of iatrogenic and spontaneous delivery at different gestations and sensitivity for spontaneous delivery according to cervical length in twin gestations. Reproduced with permission from Souka et al.[72]*

Gestational age (weeks)	n	Iatrogenic delivery	Spontaneous delivery	Cervical length (mm)			
				≤ 15	≤ 25	≤ 35	≤ 45
≤ 28	10	2 (0.9%)	8 (3.8%)	4 (50%)	8 (100%)	8 (100%)	8 (100%)
≤ 30	13	3 (1.4%)	10 (4.7%)	4 (40%)	8 (80%)	9 (90%)	10 (100%)
≤ 32	25	8 (3.8%)	17 (8.0%)	4 (24%)	8 (47%)	12 (71%)	16 (94%)
≤ 34	59	22 (10.4%)	37 (17.5%)	4 (11%)	13 (35%)	21 (57%)	34 (92%)

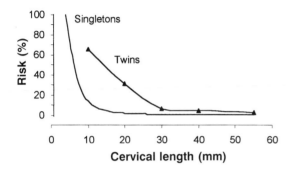

Figure 9 *Rate of spontaneous delivery at ≤ 32 weeks according to cervical length at 23 weeks of gestation in twin and singleton pregnancies. From reference 72, with permission*

Sonographic evaluation of cervical length in triplet pregnancies

One study has examined the value of cervical ultrasound in 32 triplet gestations. Progressive shortening of the cervix occurred with advancing gestational age. Cervical length in patients who delivered before 33 weeks was significantly shorter at 20, 29 and 31 weeks than in patients who delivered after ≤ 33 weeks[75].

Guzman et al.[76] conducted a prospective cohort study including 51 triplet gestations evaluated longitudinally between 15 and 28 weeks of gestation. Cervical assessment included cervical length, funnel width and length, percentage of funnelling and cervical index at rest and with transfundal pressure. A cervical length of 25 mm or less between 15 and 20 weeks' gestation had both a specificity and positive-predictive value of 100% and a sensitivity of 50% in predicting delivery at less than 28 weeks of gestation. The sensitivity, specificity, positive-predictive value and negative-predictive value of a short cervical length measured between 21 and 24 weeks and between 25 and 28 weeks were 86%, 79%, 40%, 97% and 100%, 57%, 18%, 100%, respectively. The authors suggested that a cervical length of 25 mm or less between 15 and 24 weeks' gestation and 20 mm or less between 25 and 28 weeks' gestation were at least as good as other ultrasonographic cervical parameters for the prediction of spontaneous preterm birth in triplet gestation.

To et al.[77] measured the cervical length at 23 weeks of gestation in 38 triplet pregnancies. The rate of spontaneous preterm birth at less than 33 weeks was 16% (6/38). The shorter the cervix (at 23 weeks), the higher was the rate of preterm delivery. Cervical length of 25 mm or less was present in 16% (6/38) of the patients. The sensitivity and positive-predictive values for this cut-off were both 50% (3/6). The corresponding figures for cervical length of 15 mm or less were 8%, 33% and 67%, respectively.

Maymon et al.[78] evaluated 45 triplet pregnant women longitudinally from 26 weeks of gestation. The prevalence of preterm delivery was 50% (spontaneous and indicated). Cervical length at 26 weeks' gestation was found to be a risk factor for preterm delivery (<33 weeks). A cervical length of 25 mm or less had a sensitivity, specificity, positive- and negative-predictive value of 94%, 45%, 91% and 70%, respectively. This study also indicated that the later the examination, the higher the sensitivity and positive-predictive value.

Funnelling in screening for preterm birth

Funnelling is the protrusion of no less than 3 mm of amniotic membranes into the internal os and the size of the funnel frequently changes during the course of the scan. Funnelling can be considered as effacement in progress[44]. Two types of funnelling have been described, the 'V' and 'U' shaped. In the 'V' shaped pattern, the membranes protrude into the cervical canal to form a triangular-shaped funnel. In the 'U shaped' pattern, the membranes protruding into the endocervical canal form a curvilinear image (Figures 2 and 10). Zilianti et al.[30] described the normal progression of the morphology of the upper cervix during the course of labor at term with transperineal sonography and coined the acronym of TYVU to describe the morphological changes. Figure 11 displays such an evolution. Similar findings can be demonstrated with endovaginal sonography. However, it should be noted that the work was conducted in term labor and that it remains to be determined whether preterm labor has a similar progression.

Figure 12 illustrates the morphology of the cervix, including the funnel length and funnel width, which are used to calculate the cervix index. The cervical index is equal to (funnel length + 1)/endocervical length[45]. This parameter was derived to take into account both remaining endocervical length and the length of the funnel, as they are both part of the original endocervical canal before effacement begins. Several authors have demonstrated that the cervical index and funnelling are strong predictors of the risk of preterm delivery in patients with and without preterm labor (Tables 7 and 8). Some authors have described the dimensions of the funnel as a percentage of the endocervical length. This is fundamentally a similar concept to the cervical index. For example, a funnel representing 40–50% or more of the total cervical length has been associated with an increased risk of

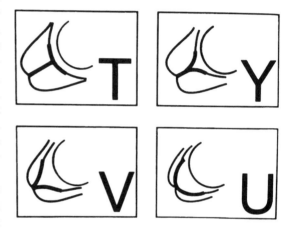

Figure 11 *Schematic representation of the correlation between the length of the cervix and the changes of the internal cervical os; the letters T, Y, V and U illustrate these changes graphically. From reference 30, with permission*

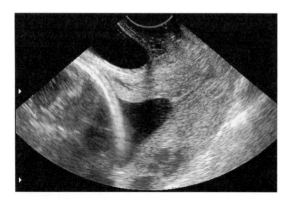

Figure 10 *U-shaped funnel*

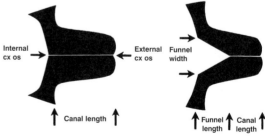

Figure 12 *Morphology of the cervix (cx), including the funnel length and funnel width. The cervical index is equal to (funnel length + 1)/endocervical length. From reference 45, with permission*

Table 7 *Cervical funnelling and preterm delivery risk in asymptomatic patients*

Authors	n	Gestational age (weeks)	Cut-off	Definition of PTD (weeks)	Prevalence of PTD (%)	Sensitivity (%)	Specificity (%)	PPV (%)	NPV (%)
Iams *et al.* (1996)[34]	2915	24	3 mm	<35	4.3	25	94	17	97
Iams *et al.* (1996)[34]	2915	28	3 mm	<35	4.3	32	92	12	98
Berghella *et al.* (1997)[35]	43	16–28	≥ 40%	<37	42	78	76	70	83

PTD, preterm delivery; PPV, positive-predictive value; NPV, negative-predictive value

Table 8 *Cervical funnelling and preterm delivery risk in symptomatic patients*

Authors	n	Gestational age (weeks)	Cut-off	Definition of PTD (weeks)	Prevalence of PTD (%)	Sensitivity (%)	Specificity (%)	PPV (%)	NPV (%)
Okitsu *et al.* (1992)[52]	77	12–30	5 mm	<37	17	69	72	33	92
Gomez *et al.* (1994)[45]	59	20–35	≥ 9 mm	<36	37	71	91	83	83
Timor Tritsch *et al.* (1996)[49]	70	20–35	wedging	<37	27	100	74	59	100
Rizzo *et al.* (1996)[46]	108	24–36	>5 mm	<37	43.5	70	67	62	74

PTD, preterm delivery; PPV, positive-predictive value; NPV, negative-predictive value

preterm birth when noted before 30 weeks in a population with a high prevalence of pre-term delivery (42%)[35].

In the NICHHD Prematurity Prediction Study, Iams *et al.* reported that the value of funnelling (defined as 3 mm in width) as a predictor of delivery was similar to the value of cervical length, but the data showed substantial variations among centers. The relative risk of funnelling for preterm delivery before 35 weeks was 5.0 at 24 weeks and 4.78 at 28 weeks[34]. The diagnostic indices are displayed in Table 5. It is of interest that in the study of Taipale and Hiilesmaa[62], funnelling, defined as dilatation of the internal os of 5 mm or more, was a stronger predictor of preterm delivery before 35 weeks than endocervical canal length. This study enrolled 3694 patients between 18 and 22 weeks of gestation. A dilated interval os (funnelling) had a relative risk of 28 for preterm delivery before 35 weeks while a short cervix (defined as <30 mm) had a relative risk of only 8. Logistic regression analysis demonstrated that the adjusted odds ratio for delivery before 35 weeks for funnelling was 20 and for a short cervix was 6.5. We believe that the most likely

explanation for the better performance of funnelling compared to cervical length in this study is that the definition of a short cervix was <30 mm. Most studies indicate that such cervical length has a low positive-predictive value for preterm delivery. Results may be different if a cervical length of 15 mm or 20 mm was used for analysis. Recently, Guzman *et al.*[79] and To *et al.*[80] concluded that funnelling does not provide any additional diagnostic information over that provided by cervical length in the prediction of preterm birth.

Cervical length in the prediction of preterm delivery in high-risk singleton gestations

Cook *et al.*[81] conducted a prospective cohort study in 120 women considered to be at risk for preterm delivery. The patients at risk included patients with a history of recurrent first-trimester loss, second-trimester loss, previous preterm delivery (<34 weeks), previous cervical surgery and uterine anomaly. Initial cervical assessment was made between 9 and 29 weeks' gestation. Further assessment varied from weekly to monthly according to cervical findings and obstetric history. The cervical parameters measured were cervical length, diameter and internal os dilatation. Twenty-four patients (20%) delivered before 34 weeks of gestation. Cervical length was the only factor found to be of value in the prediction of preterm delivery. A cervical length of 20 mm or less before 20 weeks was associated with delivery before 34 weeks in 95% of women.

Owen et al.[82] performed an observational study including 183 patients who had a history of spontaneous preterm birth before 32 weeks of gestation. The patients were enrolled between 16 and 19 weeks of gestation and followed every 2 weeks until 24 weeks of gestation. Forty-eight (26%) women delivered before 35 weeks of gestation. A short cervix (<25 mm) at the first scan was associated with a relative risk of 3.3 (2.1–5.0) for spontaneous preterm birth (<35 weeks). The sensitivity, specificity and positive-predictive values were 19%, 98% and 75%. After controlling for cervical length, neither funnelling nor dynamic shortening was an independent predictor of spontaneous preterm birth. However, using the shortest cervical length on serial evaluations, after any dynamic shortening, the relative risk of a cervical length of less than 25 mm increased to 4.5 (2.7–7.6) with a sensitivity, specificity and positive-predictive value of 69%, 80% and 55%, respectively. In conclusion, a serial measurement at up to 24 weeks significantly improved the sensitivity but lowered the positive-predictive value of the test.

Guzman et al.[83] enrolled 469 high-risk patients between 15 and 24 weeks of gestation. High-risk was defined as the presence of a history of spontaneous preterm birth before 37 weeks' gestation, prior mid-trimester loss, more than two terminations of pregnancy, cone biopsy, uterine malformation, previous cerclage and diethylstilbestrol exposure. Transvaginal cervical sonography and transfundal pressure were performed and the shortest cervical length, funnel width, funnel length and cervical index were recorded

serially. A cervical length of 25 mm or less had a sensitivity, specificity, positive-predictive value and negative-predictive value of 76%, 68%, 20% and 96%, respectively, to identify preterm birth at less than 34 weeks of gestation. Cervical length was the best parameter in the prediction of preterm birth in women with prior mid-trimester losses. The authors suggested that using a cervical length of 15 mm or less had a sensitivity, specificity, positive-predictive value and negative-predictive value of 81%, 72%, 29% and 96%, respectively, in predicting spontaneous preterm delivery at less than 34 weeks. Cervical length was better at predicting earlier forms of prematurity (at <28 and <30 weeks) than later forms (<32 and <34 weeks).

Odibo et al.[84] demonstrated the relationship between a short cervix and preterm premature rupture of membranes leading to preterm birth in a high-risk population. They studied 69 women at high risk for preterm birth (by obstetric history and transvaginal cervical length <25 mm) between 14 and 24 weeks of gestation. The incidence of preterm PROM was 39% (27/69). Cervical length of less than 10 mm had a sensitivity, specificity, positive- and negative-predictive value of 33%, 90%, 69% and 68%, respectively, in predicting preterm PROM at less than 35 weeks of gestation.

Collectively, the evidence suggested that patients with a previous history of preterm birth of mid-trimester loss require a longer cervix than patients without such history to prevent preterm delivery.

CERVICAL INCOMPETENCE

The ability of the cervix to retain the conceptus during pregnancy has been referred to as 'cervical competence' and the condition in which the cervix fails to fulfil its physiological role is designated by default as 'cervical incompetence'. Obstetricians have traditionally made this diagnosis based upon obstetric history.

Cervical incompetence is a clinical diagnosis often applied to patients with a history of one or more mid-trimester spontaneous abortions and/or early preterm deliveries in which the basic process is thought to be the failure of the cervix to remain closed during pregnancy. The basic assumption is that cervical dilatation and effacement have occurred in the absence of a significant increase in the uterine contractility. The presenting symptom is often a feeling of vaginal pressure caused by the distension of this organ by the protruding membranes or rupture of membranes in the mid-trimester of pregnancy. Typically, there is no vaginal bleeding, the fetuses are born alive, and labor is short and pain free. A history of repeated mid-trimester abortions at similar gestational age is highly suggestive of the condition.

Cervical incompetence can be due to congenital Mullerian duct abnormalities or diethylstilbestrol (DES) exposure or be secondary to cervical surgical trauma (e.g. conization or operations requiring dilatation of the canal). However, some patients will present with the typical picture in their first pregnancy without any apparent cause. Although the existence of cervical incompetence is widely accepted among obstetricians, there is no objective diagnostic test for this condition. Several methods have been proposed for the evaluation of a patient after a pregnancy loss (e.g. a hysterosalpingogram and passage of a #8 Hegar cervical dilator). However, there is a paucity of scientific evidence to support the value of these tests.

It is noteworthy that cervical incompetence is thought to result in mid-trimester spontaneous abortion. However, cervical disease (e.g. hypoplastic cervix, DES exposure or a weakened cervix after conization) is also associated with an increased risk of preterm premature rupture of membranes and preterm labor. Therefore, there is a need to revisit the traditional definition of cervical incompetence.

The hypothesis that there is a spectrum of cervical competence has been examined by Iams et al.[56]. A cross-sectional study was conducted in which cervical length was measured in patients with (1) a typical history of cervical incompetence, (2) a previous preterm delivery at <26 weeks, (3) a previous preterm delivery <27–32 weeks, and (4) a control group of women with previous term delivery. A strong relationship was found between cervical length in the index pregnancy and previous obstetric history. This relationship appears linear and patients considered to have a typical history of an incompetent cervix did not constitute a unique group. Similar results have been reported by Guzman et al.[85] who reported a strong relationship between previous obstetric history and cervical length in the subsequent pregnancy. Specifically, they observed that the frequency of a short cervix (cervical length <2 cm) or progressive shortening of the cervix to a length of <2 cm was associated with the gestational age at delivery in the previous pregnancy. Collectively, these studies suggest that there is a relationship between a history of preterm delivery and the cervical length in a subsequent pregnancy. Inasmuch as patients with a short cervix are at increased risk for a mid-trimester pregnancy loss (clinically referred to as 'cervical incompetence') or spontaneous preterm delivery with intact or rupture of membranes, a short cervix must be considered as the expression of a spectrum of cervical disease. However, further investigation is required to determine why some women with a short cervix have an adverse pregnancy outcome and others have a term uncomplicated delivery. Indeed, approximately 50% of women with a cervix of 15 mm or less deliver after 32 weeks without a cerclage[86]. This suggests that cervical length is only one of the factors determining the degree of cervical competence for a certain patient.

Sonographers have used the term 'cervical incompetence' to refer to a mid-trimester condition in which the cervix is open and the membranes bulge into the vagina. Figures 13 and 14 display the sonographic appearance of a grossly incompetent cervix. This diagnosis has clinical implications because its treatment consists of emergency cerclage. The standard management for such a patient in a subsequent pregnancy is to place a cerclage electively after 14 weeks.

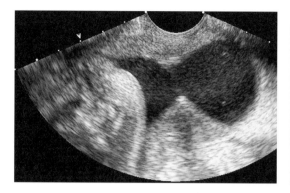

Figure 13 *Sonographic appearance of a grossly incompetent cervix, with bulging of the membranes in the vagina*

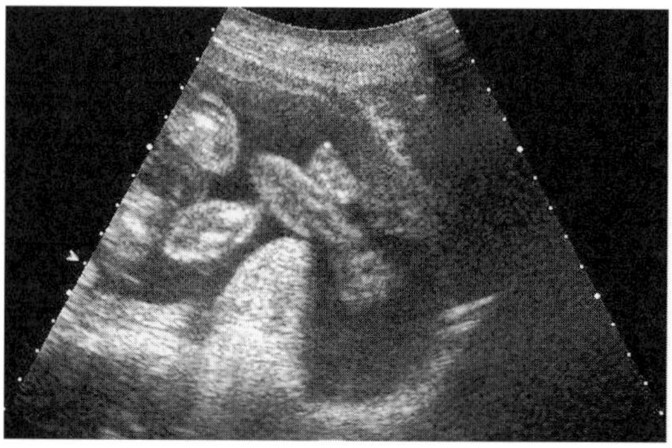

Figure 14 *Sonographic appearance of a grossly incompetent cervix, with bulging of the membranes in the vagina. The fetal lower extremities protruded into the vagina*

A common clinical problem is the management of the patient with an equivocal history for cervical incompetence. Sonographic examination of the cervix is currently being used in clinical practice to monitor cervical changes in the mid-trimester in order to determine the need for a cervical cerclage. Surveillance can be conducted by determining cervical length and detecting funnelling before and after a cervical stress test. Under normal circumstances, the cervical length does not change between 12 and 24 weeks. However, in patients who eventually develop a short cervix, the rate of cervical shortening may vary dramatically. For example, Guzman et al.[87] reported that the weekly shortening of the cervix in some patients is as much as 5 mm per week, as shown in Figure 15.

A cervical stress test is a method to identify a compliant cervix: one that has prematurely ripened. The stress is to increase intrauterine pressure and monitor cervical length and the appearance of funnelling. Intrauterine pressure can be increased by applying transfundal pressure, a Valsalva maneuver or the change in position of the patient from supine to standing position[88,89]. Guzman et al. compared different methods and concluded that transfundal pressure is the most sensitive method to elicit cervical changes in patients who will eventually demonstrate cervical changes[90]. By far the most commonly used

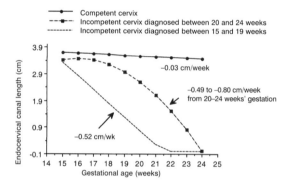

Figure 15 *Multivariable linear regression models of the endocervical lengths of women at risk for pregnancy loss and preterm birth between 15 and 24 weeks of gestation in cases of competent and incompetent cervix. From reference 83, with permission*

method is the application of moderate pressure on the maternal abdomen in the direction of the uterine axis for about 15 s[88]. Under normal circumstances, application of fundal pressure does not affect cervical length or funnelling. In contrast, if pressure results in funnelling or shortening of the cervix, premature ripening of the cervix is thought to have occurred.

The basis for the transfundal pressure stress test is a study conducted by Guzman et al.[88] in which fundal uterine pressure was applied to 150 pregnant women without risk factors at 16–24 weeks. No changes in cervical length or funnelling were detected. The rate of preterm delivery and mid-trimester loss was 6% (9/150). Of the nine patients who had a normal response to transfundal pressure and had adverse pregnancy outcome, two had spontaneous mid-trimester abortions at 22 and 23 weeks and the remainder had preterm deliveries. The same stress test was applied to 31 women at risk for cervical incompetence on the basis of history (i.e. mid-trimester spontaneous abortions, early preterm labor, previous cone biopsy, DES exposure, uterine anomaly or requirement for emergency cerclage in previous pregnancy, etc.). Transfundal pressure resulted in opening of the internal os in 45% (14/31) of patients. All patients, but one, with a positive response were treated with a cervical cerclage. The patient managed expectantly had a spontaneous abortion while of the treated patients 64% (9/14) delivered at term, 21% (3/14) had a preterm delivery and 14% (2/14) had a spontaneous abortion (<24 weeks).

Subsequently, Guzman et al.[91] followed prospectively ten patients at risk for cervical incompetence who had a positive cervical stress test at the first examination in the mid-trimester. In this study, a positive stress test was defined as a decrease in endocervical length equal to or greater than 2.0 mm. Nine of these ten patients (one case was lost to sonographic follow-up) were followed with serial scans until the cervical length was less than 10 mm or a digital examination revealed a dilated cervix at which point a cervical cerclage was placed. The patient with a positive stress test lost to follow-up had a spontaneous abortion at 23 weeks. All patients with a positive test were treated with a cervical cerclage, 66% (6/9) had a delivery after 36 weeks; two patients delivered preterm (at 27 and 34 weeks) and one patient lost her pregnancy at the time of cerclage placement (18 weeks). This study shows that a positive response to transfundal pressure in the mid-trimester is followed by progressive cervical changes.

Macdonald et al.[92] conducted an observational study of patients with a positive cervical stress test to determine the natural history of this condition. They studied 106 patients at risk for preterm delivery. All patients underwent cervical monitoring between 12 and 41 weeks of gestation. Eleven patients who demonstrated opening of the cervical canal (beaking of the internal os >5 mm or shortening of cervical length >5 mm) at rest or with fundal pressure before 24 weeks of gestation progressively shortened their cervix to less than 10 mm over a period of 2–17 days.

A frequent clinical question is whether patients with an equivocal history of cervical incompetence should have an elective cerclage placed at 14–16 weeks or rather be followed with serial measurements until there is evidence of increased cervical compliance. The literature suggests that the outcome of pregnancy is better in patients undergoing an elective cerclage rather than an emergency procedure. However, Guzman et al. compared the outcome of pregnancy in 138 patients at risk for pregnancy loss who were treated with an elective cerclage (n = 81) or monitored with serial examinations and treated when ultrasound showed signs of cervical abnormalities (n = 57). No differences in outcome were observed[93]. This finding has been confirmed in another study[94] conducted in 199 women with prior history of mid-trimester loss. The study included 114 women who were managed with serial cervical ultrasound between 15 and 24 weeks of gestation and 85 women who had an elective cerclage. While the rate of preterm delivery less than 37 weeks was not different between groups, the cerclage rate was reduced from 100% to 35% in the group managed using cervical ultrasound.

Ultrasound can be helpful in assisting in the intra-operative placement of a cerclage, in particular in patients with severe cervical hypoplasia. Using continuous transabdominal ultrasound guidance, it is possible to monitor the precise placement of the cerclage to ensure placement of the stitch as close as possible to the internal cervical os[95].

Transvaginal ultrasound can be used in the evaluation of the cervix after cerclage placement. Several studies have demonstrated that cerclage placement results in an increased cervical length. Althuisius *et al.*[96] demonstrated that the placement of an elective McDonald suture resulted in an increased mean endocervical length from 21 mm (95% CI 19–23) to 34 mm (95% CI 30–38). Similar findings have been reported after the placement of Shirodkar cerclages resulted in an increase of cervical length from 27 ± 9 mm to 36 ± 9 mm[97]. Guzman *et al.* have reported that the risk for preterm delivery is six times greater if the difference between preoperative and post-operative cervical length is less than 10 mm[98].

Transvaginal sonography may be used for the post-operative monitoring of patients who have undergone cervical cerclage. Quinn[99] reported that all patients who developed a dilated internal os and herniation of the membranes after placement of a Shirodkar cerclage had preterm birth (between 5 and 7 weeks after the detection of sonographic abnormalities). Similar findings were reported by Rana *et al.*[100] with transabdominal sonography in a small number of patients. Andersen *et al.*[101] observed 32 patients with endovaginal sonography following cerclage placement. The risk of preterm delivery was significantly increased in those patients who developed shortening of the upper cervix (above the suture) to ≤ 10 mm, as compared to patients whose upper cervical length was >20 mm (58% versus 10%, $p = 0.006$). A short upper cervix (10 mm) had a sensitivity, specificity, positive-predictive value and negative-predictive value of 86%, 76%, 50% and 95%, respectively, for the prediction of delivery before 34 weeks of gestation.

Randomized clinical trials of cervical cerclage before cervical ultrasound era

The clinical value of cervical cerclage has been a subject of debate in the obstetric literature for many years. Three randomized clinical trials have been conducted so far in singleton pregnancies. Table 9 summarizes the details of the clinical trials. All studies were conducted before sonographic evaluation of the cervix became widely available.

Rush *et al.*[102] reported a study conducted in 194 women at high risk for late spontaneous abortion or preterm delivery. Patients were randomly allocated to either cerclage ($n = 96$) or expectant management ($n = 98$) between 15 and 21 weeks. The overall rate of preterm delivery was 33% but there was no difference in the rate of preterm delivery between patients treated with a McDonald cerclage or expectant management (preterm delivery <37 weeks; expectant management 32% versus cerclage 34%). The duration of pregnancy was slightly longer in patients managed expectantly than in the cerclage group, but this difference was attributed to days gained after the 37th week. Rupture of membranes was more frequent in patients who had a cerclage than in the control group (18.7% (18/96) vs. 12.3% (12/98)), but this difference did not reach statistical significance. There was no difference in neonatal outcome. However, fever during the puerperium was more common in patients managed with cerclage (cerclage 10.4% (10/96) versus expectant 3% (3/98); $p = 0.07$).

Lazar *et al.*[103] reported a trial of 506 women considered to be at moderate risk for preterm

Table 9 *Randomized studies of cervical cerclage before cervical ultrasound era*

Reference	n	Indication	Weeks at cerclage	Delivery <37 weeks Cerclage (%)	Controls (%)
Rush *et al.* (1984)[102]	194	high risk of cervical incompetence	18	34	32
Lazar *et al.* (1984)[103]	506	moderate risk of cervical incompetence	<28	6.7	5.5
MRC/RCOG (1993)[104]	1292	obstetrician uncertainty	16	26	31

delivery based upon a scoring system which considered obstetric history, state of the cervix (i.e. open internal os, a short cervix at digital examination, etc.). Two hundred and sixty-eight patients were allocated to McDonald cerclage placement with number 3 nylon and 238 to expectant management. The rate of preterm delivery was 6.7% (18/268) in the cerclage group and 5.5% (13/238) in the control group (overall rate was 6.1%). Patients in the cerclage group had more admissions to the hospital (excluding the hospitalization for cerclage or birth) and received oral tocolysis more frequently than those in the control group ($p < 0.01$ for each). However, there were no differences in perinatal mortality between the two groups.

The largest trial conducted to date was organized by the Medical Research Council of the United Kingdom and the Royal College of Obstetricians and Gynaecologists[104]. The criteria for enrolment was uncertainty on the part of the obstetricians as to whether to recommend a cerclage. The main reason for enrolment was a past history of one or more second-trimester spontaneous abortions or preterm deliveries (71% of patients) and a history of cervical operation. The type of operation and surgical material was left to the discretion of the caregiver and the study was conducted in multiple countries. Of patients allocated to cerclage, only 92% had the suture inserted, while 8% of those in the control group had a cerclage. The mean gestational age at cerclage was 15.9 weeks (interquartile range 14.3–18.4). The primary outcome was delivery at less than 33 completed weeks. The rate of deliveries before 33 weeks (range 20–33 weeks) was significantly lower in the cerclage group than in the control group (cerclage 13% versus control group 17%; odds ratio 0.72; 95% CI 0.53–0.97; $p = 0.03$). Fever attributed to uterine infection was more common in patients allocated to the cerclage group (6% vs. 3%; odds ratio 2.12; 95% CI 1.08–4.16; $p = 0.03$). The authors estimated that 25 cerclages would need to be inserted to prevent one preterm delivery <33 weeks. The overall rate of preterm delivery was 28%

(<37 weeks). A subgroup analysis suggested that patients with a history of three spontaneous mid-trimester abortions or preterm deliveries seemed to benefit the most from the procedure. The authors call for research in methods to identify the patients who may benefit from this operation.

One small study has examined the value of cervical cerclage in twin gestation. There was no evidence of benefit in this condition[105].

In conclusion, results of randomized clinical trials suggest that cerclage had either a modest effect on reducing the rate of preterm delivery or no effect whatsoever. We believe that the fundamental problem is that preterm labor is a syndrome with multiple etiologies and the operation can only benefit those patients who have a primary or important cervical process responsible for preterm delivery. It is clear that obstetric history is insufficient to identify such a patient. We believe that future studies in which patient selection for cerclage is based upon results of cervical ultrasound or non-invasive determination of collagen content may uncover a role for cerclage in modern obstetrics.

Cervical cerclage after cervical ultrasound assessment

Observational studies

The prediction of spontaneous preterm birth with cervical sonography has clinical relevance, given the hope that an intervention would reduce the rate of prematurity in patients with a short cervix. The nature of the intervention could encompass medical treatment with agents preventing cervical ripening, mechanical devices such as pessaries or a cervical cerclage. Most effort to date has focused on the role of a cervical cerclage.

Heath et al.[86] reported that patients with a short cervix who underwent placement of a cerclage had a ten-fold reduction in the rate of preterm birth. Clinicians responsible for the care of the patients with a short cervix (defined as 15 mm or less) were informed of the results and allowed to use their preference for further management. Of the 43 patients with a short cervix, 22 were treated with the placement of Shirodkar cerclage and 21 were managed expectantly. Although there were no differences in the clinical characteristics of the two groups, the rate of preterm delivery (<32 weeks) was 52% (11/21 in the group managed expectantly and only 5% (1/22) in the group managed with a cervical cerclage) (Figure 16). Similarly, Hibbard et al.[106] reported that patients with a short cervix undergoing cervical cerclage delivered later in gestation than patients managed expectantly. Eighty-five patients with a cervical length of less than 30 mm were included. Some women had a history of a previous preterm birth. A cervical cerclage was placed in 43 patients at the discretion of the treating physician. Although the mean cervical length measurements were similar in both groups (cerclage, 22 mm vs. non-cerclage, 20 mm; $p = 0.32$), the mean gestational age at delivery and birth weight in the cerclage group were higher than in the group managed without the placement of a cerclage (34 weeks vs. 32 weeks; $p = 0.04$ and 2530 g vs. 2084 g; $p \leq 0.04$, respectively). Guzman et al.[88] also reported that cerclage improved pregnancy outcome in patients with a history of a spontaneous abortion or preterm delivery who shortened their cervix (defined as 20 mm or less) between 20 and 24 weeks of gestation. The decision to treat or not to treat was also left at the discretion of the treating physician. Seventy-nine per cent (22/28) of women treated with cerclage delivered at term (37 weeks or more) while only 35% (6/17) of those in the bed rest group delivered at term ($p = 0.04$).

In contrast to the studies suggesting that cerclage may be beneficial, two studies did not find cerclage to be beneficial. Berghella et al.[108] studied 168 women at risk for preterm delivery who underwent serial sonography between 14 and 23 weeks. Patients with a cervical length of less than 25 mm or funnelling greater than 25% of the cervical length were offered either a McDonald cerclage or expectant management. Sixty-three patients had an abnormal cervix, 39 underwent cerclage and 24 were

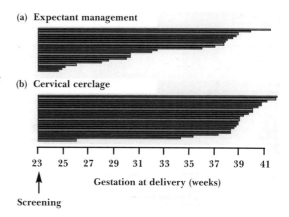

(a) Expectant management

(b) Cervical cerclage

23 25 27 29 31 33 35 37 39 41

Gestation at delivery (weeks)

↑
Screening

Figure 16 *Interval between gestational age at screening and gestational age at delivery in patients treated with expectant management (a) and cervical cerclage (b). From reference 86, with permission*

managed expectantly. Patients in the two groups were similar in clinical characteristics, cervical length and funnelling but those who were treated with a cerclage had a lower gestational age when the cervical changes were identified (18 weeks vs. 21 weeks) than those in the control group. Placement of cervical cerclage did not reduce the rate of preterm delivery (cerclage 27% vs. expectant management 23%) or the duration of pregnancy after the identification of abnormal cervical findings. Similarly, Hassan et al.[109] found cerclage to have no demonstrable beneficial effect in an observational study of 70 patients who had cervical length of less than 15 mm between 14 and 24 weeks' gestation. Fifteen (21%) patients had a previous history of preterm delivery. McDonald cerclage was placed in 25 patients (36%). The rate of preterm delivery (<34 weeks) was not different between groups (cerclage group 68% (17/25) vs. no cerclage group 53% (24/45); $p = 0.2$). Patients with cerclage placement had a higher rate of preterm PROM than those without cerclage (65% (15/23) vs. 36% (16/44); $p < 0.05$).

Randomized clinical trials

At present, there are three randomized control trials to assess the clinical value of the cerclage by using the information from cervical ultra-sound examination. The results of these trials are summarized in Table 10.

In the cervical incompetence prevention randomized cerclage trial (CIPRACT) study, Althuisius et al.[110,111] randomized 73 pregnant women at less than 15 weeks of gestation with risk factors for cervical incompetence to have a prophylactic cerclage ($n = 23$) or be observed ($n = 44$). Four patients had a spontaneous abortion during the first trimester and two were lost for follow-up. The risk factors for cervical incompetence included the history of preterm delivery before 34 weeks' gestation, previous preterm premature rupture of membranes before 32 weeks' gestation, history of cold knife conization, diethylstilbestrol exposure and a Mullerian duct abnormality. Prophylactic cerclages (i.e. McDonald) were generally placed between 10 and 12 weeks or later if enrolled at a later gestational age using a braided polyester thread. In both groups, the cervical length was evaluated every 2 weeks after randomization. The rate of preterm delivery (<34 weeks) was similar in both groups (prophylactic cerclage 13% (3/23) vs. observation 14% (6/44); $p > 0.05$) and neonatal survival (prophylactic cerclage 91% (21/23) vs. observation 93% (41/44); $p > 0.05$). Patients allocated to the observation group were followed with serial sonography. If the cervical length shortened (<25 mm) before the 27th week of gestation, they were randomized to either therapeutic cerclage with bed rest ($n = 20$) or bed rest ($n = 16$). Placement of a therapeutic cerclage reduced the rate of preterm delivery at less than 34

weeks and the composite neonatal morbidity (neonatal intensive care unit (NICU) admis-sion or neonatal death) (0% vs. 44% (7/16), $p = 0.002$; 5% (1/19) vs. 50% (8/16), $p = 0.005$, respectively).

In contrast, Rust et al.[112,113] randomized 113 patients with a short cervix (<25 mm) or funnelling (≥ 25%) between 16 and 24 weeks into the therapeutic cerclage group ($n = 55$) and the no cerclage group ($n = 58$). The population included patients with and without risk factors for preterm birth. All patients underwent amniocentesis to exclude intra-amniotic infection and received 48 h of therapy with indomethacin and antibiotics. There was no significant difference between the two groups with respect to the rate of preterm delivery <34 weeks' gestation (35% vs. 36.2%), re-admission for preterm labor (52% vs. 53%), placental abruption (11% vs. 14%), chorio-amnionitis (20% vs. 10%) and the perinatal death rate (13% vs. 12%).

The CIPRACT study enrolled only patients at risk for preterm delivery, while in the trial of Rust et al. 13% of patients were at low risk. The positive-predictive value for short cervix to predict preterm delivery tends to be higher in patients with a previous history of preterm birth. The fact that the rate of preterm delivery in the control group of the CIPRACT study is higher than that of Rust's study (43.8% vs. 36.2%) may explain, at least in part, the different results between these two studies.

The largest randomized clinical trial reported so far was conducted by the Fetal Medicine Foundation of the United

Table 10 *Randomized control trial of cervical cerclage using cervical ultrasound*

| Reference | n | Indication | Weeks at cerclage | Delivery <34 weeks | |
				Cerclage (%)	Controls (%)
Althuisius et al. (2001)[110,111]	35	previous PTD, high-risk obstetric history, cervix <25 mm	<24 <27	0 0	50 (7/14) 43.8 (7/16)
Rust et al. (2001)[112,113]	113	sonographic criteria, cervix <25 mm or funnelling ≥ 25%	16–24	34.9	36.2 ns
Liao et al. (2001)[114]	198	cervix <15 mm	23	23 (23/101)	27 (26/98)

Kingdom[114]. Cervical length was determined in low-risk patients at median gestational age of 23 weeks of gestation and those with a cervix of less than 15 mm were randomized to either expectant management ($n = 98$) or cerclage group ($n = 101$). The rate of preterm delivery at less than 33 weeks' gestation was not significantly different (27% (26/98) vs. 23% (23/101)). The conclusion of this study is that cerclage placement in patients with a short cervix but without risk factors for preterm delivery does not reduce the rate of spontaneous preterm birth or the rate of perinatal death.

FUTURE CHALLENGES

Future challenges include:

(1) Three-dimensional ultrasound;
(2) Non-invasive assessment of collagen content:
  (a) Fluorescence spectroscopy (collascope);
  (b) Quantitative ultrasonic tissue characterization of the cervix;
(3) Cervical artery Doppler velocimetry;
(4) Cervical mucus.

Three-dimensional ultrasound imaging of the cervix

In most circumstances, cervical assessment can be adequately performed by two-dimensional ultrasound. However, there are limited scan planes that can be obtained due to the anatomic limitations of the transvaginal approach. Three-dimensional ultrasound can provide innumerable planes that cannot be obtained by conventional two-dimensional ultrasound. From a stored data set, it is possible to reconstruct any plane required for examination.

Hoesli et al.[115] compared the three-dimensional volume assessment of the cervix with the two-dimensional cervical length measurement in low- and high-risk patients for cervical incompetence. The high-risk patients were 27 in-patients with preterm contraction and/or premature rupture of membranes between 22 and 34 weeks of gestation. The low-risk patients included 28 out-patients with an uncomplicated pregnancy without contraction, vaginal infection and history of preterm contractions. Patients in the high-risk group delivered earlier than patients in the low-risk group (mean 37.9 ± 3.6 vs. 39.2 ± 1.7; $p = 0.04$). Using the two-dimensional technique, the mean cervical length in high-risk patients was shorter than that in low-risk patients, but three-dimensional volume measurement did not show a statistically significant difference. In contrast, Bega et al.[116] studied 21 multiparous patients at-risk for preterm delivery with 37 cervical assessments by two- and three-dimensional ultrasound between 11 and 32 weeks of gestation. The author reported that in ten instances (27%) the cervical length measurement was different between the two techniques. Interestingly, of 21 examinations showing funnelling, six (29%) funnellings were detected only by three-dimensional ultrasound. The mean funnel width as measured in the coronal three-dimensional ultrasound plane was wider than that as measured obtained by two-dimensional ultrasound (15.9 mm vs. 13.0 mm; $p < 0.05$) and that obtained by sagittal plane (15.9 mm vs. 12.9 mm; $p < 0.05$).

Non-invasive assessment of collagen content

A decrease in total collagen content and an increase in collagen solubility and collagenolytic activity characterize cervical ripening during pregnancy. A quantitative method to determine cervical ripening analyzing the collagen content of the cervix through fluorescent spectroscopy has been proposed recently by Garfield et al.[117]. The collascope is an optical device that determines cervical collagen content by means of a fluorescent signal generated whenever collagen cross-links are excited by light whose wavelength is about 340 nm. The system has been used in rats and in humans at different stages of pregnancy, and has shown that cervical ripening occurs progressively in the last trimester of pregnancy[117]. Further studies are required to determine the value of this technology in obstetrics and if it adds information not provided by ultrasound.

Tekesin et al.[118] reported the use of quantitative ultrasonic tissue characterization in 46 pregnant women to assess the texture features of the uterine cervix. In patients with premature contraction and shortening of cervix ($n = 16$), the average Gray scale values were lower than those obtained from asymptomatic patients ($n = 30$) at the same gestational age.

References

1. Schwalm H, Dubrauszky V. The structure of the musculature of the human uterus – muscles and connective tissue. *Am J Obstet Gynecol* 1966; 94:391

2. Danforth D. The distribution and functional activity of the cervical musculature. *Am J Obstet Gynecol* 1954;68:1261

3. Yu SY, Tozzi CA, Babiarz J, et al. Collagen changes in rat cervix in pregnancy – polarized light microscopic and electron microscopic studies. *PSEBM* 1995;209:360-9

4. Uldbjerg N, Forman A, Peterson LK, et al. Biochemical changes of the uterus and cervix during pregnancy. In Reece EA, Hobbins JC, Mahoney MJ, Petrie RH, eds. *Medicine of the Fetus and of the Mother*. Philadelphia: J.B. Lippincott Co., 1992:849–68

5. Leppert FC. Proliferation and apoptosis of fibroblasts and smooth muscle cells in rat uterine cervix throughout gestation and the effect of the antiprogesterone onapristone. *Am J Obstet Gynecol* 1998;178:713–25

6. Uldbjerg N, Ekman G, Malmstrom A, et al. Ripening of the human uterine cervix related to changes in collagen, glycosaminoglycans, and collagenolytic activity. *Am J Obstet Gynecol* 1983; 147:662–6

7. Petersen LK, Uldbjerg N. Cervical hydroxyproline concentration in relation to age and parity. In Leppert P, Woessner F, eds. *Extracellular Matrix of the Uterus, Cervix and Fetal Membranes*. Ithaca: Perinatology Press NY, 1991

8. Liggins GC. Cervical ripening as an inflammatory reaction. In Ellwood DA, Anderson ABM, eds. *The Cervix in Pregnancy and Labour: Clinical and Biochemical Investigations*. Edinburgh, UK: Churchill Livingstone, 1981

9. Ito A, Hiro D, Ojima Y, et al. The role of leukocyte factors in uterine cervical ripening and dilatation. *Biol Reprod* 1987;37:511

10. Ito A, Hiro D, Ojima Y, et al. Spontaneous production of interleukin-1 factors from pregnant rabbit uterine cervix. *Am J Obstet Gynecol* 1988;159:261

11. Ito A, Leppert PC, Mori Y. Human recombinant interleukin-1 increases elastase-like enzyme in human uterine cervical fibroblasts. *Gynecol Obstet Invest* 1990;30:239

12. Osmers RG, Adelmann-Grill BC, Rath W, et al. Biochemical events in cervical ripening dilatation during pregnancy and parturition. *J Obstet Gynaecol* 1995;21:185–94

13. Kelly RW. Pregnancy maintenance and parturition: the role of prostaglandin in manipulating the immune and inflammatory response. *Endocr Rev* 1994;15:684–706

14. Chwalisz K, Benson M, Scholz P, et al. Cervical ripening with the cytokines interleukin 8, interleukin 1beta and tumor necrosis factor alpha in guinea pigs. *Hum Reprod* 1994;9:2173–81

15. Sennstrom MK, Brauner A, Lu Y, et al. Interleukin-8 is a mediator of the final cervical ripening in humans. *Eur J Obstet Gynecol Reprod Biol* 1997;74:89–92

16. Osmers RG, Blaser J, Kuhn W. Interleukin-8 synthesis and the onset of labor. *Obstet Gynecol* 1995;86:223–9

17. Rajabi MR, Dodge GR, Soloman S, et al. Immunochemical and immunohistochemical evidence of estrogen-mediated collagenolysis as a mechanism of dilatation in the guinea pig at parturition. *Endocrinology* 1991;128:371

18. Granström L, Ekman GE, Malmstrom A, et al. Serum collagenase levels in relation to the state of the human cervix during pregnancy and labor. *Am J Obstet Gynecol* 1992;167:1284–8

19. Pinto RM, Raboa W, Votta RA. Uterine cervix ripening in term pregnancy due to the action of estradiol-17. *Am J Obstet Gynecol* 1965;92:319

20. Chwalisz K, Shi S, Neef G, et al. The effect of antigestagen ZK 98 299 on the uterine cervix. *Acta Endocrinol* 1987;283:113

21. Shi S-Q, Beier HM, Garfield RE, et al. The specific cyclooxygenase inhibitor flosulide inhibits antiprogestin-induced preterm birth. *J Soc Gynecol Invest* 1996;3(Suppl):540

22. Chwalisz K, Kosub B, Garfield RE, et al. Estradiol inhibits the onapristone (ZK 98 299) induced preterm parturition in guinea pigs by blocking cervical ripening. *J Soc Gynecol Invest* 1995;2:267

23. Chwalisz K, Garfield RE, *et al.* Antiprogesterones in the induction of labor. *Ann NY Acad Sci* 1994;734:387–413

24. Chwalisz K, Shao-Qing S, Garfield RE, *et al.* Cervical ripening in guinea pigs after a local application of nitric oxide. *Hum Reprod* 1997;12:2093–101

25. Thomson AJ, Lunan CB, Cameron AD, *et al.* Nitric oxide donors induce ripening of the human cervix: a randomized controlled trial. *Br J Obstet Gynaecol* 1997;104:1054–7

26. Mason GC, Maresh MJ. Alterations in bladder volume and the ultrasound appearance of the cervix. *Br J Obstet Gynaecol* 1990;97:457–8

27. Andersen HF. Transvaginal and transabdominal ultrasonography of the uterine cervix during pregnancy. *J Clin Ultrasound* 1991;19:77–83

28. Jackson GM, Ludmir J, Bader TJ. The accuracy of digital examination and ultrasound in the evaluation of cervical length. *Obstet Gynecol* 1992;79:214–18

29. Jeanty P, D'Alton M, Romero R, *et al.* Perineal scanning. *Am J Perinatol* 1986;3:289

30. Zilianti M, Azuaga A, Calderon F, Pages G, Mendoza G. Monitoring the effacement of the uterine cervix by transperineal sonography: a new perspective. *J Ultrasound Med* 1995;14(10):719–24

31. Cicero S, Skentou C, Souka A, To MS, Nicolaides KH. Cervical length at 22–24 weeks of gestation: comparison of transvaginal and transperineal-translabial ultrasonography. *Ultrasound Obstet Gynecol* 2001;17:335–40

32. To MS, Skentou C, Chan C, Zagaliki A, Nicolaides KH. Cervical assessment at the routine 23-week scan: standardizing techniques. *Ultrasound Obstet Gynecol* 2001;217–19

33. O'Brien JM, Allen AA, Barton JR. Intravaginal saline as a contrast agent for cervical sonography in the obstetric patient. *Ultrasound Obstet Gynecol* 1999;13:137–9

34. Iams JD, Goldenberg RL, Meis PJ, *et al.* The length of the cervix and the risk of spontaneous premature delivery. *N Engl J Med* 1996;334:567–72

35. Berghella V, Kuhlman K, Weiner S, *et al.* Cervical funneling: sonographic criteria predictive of preterm delivery. *Ultrasound Obstet Gynecol* 1997;10:161–6

36. Sonek JD, Iams JD, Blumenfeld M, *et al.* Measurement of cervical length in pregnancy: comparison between vaginal ultrasonography and digital examination. *Obstet Gynecol* 1990;76:172–5

37. Yost NP, Bloom SL, Twickler DM, *et al.* Pitfalls in ultrasonic cervical length measurements for predicting preterm birth. *Obstet Gynecol* 1999;93:510–16

38. Romero R, Gomez R, Mazor M, Ghezzi F, Yoon BH. The preterm labor syndrome. In Elder MG, Lamont RF, Romero R, eds. *Preterm Labor.* New York: Churchill Livingstone, 1997:29

39. Dyson DC, Danbe KH, Bamber JA, *et al.* Monitoring women at risk for preterm labor. *N Engl J Med* 1998;338:15–19

40. Brown HL, Britton KA, Brizendine EJ, *et al.* A randomized comparison of home uterine activity monitoring in the outpatient management of women treated for preterm labor. *Am J Obstet Gynecol* 1999;180:798–805

41. Andrews WW. Randomized clinical trial of metronidazole plus erythromycin to prevent spontaneous preterm delivery in fetal fibronectin positive women. *J Soc Gynecol Invest* 2001;8:47A

42. King JF, Grant A, Keirse MJ, *et al.* Betamimetics in preterm labor: an overview of the randomized controlled trials. *Br J Obstet Gynaecol* 1988;5:211–22

43. Murakawa H, *et al.* Evaluation of threatened preterm delivery by transvaginal ultrasonographic measurement of cervical length. *Obstet Gynecol* 1993;82:829–32

44. Iams JD, Paraskos J, Landon MB, *et al.* Cervical sonography in preterm labor. *Obstet Gynecol* 1994;84:40–6

45. Gomez R, Galasso M, Romero R, *et al.* Ultrasonographic examination of the uterine cervix is better than cervical digital examination as a predictor of the likelihood of premature delivery in patients with preterm labor and intact membranes. *Am J Obstet Gynecol* 1994;171:956–64

46. Rizzo G, *et al.* The value of fetal fibronectin in cervical and vaginal secretions and of ultrasonographic examination of the uterine cervix in predicting premature delivery for patients with preterm labor and intact membranes. *Am J Obstet Gynecol* 1996;175:1146–51

47. Rozenberg P, *et al.* Evaluating the risk of preterm delivery: a comparison of fetal fibronectin and transvaginal ultrasonographic measurement of cervical length. *Am J Obstet Gynecol* 1997;176:196–9

48. Gomez R, Zajer C, Terra R, *et al.* Patients with preterm labor and a short cervix are at increased risk for intrauterine inflammation and preterm delivery. *Am J Obstet Gynecol* 2001;184:S31

49. Timor Tritsch IE, Boozarjomehri F, Masakowski Y, *et al.* Can a snapshot sagittal view of the cervix by transvaginal ultrasonography predict active preterm labor? *Am J Obstet Gynecol* 1996;174:990–5

50. Andersen HF, Nugent CE, Wanty SD, *et al.* Prediction of risk for preterm delivery by

ultrasonographic measurement of cervical length. *Am J Obstet Gynecol* 1990;163:859–67

51. Kushnir O, Vigil DA, Izquierdo L, *et al*. Vaginal ultrasonographic assessment of cervical length changes during normal pregnancy. *Am J Obstet Gynecol* 1990;162:991–3

52. Okitsu O, Minura T, Nakayama T, *et al*. Early prediction of preterm delivery by transvaginal ultrasonography. *Ultrasound Obstet Gynecol* 1992; 2:402–9

53. Ayers JW, *et al*. Sonographic evaluation of cervical length in pregnancy: diagnosis and management of preterm cervical effacement in patients at risk for premature delivery. *Obstet Gynecol* 1988;71:939–44

54. Podobnik M, *et al*. Ultrasonography in the detection of cervical incompetence. *J Clin Ultrasound* 1988;13:383–91

55. Zorzoli A, *et al*. Cervical changes throughout pregnancy as assessed by transvaginal sonography. *Obstet Gynecol* 1994;84:960–4

56. Iams JD, *et al*. Cervical competence as a continuum: a study of ultrasonographic cervical length and obstetrical performance. *Am J Obstet Gynecol* 1995;172:1097–106

57. Cook CM, *et al*. A longitudinal study of the cervix in pregnancy using transvaginal ultrasound. *Br J Obstet Gynaecol* 1996;103(1):16–18

58. Tongsong T, *et al*. Cervical length in normal pregnancy as measured by transvaginal sonography. *Int J Gynaecol Obstet* 1997;58(3): 313–15

59. Heath VCF, *et al*. Cervical length at 23 weeks of gestation: prediction of spontaneous preterm delivery. *Ultrasound Obstet Gynecol* 1998;12:312–17

60. Riley L, Frigoletto FD Jr, Benacerraf BR. The implications of sonographically identified cervical changes in patients not necessarily at risk for preterm birth. *J Ultrasound Med* 1992; 11:75–9

61. Tongsong T, Kamprapanth P, Srisomboon J, *et al*. Single transvaginal sonographic measurement of cervical length early in the third trimester as a predictor of preterm delivery. *Obstet Gynecol* 1995;86:184–7

62. Taipale P, Hiilesmaa V. Sonographic measurement of uterine cervix at 18–22 weeks' gestation and the risk of preterm delivery. *Obstet Gynecol* 1998;92:902–7

63. Heath VC, Southall TR, Souka AP, *et al*. Cervical length at 23 weeks of gestation: relation to demographic characteristics and previous obstetric history. *Ultrasound Obstet Gynecol* 1998; ??:304–65

64. Hassan SS, Romero R, Berry SM, *et al*. Patients with a sonographic cervical length ≤ 15 mm have a 50% risk of early spontaneous preterm delivery. Presented at the *6th Annual Meeting of*

the Central Association of Obstetricians and Gynecologists, Maui, Hawaii, October 1999

65. Mercer BM, Goldenberg RL, Meis PJ, *et al*. The preterm prediction study: prediction of preterm premature rupture of membranes through clinical findings and ancillary testing. *Am J Obstet Gynecol* 2000;183:738–45

66. Bergelin I, Valentin L. Patterns of normal change in cervical length and width during pregnancy in nulliparous women: a prospective, longitudinal ultrasound study. *Ultrasound Obstet Gynecol* 2001;18:217–22

67. Michaels WH, Scheiber FR, Padgett RJ, *et al*. Ultrasound surveillance of the cervix in twin gestations: management of cervical incompetence. *Obstet Gynecol* 1991;78:739–44

68. Goldenberg RL, Iams JD, Miodovnik M, *et al*. The preterm prediction study: risk factors in twin gestations. *Am J Obstet Gynecol* 1996;175: 1047–53

69. Kushnir O, Izquierdo LA, Smith JF, *et al*. Transvaginal sonographic measurement of cervical length: evaluation of twin pregnancies. *J Reprod Med* 1995;40:380–2

70. Crane JM, Van den Hof M, Armson BA, *et al*. Transvaginal ultrasound in the prediction of preterm delivery: singleton and twin gestations. *Obstet Gynecol* 1977;90:357–63

71. Imseis HM, Albert TA, Iams JD. Identifying twin gestations at low risk for preterm birth with a transvaginal ultrasonographic cervical measurement at 24–26 weeks' gestation. *Am J Obstet Gynecol* 1997;177:1149–55

72. Souka AP, Heath V, Flint S, *et al*. Cervical length at 23 weeks in twins in predicting spontaneous preterm delivery. *Obstet Gynecol* 1999;94:450–4

73. Guzman ER, Walters C, O'Reilly-Green C, *et al*. Use of cervical ultrasonography in prediction of spontaneous preterm birth in twin gestations. *Am J Obstet Gynecol* 2000;183:1103–7

74. Yang JH, Kuhlman K, Daily S, Berghella V. Prediction of preterm birth by second trimester cervical sonography in twin pregnancies. *Ultrasound Obstet Gynecol* 2000;4:288–91

75. Ramin KD, Ogburn PL Jr, Mulholland TA, *et al*. Ultrasonographic assessment of cervical length in triplet pregnancies. *Am J Obstet Gynecol* 1999;180:1442–5

76. Guzman ER, Walters C, O'Reilly-Green C, Meirowitz NB, Gipson K, Nigam J, Vintzileos AM. Use of cervical ultrasonography in prediction of spontaneous preterm birth in triplet gestation. *Am J Obstet Gynecol* 2000;183: 1108–13

77. To MS, Skentou C, Cicero S, Liao AW, Nicolaides KH. Cervical length at 23 weeks in triplets: prediction of spontaneous preterm delivery. *Ultrasound Obstet Gynecol* 2000;16:515–18

78. Maymon R, Herman A, Jauniaux E, Frenkel J, Ariely S, Sherman D. Transvaginal sonographic assessment of cervical length changes during triplet gestation. *Hum Reprod* 2001;16:956–60

79. Guzman ER, Walters C, Ananth CV, O'Reilly-Green C, Benito CW, Palermo A, Vintzileos AM. A comparison of sonographic cervical parameters in predicting spontaneous preterm birth in high-risk singleton gestations. *Ultrasound Obstet Gynecol* 2001;18:204–10

80. To MS, Skentou C, Liao AW, Cacho A, Nicolaides KH. Cervical length and funneling at 23 weeks of gestation in the prediction of spontaneous early preterm delivery. *Ultrasound Obstet Gynecol* 2001;18:200–3

81. Cook CM, Ellwood DA. The cervix as a predictor of preterm delivery in 'at-risk' women. *Ultrasound Obstet Gynecol* 2000;15:109–13

82. Owen J, Yost N, Berghella V, Thom E, Swain M, Dildy GA, Miodovnik M, Langer O, Sibai B, McNellis D. Mid-trimester endovaginal sonography in women at high risk for spontaneous preterm birth. *J Am Med Assoc* 2001;286:1340–8

83. Guzman ER, Mellon R, Vintzileos AM, *et al.* Longitudinal assessment of endocervical canal length between 15 and 24 weeks' gestation in women at risk for pregnancy loss or preterm birth. *Obstet Gynecol* 1998;92:31–7

84. Odibo AO, Berghella V, Reddy U, Tolosa JE, Wapner RJ. Does transvaginal ultrasound of the cervix predict preterm premature rupture of membranes in a high-risk population? *Ultrasound Obstet Gynecol.* 2001;18:223–7

85. Guzman ER, Mellon R, Vintzileos AM, *et al.* Relationship between endocervical canal length between 15–24 weeks gestation and obstetric history. *J Matern Fetal Med* 1998;7:269–72

86. Heath VC, Souka AP, *et al.* Cervical length at 23 weeks of gestation: the value of Shirodkar suture for the short cervix. *Ultrasound Obstet Gynecol* 1998;12:318–22

87. Guzman ER, *et al.* Longitudinal assessment of endocervical canal length between 15 and 24 weeks' gestation in women at risk for pregnancy loss or preterm birth. *Obstet Gynecol* 1998;92:31–7

88. Guzman ER, Rosemberg JC, Houlihan C, *et al.* A new method using vaginal ultrasound and transfundal pressure to evaluate the asymptomatic incompetent cervix. *Obstet Gynecol* 1994;83:248–52

89. Arabin B, Aardenburg R, van Eyck J. Maternal position and ultrasonic cervical assessment in multiple pregnancy. *J Reprod Med* 1997;42:719–24

90. Guzman ER, Pisatowski DM, Vintzileos AM, *et al.* A comparison of ultrasonographically detected cervical changes in response to transfundal pressure, coughing, and standing in predicting cervical incompetence. *Am J Obstet Gynecol* 1997;177:660–5

91. Guzman ER, Vintzileos AM, McLean DA, *et al.* The natural history of a positive response to transfundal pressure in women at risk for cervical incompetence. *Am J Obstet Gynecol* 1997;176:634–8

92. Macdonald R, Smith P, Vyas S. Cervical incompetence: the use of transvaginal sonography to provide an objective diagnosis. *Ultrasound Obstet Gynecol* 2001;18:211–16

93. Guzman ER, Forster JK, Vintzileos AM, *et al.* Pregnancy outcomes in women treated with elective versus ultrasound-indicated cervical cerclage. *Ultrasound Obstet Gynecol* 1998;12:323–7

94. Guzman ER, Benito CW, Walters C, Vintzileos AM. Elective cerclage versus cervical sonography in the management of women with prior midtrimester loss. *Obstet Gynecol* 2001;97:S30

95. Ludmir J, Jackson GM, Samuels P. Transvaginal cerclage under ultrasound guidance in cases of severe cervical hypoplasia. *Obstet Gynecol* 1991;78:1067–72

96. Althuisius SM, Dekker GA, van Geijn HP, *et al.* The effect of therapeutic McDonald cerclage on cervical length as assessed by transvaginal ultrasonography. *Am J Obstet Gynecol* 1999;180:366–9

97. Funai EF, Paidas MJ, Rebarber A, *et al.* Change in cervical length after prophylactic cerclage. *Obstet Gynecol* 1999;94:117–19

98. Guzman ER, Lazarou G, Ananth CV, *et al.* The relationship of peri-operative cervical ultrasound parameters with pregnancy outcome in women treated with ultrasound-indicated cerclage. *Ultrasound Obstet Gynecol* 1998;12(S1):abstr 77

99. Quinn MJ. Vaginal ultrasound and cervical cerclage: a prospective study. *Ultrasound Obstet Gynecol* 1992;2:410–16

100. Rana J, Davis SE, Harrigan JT. Improving the outcome of cervical cerclage by sonographic follow-up. *J Ultrasound Med* 1990;9:275

101. Andersen HF, Karimi A, Sakala EP, *et al.* Prediction of cervical cerclage outcome by endovaginal ultrasonography. *Am J Obstet Gynecol* 1994;171:1102–6

102. Rush RW, Isaacs S, McPherson K, *et al.* A randomized controlled trial of cervical cerclage in women at high risk of preterm delivery. *Br J Obstet Gynaecol* 1984;91:724–30

103. Lazar P, Gueguen S, Dreyfus J, *et al.* Multicenter controlled trial of cervical cerclage in women at moderate risk of preterm delivery. *Br J Obstet Gynaecol* 1984;91:731–5

104. MRC/RCOG Working Party on Cervical Cerclage. Final report of the Medical Research Council/Royal College of Obstetricians and

Gynaecologists Multicentre Randomized Trial of Cervical Cerclage. *Br J Obstet Gynaecol* 1993;100:516–23

105. Dor J, Shalev J, Mashiach S, *et al*. Elective cervical suture of twin pregnancies diagnosed ultrasonically in the first trimester following induced ovulation. *Gynecol Obstet Invest* 1982; 13:55–60

106. Hibbard JU, Snow J, Moawad AH. Short cervical length by ultrasound and cerclage. *J Perinatol* 2000;3:161–5

107. Guzman ER, Benito CW, Yeo L, Vintzileos AM, Walters C, Meirowitz N. Bed rest versus cervical cerclage in the treatment of cervical incompetence manifested by ultrasound around the time of fetal viability. *Am J Obstet Gynecol* 1999; 180:S78

108. Berghella V, Daly SF, Tolosa JE, DiVito MM, Chalmers R, Garg N, Bhullar A, Wapner RJ. Prediction of preterm delivery with transvaginal ultrasonography of the cervix in patients with high-risk pregnancies: does cerclage prevent prematurity? *Am J Obstet Gynecol* 1999;181:809–15

109. Hassan SS, Romero R, Maymon E, Berry SM, Blackwell SC, Treadwell MC, Tomlinson M. Does cervical cerclage prevent preterm delivery in patients with a short cervix? *Am J Obstet Gynecol* 2001;184:1325–31

110. Althuisius SM, Dekker GA, van Geijn HP, Bekedam DJ, Hummel P. Cervical incompetence prevention randomized cerclage trial (CIPRACT): study design and preliminary results. *Am J Obstet Gynecol* 2000;183:823–9

111. Althuisius SM, Dekker GA, Hummel P, Bekedam DJ, van Geijn HP. Final results of the cervical incompetence prevention randomized cerclage trial (CIPRACT): therapeutic cerclage with bed rest versus bed rest alone. *Am J Obstet Gynecol* 2001;185;1106–12

112. Rust OA, Atlas RO, Jones KJ, Benham BN, Balducci J. A randomized trial of cerclage versus no cerclage among patients with ultrasonographically detected second-trimester preterm dilatation of the internal os. *Am J Obstet Gynecol* 2000;183:830–5

113. Rust OA, Atlas RO, Reed J, van Gaalen J, Balducci J. Revisiting the short cervix detected by transvaginal ultrasound in the second trimester: why cerclage therapy may not help. *Am J Obstet Gynecol* 2001;185:1098–105

114. Liao A, Nicolaides K. Presented at the *Annual Meeting of the International Society of Ultrasound in Obstetrics and Gynecology*, Melbourne, Australia, 2001

115. Hoesli IM, Surbek DV, Tercanli S, Holzgreve W. Three dimensional volume measurement of the cervix during pregnancy compared to conventional 2D-sonography. *Int J Gynecol Obstet* 1999;115–19

116. Bega G, Lev-Toaff A, Kuhlman K, Berghella V, Parker L, Goldberg B, Wapner R. Three-dimensional multiplanar transvaginal ultrasound of the cervix in pregnancy. *Ultrasound Obstet Gynecol* 2000;16:351–8

117. Garfield RE, Saade G, Buhimschi C, *et al*. Control and assessment of the uterus and cervix during pregnancy and labour. *Hum Reprod Update* 1998;4(5):637–95

118. Tekesin I, Meyer-Wittkopf M, Heller G, Steinfeldt B, Sierra F, Schmidt S. Quantitative ultrasonic tissue characterization of the cervix – a new predictor for prematurity? *Ultrasound Obstet Gynecol* 2001;18(S1):54

Medical and ethical aspects of pre-embryo research

10

J. G. Schenker

INTRODUCTION

Recent scientific and medical advances have made it possible to obtain pre-embryos and to use them for many research applications. Potential scientific and medical benefits from pre-embryo research are enormous. However, many moral and ethical issues and reservations exist, and any potential benefits may be outweighed by the risks involved. Most societies share the fears of the threatening social results of free, unrestricted research on potential human beings. Emotional responses sometimes cloud the objective consideration of moral and social issues.

Pressure groups seek to hasten governments into legislation or other means of control. Even if research were to be permitted as a means to gain knowledge, there would be the question of the ethical use of the knowledge so attained.

The status of the human embryo can be understood based on embryological principles, from fertilization until the formation of the embryo. The gametes, ova and sperm, are derived from the germinal epithelium of the ovary and testis. Meiosis occurs, reducing the total chromosome number by half, and a random recombination of the genetic elements is achieved. Fertilization usually occurs in the ampler end of the Fallopian tube, beginning with the penetration of spermatozoa in to the ovum, followed by the formation of male and female pronuclei. Pronuclei fusion occurs between 22 and 30 h after the start of fertilization, resulting in a zygote containing 46 chromosomes. The zygote has the theoretical potential to become an adult, but only about one in three human zygotes actually accomplish this. The zygote cleaves to form two blastomeres by the second day. By the fourth day, the four blastomeres are closely packed creating a multicellular entity called the morula[1]. The blastomeres become progressively smaller, whereas the size of the total aggregate remains approximately the same. After three divisions, there are eight cells in loose association. Each blastomere at this stage, if separated from the others, has the potential to develop into a complete adult.

Furthermore, if two eight-cell blastomeres are fused a single adult is produced. Thus, at the eight-cell stage the developmental singleness of one person has not yet been established[2]. Compaction follows, during which the cells adhere to one another and one or two cells are pushed to the inside of the mass. The inner cells contribute to the development of the embryo, whereas the outer cells become flattened to form trophoblast cells. By the fifth day, a blastocyst is formed, characterized by a continuous peripheral layer of cells and an inner cell mass within a central cavity (blastocoele). The blastocyst completes its passage through the Fallopian tube into the uterine cavity, where it remains unattached to the uterus for another 2 days. As cell division continues, the blastocyst enlarges both in cell number and blastocyst volume, while implanting into the uterine wall. This constitutes the first physiological interaction with the mother, early in the second post-fertilization week, the result of which is the placenta. By the tenth day, implantation is complete. The inner cell mass organizes into two layers, which together make up the bilaminar embryonic disc. A third layer of cells appears in between the first two, simultaneously with the formation of the embryonic axis. The primitive streak, a linear region where cells from the upper layer of the embryonic disc migrate into the new middle layer, appears at this stage. With the appearance of the primitive streak, around the 14th post-fertilization day, the embryonic disc is committed to forming a single human being. Twinning does not occur beyond this point, either naturally or experimentally. The three cell layers are the primary germ layers from which all tissues and organs will be derived during the period of organogenesis that follows. The term pre-embryo refers to the period of development that begins with fertilization and ends with the appearance of the primitive streak 14 days later. The embryo stage begins approximately 16 days after the beginning of fertilization and continues until the end of 8 weeks after fertilization, when organogenesis is complete.

The status of the pre-embryo must be different from that of either the earlier gamete or the last stages of fetal development. Two factors influence the evaluation of the moral status of the pre-embryo: the lack of individuation of the pre-embryo, and the high natural failure rate of zygotes to develop into pre-embryos. Developmental individuality in the sense of singleness is not established until the formation of the primitive streak[3], corresponding roughly with the time of implantation and the initiation of physical pregnancy in the mother. Up until the eight-cell stage of pre-embryonic development, one or more blastomeres can be removed from the aggregate and the remainder can still produce a complete adult. Individual blastomeres can develop into a complete individual. Cells derived from two pre-embryos of different genetic origin can aggregate into one larger cell mass and develop into one individual called a chimera. Once the primitive streak has developed, the differentiation of embryonic cells has advanced to the point that separation can no longer result in entirely separate individuals. If twinning were to occur at this point, the separation would be incomplete creating conjoined twins. Although the pre-embryo possesses a unique human genotype, it does not possess the biological individuality

to become a single human being. There is a natural percentage of pre-embryo loss[4]. Ten to 15% of clinically recognized pregnancies terminate in spontaneous abortion.

Data based on the use of highly sensitive assays for human chorionic gonadotropin, reveal that up to 60% of fertilizations do not survive beyond the first 14 days after fertilization. These facts may lead to the conclusion that the moral status of the pre-embryo must be different from that of the embryo. The pre-embryo must be treated with respect because it may become a human. It is genetically unique and therefore, with established kinship involves other interested parties. Furthermore, it is potentially a person and therefore has an anticipatory claim to some level of societal protection under the guarantees of human rights.

POTENTIAL SOURCES OF PRE-EMBRYOS FOR RESEARCH

There are several potential sources that cause great controversy. Existing surplus pre-embryos from *in vitro* fertilization (IVF), or 'spare pre-embryos' are the preferred source. However, the question arises whether it would be preferable or more beneficial to donate the spare pre-embryos, rather than to perform research on them. Defective pre-embryos from IVF may be used, but these may not apply for some areas of research where normal pre-embryos are required.

Aborted pre-embryos or embryos obtained by flushing methods (induced or spontaneous abortions) are another possible source. These may lead to the creation of pregnancies for the sole purpose of abortion. Furthermore, these methods may not succeed in extracting the pre-embryos which may be left behind only to implant in the uterus and result in an unwanted pregnancy. Creating pre-embryos for the sole purpose of research is a highly controversial issue. It is important to keep in mind the fact that present day IVF would not exist if pre-embryos had not intentionally been created for research. The United Kingdom Human Fertilization and Embryo Authority (HFEA), for example, will not license the use of cadaver or abortive ovarian tissue or oocytes for infertility treatments, but only for research[5].

Therapeutic stem cell research

Stem cells have the ability to divide for indefinite periods in culture and to give rise to specialized cells. In the first hours after fertilization, this cell divides into identical totipotent cells. This means that either one of these cells, if placed into a woman's uterus, has the potential to develop into a fetus.

Approximately 4 days after fertilization and after several cycles of cell division, these totipotent cells begin to specialize, forming a hollow sphere of cells, called a blastocyst. The blastocyst has an outer layer of cells and inside the hollow sphere, there is a cluster of cells called the inner cell mass. The outer layer of cells will go on to form the placenta and other supporting tissues needed for fetal development in the uterus. The inner cell mass cells will go on to form all of the tissues of the human body. The inner cell mass cells cannot form an organism because they are unable to give rise to the placenta and supporting tissues necessary for development in the human uterus. These inner cell mass cells are pluripotent, they can give rise to many types of cells but not all types of cells necessary for fetal development.

The pluripotent stem cells undergo further specialization into stem cells that are committed to give rise to cells that have a particular function. These more specialized stem cells are called multipotent. At present, human pluripotent cell lines have been developed from two sources. Investigators from ten laboratories in the United States, Australia, India, Israel and Sweden reported to the National Institutes of Health (NIH) that they have derived stem cells from 64 individual, genetically diverse blastocysts. The scientists who developed these stem cell lines report that the cells are viable, show characteristic stem cell morphology, can be maintained frozen, as well as in culture, and have undergone at least several population doublings.

The majority of these cells were reported to express all of the markers known to be associated with human embryonic stem cells, including stage-specific embryonic antigens (SSEA-3 and SSEA-4), the alkaline phosphatase enzyme and tumor rejection antigen 1 (TRA-1-60 and TRA-1-81). The scientists reported to the NIH that the cells could be frozen and thawed, and continue to grow while maintaining their karyotype. They also reported that in many cases they had assayed the cells for pluripotency by injecting the cells into immune-deficient mice.

Pluripotent stem cells were isolated directly from the inner cell mass of human embryos at the blastocyst stage, embryos received from IVF. Isolated pluripotent stem cells were obtained also from fetal tissue obtained from terminated pregnancies. In animal studies pluripotent stem cells were isolated by the use of somatic cell nuclear transfer. There are several reasons why the isolation of human pluripotent stem cells is important. Pluripotent stem cells could be beneficial to understand the complex events that occur during human development, and identification of the factors involved in cell specialization[6]. Cancer and birth defects are due to abnormal cell specialization and cell division. Human pluripotent stem cell research could be applied in developing new drugs and testing them for safety. Human pluripotent stem cell research could also dramatically change the way we develop drugs and test them for safety. Pluripotent stem cells, stimulated to develop into specialized cells, offer the possible source of treating several chronic medical conditions, like Parkinson's and Alzheimer's diseases, spinal cord injury, stroke, burns, heart disease, diabetes, osteoarthritis and rheumatoid arthritis. The use of somatic cell nuclear transfer would be another approach to overcome medical problems of tissue incompatibility for some individuals by using embryonic or fetal stem cells for therapy.

EARLY PREGNANCY LOSS

The high rate of early pregnancy losses may be due to errors in gametogenesis, defects in the fertilization process, developmental abnormalities after fertilization, or a delay in implantation; the exact cause is unknown. The failures present as chemical pregnancies, early miscarriages and missed abortions. Because the highest rate of loss is in the pre-embryo stage, research in this field may bring about important solutions.

IMPROVING METHODS OF IVF TREATMENT

Clinical use of IVF is not as successful as might be hoped. The pregnancy rate per one embryo transfer is 9.8%[7]. The total worldwide rate of live-birth delivery per cycle is 18.8%[8]. Improvement of clinical results can be obtained by better laboratory techniques, which can be achieved by pre-embryo research in the following directions: biochemical analysis of pre-embryos; metabolic studies of the nutritional requirements of the pre-embryo; and determination of enzymatic activity. Pre-embryo research may reveal factors that are involved in successful implantation of the transferred pre-embryo.

It is difficult to assess which aspects of the procedures of IVF contribute most to embryonic loss. One possible influence may be the use of superovulation, which has been reported to be associated with birth defects. The detrimental effect could be directly on the pre-embryo itself or indirectly by altering the hormonal balance in the woman. Differentiating between these would entail pre-embryo research. Another important research area concerns the culture conditions of the pre-embryos, such as temperature, oxygen concentrations, pH and metabolic requirements. It is, for example, possible to measure accurately the oxygen and pyruvate uptake and lactic production by the human pre-embryo, without affecting further development *in vitro*. Techniques of cryopreservation of the pre-embryo can be used in order to avoid the indirect effects of superovulation, and in order to prevent multiple pregnancies, although not discarding the pre-embryos. Current IVF practice is to limit the number of transferred pre-embryos to three or less, as is the practice in the United Kingdom. Excess pre-embryos are preserved for future treatment cycles, without the need for additional superovulation or maintained for donation. Transferring the frozen pre-embryos in a later cycle may improve the chance of a pregnancy. Previous research has shown that pregnancies may occur even when less than half of the blastomeres are intact after thawing[8], although there may be a higher risk of abortion (30%). No morphological markers have been identified that could be prognostic for survival or implantation. Additional studies of pre-embryo cryopreservation are required, into the following aspects: type of culture or cryoprotectant; pre-embryonic stage at freezing; freezing method; and methods of cryostorage and thawing. All of these must be performed on the human pre-embryos themselves, as studies in other species would not supply the appropriate answers.

MALE INFERTILITY

Recent advances in infertility research and therapy have led to significant improvement in results in cases of male infertility, which is responsible for 40% of the causes of infertility[8]. Intracytoplasmic sperm injection (ICSI) and other methods would never have been developed had it not been for pre-embryo research. The development and testing of this technique required that pre-embryos were created in the laboratory as a measure of the technique's success. Not only would these pre-embryos not be killed, but also theoretically, more might be formed from oocytes that would otherwise not be fertilized. ICSI is now in wide clinical use and many births have resulted. Recent data show that there is a slightly increased risk of sex chromosomal abnormalities after ICSI compared with the general population. Patients undergoing ICSI are consulted to undergo prenatal diagnosis.

CONTRACEPTIVE RESEARCH

Improved contraceptive methods can contribute to the world problem of population control, as well as to decreasing the use of pregnancy termination. Some contraceptive methods may be associated with side-effects if used for a prolonged period. Research has shown that the sperm surface is covered by several specific antigens, some of which are known to be significant in the reproductive process. The development of a vaccine composed of anti-sperm antibodies may offer a new method of contraception, provided that sufficient research to identify and isolate these antigens could be performed. Use of a vaccine composed of anti-zona pellucida antibodies has been successfully tested in several animal species[9]. In order to find a similar vaccine that could be used in the human, species-specific research must be performed, meaning human pre-embryo research.

PRE-EMBRYO RESEARCH – HUMAN DEVELOPMENT AND SOME MEDICAL CONDITIONS

An understanding of early human development can be obtained from the study of human *in vitro* pre-embryos, and can be applied to understanding later development. The study of normal pre-embryonic development will shed light on abnormalities such as spina bifida, cleft lip and palate, congenital heart defects and other malformations. Such studies would involve analysis of the initiation of gene expression and gene regulation, biochemical aspects of development, cell metabolism and cell-to-cell interaction. The incidence of chromosomal abnormalities in *in vitro* human pre-embryos has been estimated to be around 30%[10]. A similar incidence may occur *in vivo*, but would result in spontaneous abortion before pregnancy detection. Chromosomal abnormalities account for 50% of recognizable early miscarriages. These are mainly trisomies and monosomies, but translocations may also occur. Some may survive to term, such as trisomy 21, trisomy 13, trisomy 18 and

monosomy X. The other aberrations must be virtually lethal, because they are hardly ever found. To elucidate the actual incidence of these anomalies, their range, or how much development each will allow, studies must be performed on human pre-embryos. Aberrant zygotes with three pronuclei can be suitable for such studies, without the need to destroy pre-embryos that could develop into viable infants. Pre-embryo research is also required to ensure that *in vitro* fertilization does not contribute to additional increase in the incidence of chromosomally abnormal pre-embryos.

Delayed fertilization may result in a chromosomally abnormal pre-embryo[11]. Fertilization by multiple spermatozoa results in a pre-embryo with an abnormal chromosome number. Triploid pre-embryos occur at a rate of 3–4% *in vivo* and up to 10% *in vitro*, usually resulting in death of the fetus or newborn due to the multiple abnormalities associated with this condition. Some diseases are believed to be caused by errors in the fertilization process, for example trophoblastic disease, which is known to contain an abnormal chromosomal composition. The human genome is found in the pre-embryo at the eight-cell stage. This is the earliest possible time to assess the quality of the pre-embryo or to perform prenatal diagnosis.

PRE-EMBRYO RESEARCH FOR THE DIAGNOSIS OF GENETIC ABERRATIONS AND THERAPY

Approximately 1–2% of newborns are born with severe genetic defects. The pre-embryo in *in vitro* fertilization may be used as a diagnostic tool for early detection of genetic aberration, thus precluding the need for invasive examinations later in pregnancy. Early diagnosis of genetic aberrations before pre-embryo transfer can save an infertile couple from the distress involved in making the choices associated with a later diagnosis, and can decrease the necessity for therapeutic abortions. Remarkable advances in genetics were made by molecular biology.

Pre-implantation diagnosis

Successful pre-implantation diagnosis requires easy access to the pre-embryo, improved biopsy techniques and sensitive analytical assays that can be performed on a few cells. Biopsy of cells from human pre-embryos would allow the diagnosis of genetic abnormalities by karyotyping, DNA analysis, or enzyme micro assay, without adversely affecting development. Pre-implantation diagnosis is currently applied mainly to sex pre-selection in X-linked, inherited diseases and in the diagnosis of single genes. Many couples request pre-implantation diagnosis of their *in vitro* pre-embryos when at risk for sex-linked disorders. This method has been applied mainly in the cases of families at risk for Duchenne muscular dystrophy, fragile X syndrome and Lesch-Nyhan syndrome. The first reports of sex pre-selection were in 1988[12], and later in 1990[13], successful pregnancies after pre-implantation diagnosis were achieved. Initially, this was performed using cleavage-stage biopsy and DNA amplification of X and Y specific sequences by polymerase chain reaction (PCR). Later, fluorescent *in situ* hybridization (FISH) with X and Y chromosome-specific probes was used, to reduce misdiagnosis rates. In addition, the use of an 18 chromosome-specific probe in combination with X and Y probes has been recommended to minimize misdiagnosis due to mosaics. Recent advances enable an answer to be obtained within several hours by FISH. PCR has also been applied for diagnosis of known single gene defects, such as cystic fibrosis, Tay-Sachs disease, hemophilia, retinitis pigmentosa and others. In 1992, the birth of a normal girl after *in vitro* fertilization and pre-implantation diagnosis testing for cystic fibrosis was reported[14]. Early diagnosis of genetic disease will enable practitioners not to implant the stored pre-embryo into the uterus, if that were the chosen option, rather than to terminate the pregnancy later, at the stages when the remaining diagnostic options are chorionic villous sampling or amniocentesis. The Human Genome Project is expected to advance this field further, which will enable pre-embryo biopsy to be used to its full potential.

Gene therapy

Gene therapy may be applied for therapeutic purposes in the pre-embryonic stage by using genetic engineering. The range of methods includes somatic gene therapy, germ-line therapy and eugenic genetic engineering, of which only the first is practised. Somatic gene therapy results in the correction of genetic disorders in somatic cells and can be beneficial to replace defective or missing enzymes in some metabolic disorders. This method has already been applied in humans for the treatment of severe combined immuno-deficiency in children for bone marrow transplantation to the fetus *in uteri*[15] and for the treatment of thalassemia. The technique involves the removal of the patient's bone marrow, introduction of a normal gene, using a retrovirus vector and re-implantation of the corrected bone marrow cells to the patient. The use of a retrovirus carries the potential risk of serious infective disease or the development of malignant diseases. Germ-line therapy has only been performed in mammalian species. A gene is inserted into the gametes or zygotes by micromanipulation methods and injection of DNA. The foreign genes may integrate into the germ lines and, hence, into future generations. A high failure rate has been observed and deleterious results may occur, because there is no control over the injected DNA. This procedure is of limited applicability to the prevention of genetic disorders. Eugenic genetic engineering involves the insertion of a gene into a normal individual with the intention of enhancing a normal characteristic. It may endanger the individual by changing the balance of the cells or the entire body. Genetic engineering can potentially be introduced for eugenic selection resulting in altering human traits. This introduces many ethical issues that are not relevant to the present discussion.

EMBRYONIC ANTIGENS AND THE STUDY OF MALIGNANT DISEASE

Cleaving pre-embryos express unusual antigens on their cell surfaces, many of which are also found on tumors. Research in the early pre-embryonic stages may help our understanding of the mechanisms involved in cancerous growth, and may lead to a potential cure. The difference in the timing of developmental events between species indicates that, in order to understand human cancers, research may need to use human pre-embryos.

RISKS OF PRE-EMBRYO RESEARCH

Some of these research suggestions may result in damage to the pre-embryo or in its destruction. As in all cases of research it is imperative to balance the value of knowledge to be gained with the risk and harm that is incurred. Some pre-embryo research such as *in vitro* testing and genetic therapy, can be validated and beneficial only if the pre-embryo is subsequently transferred to a woman's uterus in an attempt to achieve a pregnancy. Pre-embryo research may be performed in such a way that risks infringement of the rights of donors of ovum and sperm. There may be potential harm to the pre-embryo itself of damage and possible destruction. The pre-embryo may be subjected to research that is not for its own benefit. The manipulation of pre-embryos may diminish society's respect for human life in general. Adverse effects may occur, such as interspecies fertilization using human sperm or ovum, or cloning of human beings.

ETHICAL ASPECTS

Modern medical ethics is based on a multi-disciplinary and a pluralistic approach. The pluralistic nature of modern ethics results in the impossibility to achieve a consensus on almost any moral statement. When considering an ethical argument concerning human subjects, some generally universal principles are accepted, such as respect for human dignity, doing no harm, the 'slippery slope' argument, the autonomy rights of the patients and beneficence.

MORAL STATUS OF THE HUMAN PRE-EMBRYO

The central question regarding therapeutic approaches to the pre-embryo is its moral status. There are three options with which to consider the moral status of a human pre-embryo[16]:

(1) The pre-embryo has no moral status. It is merely a collection of undifferentiated cells lacking individuality. Its status is not different from that of any other human tissue or cluster of cells. As medical professionals, we have no obligation to treat the pre-embryo. Furthermore, because the pre-embryo is an integral part of the mother's body, she has the full right to abort it or to permit pre-embryo research, if she wishes to do so.

(2) The pre-embryo has the full status of a human being. A new genotype is established during fertilization and some of the pre-embryos have the potential to become full-term fetuses, children and adults. The pre-embryo has its own rights, and the gamete donors are only its guardians. The interests of the mother are irrelevant to the future of the pre-embryo. Society is obligated to apply therapeutic measures to the pre-embryo as an individual patient.

(3) The pre-embryo is a potential human being. This definition is a relatively new philosophical entity, representing a compromise between the above two approaches. It is this opinion which is generally accepted today by most scientists, physicians and ethicists. Inasmuch as the pre-embryo is a potential human being, it should be handled with dignity and its rights should be respected as long as they do not conflict with major social, maternal, or other ethical interests. Yet, it should not be treated as a person, because it

has not yet developed the features of personhood, is not yet established as developmentally individual, and may never realize its biological potential.

The origin of human life

The question arises as to when the status of a potential human being is acquired. This issue has not yet been resolved by the many sides involved in the argument. There are different religious and ethical views regarding the origin of human life. The view of the Roman Catholic Church is that life begins at conception. Another view is that life begins with the implantation of the pre-embryo. According to another opinion, life begins when brain activity starts. This could be interpreted as being 8 weeks after conception at the point when the embryo is responsive to stimuli, or later in gestation when there is evidence of higher brain activity. Some consider human life to begin when the human conceptus becomes a 'person', has some degree of sentience or even active volition.

According to Grobstein[17], there are six aspects of individuality that become identifiable during a human life and are important to the determination of status. These are in order of their appearance during development: genetic, developmental, functional, behavioral, psychic and social. The emphasis of this notion of individuality is the development of sentience and self-awareness. Therefore, the individual does not come into existence until about 26 weeks' gestation. However, the moral status of the unborn human at different stages cannot be answered by scientific facts alone.

In the common law system, the question of the status of the human pre-embryo has arisen in criminal as well as civil law. It is necessary to define the person in order to determine offences against the person. Laws pertaining to succession, marriage, domestic relations and the area of negligence in recovery for prenatal injuries stand to gain from specific definitions of status. Surprisingly, most legal actions have not been able to supply a definite answer.

Human life cannot be attributed to the pre-embryo in the *in vitro* status. There are three main views concerning when the status of a potential human being is achieved:

(1) The status of a potential human being is achieved at conception with the fusion of human gametes, at which point the zygote acquires the entire genetic information for human development.

(2) The status of a potential human being is acquired at implantation, when no active procedure is required to maintain growth, and the chances of the pre-embryo reaching the neonatal stage are increased to exceed 50%. Acceptance of this concept resolves many arguments against IVF.

(3) The status of a potential human being is acquired with the appearance of the primitive streak. Acceptance of this concept resolves most of the ethical questions that concern pre-embryo research.

Respect for human dignity

A pre-embryo should be treated with respect for its potential to become a person. The creation of embryos or their abortion for the purpose of contributing their tissue would demean the potential or actual humanity of the embryo and would harm the principle of respect for human dignity. Pre-embryo and embryo research can be performed as long as the pre-embryos were not created or aborted for research purposes alone, according to this principle. Doing no harm – pre-embryonic or embryonic tissue often becomes available as a result of pregnancy termination.

The legality of induced abortions remains controversial in the Western culture. It is possible that the subsequent use of pre-embryonic or embryonic tissue for research will encourage abortions that would otherwise not occur. This would make the issue of pre-embryo research unseparable from the issue of abortion, thus causing much greater controversy than exists already. Many women are ambivalent about abortion. This ambivalence may be tipped in favor of pregnancy termination if the women are informed that some good may come of it, i.e. given some incentive. This argument dictates that the use of pre-embryonic or embryonic tissue should not be allowed if it stimulates abortions that would otherwise not take place. Similarly, the subsequent use of IVF pre-embryos might encourage their intentional production for research purposes. A clear distinction must be made between pre-embryos from spontaneous abortion, where the incentive argument does not apply, and pre-embryos from induced abortions.

The use of pre-embryos from spontaneous abortion would only partially solve the problem, because 50% of these pre-embryos are chromosomally abnormal and thus their use may be limited. A distinction can be made as to the cases when tissue from induced abortion could be used:

(1) Induced abortion in order to save the mother's life is a generally acceptable procedure, except by those who believe that the pre-embryo acquires full human status on conception. The use of pre-embryonic tissue from these abortions may not be more questionable than the use of pre-embryos from spontaneous abortions. In order to prevent conflict of interests from affecting the advice given to patients on the issue, it is proposed that the mother, as well as the medical personnel who perform induced abortions, should not be allowed any direct or indirect benefit from the subsequent use of tissue.

(2) Induced abortion for maternal reasons other than life-saving procedures. A physician or medical center should not feel obligated to participate in research or therapy involving such tissue, if morally incapable of doing so.

(3) Induced abortion for contributing embryonic tissue is unacceptable and harms the principle of respect for human dignity. However, if we accept the idea that the pre-embryo is an integral part of the mother's body she may be able to do with

it as she wishes. Pre-embryo research could apply for the first category.

Slippery slope argument

The slippery slope argument claims that if a given act is allowed, it may end with unacceptable results. This is because there is a series of acts in between the original act and the unacceptable outcome that cannot be distinguished one from another. This argument claims that it is difficult to find the cut-off point between a pre-embryo and a human being. Starting with pre-embryo research, we might end up with research on human beings, similar to the monstrous experiments conducted by the Nazis in World War Two. Creating IVF pre-embryos solely for research purposes might similarly lead to creating neonates for medical experiments. Only a broad consensus regarding the cut-off point may give an answer to the slippery slope argument.

Autonomy rights of the patients

The demand for obtaining informed consent is derived from this principle. Autonomy, or the right to choose, is dependent on three conditions: the status of a human being; the actual ability to choose in a fully autonomous manner; and the moral right to act according to the chosen will. The first condition depends on our view of the moral status of the pre-embryo. The last condition could be naturally fulfilled. The pre-embryo is not able to voice its choice, so the second condition would not apply.

If 'substitute judgement' is to be accepted, then the lack of authentic pre-embryonic consent is not an ethical contraindication to performing pre-embryo research. An agreement for the use of pre-embryonic tissue for essential research can be based on the assumption that the pre-embryo is endowed with the natural goodness and the fine qualities of humanity. If the pre-embryo is considered an integral part of the mother, then it is her informed consent that should be acquired.

The many benefits of pre-embryo research have been outlined. There can be little dispute as to the worthiness as research subjects because they confer great benefits for the human race. Thus, the principle of beneficence is in favor of pre-embryo research.

Control of pre-embryo research

Licensing embryo research does not imply moral indifference. However, licensing without regulating does. It is obvious that cloning, placing of human embryos in other species and altering the genetic structure must be explicitly forbidden. A high respect for the nature of their research is the fundamental characteristic of scientists. Within the ethical restraint imposed by statute and regulation, there is no convincing reason why embryo research should not be performed for ends sufficiently serious. 'In communities which, while putting a very high value on human life (a value which impels them to take so much trouble to foster it) do not attribute value to undifferentiated embryonic cells, embryo research may be performed'. Embryo research must be subject to all the ethical restraints that are applied to any medical relationship. Informed consent must be obtained. The physician must not yield to a patient's demand to perform research or supply treatment if the physician renders it medically inadvisable.

Pre-implantation diagnosis causes a dilemma of sex disclosure. When pre-implantation diagnosis is performed for diagnosing a sex-linked disorder, disclosure of the sex of the embryo is legitimate. Sex selection based on personal wish is unethical. It is not part of medical duty to support the devaluing of the female sex, which is most commonly discriminated against, or to promote an unbalanced population structure.

Considering the use of embryos acquired from pregnancy termination links us with the heated issue of abortion. Those who argue that induced abortion is completely wrong in all circumstances, argue that the use of the products of abortion, even for good purposes, compound the wrong and should be prohibited.

Discussion of the use of the embryo for research should not be opened with the pregnant woman until after she has made the decision to abort. Obtaining consent for each procedure must be entirely separate. Medical teams involved in abortions and in research should be separated, the research must be approved by a local research ethics committee and the passage of tissue should go through an intermediate tissue bank.

In *in vitro* fertilization, in order to enhance the probability that an adequate number of normally developing embryos will result, more oocytes are fertilized than will be transferred to the woman. Sometimes the number of resulting embryos exceeds expectations. They become 'spare' embryos and may be cryopreserved for the couple's future use, donated to a recipient, donated for research, or disposed of. The persons who should decide the disposition of the embryos are those who provide the gametes, through the process of informed consent. Their choices should be made devoid of financial or other coercion. 'Spare' embryos are preferable to embryos generated specifically for research because of the concern that women will be placed at unnecessary risk during the required ovulation induction process, and the preference for a process that is less vulnerable to the commercialization of gametes. Research, which is not intended to benefit the subject on whom it is performed, requires more justification, especially if it involves a risk of harm to the subject. Neither medical practice nor biomedical research is static. Procedures move over time from being experimental to innovative treatments to becoming accepted as part of orthodox medical practice.

The judgement of whether a research project is ethically acceptable must be made on the basis of a proposal preceding the project, and not after its completion in light of its success or failure to provide the anticipated results. Validation must be found in the results of previous research or clinical application, which provide a basis for the reasonable expectation, and must be seen as a matter of professional opinion. Embryo research is argued to be justified as therapeutic research, because it is necessary to improve the success rate of IVF for the benefit of the women undergoing the treatment.

Human embryo research is subject to ethical controls that are generally not imposed on other areas of clinical practice.

The reason behind this is that human life is sacred and possesses unique dignity, a principle that must not be eroded under any circumstances. Research must be performed with the integrity proper to all scientific endeavors. Research must be performed with the constant reminder of ethical limitations, which must not be forsaken. To prevent misuse, strict guidelines for regulation must be applied. Setting and monitoring guidelines should help clarify acceptable versus unacceptable.

CONCLUSION

It is undeniable that the human condition has been generally improved through systematic biological and medical research. The new reproductive era introduces new considerations, involving simultaneously formidable risks as well as substantial benefits. Human pre-embryos deserve special respect because some possess the potential to become human beings.

There are dilemmas in setting and monitoring guidelines to help clarify acceptable versus unacceptable on human pre-embryos. Pre-embryo research should be conducted under restrictions and supervision by the society.

References

1. Sadler TW. *Langman's Medical Embryology*, 6th edn. Baltimore: Williams & Wilkins, 1990
2. Monk M. A stem-line model for cellular and chromosomal differentiation in early mouse development. *Differentiation* 1981;19:71–6
3. Grobstein C. *Science and the Unborn*. New York: Basic Books, 1988:21–39
4. Chard T. Frequency of implantation and early pregnancy loss in natural cycles. *Baillieres Clin Obstet Gynaecol* 1991;5:179–89
5. Human Fertilization and Embryo Authority (HFEA). *Donated Ovarian Tissue in Embryo Research and Assisted Conception*. London: Public Consultation Document, Jan 1994, report July 1994
6. Schenker JG. Medical and ethical aspects of advance technology in reproduction. Presented at the *European Congress of Obstetrics and Gynaecology*, Malmo, 2001
7. Schenker JG. Preembryo: therapeutic approaches. *Ann Med* 1993;25:265–70
8. Fasoulitis S, Schenker JG. Failures in assisted reproductive technology, in press
9. Cohen J, Simons RS, Fehilly CB, *et al.* Factors affecting survival and implantation of cryopreserved human blastocysts. *J In Vitro Fertil Embryo Transfer* 1986;3:46–52
10. Shushan A, Eisenberg VH, Schenker JG. Subfertility in the era of assisted reproduction: changes and consequences. *Fertil Steril* 1995;64:459–69
11. Plachot M, de Grouchy J, Junca AM, *et al.* Chromosome analysis of human oocytes and embryos: does delayed fertilization increase chromosome imbalance? *Hum Reprod* 1988;3:125–7
12. West JD, Gosden JR, Angell RR, *et al.* Sexing whole human preembryos by *in situ* hybridization with a Y-chromosome specific DNA probe. *Hum Reprod* 1988;3:1010–19
13. Handyside AH, Kontogianni EH, Hardy K, *et al.* Pregnancies from biopsied preimplantation embryos sexed by Y specific DNA amplification. *Nature* 1990;344:768–70
14. Handyside AH, Pattison JK, Penketh RJA, *et al.* Biopsy of human pre-implantation embryos and sexing by DNA amplification. *Lancet* 1989;1:347–9
15. Slavin S, Naparstek B, Bach S, *et al.* Intrauterine bone marrow transplantation as a means for correction of genetic disorders through induction of prenatal transplantation tolerance. In Hobbs JR, ed. *Correction of Certain Genetic Diseases*

by Transplantation. London: COGNET, 1989: 54–63

16. Schenker JG. Women's reproductive health: monotheistic religious perspectives. *Int J Obstet Gynecol* 2000;70:77–88

17. Grobstein C. *Science and the Unborn: Choosing Human Features*. New York: Basic Books, 1988

Change in public demand for genetic counselling in the past 25 years

11

Z. Papp

Genetic counselling is a field of professional expertise that involves diagnosis, provision of information and consultation with individuals about their genetic make-up and chances of bearing a child with a severe birth defect. Genetic counselling units are usually headed by medical geneticists and are located in large university hospitals or medical centers.

Genetic counsellors typically consult with couples who have previously borne a child with a defect, have one or more relatives suffering from a disease, or have a pregnancy in which they are afraid of preconceptual or prenatal damage to the embryo or fetus. Most clients are referred by other physicians, though increasing numbers are self-referred. Couples who just want to obtain information about their genetic make-up are also considered legitimate clients.

Genetic counselling developed from two different occupational groups[1]: the early pioneers, the biologists and geneticists, belonging to the profession of natural science, and the medical doctors, mainly pediatricians and obstetricians, who later assumed control over the field, belonging to the old established professions.

The pioneers in human genetics were mainly self-trained biologists and geneticists. Their high status as scientists was derived from working in areas involving mysteries, elements considered sacred by society. They worked within academic departments, isolated from the fields of psychology and medicine. Geneticists dealt with population genetics and often were more interested in the effects on human evolution than on the individual[2].

During the first third of the 20th century, genetic counselling services offered premarital, preconception and postconception heredity counselling. The counsellor proffered highly directive advice as to whether or not to marry or reproduce[3]. The typical genetic counselling process consisted of a sole interview in which a pedigree was taken and a recurrence risk estimate presented. This approach fitted with the eugenics movement's interest in bringing about a decrease in harmful genes and an increase in desirable genes[4,5]. Even as late as 1960, Curt Stern, in his textbook[6], used the term genetic counselling interchangeably with eugenics counselling.

By the 1950s, important breakthroughs in the study of hereditary diseases involving enzyme deficiencies and the study of cyto-logical and chromosomal genetics broadened the clinical applications of human genetics, allowing for the permanent linkage of genetics and medicine[7]. The entrance of medicine as a discipline substituted concern about the future of the gene pool for an emphasis on the prevention of the birth of individuals who might have a severe birth defect. The service orientation of the doctor, aimed at helping the individual patient/client, overrode the social implications in many physicians' minds as well as in the public's mind.

OBSTETRIC GENETICS

The neonate is no longer our youngest patient. Fetal medicine has emerged as a scientific discipline and the fetus, its chromosomes, enzymes and individual genes can be examined *in utero*. Currently employed prenatal tests include amniocentesis, chorionic villus sampling, cordocentesis and ultrasound, the latter enabling us to recognize major anatomical defects in the fetus[8].

With the wider availability of genetic counselling there are four main roads to the prevention of genetic disease[8]:

(1) Individuals can be identified as being at high risk of transmitting harmful mutant genes, and may be informed of this (classical genetic counselling). Their options may include various forms of contraception, sterilization, adoption, artificial insemination by donor, *in vitro* fertilization (egg donation), preimplantation diagnosis (preferential selection of unaffected pre-embryos for transfer) and taking the risk of a normally conceived pregnancy, with or without prenatal diagnosis.

(2) Preconceptual damage to the gametes (mutagens, clastogens) can be avoided by improvements in public health and hygiene, by more intensive programs of immunization (rubella), by reduced exposure to viruses, ionizing radiation, unnecessary medication and other potentially harmful factors, by provision, where appropriate, of some vitamins, and by generally raising the standards of antenatal care.

(3) The increased use of prenatal or neonatal screening, or prenatal diagnosis, to allow measures to be taken earlier which are specially designed to support the genetically or environmentally damaged fetus or neonate (fetal/neonatal therapy).

(4) Where there are no real prospects for treatment, and for major malformations or highly damaging or deleterious genetic disease, interruption of pregnancy may be offered by means of induced abortion or premature induction of labor.

As a result of the many recent fundamental advances in medicine and science, there are now these four modes of prevention (genetic counselling, pre- and periconceptual care,

fetal therapy and abortion), but they cannot be put into practice without the goodwill and collaboration of the parents. Often, they also require the assistance or intervention of an obstetrician. In this respect, we should not expect geneticists to become obstetricians, but rather that obstetricians master fetal diagnosis and understand basic genetics, in theory and practice.

Obstetrics must not only be concerned with preserving what has already been achieved – the ability to ensure that a healthy fetus be born healthy and not die or suffer permanent damage as a result of obstetric complications – but must also strive to bring children into the world who are well endowed mentally and physically, like their parents. Many embryos, carriers of mutant and/or defective genes, or badly damaged by malformation, will inevitably die *in utero*, as a result of biological selection. However, where they survive to be born alive, despite the natural screening process, families and individuals may experience many years of suffering.

PRENATAL GENETIC COUNSELLING

I received my basic knowledge in genetics from my university professor of biology and genetics when I was a medical student in 1960. In 1964, I decided to become an obstetrician who was capable of understanding basic genetics and of serving the interest of seeing fetuses unaffected by any disease[9]. I graduated in 1966 and started my career at the University Department of Obstetrics and Gynecology in Debrecen. With my director's support, I established a genetic counselling service within the obstetric department. During the first 10 years, I worked to introduce new techniques applicable in pregnancy, such as amniocentesis, chromosome analysis from amniotic fluid cells, post-mortem cord blood lymphocytes, etc.[10-13]. The program was officially confirmed in 1976.

I also have experience in classical genetic counselling and, in 1976, I combined this with the prenatal diagnosis and screening. This approach is called 'obstetric genetics'[8]. The main components of a prenatal genetic counselling service are given below[8].

Consultation (interview) with the couple

The counsellor must answer four questions for the couple:

(1)   What is the disease in question?
(2)   How severe is it and what can be done to treat the affected child?
(3)   How is it caused/inherited?
(4)   What can be done to avoid or prevent the disease in the future?

It is essential to present a clear and full description of the relevant disorder and to answer all questions honestly and promptly. A good and harmonious relationship should develop or be developed between the counsellor and the couple. The physician–patient relationship, always important in medicine, is thus replaced by a physician/counsellor–family relationship, which deepens through the course of counselling. This sort of relationship is necessary for the proper help and management of high-risk couples receiving counselling. A great deal depends on the character of the individual physician.

The physician/counsellor gives information, and the parents, in the light of their own individual circumstances and attitudes, make the decision. We call our practice non-directive prenatal genetic counselling[14].

Cytogenetic, enzyme and molecular genetics laboratories

The diagnosis, in an affected child or adult, or in the fetus *in utero*, must be made with the most up-to-date methods available. Obtaining old or recent medical records, special laboratory tests and other investigations (maybe involving referral to other specialist departments) can all be relevant or necessary procedures. All units, including the genetic laboratory, should be in the same building, which makes communication between the units and the transportation of patients and various tissue samples from the operating room to the laboratories easier.

Ultrasound laboratory with diagnostic techniques for sampling

Fetal ultrasound has a fundamental role in prenatal diagnosis. Unlike radiography, ultrasound diagnosis is risk-free for the mother, fetus and the person performing the examination. It is atraumatic, non-invasive and does not produce discomfort. Prolonged examinations may be performed, and may be repeated as often as necessary. Ultrasound examination provides an emotional experience for both parents, who see the fetus for the first time as it moves *in utero*, and the parental relationship gains in strength, as does the 'bonding' between parents and unborn child. Invasive procedures, such as amniocentesis, chorionic villus sampling and cordocentesis, start with and are guided by ultrasound examination.

Screening of fetal anomalies

After showing that, in pregnancies with a high risk of neural tube defects, the previously recommended amniocentesis may be omitted if the sonogram is performed by experienced personnel[15], and following our positive experiences in ultrasound screening[16,17], on January 1, 1988 in Eastern Hungary, we introduced non-selected, second-trimester ultrasound screening for fetal anomalies in low-risk women. Since I became the head of the First Department of Obstetrics and Gynecology at Semmelweis University in Budapest in 1990, we have been able to introduce this screening protocol throughout the whole of Hungary over the past 10 years. The Hungarian Society of Ultrasound in Obstetrics and Gynecology, founded in 1992, oversees quality assurance and carries out annual testing of obstetricians, gynecologists and sonographers working in the field of ultrasound[18,19]. In Hungary, four screening ultrasounds are offered for low-risk pregnant women (in the 8th, 18th, 28th and 38th weeks of gestation).

When an abnormal or suspicious prenatal ultrasound finding is obtained, most cases are referred to our department. In this way, we are able to gather extensive experience in the prenatal diagnosis and fetopathological evaluation of congenital anomalies[20].

Termination ward

Ideally, induction of abortion should be effective, without causing danger to the mother or damage to the fetus, and should allow confirmation of the pre-termination diagnosis, full histopathological examination and further investigations where appropriate[21,22]. Cervical ripening in first-trimester abortion can be achieved with medical management using laminaria, prostaglandins, progesterone agonists and/or prostaglandin analogs such as sulprostone, gemeprost, misoprostol and methotrexate[23]. These methods of pregnancy termination cannot be used after the 12th week, when labor must be induced. Although the fetus is usually expelled completely, instrumental emptying of the uterus is often required because of incomplete expulsion of placenta and membranes. In second-trimester terminations, prostaglandins are widely used. We have also had good experience with transcervical extra-amniotic instillation of ethacridine lactate (a myometrium-stimulating acridine dye)[21].

Fetopathological unit

Fetopathology has been, and continues to be, an important issue and an integral part of the genetic counselling process. Post-termination pathological and special laboratory examinations can confirm the prenatal diagnosis. Diagnosis is not simply a question of terminology, because the diagnosis and the estimated risk of recurrence depend on the final opinion presented by the fetopathologists. Only fetopathology can answer all the questions of differential diagnosis.

Currently, fetal pathology, the publicity of fetal pathology and the retaining of fetal organs raise sensible medico-legal issues in terms of informed consent and human rights. We are still convinced, however, that within certain limits fetopathological examination must be a part of the graduate, the post-graduate and specialist's education. This can be achieved by participating in autopsies or demonstrations of typical or rare developmental abnormalities. We believe that this specialty must be a part of the specialist and sonographer's training. Nothing can compare with *in situ* fetal demonstration in terms of effectiveness. It serves to better the specialist's education, for the benefit of society.

Post-termination (bereavement) counselling with availability of a psychologist

Pregnant women, even those not burdened by genetic problems, often become anxious when thinking of their unborn child. Women at high risk of having a malformed fetus may feel shame and remorse in addition to anxiety. The genetic counsellor must understand and attempt to satisfy the psychological needs and demands of the couple.

It is very important to provide follow-up for women who have had a termination for fetal reasons. These women may become very depressed immediately after termination and require support that is difficult to get from their own general practitioners. A clinical psychologist and a social worker have always been available in our department to help patients deal with their loss in complicated cases of abortion, and to provide counselling or care following unsuccessful pregnancies. They also need a chance to discuss the 'genetics' again at a later time. This includes discussing the recent termination and the specific fetal malformations/aneuploidy, and also the prospects for future pregnancies and how the next pregnancy might be managed[24].

Assisted reproduction unit with capability of blastomere biopsy, nuclear transfer and cytoplasmic transfer

In the past few decades, scientifically based procedures have been developed which enable children to be born independently of sexual intercourse and, as a result, thousands of people are alive today who were conceived with the help of such techniques. At the beginning, assisted reproductive technologies gained ground all over the world as a treatment for sterility and infertility. Later, they acquired a role in the prevention of certain genetic diseases.

Blastomere biopsy is an important part of the preimplantation genetic diagnostic procedure for monogenically inherited diseases such as cystic fibrosis. At this time, nuclear transfer and cytoplasmic transfer are the most promising methods in the prevention of mitochondrially determined disorders. Mitochondrial genetics is quite different from Mendelian genetics, and it is important to recognize this when attempting diagnosis and counselling for this group of disorders[25].

Ethical and legal background

The couple may choose to attempt or continue a pregnancy, or they may choose to terminate. A free decision is made by the parents and actions taken are within the law. Society creates the laws that regulate the termination of pregnancy. The legal rules and the professional codes and regulations provide a framework by which each case must be individually evaluated.

In Hungary, there is a legal framework for abortion, based on genetic indications. We have also contributed to the development of this system[26,27]. Legally, pregnancies with a prenatal diagnosis of genetic or anatomical defects that are compatible with postnatal life (such as trisomy 21 and spina bifida) can be terminated until the 24th week of gestation, at the request of the couple. If the defects are incompatible with postnatal life (such as anencephaly and bilateral renal agenesis),

pregnancies may be terminated in any subsequent week of gestation. In Hungary, following the prenatal diagnosis of severe conditions, 99% of married couples request termination of pregnancy or the induction of premature delivery, and opt for reproductive compensation[8,28].

Computer database and follow-up

All cases from our genetic counselling service have been recorded in our computer since 1976[29]. We implemented non-directive counselling from the start of this service, so we have over 50 000 counselling situations from which to study patients' views and reproductive decisions. We also obtain follow-up information on children born following a pathological prenatal diagnosis.

PRENATAL GENETIC COUNSELLING SERVICE DATA

The genetic counselling service founded in Debrecen was accepted and supported officially by the government in 1976. Since then, all cases have been registered and stored in the computer database system. Data from the first 15 years (1976–1990) were collected in Debrecen. In 1990, I organized a genetic counselling unit in Budapest, as well. I also collected data from the first decade of the period 1991–2000.

When registering cases, in addition to personal identification data, we always note: the main reasons for genetic counselling (at least three in every case); the established specific risk; the attitude of the couple; the examinations performed, including prenatal diagnosis; and the outcome of the pregnancy. Possible attitudes of the couples involved are presented in Table 1.

In the present study, I collected experiences from the past 25 years (1976–2000) and, in order to demonstrate the changing demands, differentiated five 5-year subgroups (1976–1980, 1981–1985, 1986–1990, 1991–1995 and 1996–2000). During these 25 years, 51 385 couples were counselled regarding 54 018

Table 1 *Possible attitudes of married couples regarding genetic counselling*

Genetic counselling	Attitude
Pregnancy can be attempted or carried to term (genetic risk <10%, no prenatal diagnosis)	genetic counselling was followed
Pregnancy can be attempted or carried to term (genetic risk <10%, no prenatal diagnosis)	genetic counselling was not followed (no pregnancy was attempted or termination of pregnancy was requested based on other reasons)
Pregnancy can be attempted or carried to term (genetic risk <10%, prenatal diagnosis available)	genetic counselling was followed, and prenatal diagnosis was performed
Pregnancy can be attempted or carried to term (genetic risk <10%, prenatal diagnosis available)	genetic counselling was followed partially (the pregnancy was achieved, but no prenatal diagnosis was performed)
Pregnancy can be attempted or carried to term (genetic risk <10%, prenatal diagnosis available)	genetic counselling was not followed (no pregnancy was attempted, or termination of pregnancy was requested based on other reasons)
Pregnancy can be attempted or carried to term under the protection of prenatal diagnosis (genetic risk 10–99%)	genetic counselling was followed and prenatal diagnosis was performed
Pregnancy can be attempted or carried to term under the protection of prenatal diagnosis (genetic risk 10–99%)	genetic counselling was followed partially (pregnancy was achieved, but no prenatal diagnosis was performed)
Pregnancy can be attempted or carried to term under the protection of prenatal diagnosis (genetic risk 10–99%)	genetic counselling was not followed (no pregnancy was attempted or termination of pregnancy was requested based on other reasons)
It is not advisable to attempt pregnancy or to carry the pregnancy to term (genetic risk ≥ 25%, no prenatal diagnosis)	genetic counselling was followed (no pregnancy was attempted or termination of pregnancy was requested)
It is not advisable to attempt pregnancy or to carry the pregnancy to term (genetic risk ≥ 25%, no prenatal diagnosis)	genetic counselling was not followed (pregnancy was attempted or termination of pregnancy was not requested)
The decision of the married couple will be based on the knowledge of the genetic risk of medium value (≥ 10 and <25%)	
Genetic counselling because of sterility	
Other cases of genetic counselling	

pregnancies or before planned pregnancies in 65 934 situations (requests to be answered) (Table 2, Figure 1).

Table 3 shows the distribution of the various genetic situations addressed during genetic counselling. The couples' decisions in cases where the Mendelian inherited disease or condition was the main reason for genetic counselling and where the risk was ≥ 25%, are shown in Table 4. In Tables 5 and 6 the maternal age distribution at time of counselling and the number of genetic amniocenteses performed because of advanced maternal age can be seen.

COUNSELLING TOPICS

The number of couples requesting genetic counselling has continuously increased since the establishment of our genetic counselling service (Table 2, Figure 1). This increase had a transient decrease in the beginning of the 1990s, because of the transfer of staff from Debrecen to Budapest. Independent of this slight decrease, more and more couples (mainly pregnant women) demand genetic counselling. The distribution of genetic diseases or congenital anomalies as indicators for counselling is influenced mainly by the

Table 2 *Genetic counselling data*

	1976–1980	*1981–1985*	*1986–1990*	*1991–1995**	*1996–2000*	*Total*
Number of couples	2088	9226	10 877	10 214	18 980	51 385
Number of preconceptional or prenatal counselling sessions	2498	9721	11 761	10 480	19 558	54 018
Number of requests to be answered	3166	11 970	14 474	11 881	24 443	65 934

*The Budapest genetic counselling service was established in 1990. This is the reason for the decline in numbers

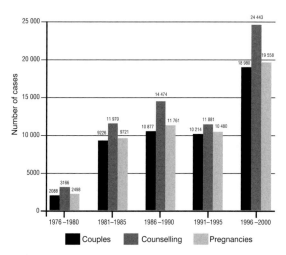

Figure 1 *Data from the Genetic Counselling Service, Debrecen, Budapest (1976–2000)*

continuous improvement of pre- and post-natal imaging, ultrasound techniques and the availability of molecular genetic methods (Table 3). Therefore, the detected cases of corpus callosum agenesis, Dandy–Walker anomaly, thoracic malformations (such as Ivemark syndrome), congenital heart defects and some monogenically inherited disorders with known gene localization, such as adult polycystic kidney disease, Huntington disease, neurofibromatosis and intestinal polyposis are increasing. The detected cases of some conditions, such as metachromatic leukodystrophy and Sanfilippo syndrome, are decreasing, because of the difficulties in diagnosing enzyme disorders in pediatric practice in Hungary.

The demand for counselling from couples at high risk for cystic fibrosis, Duchenne muscular dystrophy, hemophilia, osteogenesis imperfecta and Werdnig–Hoffmann disease has been extensive during the past 25 years. Despite improving prospects, these are still crippling disorders with a relatively high prevalence, and many parents of affected children seek prenatal diagnosis for subsequent pregnancies. When prenatal diagnosis was not available, the reproductive decision was strongly influenced by the 25–50% genetic risk of disease in future offspring. A considerable proportion of parents with an affected child changed their intended family size or abstained from further childbearing. The availability of prenatal diagnosis induced a change in reproductive planning in a majority of parents with one or more children affected by such diseases[30]. Our experiences confirm that the availability and reliability of prenatal diagnosis are the most decisive factors in the reproductive planning of couples at high risk for such diseases[28]. The strength of the desire to have children can be inferred from the number of affected and healthy children the couples had during the decision-making period[30].

The desire to have children is also reflected by the position the affected child holds in the birth order. Our experience shows that couples were more likely to plan a subsequent pregnancy when the affected child was the first-born[28].

When a Mendelian inherited disease or condition was the main reason for genetic counselling, the risk was high and prenatal diagnosis was available, only 15% of the couples requested termination or did not attempt a pregnancy (Table 4). The majority

Table 3 *Distribution of the indications for counselling from 1976 to 2000*

Indication	1976–1980	1981–1985	1986–1990	1991–1995	1996–2000	Total
Mendelian inherited disease or						
condition	132	415	668	412	584	2211
autosomal dominant trait	22	81	108	103	159	473
autosomal recessive trait	88	227	420	220	290	1245
X-linked recessive trait	22	104	136	87	131	480
X-linked dominant trait	0	3	4	2	4	13
Consanguinity	29	70	77	38	71	285
Chromosome aberrations	101	178	279	294	678	1530
Multifactorially determined						
common chronic diseases	210	1002	1001	342	720	3275
Congenital anomalies	602	1793	1959	843	1727	6924
pathology of placenta and membranes	4	33	47	21	10	115
multiple malformation syndrome	126	338	302	154	316	1236
thoracic malformation	94	341	403	196	468	1502
abdominal malformation	38	130	128	48	72	416
cystic kidney disease	10	52	65	50	78	255
obstructive uropathy	3	17	31	13	16	80
skeletal malformation	39	125	119	69	106	458
craniospinal malformation	279	709	774	246	568	2576
immune and non-immune hydrops	8	38	71	44	44	205
pathology of multiple pregnancy	1	10	19	2	49	81
Maternal serum AFP screening	14	1493	1255	1193	4805	8760
high AFP level	1	33	137	591	2013	2775
low AFP level	0	0	18	585	2682	3285
MSAFP + ultrasound screening						
organized by the service	13	1460	1100	17	110	2700
Abnormal sonographic finding	16	227	489	1721	3245	5698
fetal anatomy	5	200	443	1704	2806	5158
amniotic fluid volume (poly- and						
oligohydramnios)	11	27	46	17	439	540
Unsuccessful previous pregnancies	422	1371	1230	508	1042	4573
recurrent abortion and/or perinatal						
death (stillbirth or infant death)	412	1356	1217	507	1032	4524
hydatidiform mole	10	15	13	1	10	49
Perinatal damage, mental handicap						
(not classified)	126	302	282	139	239	1088
Teratogenic exposition during pregnancy	1065	3426	3747	1539	3150	12 927
drug (medicine) and/or chemical	559	2185	2466	1047	2092	8349
bacterial, viral, protozoon	333	836	797	273	550	2789
others	173	405	484	219	508	1789
Advanced maternal age						
(as a main request)	86	777	2598	4338	6710	14 509
Infertility	298	547	536	210	701	2292
sterility	126	306	296	70	83	881
pregnancy conceived by assisted						
reproduction technology	1	5	3	35	444	488
amenorrhea, intersexuality	171	236	237	105	174	923
Trivial complaint	65	369	353	304	771	1862
TOTAL	3166	11 970	14 474	11 881	24 443	65 934

AFP, α-fetoprotein; MSAFP, maternal serum AFP

Table 4 *Decisions made by couples in cases where a Mendelian inherited disease or condition was the main indicator for genetic counselling (risk ≥ 25%)*

Inheritance	Prenatal diagnosis available			Prenatal diagnosis not available	
	Prenatal diagnosis performed	Prenatal diagnosis not requested	Terminated without prenatal diagnosis	Termination requested	Pregnancy continued
Autosomal dominant	12	23	12	69	90
Autosomal recessive	265	102	55	64	131
X-linked recessive	124	59	38	10	17
X-linked dominant	2	2	0	3	0
Total	403	186	105	146	238

Table 5 *Maternal age distribution at time of counselling*

Maternal age (years)	1976–1980		1981–1985		1986–1990		1991–1995		1996–2000		Total	
	n	%	n	%	n	%	n	%	n	%	n	%
<35	2295	92.0	8406	86.5	8755	74.4	6117	58.4	13 595	69.5	39 168	72.5
35–37	96	3.8	568	5.8	1277	10.9	1838	17.5	2890	14.8	6669	12.3
38–40	66	2.6	405	4.2	1104	9.4	1678	16.0	2035	10.4	5288	9.8
41–43	30	1.2	250	2.6	517	4.4	709	6.8	864	4.4	2370	4.4
>43	11	0.4	92	0.9	108	0.9	138	1.3	174	0.9	523	1.0
Total	2498	100.0	9721	100.0	11 761	100.00	10 480	100.0	19 558	100.0	54 018	100.0

Table 6 *Number of prenatal chromosome analyses requested and performed. Values in parentheses are the numbers of patients of advanced maternal age (≥ 35 years)*

1976–1980		1981–1985		1986–1990		1991–1995		1996–2000	
Year	n	Year	n	Year	n	Year	n	Year	n
1976	5	1981	59	1986	120	1991	288	1996	1033
1977	6	1982	84	1987	149	1992	471	1997	1313
1978	5	1983	101	1988	209	1993	755	1998	1339
1979	11	1984	104	1989	304	1994	823	1999	1564
1980	27	1985	118	1990	146	1995	867	2000	1769
Total	54 (48)		466 (428)		928 (903)		3204 (2050)		7018 (3011)

of women (85%) decided to attempt or continue a pregnancy, and nearly 70% of them requested prenatal diagnosis. This distribution of decision-making behavior was consistent throughout the past 25 years and was mainly influenced by the psychological and emotional attitudes of the couples.

Maternal serum α-fetoprotein (AFP) screening for the detection of neural tube defects has been a routine practice in Hungary for many years. Similarly, ultrasound screening for fetal anomalies is another option which has been accepted by the majority of pregnant women. The biochemical screening for trisomy 21 is not widely used in our country, but, because of the anxiety and concern caused by 'low maternal serum AFP level' many pregnant women are referred to our center (Table 3). Consequently, there are a great number of unnecessary genetic amniocenteses and prenatal chromosome analyses. Conversely, most abnormal sonographic findings in women referred to our department are confirmed, resulting in many prenatally diagnosed cases of fetal anomalies and pathological pregnancy cases. The number of patients seeking advice because of unsuccessful previous pregnancies is decreasing slightly, because most recurrent miscarriages are not genetic in origin.

Anxiety because of teratogenic exposure during pregnancy is still a frequent counselling issue, because the administration of drugs during pregnancy is still unnecessarily high even though a large proportion of drugs have no real clinical indication during pregnancy. By analyzing the outcome of pregnancies with drug exposure during early gestation, it is relevant that no significant increase in congenital anomalies can be observed in these cases. In this respect, the large number of pregnant women afraid of the consequences of teratogenic exposure is not justified and public health education is required.

The age distribution of women receiving counselling has changed over the past 25 years: the number of women 35–43 years of age and their requests for prenatal chromosome analysis are continuously increasing (Tables 5 and 6). Between 1976 and 1980, 25% of women over 34 years of age requested genetic amniocentesis. Since 1990, this proportion has risen to nearly 50%. The indication for prenatal chromosome analysis has justifiably changed in favor of abnormal ultrasound findings and the large number of positive biochemical screening test results.

At the beginning, our genetic counselling service dealt with infertile couples and amenorrhea patients as well, but new assisted reproductive technology has changed the management of infertility and a modern endocrine laboratory has also been established. These couples now look to the genetic counselling service for prenatal chromosome analysis (Table 3).

NON-DIRECTIVE OR DIRECTIVE GENETIC COUNSELLING?

The information to be given in the context of genetic counselling should include:

(1) The purpose and nature of the intervention;
(2) The possible risks;
(3) The diagnosis and prognosis for the person concerned;
(4) The risk of disease for future children or other family members;
(5) The consequences and choices available for the person concerned.

There is widespread support among medical geneticists and genetic counsellors for non-directiveness and value neutrality in genetic counselling[31,32]. Such support arises from concern about early abuses in the eugenics movement and recognition of the right to privacy and autonomy in reproductive decisions. Recently, discussions have focused on the desirability and practicality of non-directive and value-neutral counselling, with a number of authors questioning whether it is ever possible to achieve[33–35]. Despite the ethos of non-directiveness that has prevailed in genetic counselling, there have been few empirical studies of directiveness, and no method of measuring it has been suggested or tested.

Michie and colleagues have presented a methodology for quantifying directiveness in a clinical genetics setting[36]. What can we learn from this study? First, as stated by the authors, the practice of genetic counselling 'is not characterized … as uniformly non-directive'. Kessler[34] has suggested that directive counselling that supports the client's decision direction is often helpful, but requires 'greater flexibility than dogmatism in genetic counselling practices'.

Genetic counsellors always have the power to influence clients by choosing to discuss one aspect of a situation while ignoring or down-playing another. Through interviews with genetic counsellors and genetic-counselling students, Brunger and Lippman have shown how a genetic-counselling session is context dependent[37]. For example, the information on Down syndrome that is included in a pre-amniocentesis counselling session differs greatly from that in a session concerning a neonate with Down syndrome[38].

A partnership model has evolved that incorporates high levels of both provider and patient participation in decision making[39]. This model acknowledges that the patients' needs and desires be considered and that patients play a role in decision making, but it does not go so far as to advocate that physicians abdicate their role in providing recommendations[40].

A review of the literature provides no evidence that a non-directive approach benefits the clients[41]. On the contrary, there is an indication that genetic-counselling clients may welcome exactly the opposite. Shiloh and Saxe[42] have shown that genetic-counselling clients reported a higher perceived risk associated with more neutral counselling, perhaps stemming from client belief that the counsellor must be concealing bad news. In another study, Furu and colleagues[43] have reported that among individuals with retinitis pigmentosa or choroideremia and their relatives, 80% would like to know the opinion of the genetic counsellor with regard to whether they should have children or undergo abortion after a positive prenatal diagnosis result.

One of the most significant contributions of the Michie study[36] relates to the lack of association of rated directiveness with client satisfaction, fulfilment of client expectation and self-reported client anxiety and concern. The study shows that, even when clients knew the counsellor had an opinion as to what decision they should make, many clients did not feel steered by this opinion. The impli-cation that provider directiveness may not really matter to clients forces us to consider whether focusing on non-directiveness as the

sine qua non of current genetic counselling practice diverts attention from other important goals, process measures or outcomes of genetic counselling. Such consideration is especially timely, given the need for outcome-based measures[44]. In the majority of counsel-ling sessions, there is a lack of agreement between the counsellor and the client as to the agenda items that each wants to address. Without agreement between counsellor and counsellee as to what outcomes to expect, measurements will be meaningless.

Not all individuals at risk for transmitting a genetic defect wish to prevent its occurrence if it means relinquishing biological parenthood; some do not even agree with the counsellor's view that a specific genetic disease ought to be prevented.

I think that the most important principle is to transmit the information in a non-directive manner and adapt it to the needs of each person. As Table 4 shows, we prefer the non-directive approach to genetic counselling. This approach is a logical consequence of the principle that consultants must be assisted in reaching an informed and autonomous decision that is appropriate to their life situ-ation. The options of attempting a pregnancy and requesting prenatal diagnosis belong to the parents. That is the principle of non-directive prenatal genetic counselling. Nevertheless, supportive counselling by social workers and clinical psychologists affiliated with prenatal genetic counselling centers can be essential in helping consultants in their decision-making process. This principle has remained unchanged in our practice for the last 25 years.

Most discussions of non-directiveness have focused on prenatal testing and reproductive decision making, areas in which genetic counselling has been focused for at least 25 years. Genetic counselling will increasingly be provided in conjunction with the offering of presymptomatic or predisposition testing. Because early treatment might be effective for some disorders for which predisposition testing is available, providers arguably should recommend that clients be tested. How likely is it that the doctrine of non-directiveness will or should be upheld in the era of predictive testing for common adult-onset disorders?

For several reasons, it is likely that most clients seeking genetic counselling in conjunction with predictive testing will be given directive counselling. Genetic counselling and testing will increasingly move into the primary care arena and be provided by non-geneticists. There is a perception on the part of non-geneticist physicians that patients want direction. Many physicians believe that opinion seeking on the part of patients is a sign of trust and that not rendering an opinion is irresponsible[45]. The ethicist Caplan believes that primary-care physicians are unlikely to 'warm to suggestions' that conversations become non-directive when the subject turns to heredity. Moreover, he suggests that their patients are unlikely to accept non-directiveness with regard to genetic discussions when the said 'ethos does not prevail in other aspects of their relationships with providers'[46].

PREDICTIVE GENETIC TESTING

Predictive genetic testing is the use of a genetic test in an asymptomatic person to predict future risk of disease. The presymptomatic test is a predictive test with a high risk (almost 100%) for the development of the tested disease. These tests represent a new and growing class of medical tests, differing in fundamental ways from conventional medical diagnostic tests. The hope underlying such testing is that early identification of individuals at risk of a specific condition will lead to reduced morbidity and mortality through targeted screening, surveillance and prevention. Yet the clinical utility of predictive genetic testing for different diseases varies considerably.

A predictive genetic test informs us only about a future condition that may (or may not) develop. The identified risk is sometimes high, as in a positive test for Huntington's disease, but always contains a substantial component of uncertainty, not only regarding whether a specific condition will develop, but

also when it may appear and how severe it will be. Predictive genetic tests often carry a further element of uncertainty: the interventions available for individuals at risk are often untested and recommendations may be based on presumed benefit rather than observations of outcomes.

These uncertainties contrast with the presentation of predictive genetic testing in the popular media, which often fosters an illusion that genetic risk is highly predictable and determinative. In fact, inherent uncertainties in most genetic tests represent a major limitation to their clinical utility.

Whereas conventional diagnostic testing rarely has medical importance for anyone other than the person tested (except in the case of communicable diseases), predictive genetic testing typically has direct implications for family members. Concern for relatives may be an important motivating factor for a patient's desire to undergo such testing. Some family members, however, may resist participating in the testing because they would rather not have information about their genetic risk. The utility of a predictive genetic test will, therefore, depend on whose point of view is considered.

About 5–10% of breast and ovarian cancers result from the inheritance of mutations in the BRCA1 or BRCA2 gene. Predictive genetic testing for breast and ovarian cancer, as for hereditary non-polyposis colon cancer, can be useful to identify those at increased risk. In both breast and ovarian cancer, however, utility is limited because of considerable uncertainty about the predictive value of the test.

A woman carrying a mutation in the BRCA1 or BRCA2 gene may develop breast cancer, ovarian cancer, breast and ovarian cancers, or no cancer at all. Penetrance estimates range from 36 to 85% for breast cancer and 10–44% for ovarian cancer. Moreover, the age at which cancer occurs is widely variable. These uncertainties probably reflect a combination of factors, including the environment, modifying genes, the nature of a woman's specific mutation and purely stochastic processes.

Predictive genetic testing should be accompanied by genetic counselling. In the study by Holtzman and colleagues[47] which explored women's decision-making preferences with regard to genetic testing for susceptibility to breast cancer, they found that most women wanted to hear their providers' recommendation about testing. Women still wanted to make their own decisions, either by choosing to follow their provider's recommendation or by choosing to veto it. If a provider did not give a recommendation based on her expertise, women believed either that the provider was not fulfilling her duty or that they were not getting their money's worth. It has been suggested that concerns about autonomy should shift from focusing on whether the decision was made voluntarily to whether the decision-making process was entered voluntarily. Such a shift would preserve autonomy and empower patients, as they are able to play their preferred role in decision making.

Genetic screening is changing from Mendelian disease ascertainment to predictive testing. We are also learning that the pheno-types of even simple Mendelian disorders are influenced by complex genetic and environmental factors[48–51]. The observations that genotypes rarely predict phenotypes absolutely have significant ramifications for counselling. We must recognize that for single-gene disorders with high penetrance, the information derived from such testing may be relatively easy to interpret and apply. For complex diseases, however, the populations studied and their demographic characteristics are extremely important for extrapolation to counselling of individual patients[52].

It is likely that the goals of genetic counselling vary according to individual client needs and should be established or re-established as each session begins. From the client's point of view, the goal might involve soliciting the counsellor's expert opinion. We need to accept that there are times when the recent challenges of genetics make directiveness permissible or even positive, and elucidate better ways to make our services more responsive to the needs of our clients and their families.

References

1. Reiss A Jr. Occupational mobility of professional markers. *Am Sociol Rev* 1955;20: 693–700

2. Kenen RH. Genetic counseling: the development of a new interdisciplinary occupational field. *Soc Sci Med* 1984;18:541–9

3. Fraser FC. Current issues in medical genetics. *Am J Hum Genet* 1974;26:636–59

4. Dice LR. Heredity clinics, their value for public service and for research. *Am J Hum Genet* 1952; 4:1

5. Herndon CN. Heredity counseling. *Eugenics Q* 1955;2:88–9

6. Stern C. *Principles of Human Genetics*, 2nd edn. San Francisco, CA: W.H. Freeman, 1960

7. Ludmerer K. *Genetics and American Society*. Baltimore: Johns Hopkins, 1972:174–93

8. Papp Z. *Obstetric Genetics*. Budapest: Hungarian Academic Press, 1990

9. Papp Z. The history of fetal diagnosis and therapy: the Semmelweis University experience. *Fetal Diagn Ther* 2002;in press

10. Papp Z, Gardó S, Herpay G, Arvay A. Prenatal sex determination by amniocentesis. *Obstet Gynecol* 1970;36:429–32

11. Papp Z, Gardó S. Cytogenetic analysis of cord-blood lymphocytes. *Lancet* 1970;1:1401–2

12. Papp Z, Gardó S, Méhes K. Intrauterine Diagnose von G/G-Translokation. *Z Geburtshilfe Perinatol* 1972;176:409–12

13. Papp Z, Gardó S, Dolhay B. Chromosome study of couples with repeated spontaneous abortion. *Fertil Steril* 1974;25:713–17

14. Papp Z, Tóth-Pál E, Papp CS. Non-directive prenatal genetic counseling. In Kurjak A, Chervenak FA, eds. *The Fetus as a Patient*. Carnforth, UK: Parthenon Publishing, 1994: 71–7

15. Papp Z, Tóth Z, Török O, Szabó M. Prenatal diagnosis policy without routine amniocentesis in pregnancies with a positive family history for neural tube defects. *Am J Med Genet* 1987;26:103–10

16. Papp Z, Tóth Z, Szabó M, Csécsei K, Török O. Prenatal screening for neural tube defects and

other malformations by both serum AFP and ultrasound. In Kurjak A, ed. *The Fetus as a Patient.* Amsterdam, New York, Oxford: Elsevier Science Publishers, 1985:167–80

17. Papp Z, Tóth-Pál E, Papp CS, Tóth Z, Szabó M, Veress L, Török O. Impact of prenatal mid-trimester screening on the prevalence of fetal structural anomalies: a prospective epidemiological study. *Ultrasound Obstet Gynecol* 1995;6: 320–6

18. Papp Z. Quality assurance in obstetric and gynecological ultrasound in Hungary [Editorial]. *Ultrasound Obstet Gynecol* 1996;7:305–6

19. Szabó I, Csabay L, Tóth Z, Török O, Papp Z. Quality assurance in obstetric and gynecologic ultrasound: the Hungarian model. *Ann NY Acad Sci* 1998;847:99–102

20. Papp Z, Csécsei K, Lindenbaum RH, Szeifert GT, Tóth Z, Váradi V. *Atlas of Fetal Diagnosis.* Amsterdam, London, New York, Tokyo: Elsevier, 1992

21. Papp Z. Spontaneous and indicated abortions. In Iffy L, Apuzzio JJ, Vintzileos AM, eds. *Operative Obstetrics.* New York: McGraw-Hill, Inc., 1992:29–49

22. Marton T, Tankó A, Gávai M, Papp Z. Pathological evaluation in the first trimester. In Kurjak A, Chervenak FA, Carrera JM, eds. *The Embryo as a Patient.* Carnforth, UK: Parthenon Publishing, 2001:213–21

23. Gávai M, Papp Z. Management of early abortion. In Kurjak A, Chervenak FA, Carrera JM, eds. *The Embryo as a Patient.* Carnforth, UK: Parthenon Publishing, 2001:121–8

24. Gávai M, Papp Z. Post-termination counselling after abnormal prenatal genetic diagnosis. In Cosmi EV, ed. *The Fetus as a Patient.* Bologna: Monduzzi Editore, 2000:43–6

25. Thorburn DR, Dahl H-HM. Mitochondrial disorders: genetics, counseling, prenatal diagnosis and reproductive options. *Am J Med Genet* 2001;106:102–14

26. Papp Z. Genetic counseling and termination of pregnancy in Hungary. *J Med Philos* 1989;14: 323–33

27. Papp Z, Gávai M, Görbe É. Is third trimester abortion justified? *Br J Obstet Gynaecol* 1996;103: 187–9

28. Papp Z, Németi M, Papp CS, Tóth-Pál E. Reproductive decisions after genetic counseling of couples at high risk for cystic fibrosis: a perspective from the last two decades. In Kurjak A, Chervenak FA, eds. *The Fetus as a Patient.* Carnforth, UK: Parthenon Publishing, 1994: 107–15

29. Tóth-Pál E, Papp CS, Papp Z. Computer follow-up system for obstetric, genetic and neonatal care in Hungary. *Int J Gynecol Obstet* 1993;43:323–4

30. Frets PG, Niermeijer MF. Reproductive planning after genetic counselling: a perspective from the last decade. *Clin Genet* 1990;38:295–306

31. Wertz DC, Fletcher JC. Attitudes of genetic counselors: a multinational survey. *Am J Hum Genet* 1988;42:592–600

32. Penchrinha DF, Bell NK, Edwards JG, Best RG. Ethical issues in genetic counseling: a comparison of M.S. counselor and medical geneticist perspectives. *J Genet Couns* 1992;1:19–30

33. Clarke A. Is non-directive genetic counselling possible? *Lancet* 1991;338:998–1001

34. Kessler S. Psychological aspects of genetic counseling. VII. Thoughts on directiveness. *J Genet Couns* 1992;1:9–18

35. Burke BM, Kolker A. Directiveness in prenatal genetic counseling. *Women Health* 1994;22:31–53

36. Michie S, Bron F, Bobrow M, Marteau TM. Nondirectiveness in genetic counseling: an empirical study. *Am J Hum Genet* 1997;60:40–7

37. Brunger F, Lippman A. Resistance and adherence to the norms of genetic counseling. *J Genet Couns* 1995;4:151–67

38. Bernhardt BA. Empirical evidence that genetic counseling is directive: where do we go from here? *Am J Hum Genet* 1997;60:17–20

39. Roter D. An exploration of health education's responsibility: a partnership mode of client-provider relations. *Patient Educ Couns* 1987;9: 25–31

40. Thompson SC, Pitts JS, Schwantovsky L. Preferences for involvement in medical decision-making: situational and demographic influences. *Patient Educ Couns* 1993;22:133–40

41. Wolff G, Jung C. Nondirectiveness and genetic counseling. *J Genet Couns* 1995;4:3–25

42. Shiloh S, Saxe L. Perception of risk in genetic counseling. *Psychol Health* 1989;3:45–61

43. Furu T, Kaariainen H, Sankila E-M, Norio R. Attitudes towards prenatal diagnosis and selective abortion among patients with retinitis pigmentosa or choroideremia as well as among their relatives. *Clin Genet* 1993;43:160–5

44. Mariner W. Outcomes assessment in health care reform: promise and limitations. *Am J Law Med* 1994;20:37–57

45. Geller G, Holtzman NA. A qualitative assessment of primary care physicians' perceptions about the ethical and social implications of offering genetic testing. *Qual Health Res* 1995;5: 97–116

46. Caplan AL. Neutrality is not morality: the ethics of genetic counseling. In Bartels DM, Le Roy BS, Caplan AL, eds. *Ethical Challenges in Genetic Counseling.* Hawthorne, NY: Aldine De Gruyter, 1993:149–65

47. Holtzman NA, Bernhardt BA, Doksum T, Helzlsouer KA, Geller G. Education about

BRCA1 testing decreases women's interest in being tested. *Am J Hum Genet* 1996;(Suppl 59):A56

48. Dipple KM, McCabe ERB. Modifier genes convert 'simple' Mendelian disorders to complex traits. *Mol Genet Metab* 2000;71:43–50

49. Dipple KM, McCabe ERB. Phenotypes of patients with 'simple' mendelian disorders are complex traits: thresholds, modifiers and systems dynamics. *Am J Hum Genet* 2000;66:1729–35

50. Scriver CR, Waters PJ. Monogenic traits are not simple: lessons from phenylketonuria. *Trends Genet* 1999;15:267–72

51. Vladutiu GD. Complex phenotypes in metabolic muscle diseases. *Muscle Nerve* 2000;23:1157–9

52. McCable LL, McCabe ERB. Postgenomic medicine. Presymptomatic testing for prediction and prevention. *Clin Perinatol* 2001;28:425–34

Prenatal informed consent for sonogram: the time for first-trimester nuchal translucency has come

12

S. T. Chasen, D. W. Skupski, L. B. McCullough and F. A. Chervenak

Ultrasound screening in pregnancy has been and continues to be a matter of controversy. For the past 20 years, second-trimester ultrasound screening has been debated. Even today, the ACOG does not endorse this as a standard of care in low-risk pregnancies. Nonetheless, offering second-trimester ultrasound is widely practiced. In 1989, two of us (FAC, LBM) made the argument that 'the standard of care demands that prenatal informed consent for sonogram be accepted as an indication for the prudent use of obstetric ultrasonography performed by qualified personnel'[1]. We seek to extend this argument to first-trimester ultrasound screening for aneuploidy using nuchal translucency determination.

THE RELIABILITY OF FIRST-TRIMESTER ULTRASOUND SCREENING FOR ANEUPLOIDY

The term 'nuchal translucency' refers to the sonographic measurement of nuchal skin late in the first trimester. A specific feature of newborns with Down syndrome is redundant nuchal skin. This has also been noted with other autosomal trisomies and Turner syndrome[2]. Nuchal edema occurs in the fetus as well, and varying degrees of this are visible sonographically. This ranges from slight thickening of nuchal skin to cystic hygromas, congenital malformations in which dilated lymphatic channels form a soft tissue mass, typically in the posterior neck.

Benacerraf *et al.* described an association between increased nuchal skin fold thickness in the second trimester and Down syndrome, in 1985[3]. Although this is a useful second-trimester marker for Down syndrome, a minority of second-trimester fetuses with Down syndrome will have increased nuchal skin fold thickness[4].

Pandya *et al.* described an association with first-trimester nuchal edema and aneuploidy in 1992[5]. Subsequently, many studies described increased nuchal translucency in fetuses with Down syndrome and other forms of aneuploidy between 10 and 14 weeks. Most early studies defined increased nuchal translucency using a single cut-off, usually 3.0 mm[5].

A problem with using a single cut-off in defining abnormal nuchal translucency is the fact that nuchal translucency increases with gestational age in normal fetuses[6]. Thus, sensitivity rates for aneuploidy with a single cut-off would be lower at earlier gestational ages, and false-positive rates would be higher at later gestational ages.

Another problem with ultrasound screening for aneuploidy in the first trimester concerns operator technique in measuring nuchal translucency. Nuchal translucency must be measured with a fetus in the optimal position, with appropriate image magnification and caliper placement[7]. When appropriate techniques are not used, harm may result from lower detection rates and higher false-positive results.

Finally, maternal age is an integral part in the estimation of risk in any screening test for aneuploidy. The relative risk of Down syndrome in a fetus with an abnormal nuchal translucency is independent of maternal age. It must be noted, however, that an abnormal nuchal translucency measurement with a maternal-age-related risk of 1 in 100 would reflect a much higher absolute risk of Down syndrome than with an age-related risk of 1 in 1000[6].

Many studies evaluating nuchal translucency screening for Down syndrome, including those performed in the United States, were performed using single cut-offs, without standardized techniques, and did not consider maternal age. Not surprisingly, wide ranges of sensitivity and false-positive rates have been described[8].

In 1998, Snijders *et al.* published the results from the Fetal Medicine Foundation (FMF) multicenter study assessing nuchal translucency screening for Down syndrome. Over 100 000 pregnancies at 22 centers in the United Kingdom were screened from 10 to 14 weeks. All participating centers had demonstrated the ability to obtain appropriate nuchal translucency measurements by submitting images to a centralized auditing agency. The criteria for an appropriate image were magnification such that the fetus occupied at least 75% of the image; that the skin could be distinguished from the amnion; and that the maximum thickness of subcutaneous translucency between the skin and soft tissue overlying the cervical spine was measured. Risks for Down syndrome were calculated based on crown–rump length, nuchal translucency and maternal age[7].

In 22 centers, 100 311 singleton pregnancies were screened from 10 to 14 weeks. In 96 127 cases, prenatal or postnatal karyotype was obtained, or a birth of a phenotypically normal child was documented. To determine sensitivity of nuchal translucency, a risk threshold of 1 in 300 was used. A risk estimate of 1 in 300 or more was reported in 7907 normal fetuses (8.3%), in 268 of 326 fetuses with Down syndrome (82.2%) and 253 of 325 fetuses with other chromosomal abnormalities (77.9%)[7].

The FMF has since accredited many international sites. Centers must demonstrate expertise in measuring nuchal translucency, and images from all sonographers must be submitted for review before software for risk estimation is provided. Annual audits of all data including submission of sample nuchal translucency images from each sonographer are also required. Investigators outside the United Kingdom have described similar effectiveness of first-trimester ultrasound screening for Down syndrome using software provided by the FMF[9–14].

At New York Weill-Cornell Medical Center, referring obstetricians have been offering nuchal translucency as an option from 11 to 14 weeks' gestation. We have been estimating risk based on nuchal translucency and maternal age as part of the FMF since April 2000, and we recently published results from our first 800 patients[11]. We have now screened 1600 patients, 36.4% of whom were 35 years of age or older, and 1775 fetuses. The risk estimate based on age, gestational age and nuchal translucency was greater than 1 in 300 in 158 patients (8.9%). We have reviewed the results of all cytogenetic studies performed in our institution from CVS, amniocentesis, blood from phenotypically abnormal newborns, or tissue from spontaneous miscarriages and intrauterine fetal demises.

We have had eight documented cases of Down syndrome in our screened patients. In seven of these cases (87.5%) estimation of risk was greater than 1 in 300. In seven of eight cases of trisomy 18 (87.5%) and five of seven cases with other forms of aneuploidy (71.4%), estimation of risk was greater than 1 in 300.

In our view, data from FMF sites demonstrate that nuchal translucency should be regarded as a clearly reliable screen for aneuploidy, because of the universal standard of quality in all FMF testing sites and the large number of patients involved in published reports describing nuchal translucency screening in FMF centers.

First-trimester biochemical screening for aneuploidy has also been described. Using a combination of free β-hCG and pregnancy-associated plasma protein A with maternal age, detection rates of 60–70% for Down syndrome have been reported[15,16]. Combining first-trimester serum analytes with nuchal translucency and maternal age, detection rates of approximately 90% have been reported[17,18].

Recently, Wapner reported results from a multicenter study funded by the National Institutes of Health evaluating first-trimester nuchal translucency and biochemical screening. The techniques of measuring nuchal translucency and risk estimation were identical to those of the FMF. Not surprisingly, detection rates over 80% using nuchal translucency alone or in combination with biochemical screening were described. This NICHD study performed in multiple sites in the United States confirms that nuchal translucency performed in a quality setting is indeed a reliable screening test[19].

Ongoing studies, in which patients undergo first-trimester ultrasound screening as well as first- and second-trimester biochemical screening, may suggest ways to integrate these different screening tests. Integration could maximize sensitivity, and minimize the rate of false-positive tests[20].

While certain questions concerning aneuploidy screening remain unanswered, data overwhelmingly suggest that nuchal translucency, when performed in quality settings, is a reliable screening test. The comparative value of nuchal translucency to biochemical screening and second-trimester ultrasound, the ideal combination of tests in aneuploidy screening, and the natural history of the aneuploid fetus with abnormal nuchal translucency are investigational[21]. Nonetheless, investigation in these areas does not negate the established value of first-trimester ultrasound screening for aneuploidy, or preclude its use in a non-investigational setting.

BENEFICENCE-BASED DIMENSIONS OF FIRST-TRIMESTER ULTRASOUND SCREENING

Beneficence is a principle of medical ethics that obliges the physician to seek for patients a greater balance of clinical goods over clinical harms. This is the oldest principle of medical ethics and can be found through history from Hippocratic texts to contemporary bioethics. In order to apply beneficence to this subject, there needs to be an analysis of potential clinical benefits and harms[22].

If first-trimester screening for Down syndrome with nuchal translucency is available at a specialized center with expertise and ongoing quality control, patients may benefit in several ways. Some women at high risk based on age or history would prefer to avoid invasive testing, because of the associated risk of miscarriage, especially if pregnancy has been achieved after therapy for infertility. These women may choose to undergo invasive testing, however, if there is any evidence of an increased risk based on screening tests. One study suggests that the availability of nuchal translucency screening may decrease the rate of invasive testing in high-risk women[23]. Undergoing a combination of tests, including first-trimester ultrasound as well as second-trimester serum screening, could increase the likelihood that a fetus with Down syndrome will be identified. Ongoing studies may develop the ability to integrate these and other tests to derive a single estimation of risk in the future[20].

Other women are determined to undergo invasive testing to exclude the possibility of aneuploidy, but may use nuchal translucency to assist them in choosing between chorionic villus sampling (CVS) and amniocentesis. Although it is not clear that CVS, when performed by an experienced operator, has a significantly higher complication rate than amniocentesis, there is some evidence to suggest slightly higher miscarriage rates with CVS[24,25]. Some women would prefer to avoid CVS and undergo amniocentesis for other reasons. These include the small incidence of placental mosaicism found on CVS, which requires amniocentesis to be performed subsequently, and the ability to screen for neural tube defects by determining amniotic fluid α-fetoprotein (AFP), though the routine determination of amniotic fluid AFP has been questioned[26]. If nuchal translucency were to reveal a substantial risk of Down syndrome, however, these women could undergo CVS to achieve an earlier diagnosis.

Finally, women considered to be at low risk may be interested in first-trimester screening for Down syndrome. Informed patients are aware that women at any age can give birth to a child with Down syndrome, and have shown interest in first-trimester screening. If a sensitive first-trimester test with a relatively low false-positive rate is available, this is certainly a reasonable option, as these women could undergo invasive testing if nuchal translucency were abnormal.

Aside from screening for Down syndrome, ultrasound performed to measure nuchal translucency has other benefits. Many other congenital anomalies have been described in euploid fetuses with increased nuchal translucency as well[27]. Accurate estimation of gestational age, and accurate identification of amnionicity and chorionicity in multifetal gestations, are other well-described benefits of first-trimester ultrasound[28].

The use of nuchal translucency also has the potential to harm. Obtaining this measurement requires meticulous attention to technique; failure to do so could lead to both false-positive and false-negative results. This could lead to higher rates of invasive testing and miscarriage if risks were overestimated, or women with affected pregnancies not undergoing prenatal diagnosis if risks were underestimated. Ongoing review of data and follow-up are essential to document the quality of screening in every center providing this service.

It is also important to note that nuchal translucency does not replace second-trimester serum screening, which should be performed if nuchal translucency testing reveals a low risk of Down syndrome. Until different screening tests can be integrated to derive a single estimation of risk, it is important that women be aware that serial screening will result in higher cumulative false-positive rates, if cut-offs are not modified. This could increase the number of invasive tests performed, and lead to a higher rate of loss of normal fetuses.

In summary, it is not reasonable to conclude that the potential harms of nuchal translucency screening outweigh the potential benefits when quality testing is available. Moreover, in our view, the potential benefits clearly outweigh the potential harms.

THE RELEVANCE OF RESPECT FOR AUTONOMY

Respect for autonomy is a principle that obliges the physician to seek for the patient the greater balance for goods over harms as that balancing is judged by the patient[22]. The relevance of respect for autonomy to nuchal translucency screening is that first-trimester identification of fetuses at risk provides the option of prenatal testing and the subsequent option of early abortion, which is of considerable value to many women.

The process should involve several stages[1]. Since nuchal translucency screening must be done prior to 14 weeks' gestation, the physician should discuss this test with the pregnant woman at the initial prenatal visit. Information should be provided about the actual and theoretical benefits of nuchal translucency, including potential benefits and harms. The pregnant woman should evaluate this information in terms of her own values and beliefs; this is something every autonomous patient is able to do. The physician should be prepared to discuss his or her scientific evaluation of available data regarding nuchal translucency screening for Down syndrome.

After these steps, the pregnant woman should be able to articulate her preference regarding the use of nuchal translucency to screen for Down syndrome in the first trimester. The physician can then make a recommendation to the pregnant woman. Finally, a thoughtful and sensitive discussion of any disagreement should ensue, after which a woman can make her decision. This process provides a significant role for the judgement and experience of the physician, while maintaining respect for a pregnant woman's autonomy.

It must be noted that the physician should only offer the option of nuchal translucency with a pregnant woman if quality testing is available. It is the responsibility of the physician to ensure that the center to which he or she will refer patients for nuchal translucency screening maintains the highest standards. Without quality testing in experienced centers, the harms of testing may outweigh the benefits.

CONCLUSION

First-trimester screening for nuchal translucency when conducted according to accepted standards of quality is a reliable diagnostic screen. There is no compelling beneficence-based argument opposed to offering it, and offering it is an important autonomy-enhancing strategy. Such screening should be offered only in centers where high quality is available. In our view, the results of ongoing trials will enhance this position.

References

1. Chervenak FA, McCullough LB, Chervenak JL. Prenatal informed consent for sonogram: an indication for obstetric ultrasonography. *Am J Obstet Gynecol* 1989;161:857–60

2. Jones KL. *Smith's Recognizable Patterns of Human Malformation*, 5th edn. Philadelphia, PA: WB Saunders, 1997

3. Benacerraf BR, Barss VA, Laboda LA. A sonographic sign for the detection in the second trimester of the fetus with Down's syndrome. *Am J Obstet Gynecol* 1985;151:1078–9

4. Nicolaides KH, Azar G, Byrne D, Mansur C, Marks K. Fetal nuchal translucency: ultrasound screening for chromosomal defects in first trimester of pregnancy. *Br Med J* 1992;304:867–9

5. Pandya PP, Santiago C, Snijders RJ, Nicolaides KH. First trimester fetal nuchal translucency. *Curr Opin Obstet Gynecol* 1995;7:95–102

6. Pandya PP, Snijders RJM, Johnson SJ, Brizot M, Nicolaides KH. Screening for fetal trisomies by maternal age and fetal nuchal translucency thickness at 10 to 14 weeks of gestation. *Br J Obstet Gynaecol* 1995;102:957–62

7. Snijders RJM, Noble P, Sebire N, Souka A, Nicolaides KH. UK multicentre project on assessment of risk of trisomy 21 by maternal age and fetal nuchal translucency thickness at 10–14 weeks of gestation. *Lancet* 1998;351:343–6

8. American College of Obstetricians and Gynecologists Committee on Genetics. *First-Trimester Screening for Fetal Anomalies with Nuchal Translucency*. Committee Opinion Number 223. Washington, DC: American College of Obstetricians and Gynecologists, 1999

9. O'Callaghan SP, Giles WB, Raymond SP, McDougall V, Morris K, Boyd J. First trimester ultrasound with nuchal translucency measurement for Down syndrome risk estimation using software developed by the Fetal Medicine Foundation, United Kingdom – the first 2000 examinations in Newcastle, New South Wales, Australia. *Aust NZ J Obstet Gynaecol* 2000;40:292–5

10. Theodoropoulos P, Lolis D, Papageorgiou C, Papaioannou S, Plachouars N, Makrydimas G. Evaluation of first-trimester screening by fetal nuchal translucency and maternal age. *Prenat Diagn* 18:133–7

11. Chasen ST, Skupski DW, McCullough LB, Chervenak FA. Prenatal informed consent for sonogram. The time for first-trimester nuchal translucency has come. *J Ultrasound Med* 2001;20:1147–52

12. Gasiorek-Wiens A, Tercanli S, Kozlowski P, *et al.* Screening for trisomy 21 by fetal nuchal translucency and maternal age: a multicenter project in Germany, Austria and Switzerland. *Ultrasound Obstet Gynecol* 2001;18:645–8

13. Zoppi MA, Ibba RM, Floris M, Monni G. Fetal nuchal translucency screening in 12,495 pregnancies in Sardinia. *Ultrasound Obstet Gynecol* 2001;18:649–51

14. Brizot ML, Carvalho MHB, Liao AW, Reis NSV, Armbruster-Moraes E, Zugaib M. First-trimester screening for chromosomal abnormalities by fetal nuchal translucency in a Brazilian population. *Ultrasound Obstet Gynecol* 2001;18:652–5

15. Haddow JE, Palomaki GE, Knight GJ, Williams J, Miller WA, Johnson A. Screening of maternal serum for fetal Down's syndrome in the first trimester. *N Engl J Med* 1998;338:955–61

16. Krantz DA, Larsen JW, Buchanan PD, Macri JN. First trimester Down syndrome screening; free beta human chorionic gonadotropin and pregnancy-associated plasma protein A. *Am J Obstet Gynecol* 1996;174:612–16

17. Spencer K, Spencer CE, Power M, Moakes A, Nicolaides KH. One stop clinic for assessment of risk for fetal anomalies: a report of the first year of prospective screening for chromosomal anomalies in the first trimester. *Br J Obstet Gynaecol* 2000;107:1271–5

18. Krantz DA, Hallahan TW, Orlandi F, Buchanan P, Larsen JW Jr, Macri JN. First-trimester Down syndrome screening using dried blood

biochemistry and nuchal translucency. *Obstet Gynecol* 2000;96:207–13

19. Wapner RJ. First trimester aneuploid screening: results of the NICHD multicenter study. *Am J Obstet Gynecol* 2001;185:S70

20. Wald NJ, Watt HC, Hackshaw AK. Integrated screening for Down's syndrome on the basis of tests performed during the first and second trimesters. *N Engl J Med* 1999;12:461–7

21. Malone FD, Berkowitz RL, Canick JA, D'Alton ME. First-trimester screening for aneuploidy: research or standard of care. *Am J Obstet Gynecol* 2000;182:490

22. McCullough LB, Chervenak FA. *Ethics in Obstetrics and Gynecology.* New York, NY: Oxford University Press, 1994

23. Zoppi MA, Ibba RM, Putzolu M, Floris M, Monni G. Nuchal translucency and the acceptance of invasive prenatal chromosomal diagnosis in women aged 35 and older. *Obstet Gynecol* 2001; 97:916–20

24. Jenkins TM, Wapner RJ. First trimester prenatal diagnosis: chorionic villus sampling. *Semin Perinatol* 1999;23:403–13

25. Alfirevic Z, Gosden CM, Neilson JP. Chorion villus sampling versus amniocentesis for prenatal diagnosis. Cochrane Database Syst Rev 2000; CD000055

26. Silver RK, Leeth EA, Check IJ. A reappraisal of amniotic fluid alpha-fetoprotein measurement at the time of genetic amniocentesis and midtrimester ultrasonography. *J Ultrasound Med* 2001;20:631–7

27. Souka AP, Snijders RJ, Novakov A, Soares W, Nicolaides KH. Defects and syndromes in chromosomally normal fetuses with increased nuchal translucency thickness at 10–14 weeks of gestation. *Ultrasound Obstet Gynecol* 1998;11: 391–4000

28. Kurtz AB, Wapner RJ, Mata J, Johnson A, Morgan P. Twin pregnancies: accuracy of first-trimester abdominal US in predicting chorionicity and amnionicity. *Radiology* 1992;185:759–62

Prenatal diagnosis of fetal cells in maternal blood by comparative genomic hybridization

13

Y. H. Yang, S. H. Kim and J. E. Jung

Prenatal diagnosis of genetic diseases can be divided into invasive and non-invasive methods. Invasive methods include amniocentesis[1], chorionic villus sampling[2,3] and cordocentesis[4]. These methods give an accuracy that reaches almost 99%, but more than 2 weeks are required for the result to become available which is a long time for the pregnant woman to wait in agitation. Also, there is a possibility of trauma both to the pregnant woman and her fetus. In contrast to invasive methods, non-invasive methods such as the α-fetoprotein, dual-marker, triple-marker test are determined using maternal serum, but the accuracy of these tests reaches only 60%[5]. The above-mentioned invasive and non-invasive methods are applied after the pregnancy has already been established, rendering them inappropriate as a preventive method. The need for a safe and fast prenatal genetic diagnosis is mandated, and, recently, fetal cells in maternal blood have been isolated which has made prenatal genetic diagnosis feasible[6–8].

As a safe and fast prenatal genetic diagnostic tool, fetal cell isolation from maternal blood has been investigated[7,8]. Fetal nucleated red blood cells (nRBCs) are the most popularly used fetal cells present in the maternal blood, but they compose only one in 10^5–10^7 maternal cells[9,10], therefore effective separation and enrichment methods are crucial. Until now fetal cell surface specific antigens were used in applying magnetic-activated cell sorting (MACS) or fluorescence-activated cell sorting (FACS) for the separation and enrichment of fetal cells in maternal blood, but no definitely successive method has been elucidated yet[11–15].

The development of molecular genetics made prenatal genetic diagnosis possible using chromosome-specific DNA probes with interphase fluorescence *in situ* hybridization (FISH). This method eliminated the tedious process of cell culture in the conventional cytogenetic studies, but less than half the chromosome complement can be analyzed in any one cell, rendering FISH an inefficient method.

Comparative genomic hybridization (CGH) has emerged to solve the above-mentioned problems and, recently, it was successfully applied in clinical cytogenetics having the advantage of providing complete chromosome analysis with single hybridization[16]. Detection of whole and segmental aneuploidies on different kinds of tissues such as blastomeres, chorionic villi, cultured amniocytes and uncultured amniocytes has been applied using CGH. Kallioniemi *et al.* originally developed CGH[17,18], and Bryndorf *et al.* used CGH in clinical cytogenetics to analyze partial or complete monosomy and trisomy[19]. CGH is especially useful in single-cell analysis or in cases where only limited numbers of cells can be retrieved such as prenatal genetic diagnosis using blastomeres. For molecular analysis of such small samples it is essential to first amplify the DNA using the polymerase chain reaction (PCR). The amplification of template DNA using polymerase chain reaction is unequivocally necessary to retrieve a sufficient amount of DNA template. To date, degenerate oligonucleotide primed (DOP)-PCR is considered to be the most effective method of whole genome amplification[20].

In this chapter prenatal genetic diagnosis using fetal nRBCs in maternal blood will be introduced. Isolation of fetal nRBCs was achieved by triple density gradient centrifugation MACS using CD45 and CD71. Fetal nRBCs were microdissected and DNA was retrieved from each cell. Template DNA was amplified using DOP-PCR, and lastly CGH was applied for the final diagnosis.

HISTORICAL BACKGROUND

The presence of fetal cells in maternal blood was originally discovered by Schmorl in 1893: trophoblasts were found in the pregnant woman's lung and uterine vein[21]. Walknowska was the first person to try isolating the fetal cells in the maternal blood. He isolated lymphocytes and allegedly verified XY interphase fetal cells. Afterwards, in the 1970s fetal cells were identified by confirming the Y-chromatin using quinacrine dye. In 1999 Herzenberg et al.[15] and Yeoh et al.[16] applied the difference of human leukocyte antigen (HLA) type in flow sorting fetal lymphocytes from maternal cells[22]. This was based on the idea that in the case of a HLA antigen-positive father and a HLA antigen-negative mother, the presence of HLA antigen-positive cells in maternal blood would be identified as fetal cells. In the mid 1980s, fetal cells were identified using PCR with the identification of a Y-specific sequence. Nowadays fetal cell-specific monoclonal antibodies are used to select the required cells, and FACS and MACS are used additionally for further isolation. These isolated cells can be used for prenatal genetic diagnosis using FISH with specific DNA probes or more specifically CGH.

CGH, which was introduced by Kallioniemi et al., provides an overview of chromosomal gains and losses by scanning the entire genome in a single step[17]. This is a method that allows more genetic information to be obtained from minute DNA samples, and from a single cell in particular. This method aims to generate a non-specific amplification of all genomic sequences (whole genome amplification).

Conventional cytogenetic studies require dividing cells from the test subject, and therefore cell culture to generate metaphase chromosomes is required taking a significant length of time. Multicolor fluorescent in situ hybridization performed on interphase nuclei for the detection of specific chromosomal regions has overcome some of these problems, circumventing the need for cell culture. But specific DNA probes are required, and only a limited number of chromosomes can be screened at a time. Overcoming the above-mentioned difficulties in prenatal genetic diagnosis, CGH requires no extensive series of specific DNA probes and no prior knowledge of the genomic region to be studied.

TECHNIQUE

Materials

Samples of 20–30 ml of peripheral venous blood are collected from pregnant women for whom prenatal genetic counselling and procedures are indicated. Informed consent is obtained in all cases prior to performing this technique.

Methods

Isolation of fetal cells

For the isolation of fetal cells, a modified Gänshirt-Ahlert method is applied[23]. The maternal venous blood samples are diluted 1 : 2 with phosphate buffered saline (PBS) and preserved at room temperature. Then 6 ml of diluted blood samples are underlaid with Ficoll-Histopaque (Sigma, St. Louis, Montana, USA) 1077, 1107 and 1119 in 50 ml tubes and centrifuged for 30 min at 3000 rpm (4°C). The mononuclear cells, in the second layer from the top, are isolated. We wash these mononuclear cells with $1 \times$ PBS three to four times in the 15 ml polyethylene tube. Well-washed cells are resuspended with 20 µl/10^7 cells of anti-CD45 magnetic microbeads (DAKO, GmbH, Bergisch, Gladbach, Germany) and incubated in the refrigerator for 20 min. For CD45-negative cell separation, separation columns are designed for optimal negative selections and a MACS (Miltenyi Biotec, Bergisch Erladbach, Germany) system is used. The cells adherent to the beads are removed and the negative-selected cells are washed two to three times with 1 × PBS. After washing, the cells are centrifuged for 10 min at 1200 rpm at 4°C , the pellet is treated with 30 µl/10 cells of anti-CD71 magnetic microbeads (DAKO) and incubated for 20 min in the refrigerator (8°C). After the incubation, the CD71-positive cells in the MACS separation column are isolated using a pressure syringe in the MACS kit.

Microdissection of nRBCs

The nRBCs on the slide are dissected by the micromanupulator and transferred to the Eppendorf tube containing 10 µl of PBS (Figure 1).

DNA separation and DOP-PCR amplification from microdissected nRBCs

The separated nRBCs are washed with PBS and transferred to a PCR tube. They are then lysed with 5 µl of lysis buffer (200 mmol/l potassium hydroxide (KOH)), heated for 10 min at 65°C and cooled to 4°C. Adding 5 µl of neutralizing buffer (500 mmol/l Tris (pH 8.3) : 300 mmol/l KCl : 200 mmol/l HCl), DNA which will be the template of sequential DOP-PCR (ROCHE, Mannheim, Germany) is separated. The final concentration of reactive solution for DOP-PCR should be 2.5 U Taq DNA polymerase : 200 µmol/l dNTP : 10 mmol/l Tris-HCl : 50 mmol/l KCl : 1.5 mmol/l $MgCl_2$: 2 µmol/l DOP-PCR primer. The conditions for DOP-PCR consist of 5 min denaturation at 95°C; eight cycles of 1 min denaturation at 94°C, 1.5 min annealing at 30°C and 3 min extension at 72°C; and 35 cycles of 1 min denaturation at 94°C, 1 min annealing at 62°C and 3 min extension at 72°C. In each step of the PCR, negative (water) and positive (genomic DNA) control should be tested to confirm whether the PCR solution is contaminated or not (PTC-100 Programmable Thermal Controler, MJ Research, Inc., Massachusetts, USA). After performing PCR, a part of the amplified DNA

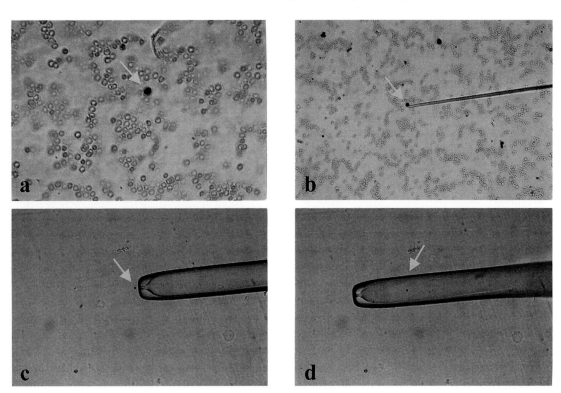

Figure 1 *Fetal nucleated red blood cell isolation using micromanipulator*

solution undergoes electrophoresis in 1% agarose gel. A photograph of the gel documentation (Amersham Biosciences, Uppsala, Sweden) stained gel is taken and interpreted.

Target metaphase slide

The slide is made from normal human peripheral blood by routine chromosomal culture technique and then selected for the performing of CGH. Before hybridization, the slide is denatured with 70% formamide, 2 × saline-sodium citrate buffer (SSC) for 3–4 min and dehydrated with 70%, 85% and 100% ethanol at each concentration for 1 min.

CGH and digital imaging analysis

The amplified genomic DNA is labelled at 15°C for 90–105 min by using the Nick translation kit (Vysis, Illinois, USA) and treated at 72°C for 10 min to stop the reaction. The reference DNA is labelled with Spectrum Red (Vysis) and the test DNA is labelled with Spectrum Green (Vysis). The suitable DNA size for CGH is 500–1500 base pairs in 1% agarose gel. After precipitation with 3 mol/l sodium acetate (0.1 vol) and 100% ethanol (2.5 vol) in a 1.5 ml microtube, the mixture (500 ng of labelled test DNA, 500 ng of reference DNA and 20 μg of Cot1 DNA (Vysis)) is vortexed and incubated in the refrigerator for 30 min. The pellet (DNA deposited by microcentrifuge at 1200 rpm for 30 min (4°C)) is dried at 37°C for 30 min and resuspended in purified H$_2$O. The hybridization buffer is added. The probe mixture denatured at 73°C for 5 min is applied to the target metaphase slide, covered by a cover slip and sealed with rubber cement. This slide put in the humidity chamber is hybridized in the incubator at 37°C for 48–72 h. After the removal of the cover slip and treatment with 0.4 × SSC/0.3% Nonidet P-40 (NP-40) (1 min) and 2 × SSC/0.1% NP-40 (1 min), it is air-dried in a dark room. Then the 4′6-diamidino-2-phenylindole 2HCl (DAPI) differential stained slide is observed under the fluorescence microscope. The image is analyzed by the Cytovision image analysis system (Applied Imaging Co.,

California, USA) for the detection of amplification or deletion of the gene.

WHOLE GENOMIC AMPLIFICATION

A single diploid human cell contains about 6 pg of DNA[24] and it is generally accepted that a DNA sample of 0.2–1.0 μg is required to perform the standard CGH technique. Consequently, in order to perform the CGH technique with a limited number of fetal erythrocytes, the process of whole genomic amplification (WGA), in which a sufficient amount of DNA is obtained via repeated cycles of PCR, is almost obligatory. The WGA could be performed through various methods such as DOP-PCR, tagged-PCR (T-PCR), primer extension preamplification-PCR (PEP-PCR) and alu-PCR.

The CGH technique performed by using the DNA concentrate obtained through the DOP-PCR was first introduced by Kuukasjärvi et al.[25], in which tumor cells were analyzed after the microdissection of cells from a fixed tissue sample, whereas Griffin et al.[26] employed the same method in the detection of genomic duplication in flow-sorted chromosomes. However, a relatively large numbers of cells were required in the analysis of both cases. Recently, Wells et al.[20] have reported that a sufficient amount of DNA could be obtained from approximately 25 duploid cells of varying types such as fibroblasts, buccal cells, amniocytes and blastomeres and that DOP-PCR was regarded as the most

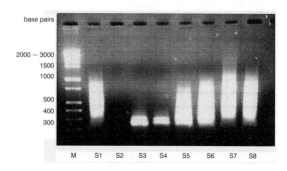

Figure 2 *Assessment of DNA quality after degenerate oligonucleotide primed polymerase chain reaction (DOP-PCR). M, DNA marker; S1, S5, S6, S7, S8, good quality after DOP-PCR; S2, S3, S4, poor quality after DOP-PCR*

outstanding method. The effort to obtain a sufficient amount of DNA sample from a smaller number of cells is still ongoing (Figure 2).

DIGITAL IMAGING ANALYSIS

Genomic DNA from cells of interest (test DNA) and genomic DNA from karyotypically normal cells (reference DNA) are respectively labelled with a green and red fluorochrome. Greater volume of unlabelled repetitive COT-1 DNA is added to the mixture to block repetitive sequence regions. Then, DNA is co-hybridized as a probe in equal amounts to well-defined normal metaphase spreads. Images of the fluorescent signals are captured, and the green-to-red signal ratios are digitally quantified for each chromosome. Chromosomal locations of copy number changes within the DNA segments of the test genome are revealed by a variable fluorescence intensity ratio (FR) along each target chromosome. A gain of chromosomal material specimen would be detected by an elevated green-to-red ratio, whereas deletions or chromosomal losses would produce a reduced green-to-red ratio[27]. As a result from the process described above, CGH enables analysis of all chromosomes in a single experiment from DNA samples and this procedure requires only 36–48 h to be completed.

In the presence of the same amount of DNA in the reference and test samples, the amount to be hybridized in the metaphase cell would be the same. This would lead to the green-to-red ratio being 1 (Figure 3a). In Figure 3b, normal female DNA was used for reference as usual, and a little deviation to the right can be noted in the chromosomes 1, 16, 19 and 20. Especially in chromosomes 1 and 16, almost normal configuration can be noted at around the centromere where abundant heterochromatic regions are present. Chromosomes 19 and 20 showed a more profound deviation to the right, almost suggesting aneuploidy, but this is probably due to the partial overexpression in the process of DOP-PCR[28]. This error happened in the process of accumulating ten chromosomes, and the ambiguity was confirmed to be a normal female by amniocentesis.

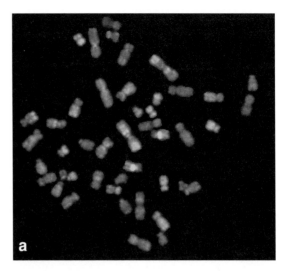

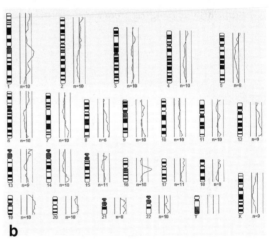

Figure 3 *Metaphase images (a) and comparative genomic hybridization fluorescent ratio profiles (b) obtained following hybridization of the degenerate oligonucleotide primed polymerase chain reaction (DOP-PCR) product from a single female fetus cell labelled with Spectrum Green together with the DOP-PCR product from normal female DNA labelled with Spectrum Red. The fluorescent ratios for all chromosomes are within the cut-off threshold of 0.8–1.2 (see Color Plates Q and R)*

In trisomy 21, an extra chromosome is added to the normally present pair of chromosomes. In this case the co-hybridized chromosome 21 will show a green fluorescence. As you can see in Figure 4a, the X chromosome gives a red fluorescence whereas chromosome 21 gives a green fluorescence. In Figure 4b this is interpreted in a DNA profile. Deviation to the left means deletion of the chromosome. If normal female DNA was used as the reference DNA, dominance of red light in the X chromosome would represent a male fetus (positive control). Analysis of 11 chromosome 21s shows a deviation to the right which can be interpreted as an amplification of the chromosome indicating trisomy 21. The slight deviation to the left in chromosomes 1 and 9 should be interpreted as a normal deviation as it was noticed in chromosomes 1 and 16 in

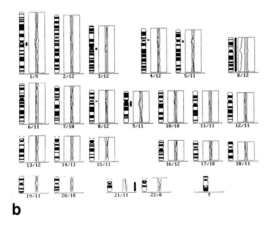

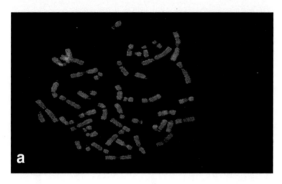

Figure 4 *Metaphase images (a) and comparative genomic hybridization fluorescent ratio profiles (b) obtained following hybridization of the degenerate oligonucleotide primed polymerase chain reaction (DOP-PCR) product from a single trisomy 21 male fetus cell labelled with Spectrum Green together with the DOP-PCR product from normal female DNA labelled with Spectrum Red. The fluorescent ratios for all chromosomes except 21 and X are within the cut-off threshold of 0.8–1.2. The profile for the X chromosome shows a deviation to the left and the profile for chromosome 21 shows a deviation to the right indicating increased copy number for 21 in the test cell (see Color Plates S and T)*

Figure 3b. The result of amniocentesis of the case shown in Figure 4 was confirmed to be male trisomy 21.

ADVANTAGES

The main advantages of the CGH analysis are the precise localization of extra or missing chromosomal material, the genome-wide screening for such unbalanced aberrations, and the fact that CGH depends on DNA isolation rather on the preparation of metaphase preparation. In cases where satisfactory metaphase preparation cannot be obtained, CGH is especially useful. It also obviates the time-consuming tissue culture of patient samples.

DISADVANTAGES

The main disadvantages of CGH for a cytogenetic service laboratory are the cost of the required image analysis equipment, the inability of CGH to evaluate some chromosomal regions and the difficulties in detecting mosaicism. Centromeric regions and heterochromatic repeat regions such as the p-arms of the acrocentric chromosomes cannot be reliably evaluated, because they are blocked, to various extents, by the unlabelled COT-1® (Life Technologies Inc., Gaithersburg, MI, USA) DNA in the hybridization. Telomeric regions are excluded because the absolute green and red fluorescence intensities gradually decrease at those regions. Unreliable ratio changes may appear as the fluorescence intensities approach the background fluorescence[16]. Difficulties also exist in detecting weak mosaicism, balanced chromosomal translocations, inversions and ploidy changes[19].

For an accurate diagnosis, hybridization signals should be uniform, smooth, intense and without high background noise and hybridization artefacts over the entire metaphase spread. In addition to that, interspersed repetitive sequences of the DNA should be suppressed and binding of the labelled DNA to chromosome centromeres and heterochromatic regions should be low.

CONCLUSION

Applying CGH in prenatal genetic diagnosis using fetal cells from maternal blood is an innovative method which is non-invasive, fast and accurate. Further studies on fetal nRBCs isolation and whole genomic amplification to retrieve enough DNA material is warranted. The progress in this field will enable prenatal genetic diagnosis using fetal nRBCs and CGH to be a popularly used screening method in the near future.

References

1. Golbus MS, Loughman WD, Epstein CJ, Halbasch G, Stephens JD, Hall BD. Prenatal genetic diagnosis in 3000 amniocenteses. *N Engl J Med* 1979;300:157–63
2. Yang YH, Kim MS, Park YW, Kim SK, Cho JS, Jeong HJ. Chorionic villus sampling: experience of first 510 cases in Korea. *Kor J Obstet Gynecol* 1993;36:906–15
3. Yang YH, Park YW, Cho JS. Chorionic villus sampling: clinical experience of the initial 750 cases. *J Obstet Gynecol Res* 1996;22(2):143–9
4. Daffos F, Capella-Pavlovsky M, Forestier F. Fetal blood sampling during pregnancy with use of a needle guided by ultrasound: a study of 606 consecutive cases. *Am J Obstet Gynecol* 1995;153:655–60
5. Spencer K, Salonen R. Muller F. Down's syndrome screening in multiple pregnancies using alpha-fetoprotein and free beta hCG. *Prenat Diagn* 1994;14:537–42
6. Simpson JL. Isolating fetal cells in maternal circulation for prenatal diagnosis. *Prenat Diagn* 1994;14(13):1229–42
7. Bianchi DW. Prenatal diagnosis by analysis of fetal cells in maternal blood. *J Pediatr* 1995;127(6):847–56
8. Bianchi DW, Flint AF, Pizzimenti MF, Knoll J, Latt SA. Isolation of fetal DNA from nucleated erythrocytes in maternal blood. *Proc Natl Acad Sci USA* 1990;87:3279–83
9. Hamada H, Arinami T, Kubo T, Hamguchi H, Iwasaki H. Fetal nucleated cells in maternal peripheral blood: frequency and relationship to gestational age. *Hum Genet* 1993;91:427–32
10. Sohda S, Arinami T, Hamada H, Nakauchi H, Hamguchi H, Kubo T. The proportion of fetal nucleated red blood cells in maternal blood: estimation by FACS analysis. *Prenat Diagn* 1997;17:743–52
11. Bhat NM, Bieber NM, Teng N. One step enrichment of nucleated red blood cells. *J Immunol Meth* l993;158:277–80
12. Milteneyi S, Muller W, Weichel W. High gradient magnetic cell separation with MACS. *Cytometry* 1990;11:231–4
13. Gänshirt-Ahlert D, Burschyk M, Garritsen H, Helmer L, Miny P, Horst J, *et al.* Magnetic cell sorting and the transferrin receptor as potential means of prenatal diagnosis from maternal blood. *Am J Obstet Gynecol* 1992;166:1350–5
14. Bianchi DW. Development of a model system to compare cell separation methods for the isolation of fetal cells from maternal blood. *Prenat Diagn* 1996;16(4):289–98
15. Gänshirt-Ahlert D. Enrichment of fetal nucleated red blood cells from the maternal circulation for prenatal diagnosis: experiences with triple density gradient and MACS based on more than 600 cases. *Fetal Diagn Ther* 1998;13(5):276–86
16. du Manoir S, Schrock E, Bentz M, Speicher MR, Joos S, Reid T, *et al.* Quantative analysis of comparative genomic hybridization. *Cytometry* 1995;19(1):27–41
17. Kallioniemi A, Kallioniemi OP, Sudar D, Rutovitz D, Gray JW, Waldman FM, *et al.* Comparative genomic hybridization for molecular cytogenetic analysis of solid tumors. *Science* 1992;258(5083):818–21
18. Kallioniemi OP, Kallioniemi A, Piper J, Isola J, Waldman FM, Gray JW, *et al.* Optimizing comparative genomic hybridization for analysis of DNA sequence copy number changes in solid tumors. *Genes Chromosom Cancer* 1994;10:231–43
19. Bryndof T, Kirchhoff M, Rose H, Maahr J, Gerdes T, Karhu R, *et al.* Comparative genomic hybridization in clinical cytogenetics. *Am J Hum Genet* 1995;57:1211–20
20. Wells D, Sherlock JK, Handyside AH, Delhanty JDA. Detailed chromosomal and molecular genetic analysis of single cells by whole genome amplification and comparative genomic hybridization. *Nucleic Acids Res* 1999;27(4):1214–18
21. Schmorl G. *Pathologisch-anatomische untersuchungen uber Publeraleklampsie.* Leipzig: Vogel, 1893
22. Herzenberg L, Bianchi D, Schroder J. Fetal cells in the blood of pregnant women: detection and enrichment by fluorescence activated cell sorting. *Proc Natl Acad Sci USA* 1979;76:1453–5

23. Gänshirt-Ahlert D, Borjesson-Stroll R, Burschyk M, Dohr A, Hemer E, Velasco M, *et al*. Detection of fetal trisomies 21 and 18 from maternal blood using triple gradient and magnetic cell sorting. *Am J Reprod Immunol* 1993;30:194–201

24. Morton NE. Parameters of the human genome. *Proc Natl Acad Sci USA* 1991;88:7474–6

25. Kuukasjärvi T, Tanner M, Pennanen S, Karhu R, Visakorpi T, Isola J. Optimizing DOP-PCR for universal amplification of small DNA samples in comparative genomic hybridization. *Genes Chromosom Cancer* 1997;18:94–101

26. Griffin DK, Sanoudou D, Adamski E, McGriffert C, O'Brien P, Weinberg J, *et al*. Chromosome specific comparative genomic hybridization for determining the origin of intrachromosomal duplications. *J Med Genet* 1998;35:37–41

27. Karhu R, Kähkönen M, Kuukasjärvi T, Pennanen S, Tirkkonen M, Kallioniemi O. Quality control of CGH: impact of metaphase chromosomes and the dynamic range of hybridization. *Cytometry* 1997;28:198–205

28. Voullaire L, Wilton L, Slater H, Williamson R. Detection of aneuploidy in single cells using comparative genomic hybridization. *Prenat Diagn* 1999;19:846–51

Prenatal diagnosis of hemoglobinopathies

14

A. J. Antsaklis

INTRODUCTION

Serious congenital disorders may be defined as conditions that arise at the time of conception or during intrauterine development. They can cause lifelong and burdensome pathology. Some of them if diagnosed in the neonatal period can be managed relatively simply with satisfactory results. However, there is no satisfactory treatment for most severe congenital disorders and the only possible active intervention is early intrauterine diagnosis followed by selective termination.

Hemoglobinopathies and especially thalassemia major constitute a typical example of inherited disease for which the indication for prenatal diagnosis is clear. The social and ethical issues involved are not unique to the hemoglobinopathies, but the hemoglobinopathies are unique among genetic diseases at present, because of their high frequency, because so much is known about their biological basis and because so much can be done to treat and to prevent them. Hemoglobinopathies are the most commonly inherited recessive diseases in humans with an estimated 240 million carriers worldwide, and 200 000 homozygotes or compound heterozygotes born each year[1–3].

The condition is chronic and practically incurable. Recent medical and scientific developments, such as bone marrow transplantation, stimulation of fetal hemoglobin synthesis by antimetabolites or other agents, gene transfer and stem cell transplantation are promising issues, but these will never be applied on a large scale, because they are extremely expensive and complicated.

In past years babies with hemoglobinopathies and especially with thalassemia major could not survive without external support. In recent years the situation has changed and blood transfusion has made life possible for most of the affected individuals, and iron chelation appears to relieve some of the deleterious effects of transfusional hemosiderosis. Optimization of care creates the hope that life expectancy of patients may reach normal levels. However, the price of this gain is heavy. Life is a misery for the patients, and an endless sadness for their families. The quantity of blood necessary, the undesirable reactions, the transmissible diseases and the increased cost of iron chelating agents are the causes for suboptimal treatment in most populations where the number of patients is high and the resources remain limited[4].

In this instance prevention of the birth of new cases appears to be the only realistic solution, and today in most countries identification of carriers, genetic counselling and prenatal diagnosis are widely accepted and practiced. This combination of action has reduced the number of affected infants born in many countries, especially in countries such as Greece, where the frequency of thalassemia is very high. Families at risk are recognized because they already have an affected child or through carrier screening. The latter is only relevant in areas or groups with high numbers (for thalassemia in Mediterraneans or Orientals, sickle cell disorders in Blacks).

Education and counselling must be provided, so that families can understand the potential severity of the disease as well as the availability, reliability and possible risk of the prenatal test. The appropriate blood or tissue sample must be obtained with safety and reliability, free of contamination by maternal blood or tissue. The risk to mother and fetus must be acceptably low, and the test must be specific and sensitive, with low overall error rate[5].

IDENTIFICATION OF CARRIERS

Prevention of thalassemia starts with the identification of carriers, and this becomes very complicated when it has to be carried out on a large scale. Identification of heterozygous carriers in a given population may be carried out on an obligatory or voluntary basis. As a rule, the former approach, applicable in schools, the army, or other population clusters, has always met with a strong reaction, despite knowledge of the risk, and should be discouraged, as it may produce negative results, especially in some ethnic groups.

A premarital medical certificate, legally required in Greece for a while, was abandoned many years ago on the grounds that it is unconstitutional. The example of Cyprus, where a certificate of blood examination is required by the church authorities before issuing permission for marriage, has in fact proven to be a realistic and most efficient solution, but it is seriously questioned at various legal, social and religious levels.

A key for success in programs for mass screening on a voluntary basis is ample sensitization of the population at risk. In areas where thalassemia is frequent, sensitization can be carried out at school, and the risk of thalassemia should be brought to the attention of all age groups. The army, youth organizations and the universities are excellent targets for sensitization. Sensitization of the population at large makes use of the mass media such as the daily press, family journals, television and radio programs. Spots of only a few seconds, advertising the benefits of prevention, prove most effective. Our experience in Greece is that the number of individuals requesting carrier identification increases consistently every time an interview or other information concerning thalassemia is shown on television[6,7].

A carrier identification program has to meet the following requirements: (1) high frequency of the deleterious genes among the involved population; (2) adequate sensitization and request for screening; (3) access to prenatal diagnosis.

When both prospective parents are found to carry such genes, they can choose to proceed to prenatal diagnosis and selectively bring to term the unaffected fetuses only. These programs require a critical mass of expert professionals and laboratory backup. The yield in screening pregnant women for hemoglobulin disorders depends on the risk profile of the population being tested.

The most definite methods for diagnosis of thalassemia trait include quantitative determinations of hemoglobin HbA_2, HbF and globin chain synthetic ratio, as well as DNA studies for special mutations. These are accurate but too expensive for mass screening. Since thalassemia is almost invariably associated with significant hypochromia (mean cell hemoglobin (MCH) < 26 pg) and microcytosis (mean cell volume (MCV) < 75 fl) determination of red cell indices has been used as a preliminary indicator of possible thalassemia trait. Microcytosis due to iron deficiency must be excluded. Serum ferritin and iron binding capacity studies are also important in the diagnosis of iron deficiency.

Most screening programs use a simple but sensitive screening test such as red cell MCV or osmotic fragility. These tests exclude the great majority of individuals who do not have thalassemia trait, but they do not differentiate precisely between thalassemia trait and iron deficiency. In one study, electrophoresis in combination with a complete blood count was performed in 298 African, American and South East Asian prenatal patients. Ninety-four patients (31.5%) had a hemoglobin disorder including sickle cell, hemoglobin E, α-thalassemia, and β-thalassemia trait, hemoglobin H and hemoglobin C[8].

HbF determinations and hemoglobin electrophoresis are necessary to diagnose δβ-thalassemia and Hb-Lepore trait in microcytotic patients. It is important to note that no simple screening procedure will detect the so-called silent carrier. α-Thalassemia, which occurs in the same population as β-thalassemia, makes screening more complicated.

Two-tier hemoglobin electrophoresis (cellulose acetate electrophoresis with confirmation by citrate agar electrophoresis) or thin layer isoelectric focusing are widely used screening tests for hemoglobin disorders. High-performance liquid chromatography (HPLC) is a newer technique that offers high resolution. Techniques employing monoclonal antibodies and recombinant DNA technology are not used widely[9]. The results are communicated to the subjects concerned by results, or by a personal interview when both parents are found to carry an abnormal gene. When pregnancy occurs, couples at risk are referred for prenatal diagnosis.

PRENATAL DIAGNOSIS

Prenatal diagnosis is the ultimate step in the process of prevention of hemoglobinopathies. However, resorting to prenatal diagnosis on a widespread basis cannot be decided upon lightly. The procedure is burdened with moral, legal, social, financial and technical problems, which must be thoroughly taken into account. There is no universal answer to the problems mentioned above, and laws in many instances coupled with religious rules range from total permissiveness to extreme severity. The social impact of the disease and acceptance of prenatal diagnosis with the prospect of elective abortion by women at risk also vary depending on available patient care and level of education and income[10,11].

Prenatal diagnosis of thalassemia is feasible at two levels:

(1) Assessment of whether the fetal blood contains an amount of βA_2-chains, HbA or HbS which is considered 'normal' for the time of pregnancy when sampling is carried out (protein level);

(2) Identification of whether the genes governing β-globin chain synthesis in the fetus have the expected normal structure and function (gene level).

Prenatal diagnosis of thalassemia and hemoglobinipathies was first achieved in 1972, following the development of fetal blood sampling, by the study of globin synthesis in a fetal blood sample. This method has proved highly successful, and several countries, in which β-thalassemia is a major public health problem, have used it effectively to control the condition. However, it suffers from the disadvantage that fetal blood sampling is not possible until about the 18th week of pregnancy, which means a long wait for the mother, and if indicated, a relatively difficult therapeutic abortion.

In 1972 Kan and associates[12] first detected sickle cell trait in a second-trimester fetus by incubating umbilical cord blood with radioactive leukine, followed by separation of the globin chains using carboxymethyl cellulose chromatography (CMC). Thalassemias are characterized by decreased production of α- or β-globin chain synthesis and fetal blood samples were used to evaluate the globin chain synthesis. CMC was used to calculate the β/γ synthetic ratio since a rise in the β/γ ratio occurs normally throughout gestation. A quantitative decrease of β-chain production was highly suggestive of the homozygous state. Diagnostic errors were known to occur in those patients with high β-globin production, β^+-thalassemia major and low β^- production or β-thalassemia[13].

Other methods for globin chain analysis have been devised including electrophoresis on polyacrylamide gels containing urea, acetic acid and Triton-X-100, as well as hemoglobin immunofluorescence. CMC was gradually replaced by HPLC by ion exchange, which can separate globin chains to provide an answer within 15 min. Isoelectric focusing is an alternative method for analysis of hemoglobin tetramers, instead of globin chain synthesis, in pure fetal samples[14–16]. Other mutant β-globin chain variants such as HbE, Hb Lepore, HbC and HbO-Arab are also detectable by CMC using fetal cells[17].

Hemoglobinopathies were the first group of single gene disorders to which techniques derived from recombinant DNA technology were applied for prenatal diagnosis. Southern blood analysis was first used in the antenatal diagnosis of sickle cell disease at the DNA level. As polymorphism of the DNA sequence adjacent to the β-globin gene was established, the normal HbA fragment was differentiated from the Hbs allele of a different length. Several altered restriction endonuclease sites have been found using the enzymes Hpa I, Dde I, Mst II, Cvn I and oxa NI. PCR techniques allow for restriction digestion and direct visualization of DNA fragments more rapidly and without the need of radioisotopes. Direct assays that detect the Hbs mutation in enzymatically amplified fetal DNA are possible with allele-specific oligonucleotide probes[18].

Routine and reliable diagnosis of thalassemia mutations can now be accomplished by using fetal DNA obtained between 8 and 18 weeks of gestation. The most reliable methods are based on identification of the abnormal gene by direct DNA analysis. With chorionic villus sampling (CVS) adequate amounts of DNA can be obtained safely at an earlier gestational age. The DNA is analyzed by a variety of PCR-based or other methods for the presence of the thalassemia mutations. The heterogenicity of thalassemia mutations complicates the approach to antenatal diagnosis. More than 125 independent mutations can cause β-thalassemia.

Although rarer alleles are expected to be identified in the future, it is estimated that the 54 known alleles account for 99% of β-thalassemia gene defects in the world. The combination of PCR and specific restriction enzymes or probes is the most commonly used method of prenatal assessment. Until recently, this required indirect analysis of DNA polymorphism in both parents, and multiple Southern blot analysis of fetal DNA. The final results were only 70–80% predictive of the genotype of the fetus.

Three major factors have improved the efficacy and the reliability of DNA diagnosis. First, extensive survey of most populations in which these alleles are frequent has revealed that about 15 β-thalassemia mutations account for > 90% of individuals affected worldwide. Within any given ethnic group, three to five mutations are usually responsible for the vast majority of severe cases. The search can then be customized for mutations according to the ethnic origin of the family at risk. Second, PCR and accurate, precise oligonucleotide

hybridization assays can now be combined to permit screening of minute DNA samples for several mutations very rapidly, even with non-radioactive probes. Third, amplification, and even sequences of the β-globin genes, can now be performed by PCR in about the time previously required to culture amniocytes and perform Southern blot analysis.

Diagnosis of most cases of severe α-thalassemia can be completed by similar approaches. Therefore, genetic counselling for antenatal diagnosis should be offered to all families at risk, for either severe α- or β-thalassemia. DNA can be extracted from trophoblastic or amniotic cells, which can be easily and safely obtained by amniocentesis and chorionic villus sampling, becoming useful for prenatal diagnosis despite the fact that they produce no globin molecules. With increasing experience, both obstetric methods have become safe enough and easily applicable.

In Greece, a nation-wide program for prevention of thalassemia and Hbs syndromes has been functioning over the past 27 years and the program is carried out through a central unit for prevention of thalassemia in Athens and another 25 similar units for prevention dispersed in various large towns of the country, mainly in areas with high frequencies of the abnormal genes[6,7].

Approximately 40 000 persons are examined every year. Carrier identification is carried out in all units following a standard schema: complete blood tests followed by electrophoresis and measurements of hemoglobin fractions, quantitative determination of HbA_2 and HbF. Our experience has shown that the number of individuals seeking the test is steadily increasing and the frequency of diagnosed heterozygotes is much higher than that determined for the general population in previous surveys (14% vs. 8%)[8,9].

Recently in our unit we have started to use new methodologies and technology in order to show molecular defects of different globin genes using non-radioactive procedures (denatured gradient gel electrophoresis (DGGE)) and direct sequencing. Of the total number of people who presented at the unit, either for prenatal diagnosis or for detection of the β-globin gene mutation, 27 different mutations were recorded whose frequency varied from 43% to 0.07%. The prevalent mutation is the IVSI-110 (43%), while the four most common mutations together with sickle cell mutation cover more than 90% of the samples examined.

Prenatal diagnosis has been adopted in Greece as the most realistic means to reduce the birth of children with thalassemia major. Prenatal diagnosis was supplemented with educational programs. The number of affected neonates expected to be born annually is estimated at approximately 150 per year. This number is lower than that previously estimated, because of the significant decrease in the birth rate (approximately 100 000 new-borns/year) in Greece over the past decade. On the basis of this estimation, each year about 500 couples at risk must be referred for counselling and prenatal diagnosis in our unit.

The total number of pregnancies examined so far in our unit is more than 9000 cases. The annual percentage of positive diagnoses did not deviate considerably from the anticipated 25%. The Thalassemia Prevention Program has reduced the birth rate of thalassemia patients dramatically in recent years.

Prenatal diagnosis was carried out by fetal blood sampling and globin chain separation until 1983. Prenatal diagnosis in the first trimester of pregnancy by restriction fragment length polymorphism (RFLP) on the DNA of chorionic villi or amniotic fluid cells was applied in 1983 and was completely replaced in 1989 by gene amplification using the PCR technique and hybridization with allele-specific oligonucleotide (ASO) probes for the direct identification of the mutation. The latter approach is being used currently in our unit for the diagnosis of 13 different mutations that cover the heterogeneity of β-thalassemia in Greece. Other hemoglobinopathies are diagnosed by the PCR technique by amplification with specific primers, which generate fragments specific for normal and recombinant DNA (δβ-thalassemia, Sicilian type, Lepore etc.) or by restriction enzyme digestion of PCR products (βδ, βo-Arab, β D-Pynjab).

During the whole period among the prenatal diagnosis cases we had 22 false-negative results. Sixteen were by fetal blood studies. Although most of them were an over-optimistic interpretation of the β to γ ratio, four may have resulted from switching of the samples during the multiple steps of the procedure. The six missed diagnoses had been from DNA studies. Two of them were due to maternal contamination of the chorionic villus sampling. Three of them were due to false diagnosis of parental mutations and one of them was a mistake in the selective termination of a twin pregnancy.

The information collected through personal contacts, from all major units transfusing patients with thalassemia and syndromes of Hbs, shows that the annual number of new cases of thalassemia has been reduced to 2–3 new cases over the past 5 years.

OBSTETRIC PROCEDURES

Fetal blood sampling

Obtaining a pure fetal blood sample is a major step in prenatal diagnosis at the protein level. Access to the fetal circulation has become less formidable in recent years through advances in obstetric techniques and with the advent of ultrasonography.

Placentocentesis or needle aspiration of intraplacental fetal blood was the first method of accessing fetal blood; this technique was used before the era of obstetric ultrasound and was associated with a high rate of contamination of the specimen with maternal blood or amniotic fluid or both, making it unreliable for determining most hematological disorders. The procedure-related fetal mortality was about 10%, mainly due to fetal exsanguination. Placentocentesis was replaced in 1973 by fetoscopic blood sampling.

Fetoscopy involved a fiberoptic endoscopic approach, first to placental surface vessels, and later to the umbilical cord itself, by passage of a very thin needle through the fetoscope. This procedure was limited to the second trimester of pregnancy (18–21 weeks) using endoscopes housed in a trocar with an outer diameter of

2.2 mm and a side arm for the sampling needle. This is a reliable method of obtaining pure fetal blood, and increasing experience and reliance on sonography for locating optimal entry sites led to a decrease in procedure-related fetal loss rates to 1%[19].

In 1983 Daffos and associates reported their experience with ultrasound-guided umbilical blood sampling using a 20-gauge needle introduced transabdominally and advanced towards the umbilical cord vein, which was punctured at approximately 1 cm from the placental insertion; 1–3 ml of blood was aspirated and the purity of the sample was assessed to exclude maternal blood/amniotic fluid contamination[20].

This technique, known as cordocentesis, or percutaneous umbilical blood sampling (PUBS), has all the advantages of specimen purity, as well as decreased fetal loss rates and relative technical simplicity. Cordocentesis is much less invasive than fetoscopy, and it can be performed from the second trimester of pregnancy until term, but it has been used to make prenatal diagnosis as early as 15 weeks' gestation[21]. Difficulty in obtaining blood samples occurs if fetal movements are frequent and strong enough to dislodge the needle. If oligohydramnios and maternal obesity are present, there is poor ultrasound visualization.

Although cordocentesis has proved to be safer than other fetal blood sampling techniques, this procedure is not without risk. Fetal bradycardia occurs in about 10% of cases and it is transient. While bleeding from the umbilical puncture site is a relatively common occurrence, noted in up to 41% of patients, it lasts for more than 2 min in only 2% of these individuals. On occasion it can lead to significant fetal anemia. Uterine contraction after the procedure, chorioamnionitis (0.6%), cord hematoma and premature rupture of the membranes (0.2%) are rare. The procedure-related fetal loss rate from several large series has been estimated to be approximately 1%, but it may be greater before 19 weeks' gestation[22–24]. When cordocentesis is technically impossible, hepatic vein sampling or cardiac puncture have been used for fetal blood sampling. With cardiocentesis the rate of transient fetal bradycardia (9%)

compares with that found in cordocentesis, but hemopericadium is a serious complication leading to a fetal loss rate of 6.5%[25].

Cordocentesis remains the most desirable way of accessing the fetal circulation. Prenatal diagnosis of the hemoglobinopathies and management of hematological conditions constitutes the main indications for cordocentesis. In addition, cordocentesis has been used for rapid karyotyping, diagnosing congenital infections, assessing fetal blood pH and acid–base status, assessment of intrauterine growth restriction and fetal pharmacological therapy[26–29].

Amniocentesis

The idea of obtaining amniotic fluid cells for diagnostic purposes had its origin in 1930[30]. In 1950 amniocentesis was introduced as a method of diagnosing and managing erythoblastosis fetalis[31,32]. In the same decade desquamated fetal cells in the amniotic fluid were used for sex chromatin analysis[33].

In the early 1960s Steele and Breg[34] first reported amniotic fluid cell cultures in sufficient quantity to be karyotyped. Although early cultures of amniotic fluid cells were difficult, in 1968 Valenti and colleagues[35] reported the first diagnosis of Down syndrome *in utero*, and Nadler the first antenatal detection of the hereditary disorders galactosemia and mucopolysaccharidosis[36]. By 1970 an estimated 10 000 procedures had been performed in a high-risk population with a fetal morbidity and mortality of <1%.

Amniotic cell sampling is carried out in the 16th week of pregnancy and in most specialist centers is now performed with continuous ultrasound guidance. The free-hand technique is preferred and this technique can be easily adapted to all ultrasound-guided diagnostic and therapeutic procedures. An ultrasound scan is performed before amniocentesis to confirm gestational age, fetal viability, fetal position and fetal anatomy. At the chosen site of entry on the maternal abdomen, 20 ml of amniotic fluid is drawn with a 20–22-gauge needle, and fetal activity observed immediately after the procedure. The identification and quantification of fetal risk have been based on large multicenter trials. A prospective randomized controlled trial reported a total fetal loss related to the procedure of 0.5%, a figure that is believed should be used for counselling. It has been demonstrated that there were significant associations between spontaneous abortion and penetration of the placenta, high maternal serum α–fetoprotein and stained amniotic fluid. Complications are rare, but may include amniotic fluid leakage, severe cramping, fetal trauma, blood-stained amniotic fluid and infection. There is no conclusive evidence for an association of positional deformation and pulmonary hypoplasia due to removal of amniotic fluid early in pregnancy[37].

Amniocentesis is a simple, accurate and safe invasive procedure, and today constitutes the method of choice in specific instances where the thalassemic defect is well defined and does not require a large quantity of DNA for gene mapping[38].

Chorionic villus sampling

Although prenatal diagnosis was shown to be feasible using fetal DNA from cultured amniotic fluid cells in 1978[39], prenatal diagnosis programs were only started when the first-trimester procedure of chorionic villus sampling (CVS) was developed and prenatal diagnosis of hemoglobinopathies using chorionic villus DNA shown to be feasible. Chromosome analysis from CVS in the first trimester became possible in the early 1980s. Since that time the method has spread rapidly and successfully in several centers. In April 1983 only eight of them, including the center in Athens, were able to report their diagnostic experience on a limited number of women at risk. In September 1985 the list of the International CVS Collaborative Study contained more than 80 centers in Europe and North America with more than 10 000 diagnostic cases; today CVS has emerged as a means of making earlier prenatal diagnosis more quickly, and is as reliable as amniocentesis.

In all CVS cases an ultrasound scan is performed before the procedure to evaluate fetal growth and fetal viability. CVS is commonly performed under ultrasound guidance between the 9th and 12th weeks of pregnancy and involves the aspiration of 20–30 mg of villus. The sample must be in good condition in order to allow an accurate diagnosis.

Transcervical CVS ultrasound guidance can be carried out with suction using special catheters, or by biopsy with a suitable forceps. If insufficient material is obtained with the initial aspiration, a total of three attempts can be made. With experience more than 99% of the cases provide adequate tissue for diagnosis with one or two insertions. The transabdominal approach under ultrasound guidance has the same yield of tissue suitable for diagnosis and no difference in risk. The method is highly acceptable and the simplicity of the procedure is apparent from its ready adoption[40]. CVS provides large amounts of metabolically active material, and DNA for enzyme and gene probe diagnosis of genetic defects[41]. Unlike standard blot techniques, when just under 1 week is required to detect a specific molecular mutation, application of PCR has shortened the time required to a few hours. Early concerns over both the safety and accuracy of CVS led to randomized trials between first-trimester CVS and second-trimester amniocentesis[42]. It appears that the fetal loss rate attributed to the procedure is not more than 1% and may be less. Some of the loss appears to be correlated with avoidable trauma to the chorionic area. CVS permits earlier diagnosis of a genetic defect and this must be weighed against a slightly poorer performance with respect to fetal loss rate and diagnostic accuracy[43].

Maternal contamination of the sample can be avoided with experience, fetal hemorrhagic lesions after CVS can occur as a result of inexperience, and the controversial link between CVS and limb and oromandibular malformations is rare and is greater in cases in which CVS is performed at < 9 weeks' gestation[44,45]. Appropriate timing of the procedure and doctors' experience can avoid this potential complication. CVS is likely to remain the optimum procedure used to diagnose several chromosomal abnormalities, inherited diseases and metabolic disorders early in pregnancy.

Both amniocentesis and chorionic villus biopsy have been used with success for the identification of the abnormal gene by direct DNA analysis. In experienced hands the latter method is preferable, because adequate amounts of DNA can be obtained safely at an earlier gestational age.

THE IMPACT OF PRENATAL DIAGNOSIS IN THALASSEMIA

The single hematological disease for which fetal diagnosis might have had an impact so far is thalassemia. The impact can be evaluated only at a local level, since clearly the number of cases examined worldwide is negligible compared to the annual birth rate of homozygotes. Birth of infants with thalassemia in Britain has declined among Greeks, Cypriots, East Africans, Asians and Pakistanis. In Greece, Sardinia, Italy and Cyprus the birth rate of thalassemic infants declined dramatically by up to 95%. These reductions are due to the combinations of screening, counselling and prenatal diagnosis.

The number of pregnancies which are required to be monitored is equal to four times the number of expected homozygotes. This is an effective program in comparison to the expense of treating each thalassemic with transfusions and iron chelation. The future of prenatal diagnosis of thalassemia lies in the improvement of diagnostic methods and intrauterine treatment. Every invasive prenatal procedure carries the risk of fetal death. Several attempts have been made to detect fetal nucleated cells in the maternal circulation[46]. Monoclonal antibodies directed at the syncytiotrophoblast antigen, the HLA antigen and the transferring receptor antigen OKT9 of fetal nucleated erythrocytes have been used to detect these cells. PCR can then be used to detect fetal DNA sequences of interest[47,48]. The high frequency of false-positive and -negative results as well as the problems associated with maternal cell contamination suggests that a non-invasive procedure has to be determined. Preimplantation genetic diagnosis is now technically feasible. The genetic structure of the embryo formed by *in vitro* fertilization may

be assessed, followed by the uterine transfer of the genetically unaffected embryo. Although strong ethical objections to this practice have been raised, preimplantation genetic determination may appeal to those who are opposed to selective termination but who are at high risk of a genetically affected offspring.

Until *in utero* stem cell transplantation can be performed, there will still be a role for prenatal testing. The immaturity of the fetal immune system and the presence of marrow space make the fetus the ideal transplantation host, requiring neither extensive preconditioning regimens nor HLA identical transfusions. *In utero* fetal stem cell transplantation offers the advantages of increased probability of engraftment and chimerism, decreased risk of acute graft versus host disease and a sterile environment, while early gestational age improves the chance for full and rapid development of transplanted fetal stem cells. The source of hematopoietic stem cells appears critical to engraftment, as isolated attempts to correct several inherited diseases including thalassemia have been unsuccessful when using paternal marrow donor cells. Fetal liver cells, alone or with syngeneic fetal thymic cells and fetal skin cells, have shown engraftment following umbilical vein and intraperitoneal transfusion. Complete cure or significant improvements have been demonstrated in conditions associated with SCID, aplastic anemia and thalassemia[49-51]. The ideal situation will be a combination of fetal monitoring to identify thalassemia, or sickle cell disorders, with *in utero* treatment with fetal stem cell transplantation. Advances in gene transfer techniques may provide yet another avenue of treatment. *In utero* gene transfer and expression of neomycin-resistant genes in fetal sheep hematopoietic cells have been demonstrated. Direct gene targeting to fetal hepatocytes as well as *in utero* genetically modified hematopoietic stem cell transplantation to treat a variety of the inherited hematological disorders can be expected.

The use of such technology may make prenatal diagnosis more palatable to individuals who would not consider termination of pregnancy the only solution.

References

1. Modell B. Prevention of the hemoglobinopathies. *Br Med Bull* 1993;39:386

2. WHO Working Group. Hereditary anaemia, genetic basis, clinical features, diagnosis and treatment. *WHO Bull* 1982;60:643

3. Modell B. Ethical and social aspects of fetal diagnosis of the hemoglobinopathies: a practical view. In Loukopoulos D, ed. *Prenatal Diagnosis of Thalassemia and the Hemoglobinopathies*. Florida: CRC Press, 1988:29–54

4. Fessas P, Loukopoulos D. The B-thalassemias. *Clin Haematol* 1974;3:411

5. WHO Working Group: Community control of hereditary anaemia. *WHO Bull* 1983;61:63

6. Loukopoulos D. Prenatal diagnosis of thalassemia and of the hemoglobinopathies: a review. *Hemoglobin* 1985;9:435

7. Antsaklis A. Prenatal diagnosis of hemoglobinopathies. The nation-wide program for the prevention of B-thalassemia in Greece. *FIGO Congress*, Rio Janeiro 1988

8. Stein J, Berg C, Jones J, *et al*. A screening protocol for a population at risk for inherited hemoglobin disorders: results of its application to a group of Southeast Asians and blacks. *Am J Obstet Gynecol* 1984;150:333–41

9. Garrick MD. Alternative methods for screening. *Pediatrics* 1989;83:855–7

10. Aleporou-Marinou B, Sakarelou-Papapetrou N, Antsaklis A, Fessas P, Loukopoulos D. Prenatal diagnosis of thalassemia major in Greece: evaluation of the first large series of attempts. *Ann NY Acad Sci* 1980;344:181–8

11. Loukopoulos D, Hadji A, Papadakis M, *et al*. Prenatal diagnosis of thalassemia and sickle cell syndromes in Greece. *Ann NY Acad Sci* 1990;612:226–36

12. Kan YW, Dozy AM, Alter BP, *et al*. Detection of the sickle gene in the human fetus. *N Eng J Med* 1972;287:1

13. Alter BP. Prenatal diagnosis of hemoglobinopathies and other hematologic diseases. *J Pediatr* 1979;95:501

14. Ferrari M, Crema A, Cautu-Rajnoldi A, *et al*. Antenatal diagnosis of haemoglobinopathies by improved method of isoelectric focusing of haemoglobins. *Br J Haematol* 1984;57:265

15. Antsaklis A. Prenatal diagnosis of thalassemia. *Prenat Neonat Med* 1997;2:73–9

16. Cao A, Leoni GB, Sardu R, Piscaeld MC. Prenatal diagnosis of inherited haemoglobinopathies. *Recent Prog Med* 1992;83:224

17. Kan YN, Valenti C, Carnazza V, *et al*. Fetal blood sampling *in utero*. *Lancet* 1974;1:79

18. Antsaklis A, Bang V, Benzie E, *et al*. Special report. The status of fetoscopy and fetal tissue sampling. *Prenat Diagn* 1984;4:79

19. Antsaklis A, Benzie R and Hughes R. Fetoscopy: fetal visualisation and blood sampling in prenatal diagnosis. In: Filkins K, Russo J, eds. *Human Prenatal Diagnosis*, New York: Marcel Dekker, 1985:109

20. Daffos F, Capella-Pavlowsky M, Forestier F. A new procedure for blood sampling *in utero*: preliminary report of 53 cases. *Am J Obstet Gynecol* 1983;146:985

21. Trapani FD, Marinou M, Dalcamo E, *et al*. Prenatal diagnosis of hemoglobin disorders by cordocentesis at 12 weeks' gestation. *Prenat Diagn* 1991;11:899

22. Boulet P, Deschamps F, Lefort G, *et al*. Pure fetal blood samples obtained by cordocentesis: technical aspects of 322 cases. *Prenat Diagn* 1990;11:899

23. Sacher RA, Falchnk JC. Percutaneous umbilical blood sampling. *Clin Rev Clin Lab Sci* 1990;28:19

24. Nicolaides KH. Cordocentesis. *Clin Obstet Gynecol*. 1988;311:123

25. Antsaklis A, Papantoniou N, Mesogitis S, *et al*. Cardiocentesis: an alternative method of fetal blood sampling for the prenatal diagnosis of hemoglobinopathies. *Obstet Gynecol* 1992;79:630

26. Shah DM, Roussis P, Ulm J, *et al*. Cordocentesis for rapid karyotyping. *Am J Obstet Gynecol* 1990;162:1548

27. Daffos F, Forestier F, Grangeot-Keros, *et al*. Prenatal diagnosis of congenital rubella. *Lancet* 1984;2:613

28. Daffos F, Capella-Pavlowsky M, Forestier F. Fetal blood sampling during pregnancy with use of guided ultrasound. A study of 606 consecutive cases. *Am J Obstet Gynecol* 1985;153:655

29. Pardi G, Buscaglia M, Ferrazzi E, *et al*. Cord sampling for the evaluation of oxygenation and acid–base balance in growth retarded human fetuses. *Am J Obstet Gynecol* 1987;157:1221

30. Menees T, Miller JP, Holly LE. Amniography: a preliminary report. *Am J Roentgenol* 1930;24:363

31. Bevis DCA. Composition of liquor amnii in haemolytic disease of the newborn. *J Obstet Gynaecol Br Common* 1953;60:244

32. Liley AW. Liquor amnii analysis in the management of pregnancy complicated by rhesus sensitization. *Am J Obstet Gynecol* 1961;82:1359

33. Fucks F, Riis D. Antenatal sex determination. *Nature (London)* 1956;177:330

34. Steele MW, Breg WR. Chromosome analysis of human amniotic fluid cells. *Lancet* 1966;1:383

35. Valenti C, Schutta EJ, Kehay T. Prenatal diagnosis of Down's syndrome. *Lancet* 1968;2:220

36. Nadler HL. Antenatal detection of hereditary disorders. *Paediatrics* 1968;42:912

37. Henry GP, Miller WA. Early amniocentesis. *J Reprod Med* 1992;37:396

38. Old JM, Ward RH, Petrou M, Karagozlu F, Modell B, Weatherall DJ. First trimester diagnosis of hemoglobinopathies: a report of 3 cases. *Lancet* 1987;1:1413

39. Kan YW, Dozy AM. Antenatal diagnosis of sickle cell anaemia on DNA analysis of amniotic fluid cells. *Lancet* 1978;2:910

40. Smidt-Jensen S, Philip S. Comparison of transabdominal and transcervical CVS and AC: sampling success and risk. *Prenat Diagn* 1991;11:529

41. Lilford RJ. The rise and fall of CVS. *Br Med J* 1991;303:936

42. Canadian Collaborative CVS – Amniocentesis Trial Group. Multicentric trial comparing CVS and AC in prenatal diagnosis. *Lancet* 1989;1:1

43. Medical Research Council. European trial of chorionic villus sampling. *Lancet* 1991;337:1491

44. Burton BK, Schulz CJ, Burd LI. Limb anomalies associated with chorionic villus sampling. *Obstet Gynecol* 1992;79:726

45. Firth HV, Boyd BA, Chamberlain P, *et al.* Severe limb abnormalities after chorion villus sampling at 56–66 days gestation. *Lancet* 1991;337:762

46. Aldinolfi M. Fetal nucleated cells in the maternal circulation. In Brock DJ, Rodeck CH, Ferguson-Smith MA, eds. *Prenatal Diagnosis Screening*. Edinburgh: Churchill Livingstone, 1991.

47. Thorpe SI, Huehns ER. A new approach for antenatal diagnosis of B-thalassemia: a double labelling immunofluorescence microscopic technique. *Br J Haematol* 1983;53:103

48. Rouyer-Fessard P, Plazza F, Blouquit Y, *et al.* Prenatal diagnosis of haemoglobinopathies by ion exchange HPLC of haemoglobins. *Prenat Diagn* 1989;9:19

49. Dinkman R, Golbuns MS. *In utero* stem cell therapy. *J Report Med* 1992;37:515

50. Touraine JL. Rationale and results of *in utero* transplants of stem cells in humans. *Bone Marrow Transplant* 1992;9:121

51. Touraine JL. The fetal liver as a source of stem cells for transplantation in fetuses *in utero*. *Cult Top Microbiol Immunol* 1992;177:187

Prenatal diagnosis of β-thalassemia: Sardinian experience of 6000 cases

15

G. Monni, M. A. Zoppi and R. M. Ibba

β-Thalassemia is a common inherited autosomal recessive disorder characterized by severe microcytic anemia, spleen and liver enlargement, and bone modifications. The disease occurs with a high frequency amongst the Mediterranean coasts and islands, the Middle East and Indian subcontinent to the Far East, and is also observed in people of African origin. World-wide there are at least 240 million heterozygotes for β-thalassemia and at least 200 000 affected homozygotes are born each year.

Through immigration, β-thalassemia has spread all over the world. In Sardinia, an Italian island in the Mediterranean sea with 1.6 million inhabitants, the disease has a carrier frequency rate of 12.6% which means that one couple out of 60 is at risk of having a child with thalassemia major, and the incidence of this disorder among newborn babies is 1 per 250 live births each year (Table 1). The traditional therapy consists of regular transfusions and iron chelation with desferrioxamine-β, resulting in a life expectancy which can reach up to the fourth decade.

Awaiting gene therapy, bone marrow transplantation from human leukocyte antigen (HLA) identical siblings in patients in a good condition is a good therapeutic alternative with a success rate of 90%. At the present time, prenatal diagnosis is the method of choice for prevention of β-thalassemia and in this study we present our Sardinian experience.

PREVENTION AND SCREENING

Prevention of β-thalassemia was based on information and sensitization of the population to identify carriers. Genetic counselling, always informative and never directive, is of paramount importance and precedes antenatal diagnosis. Information concerning carrier screening was particularly important and, in our experience, the main channels of information were the mass media (44%), general practitioners (31%), obstetricians (23%) and midwives (2%).

Screening of β-thalassemia was performed hematologically and molecularly using the following methods:

(1) Hematological identification of carrier by mean cell volume, mean cell hemoglobin and hemoglobin A$_2$ evaluation;
(2) Molecular screening for the common mutation by specific primer mutation and specific probe mutation.

For less common mutations we used denaturing gradient gel electrophoresis (DGGE), chemical mismatch, single strend conformation polymorphism (SSCP) cleavage and, lastly, direct sequencing of the gene to characterize the mutations. The most common mutations of β-thalassemia found in Sardinia were β-39 (96%), β-6, βII-745, βI-110 and β-76 (Table 2). Other couples coming from the Mediterranean area were also analyzed by different mutations.

Once the couple had been identified from a molecular point of view, genetic counselling followed to provide information about the fetal

Table 1 *Demographic characteristics and frequency of β-thalassemia in Sardinia*

Population (millions)	1.6
Couples of child-bearing age (*n*)	170 000
Target screening population (15–40 years)	700 000
Marriages/year (*n*)	10 000
Carrier frequency (%)	12.6
Couples at risk (*n*)	2700
New at risk couples/year (*n*)	160
Incidence of homozygous state	1 : 250

sampling procedures, its risk and the fetal analysis accuracy. On the basis of this information, couples were free to make a decision about fetal testing and termination of pregnancy in case of an affected fetus. With this type of genetic counselling, acceptability of prenatal diagnosis was extremely high both in pregnancy (97%) and out of pregnancy (93%).

INVASIVE PRENATAL PROCEDURES

Methods of fetal sampling, which have been used in Cagliari since 1977, are presented in Table 3. Initially we used placentacentesis, then in 1983–5 we performed fetoscopy and in 1984–5 cordocentesis and in a few cases cardiocentesis. From 1982 to 1983, thanks to progress in molecular biology we performed amniocentesis and subsequently in 1983 transcervical chorionic villus sampling (TC-CVS), and later, since 1985, transabdominal chorionic villus sampling (TA-CVS) which is the only sampling performed at the present time (Table 4).

Placentacentesis involved the aspiration of fetal blood, contaminated by maternal blood and amniotic fluid, from the placenta at 18–20 weeks' gestation. Until 1983 it was the only technique performed in Sardinia.

Thanks to recent progress in ultrasound equipment and in sampling techniques, we used an optical fiber instrument with a needle introduced into the umbilical cord at 20 weeks' gestation to perform fetoscopy. This procedure allowed a pure blood sample to be obtained, but was very traumatic for the mother and for the fetus.

Cordocentesis consisted of direct insertion of the spinal needle 20 or 22G into the umbilical cord under ultrasound monitoring at 18 weeks' gestation. This method was the only procedure used in particular cases when it was not possible to perform DNA analysis.

Cardiocentesis by direct insertion of the needle into the fetal heart at 18 weeks' gestation was performed in a few cases when cordocentesis or fetoscopy were not available.

Table 2 *Frequency of β-thalassemia mutations in Sardinia*

Mutation		%
β-39	(C->T)	95.7
β-6	(-A)	2.2
β-76	(-6)	0.7
βI-110	(G->A)	0.5
βII-745	(C->G)	0.4
β-87	(C->G)	0.2
βI-6	(T->C)	0.2
β1	(-G)	0.1
βII-1	(G->A)	0.1
βI-1	(G->A)	0.03

Table 3 *Invasive procedures for prenatal diagnosis of β-thalassemia*

Technique	Years
Placentacentesis	1977–83
Fetoscopy	1983–85
Cordocentesis	1984–85
Cardiocentesis	1984–86
Amniocentesis	1982–83
Transcervical CVS	1983–86
Transabdominal CVS	1985–2001

CVS, chorionic villus sampling

Table 4 *Invasive procedures in 6000 prenatal diagnoses of β-thalassemia*

Technique	n	Gestational age (weeks)	Failure	Loss (%)	Misdiagnoses
Placentacentesis	981	18–24	10	5.2	2
Fetoscopy	67	18–24	2	5.6	—
Cordocentesis	120	18–24	—	2.1	—
Cardiocentesis	6	18–24	—	—	—
Amniocentesis	203	16–18	6	2.6	—
Transcervical CVS	572	9–13	1	4.2	1
Transabdominal CVS	4051	6–24	—	1.3	—

CVS, chorionic villus sampling

By the end of 1981, following the advent of DNA analysis, prenatal diagnosis of β-thalassemia was done by amniocentesis at 16 weeks' gestation; 30–40 ml of amniotic fluid were sampled and the analysis was carried out by the oligomer technique.

Samples obtained by CVS at 10 weeks' gestation revolutionized fetal diagnosis and improved acceptance, safety and efficacy of prenatal diagnosis of β-thalassemia. In our experience the acceptance of prenatal diagnosis has been improved by CVS compared to the other techniques (Table 5).

In 1983 transcervical TC-CVS was performed from 9 to 13 weeks' gestation using rigid forceps under ultrasound monitoring.

In 1985, transabdominal TA-CVS using a freehand technique was done with a 20G spinal needle inserted into the placenta tangentially to the probe with an up and down movement under ultrasound monitoring. This sampling method is still used today and is the only technique performed by us for prenatal diagnosis of β-thalassemia.

ANALYSIS

The above-mentioned obstetric procedures would not have been possible without the remarkable progress made in molecular biology. Whilst at the beginning the only available method of diagnosis was fetal blood sampling and chain globin synthesis, since 1982 the majority of all diagnoses have been obtained through DNA analysis, and after 1985 all diagnoses have been made by CVS and DNA analysis.

Analysis was accomplished initially on enzymatically restricted genomic DNA using allele-specific oligonucleotide radioactive probes. Subsequently, when polymerase chain reaction (PCR) became available, fetal analysis was carried out using reverse dot blot, allelic-specific oligonucleotide primers (amplified refractory mutant system (ARMS)), denaturing gradient gel electrophoresis (DGGE) and direct sequencing which underlines the mutation type. The last two methods were used in cases of unknown or rare mutations.

The most frequent mutations of β-thalassemia in Sardinia were studied using DNA amplified with specific oligonucleotide probes using reverse dot blot analysis. ARMS, which is an extremely precise method for specific research of known mutations, was used extensively in prenatal diagnosis in couples in whom mutations were known to be present. To avoid maternal decidua contamination we carried out variable number tandem repeat (VNTR), a rapid system of analysis using multiallelic polymorphism. The most frequently used method was MCT 118.

Because the most common cause of misdiagnosis is maternal contamination in the villus sampling, we adopted the guidelines of: first, careful dissection under the inverted microscope of maternal decidua from fetal trophoblast; second, the request of a minimal amount of chorionic villi (about 3 mg) to limit the effect of maternal contamination; third, the use of a limited number of amplification cycles, which may reduce the chances to co-amplify DNA from maternal decidua; and, finally, analysis in duplicate by using two different, but overlapping amplified DNA fragments.

RESULTS AND DISCUSSION

Table 4 shows the overall results obtained in 6000 fetal diagnoses. The best results obtained with regard to sampling success, fetal loss and analysis accuracy were by transabdominal CVS, which since 1985/86 has been the only procedure used. At the beginning of our experience we had only one failure by TC-CVS and the diagnosis was achieved by amniocentesis. We had 1.7% fetal loss (24/572 by TC-CVS and 53/4051 by TA-CVS), one misdiagnosis and 1.6% fetal malformations. Our results demonstrate the high safety of the

Table 5 *Acceptance rate of prenatal diagnosis of β-thalassemia according to the invasive procedure*

Technique	Acceptance (%)
Fetal blood sampling	93.2
Amniocentesis	96.4
Chorionic villus sampling	99.3

procedures and the high accuracy of fetal analysis. With regard to the procedures, TA-CVS, which may be performed at any time from 6 to 40 weeks, is the most appropriate technique and is preferable to TC-CVS due to its simplicity, speed, better success, absence of infection and bleeding, and, particularly, better patient acceptance.

In a study carried out in our center on 72 patients who had undergone both TC- and TA-CVS in different years, all, except one woman, stated their preference for TA-CVS. Moreover, TA-CVS can be performed at any gestational period, which is particularly important for those couples who come late to our observation. We also compared TA-CVS versus amniocentesis in the second trimester of pregnancy, and once again TA-CVS was the chosen technique for better analysis and lower fetal loss rate.

FUTURE

The evaluation of prenatal diagnosis is represented by preimplantation genetic diagnosis. Preimplantation and preconception diagnosis is of considerable interest and would mean that women would not be forced to abort in the case of abnormal results. Preimplantation diagnosis is performed using *in vitro* fertilization (IVF), embryo micromanipulation and DNA amplification analysis on a single cell.

A study carried out in our center on preimplantation genetic diagnosis revealed that 100% of women who had undergone prenatal diagnosis with subsequent termination of pregnancy when fetuses were affected, would invariably have preferred to have preimplantation diagnosis rather than the traditional CVS. At the present time, several groups have performed preimplantation genetic diagnosis of β-thalassemia and the results are very promising. Our group has already set up the procedure of preimplantation diagnosis through the analysis of a single-cell embryo by *in vitro* fertilization (IVF) and polymerase chain reaction (PCR) analysis. Many difficulties are encountered in preimplantation diagnosis: first, the high costs involved and organizational aspects and, second, the need for a staff of

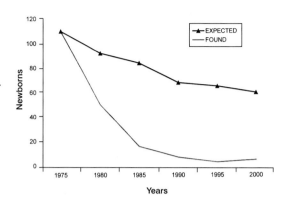

Figure 1 *Fall in the birth rate of homozygous β-thalassemia in Sardinia. The top line represents affected children born in absence of prenatal diagnosis and the bottom line the affected children born with prenatal testing*

obstetricians and molecular biologists experienced in both IVF and DNA analysis of a single cell.

We are also carrying out studies to perform the analysis of fetal cells from maternal circulation, isolating nucleated red blood cells by microdissection and non-radioactive PCR analysis.

CONCLUSION

In conclusion, to underline the social aspect of β-thalassemia control, in Sardinia in 1974, due to the absence of prevention programs, 120 children affected by thalassemia major were born. Following the introduction of prenatal diagnosis and thanks also to the change in obstetric and molecular approach (changing from fetal blood sampling and β-globin analysis at 18 weeks to CVS at 10 weeks and DNA analysis), today only three to five children with β-thalassemia are born in Sardinia instead of 70–80 per year expected (Figure 1).

The cause of the birth of these three to five affected children per year can be explained by lack of information in 57% of cases, refusal to abort in 30% of cases (thus proving our non-directive genetic counselling) and false paternity in 13%.

Bibliography

Angastiniotis M, Modell B, Boulinzhenkov V. Prevention and control of haemoglobinopathies. *Bull WHO* 1995;73:375–86

Bianchi DW, Flint AF, Pizzimenti MF, *et al*. Isolation of fetal DNA from nucleated erythrocytes in maternal blood. *Proc Natl Acad Sci USA* 1990;87:3279–83

Cao A, Galanello R, Furbetta M, Muroni PP, Garbato L, Rosatelli C, Scalas MT, *et al*. Thalassaemia types and their incidence in Sardinia. *J Med Genet* 1978; 33:592–605

Cao A, Falchi AM, Tuveri T, Scalas MT, Monni G, Rosatelli C. Prenatal diagnosis of thalassemia major by fetal blood analysis: experience with 1000 cases. *Prenat Diagn* 1986;6:159–67

Cao A, Cossu P, Monni G, Rosatelli C. Chorionic villus sampling and acceptance rate of prenatal diagnosis. *Prenat Diagn* 1987;7:531–3

Cao A, Rosatelli C, Galanello R, Monni G, Olla G, Cossu P, Ristaldi MS. The prevention of thalassemia in Sardinia. *Clin Genet* 1989;36:277–85

Cao A. 1993 William Allan Award Address. *Am J Hum Genet* 1994;54:397–402

Cheung M-C, Goldberg JD, Kan YW. Prenatal diagnosis of sickle cell anemia and thalassemia by analysis of fetal cells in maternal blood. *Nat Genet* 1996;14:264–8

De Rycke M, Van de Velde H, Sermon K, Lissens W, De Vos A, Van Vanderfaeillie A, Van Steirteghem A, Liebaers I. Preimplantation genetic diagnosis for sickle-cell anemia and thalassemia. *Prenat Diagn* 2001;21(3):214–22

Giardini C, Lucarelli G. Bone marrow transplantation for β-thalassemia. *Hematol Oncol Clin North Am* 1999; 8:1059–64

Harper J, Handyside AH. The current status of preimplantation diagnosis. *Curr Obstet Gynecol* 1994; 4:143–9

Kan YN, Valenti C, Carnazza V, *et al*. Fetal blood sampling *in utero*. *Lancet* 1974;1:79

Kan YW, Golbus MS, Trecartin RF, Furbetta M, Cao A. Prenatal diagnosis of homozygous β-thalassemia. *Lancet* 1975;2:790–2

Kan YW, Golbus MS, Trecartin RF, Filly RA, Valenti C, Furbetta M, Cao A. Prenatal diagnosis of β-thalassemia and sickle-cell anemia: experience with 1000 cases. *Lancet* 1977;1:269–71

Kan YW, Dozy AM. Antenatal diagnosis of sickle cell anaemia on DNA analysis of amniotic fluid cells. *Lancet* 19XX;2:910

Monni G, Rosatelli C, Falchi AM, Scalas MT, Addis M, Maccioni L, Di Tucci A, Tuveri T, Cao A. First trimester diagnosis of β-thalassemia in a twin pregnancy. *Prenat Diagn* 1986;6:63–8

Monni G, Ibba RM, Olla G, Rosatelli C, Cao A. Chorionic villus sampling by rigid forceps: experience with 300 cases at risk for thalassemia major. *Am J Obstet Gynecol* 1987;156:912–14

Monni G, Olla G, Cao A. Patient's choice between transcervical and transabdominal chorionic villus sampling. *Lancet* 1988;1:1057

Monni G, Ibba RM, Olla G, Rosatelli C, Cao A. Prenatal diagnosis of β-thalassemia by second trimester chorionic villus sampling. *Prenat Diagn* 1988;8:447–51

Monni G, Olla G, Rosatelli C, Cao A. Second trimester placental biopsy versus amniocentesis for prenatal diagnosis of β-thalassemia. *N Engl J Med* 1990;322: 60–1

Monni G, Ibba RM, Lai R, Olla G, Cao A. Limb reduction defects and chorionic villus sampling. *Lancet* 1997;337:1091

Monni G, Lai R, Cau G, Ibba RM, Mura S, Palomba ML, Olla G, Rosatelli C, Cao A. Acceptability of preimplantation diagnosis. *Prenat Diagn* 1992; 12S:S24

Monni G, Ibba RM, Lai R, Cau G, Mura S, Olla G, Cao A. Transabdominal chorionic villus sampling: fetal loss rate in relation to maternal and gestational age. *Prenat Diagn* 1993;12:815–20

Monni G, Ibba RM, Lai R, *et al*. Early transabdominal chorionic villus sampling for couples at high genetic risk. *Am J Obstet Gynecol* 1993;168:170–3

Monni G, Ibba RM, Zoppi MA, Floris M. *In utero* stem cell transplantation. *Croatian Med J* 1998;39(2):220–3

Old JM, Ward RH, Petrou M, Karagozlu F, Modell B, Weatherall DJ. First trimester diagnosis of hemoglobinopathies: a report of 3 cases. *Lancet* 1987;1: 1413

Palomba ML, Monni G, Lai R, Cau G, Olla G, Cao A. Psychological implications and acceptability of preimplantation diagnosis. *Hum Reprod* 1994;9(2): 360–2

Rosatelli C, Falchi AM, Tuveri T, Scalas MT, Di Tucci A, Monni G, Cao A. Prenatal diagnosis of β-thalassemia with the synthetic oligomer technique. *Lancet* 1985;2:241–3

Rosatelli C, Sardu R, Tuveri T, Scalas MT, Di Tucci A, Demurtas M, Loudianos G, Monni G, Cao A. Reliability of prenatal diagnosis of genetic diseases by analysis of amplified trophoblast DNA. *J Med Genet* 1990;27:249–51

Rosatelli C, Tuveri T, Scalas MT, *et al*. Molecular screening and fetal diagnosis of β-thalassemia in the Italian population. *Hum Genet* 1992;89:585–9

Saiki RK, Chang CA, Levenson CH, *et al*. Diagnosis of sickle cell anemia and β-thalassemia and enzymatically amplified DNA and nonradioactive allele-specific oligonucleotide probes. *N Engl J Med* 1988;319:537–41

Sorrentino BP, Nienhuis AW. Gene therapy for hematopoietic disease. In Stomatoyannopoulos G, Majerus PW, Perlmutter RM, Vormus H, eds. *The Molecular Basis of Blood Diseases*. 3rd edn. W.B. Saunders Company, 2001:963–1003

Weatherall DJ, Clegg JB. *The Thalassaemia Syndromes*, 4th edn. Oxford: Blackwell Scientific Publication, 2001

WHO Scientific Group. *Control of Hereditary Disease*. Technical Report Series 865. Geneva: WHO, 1996

Working Group on preimplantation genetics. Preimplantation diagnosis of genetic and chromosomal disorders. *Int J Assist Reprod Genet* 1994; 11(5):236–45

Amniocentesis

16

T. Stefos

HISTORICAL ASPECTS

Amniocentesis is the oldest invasive method for prenatal diagnosis. The medical literature contains reports from 100 years ago, when amniocentesis was used for various indications such as polyhydramnios, elective termination of pregnancy and amniography[1-4]. In the 1950s analysis of amniotic fluid bilirubin was found to be useful in the management of pregnancies complicated by isoimmunization[5]. In 1956, Fuchs and Riis[6] reported gender determination, by examination of the X-chromatin component in human amniotic fluid cells. In 1966 Steele and Breg[7] reported successful culture of amniotic cells and determination of a human karyotype. The first chromosomal abnormality, which was a balanced translocation, was diagnosed 1 year later[8]. Valenti *et al.*[9] were the first to report a case of trisomy 21, in 1968. Also, the first congenital metabolic disorder, an adrenogenital syndrome, was diagnosed by amniotic fluid analysis in 1965[10]. Since then, amniocentesis has become the most common invasive procedure for prenatal diagnosis. It has been used not only for karyotype determination but also for the diagnosis of a wide spectrum of disorders, by either enzymatic analysis of amniotic fluid and activity of fetal cells or analysis of fetal DNA.

INDICATIONS

There are several indications for amniocentesis. The most common indication is prenatal diagnosis. The evaluation of lung maturity as well as the diagnosis of intrauterine infection are other indications. The following are the main indications for amniocentesis:

(1) Cytogenetic analysis;
(2) Diagnosis of neural tube defects;
(3) Diagnosis of metabolic disorders;
(4) Diagnosis of fetal infections (CMV, toxoplasmosis, parvovirus B19);
(5) Evaluation of fetal lung maturity;
(6) Estimation of severity in cases of isoimmunization;
(7) Diagnosis of intrauterine, intra-amniotic infection;
(8) Therapeutic amnioreduction in polyhydramnios and twin–twin transfusion syndrome.

Cytogenetic analysis (fetal karyotyping) is the common indication in cases of:

(1) Advanced maternal age ($\geq$ 35 years at the expected time of delivery);
(2) Parental balanced translocation;
(3) Previous offspring with aneuploidy;
(4) Abnormal second-trimester triple screen or first-trimester screen;
(5) Fetal abnormality or growth restriction detected by ultrasonography;
(6) Two or more unexplained pregnancy losses;
(7) Abnormal measurement of nuchal translucency.

AMNIOTIC FLUID VOLUME AT THE TIME OF AMNIOCENTESIS

The mean volume of amniotic fluid is 30 ml at 10 weeks and increases by approximately 20 ml per week until 14 weeks, and then the rate doubles until 18 weeks[11].

CONTRAINDICATIONS TO AMNIOCENTESIS

There are no absolute contraindications to amniocentesis. Some relative contraindications such as HIV infection, hepatitis B, maternal coagulopathy, anticoagulation and fever must be discussed with patients. Some experts recommend some type of added prophylaxis before the procedure.

Technical difficulty such as in the case of bowel overlying the uterus is also a relative contraindication which must be considered before the procedure[12].

TECHNICAL ASPECTS

Some years ago, in the 1960s, amniocentesis was performed without the guidance of ultrasonography. Since the early 1970s an ultrasound examination is performed to confirm fetal viability, the number of fetuses, the placental location, the amniotic fluid volume and the gestational age, as well as to detect any fetal abnormality or uterine abnormality such as fibromas, etc.

The mid-trimester amniocentesis is usually performed between 15 and 18 weeks of gestation. Alternative procedures for earlier prenatal diagnosis are early amniocentesis, which is performed at 12–15 weeks' gestation, and chorionic villus sampling (CVS) at 11–13 weeks' gestation. The major concern with early amniocentesis is the increased risk of spontaneous fetal loss in comparison with either CVS or conventional mid-trimester amniocentesis. Therefore, it has not been accepted as a traditional method for prenatal diagnosis.

Amniocentesis should be performed with a regular spinal needle with a bore of 20–22 gauge. An increased rate of fetal loss is associated with a larger-bore needle[13,14]. Smaller-bore needles are not recommended, because of the difficulty in intraoperative manipulations, if needed, and also because of the required prolonged time in obtaining an adequate volume of amniotic fluid. The length of the needle is generally 9–10 cm. However, in some cases of obese patients, one may need a longer needle. There are also commercially available needles that optimize the sonographic visualization and have side orifices that allow fluid to flow not only through the needle tip but also through the side orifices.

Amniocentesis is a sonographically guided and monitored technique. This means that the site of the needle insertion into the amniotic cavity, the movement of the needle and the fetal movements during the procedure are under continuous sonographic surveillance[15].

It has been shown that the continuous use of ultrasound during the procedure reduces the multiple insertions and the bloody or dry taps, and allows the operator to make proper manipulations in cases with procedure difficulties. The procedure is also very well accepted by the patient and improves the psychological aspects.

Asepsis of the skin is performed after the determination of the site for the needle insertion. The selected site for the needle insertion must be far from the placenta, the umbilicus and a uterine fibroma, if it is present. An anterior placenta is not a contraindication for the procedure, but preference is given to the thinnest portion of the organ in cases of transplacental puncture. The frequency of bloody amniotic fluid is higher in such cases than with the non-transplacental needle passage[15]. The fetal loss rate does not differ between transplacental and non-transplacental insertion[16]. Under direct sonographic visualization the needle is inserted along the side of the transducer and the tip, which appears as a bright echo, is continuously monitored throughout the procedure. The stylet is removed and the amniotic fluid is aspirated and collected in a syringe. An alternative would be for the amniotic fluid to be collected in a tube attached to the hub of the needle and connected to the syringe.

The first 0.5 ml of amniotic fluid is discarded in order to reduce the possibility of maternal-cell contamination of the amniotic fluid. The volume of the amniotic fluid drawn at the time of the genetic amniocentesis varies between 10 and 30 ml. It is believed that this volume represents 10% of the total volume for 16 weeks' gestation. There have been controversial results between the Canadian study[13] and American Collaborative Study[14] in terms of fetal loss and prevalence of neonatal complications in relation to the volume of the removed amniotic fluid for genetic amniocentesis. The Canadian study revealed an increased prevalence in neonatal complications with volumes greater than 16 ml while the American study showed that there was no relation between withdrawn volume of amniotic fluid and fetal loss.

After the aspiration of the amniotic fluid the stylet is replaced and the needle is removed. Sonographic examination must be performed following the procedure in order to confirm fetal movement and fetal cardiac activity. The patient must be informed about the fetal condition and the likelihood of complications related to the procedure, especially with any signs of infection, vaginal leakage of fluid or bleeding. In cases of an unsensitized Rh-negative patient, anti-Rh immunoglobulin must be administered. Local anesthesia is not recommended. In our experience from our own institution over the past 15 years, we have never used local anesthesia. The information concerning amniocentesis, which is given to patients during genetic counselling prior to being tested, helps them undergo the procedure without anesthesia and with good co-operation with the operator.

The amniotic fluid is carried to the laboratory in a container labelled with the patient's name. According to our experience we do not recommend the transvaginal aspiration of amniotic fluid, especially in cases where an early amniocentesis (before 15 weeks' gestation) is performed. We believe that CVS is preferable for prenatal diagnosis in the first trimester of pregnancy.

The time required to obtain results of midtrimester genetic amniocentesis varies between 1 and 2 weeks. Another technique, fluorescence *in situ* hybridization (FISH), is an alternative method for the rapid diagnosis of numeric abnormalities of chromosomes 13, 18, 21, X and Y. Chromosome-specific probes are utilized on uncultured amniocytes[17]. This method requires a small amount of amniotic fluid and provides rapid and accurate diagnosis within 24–48 h from the procedure, but only for the chromosomal abnormalities for which it has been designed[18]. The American College of Medical Genetics recommends that clinical action should not be based on the results of FISH alone[19].

COMPLICATIONS

Possible complications during the procedure may be the following:

(1) *Membrane tenting* this is separation of the chorioamniotic membrane from the uterine wall during the needle insertion. It is a frequent complication in cases with multiple insertions and failure to aspirate amniotic fluid. In these cases a new procedure 1–2 weeks later is recommended.

(2) *Multiple needle insertions* these are more frequent in cases of anterior placenta or bloody and dry taps. More than two insertions may be a cause of increased fetal loss. The conclusions of different studies are controversial[13–16].

(3) *Bloody taps* maternal or fetal blood can result in bloody amniotic fluid. There are also controversial results in different collaborative studies concerning fetal loss and bloody taps[13–16].

(4) *Fetomaternal transfusion* this is more common in cases of anterior placenta or in cases with multiple needle insertions. It can lead to isoimmunization. Anti-Rh immunoglobulin is recommended in cases of Rh-negative unsensitized patients.

(5) *Discolored amniotic fluid* the appearance of brown- or green-stained amniotic fluid means intra-amniotic hemorrhage. A relative risk of 9.9 for spontaneous abortion in cases of retrieval of discolored amniotic fluid has been reported[20].

RISKS OF AMNIOCENTESIS

Maternal risks

The maternal risks are very small. The following constitute these complications:

(1) Intra-abdominal infection in cases of perforation of the intra-abdominal viscera;
(2) Bleeding;
(3) Blood group sensitization;
(4) Amniotic fluid embolism (in third-trimester therapeutic amniocentesis)[21];

(5) Hemorrhage due to laceration of the inferior epigastric vessels (in third-trimester amniocentesis)[22];

(6) Perforation of the aorta (extremely rare, in a very thin patient).

Fetal risks

(1) Fetal loss due to:
   (a) unexplained reasons during the procedure
   (b) fetal injury
   (c) fetal infection
(2) Ruptured membranes – amnionitis by *Mycoplasma hominis* or *Ureoplasma urealyticum*[23];
(3) Respiratory distress syndrome[24];
(4) Orthopedic abnormalities (talipes equinovarus, congenital dislocation of the hip, metastarsus abductus)[25,26];
(5) Leakage of amniotic fluid. This occurs in 1–2% of all cases and resolves within 48 h. In some cases there is chronic leakage. This is a rare complication. It requires bed rest, no digital vaginal examination, frequent white blood cell counts and maternal surveillance for chorioamnionitis;
(6) Fetal injuries. Most of the cases reported were prior to utilization of ultrasound guidance during the procedure. These included skin puncture, ocular lesions, limb deformities and some other fetal injuries[27].

Genetic mid-trimester amniocentesis has been used for more than 20 years. It seems to be a safe procedure concerning the long-term outcome of the newborns. A study[28] revealed that the long-term outcome of the offspring of women who had mid-trimester amniocenteses did not differ from those who did not have the procedure. They did not find a significant difference between the two groups with regard to cerebral palsy, delayed speech, hearing deficits, epilepsy or limb defects. However, an increased risk for maternal blood isoimmunization was reported in the group who underwent amniocentesis. Another controversial issue is the risk of Rh-isoimmunization in unsensitized Rh-negative mothers after mid-trimester amniocentesis. Although there is no clear evidence to support the routine administration of anti-D immunoglobulin after genetic amniocentesis, this has become standard practice. In many countries around the world there is no agreement on the dose; the WHO recommends 50 µg, whereas the ACOG recommends 300 µg[29].

AMNIOCENTESIS IN MULTIPLE GESTATION

In multiple gestations some special issues must be considered before amniocentesis is performed. The risk of chromosomal abnormalities seems to be higher in twins than in singleton pregnancies in cases with advanced maternal age (≥ 35 years). It is also known that, in cases with a previous child with a neural tube defect, the recurrence risk for the same defect in a subsequent twin pregnancy is higher than in a singleton[30]. In cases of discrepancy in results of the genetic analysis, possible management alternatives must be discussed with the parents. If one of the fetuses is affected, there are several options: abortion of both fetuses; selective feticide of the affected fetus; continuation of the pregnancy. Each system of management has its own potential complications or unfavorable long-term outcome. It is therefore critical that amniocentesis be performed with the highest accuracy, and precise identification of each fetus. A detailed ultrasound examination must be performed before amniocentesis. We need to know the number of fetuses, zygosity, sex of each one if possible, location of the placenta or placentas, fetal anatomy and biometry, and position of each fetus with regard to maternal right and left, anterior or posterior sides. The identification of each fetus is a critical issue, especially in cases where selective feticide is to be performed.

Several techniques have been used for amniocentesis in multiple pregnancies. Either a single-needle insertion, or a two-needle insertion is performed. The overall aim is to obtain fluid from the two sacs. The pregnancy loss rate in twins that undergo genetic amniocentesis does not differ statistically from the natural fetal loss rate for twins.

EARLY AMNIOCENTESIS

An alternative to the classical mid-trimester genetic amniocentesis is 'early amniocentesis', which is performed before 15 weeks' gestation. This is an attractive option, especially for women who are very anxious and prefer to have the procedure before the 15th week of gestation.

However, several disadvantages to the procedure make it unfavorable. It is well known that CVS, which is performed between 11 and 14 weeks' gestation, has replaced early amniocentesis. A Canadian study revealed that the post-procedure spontaneous loss rate, excluding stillbirths and neonatal deaths, was 2.6% for early amniocentesis and 0.8% for mid-trimester amniocentesis[31]. The same study reported that early amniocentesis was associated with more needle insertions, more cases with amniotic fluid leakage before 22 weeks' gestation and higher risk for talipes compared to mid-trimester amniocentesis.

In 1996 a new filtration technique for the aspiration and culture of amniotic fluid in cases of early amniocentesis was reported[32]. The success in obtaining and culturing fetal cells was higher and mosaicism less. In another study[33] no significant difference was found in culture success, mosaicism, problems related to technique and maternal contamination.

SUMMARY

Amniocentesis is the oldest invasive method for prenatal diagnosis. It is also used for the diagnosis of intra-amniotic infections, fetal congenital infections, evaluation of fetal lung maturity and therapeutic amnioreduction in twin–twin transfusion syndrome. Cytogenetic analysis is the most common indication in cases of advanced maternal age ($\geq$ 35 years). There are no absolute contraindications to amniocentesis. Mid-trimester genetic amniocentesis is usually performed between 15 and 18 weeks of gestation. It is a sonographically guided and monitored procedure. It is a safe procedure with rare and minor risks and complications for the mother and fetus. It is estimated that the post-procedure spontaneous fetal loss rate is 0.8% for mid-trimester amniocentesis and 2.6% for early amniocentesis (performed before 15 weeks of gestation). Chorionic villus sampling seems to be preferable for prenatal diagnosis in the first trimester of pregnancy compared to early amniocentesis. A wide spectrum of laboratory tests of the amniotic fluid are available for fetal karyotyping (cell culture, FISH, DNA analysis) for genetic studies for metabolic and enzymatic analysis.

In experienced and skilled hands, amniocentesis is a safe and reliable invasive method for prenatal diagnosis.

References

1. Prochnownick I. Bietrage zur lehre vom frachtawasser und entstehung. *Arch Gynaekol* 1877;11: 304

2. Lambl D. Ein seltener fall van hydramnios. *Zentralbl Gynaekol* 1881;5:329

3. Menees TO, Miller JD, Holly LE. Amniography. Preliminary report. *Am J Roentgenol* 1930;24:363

4. Boero E. Intra-amniotiques. *Semana Med Buenos-Aires*. 1935; August 15

5. Bevis DCA. Composition of liquor amnii in hemolytic disease of newborn. *Lancet* 1950;2:443

6. Fuchs F, Riis P. Antenatal sex determination. *Nature* 1956;177:330

7. Steele MW, Breg WR Jr. Chromosome analysis of human amniotic fluid cells. *Lancet* 1966;1:383

8. Jacobson CB, Barter RH. Intrauterine diagnosis and management of genetic defects. *Am J Obstet Gynecol* 1967;99:796

9. Valenti C, Schutta EJ, Kehaty T. Prenatal diagnosis of Down's syndrome [letter]. *Lancet* 1968;2:220

10. Jeffcoate TNA, Fliegner JRH, Russell SH, *et al.* Diagnosis of the adrenogenital syndrome before birth. *Lancet* 1965;2:553

11. Brace RA. Amniotic fluid dynamics. In Creasy R, Resnick R, eds. *Maternal and Fetal Medicine: Principles and Practice.* Philadelphia: WB Saunders, 1988:128

12. Lynch L. Second trimester prenatal diagnosis. In Reece A, Hobbins J, eds. *Medicine of the Fetus and Mother,* 2nd edn. Philadelphia: Lippincott-Raven, 1999:679

13. Simpson NE, Dallaire L, Miller JR, *et al.* Prenatal diagnosis of genetic disease in Canada: report of a collaborative study. *Can Med Assoc J* 1976;115:739

14. Lowe BY, Alexander D, Bryla D, *et al.* The NICHD Amniocentesis Registry. The safety and accuracy of midtrimester amniocentesis. DHEW Publication No. (NIH) 78-190. Washington, DC: US Department of Health, Education and Welfare, 1978

15. Romero R, Jeanty P, Reece EA, *et al.* Sonographically monitored amniocentesis to decrease intraoperative complications. *Obstet Gynecol* 1985;65:426

16. Bombard AT, Powers JF, Carter S, *et al.* Procedure-related fetal losses in transplacental versus nontransplacental genetic amniocentesis. *Am J Obstet Gynecol* 1995;172:868–72

17. D'Alton ME, Malone FD, Chelmow D, *et al.* Defining the role of fluorescence *in situ* hybridization on uncultured amniocytes for prenatal diagnosis of aneuploidies (and discussion). *Am J Obstet Gynecol* 1997;176:769–76

18. Aviram-Goldring A, Daniely M, Chaki R, *et al.* Advanced FISH with directly labeled X, Y and 18 DNA probes as a tool for rapid prenatal diagnosis. *J Reprod Med* 1999;44:497–503

19. American College of Medical Genetics. Prenatal interphase fluorescence *in situ* hybridization (FISH) policy statement. *Am J Hum Genet* 1993;53:526–7

20. Hankins GDV, Rowe J, Quirk JG, *et al.* Significance of brown and/or green amniotic fluid at the time of second trimester genetic amniocentesis. *Obstet Gynecol* 1984;64:353

21. Dodgson J, Martin J, Boswell J, *et al.* Probable amniotic fluid embolism precipitated by amniocentesis and treated by exchange transfusions. *Br Med J* 1987;294:1322

22. Galle PC, Meis PJ. Complications of amniocentesis. *J Reprod Med* 1982;27:149

23. Gray DJ, Robinson H, Malone J, *et al.* Adverse outcome in pregnancy following amniotic fluid isolation of *Ureoplasma urealyticum. Prenat Diagn* 1992;12:111–17

24. Tabor A, Madsen M, Obel EB, *et al.* Randomized controlled trial of genetic amniocentesis in 4606 low-risk women. *Lancet* 1986;1:1287

25. NICHD. National Registry for Amniocentesis Study Group. Midtrimester amniocentesis for prenatal diagnosis, safety and accuracy. *J Am Med Assoc* 1976;236:1471

26. Chayen S, ed. An assessment of the hazards of amniocentesis. Report to the Medical Research Council by their Working Party on amniocentesis. *Br J Obstet Gynecol* 1978;85(suppl 2):1

27. Maymon E, Romero R, Goncalves L, *et al.* Amniocentesis. In Fleischer A, Manning F, Jeanty P, Romero R, eds. *Sonography in Obstetrics and Gynecology: Principles and Practice,* 6th edn. McGraw-Hill, Medical Publishing Division, 2001:750

28. Baird PA, Yee IML, Sadovnick AD. Population-based study of long-term outcomes after amniocentesis. *Lancet* 1994;344:1134–6

29. American College of Obstetricians and Gynecologists. Prevention of RhD alloimmunization. ACOG Practice Bulletin 4. Washington DC: ACOG, 1999

30. Hunter AGW, Cox DM. Counseling problems when twins are discovered at genetic amniocentesis. *Clin Genet* 1979;16:34

31. The Canadian Early and Mid-trimester Amniocentesis Trial (CEMAT) Group. Randomized trial to assess safety and fetal outcome of early and midtrimester amniocentesis. *Lancet* 1998;351:242

32. Sundberg K, Lundsteen C, Philip J. Comparison of cell cultures, chromosome quality and karyotypes obtained after chorionic villus sampling and early amniocentesis with filter technique. *Prenat Diagn* 1999;19:12–16

33. Sundberg K, Lundsteen C, Philip J. Early amniocentesis for further investigation of mosaicism diagnosed by chorionic villus sampling. *Prenat Diagn* 1996;16:1121

Selective reduction

17

M. I. Evans and R. J. Wapner

INTRODUCTION

Infertility management has allowed more than a million previously infertile women to become pregnant and have their own children. However, a consequence of this remarkable success in treatment has included a virtual epidemic of multifetal pregnancies. The twin pregnancy rate, commonly quoted for generations as 1 in 90, has now doubled to more than 1 in 45. Even in the past decade, twin pregnancies have risen by 20%, and triplets or more by well over 100% (Table 1)[1]. The ratio of observed to naturally expected multifetal pregnancies shows that the twin rate is approximately double the expected rate. Quintuplets occur more than 1000-fold over expected numbers without infertility therapies (Table 2).

There is still controversy over the risks inherent with multifetal pregnancies. The major criterion for the extent of appreciated pregnancy losses relates to when in gestation one starts counting. There have been optimistic reports by some perinatologists who do not start counting until they begin to see patients at nearly 20 weeks. By that time most of the losses have already occurred[2].

We have previously calculated losses before viability from the attempts to carry twins at 10%, triplets at 18%, quadruplets at > 25% and quintuplets at 50%[2]. Serious morbidity rates also correlate with starting numbers.

In the 1980s, in about 75% of multifetal pregnancy patients seeking reduction, the pregnancies were initiated with ovulation induction agents such as Pergonal®[4]. However, we have seen quintuplets with even the first month of the lowest dose of Clomid®. Over the years, there has been a gradual shift to cases induced by assisted reproductive technologies (ART), such as IVF. At the millennium about 70% of cases came from ART.

Table 1 *Multiple births in the United States*

Year	Twins	Triplets	Quadruplets	Quintuplets and higher multiples
1998	110 670	6919	627	79
1997	104 137	6148	510	79
1996	100 750	5298	560	81
1995	96 736	4551	365	57
1994	97 064	4233	315	46
1993	96 445	3834	277	57
1992	95 372	3547	310	26
1991	94 779	3121	203	22
1990	93 865	2830	185	13
1989	90 118	2529	229	40
% Increase from 1989–1998	22.8%	173.6%	173.8%	97.5%

Data taken from *National Vital Statistics Report*, Volume 48, no. 3, page 17, 2001

Table 2 *Multiple births in the United States*

Births	Observed	Expected	Ratio
Twins	110 670	43 795	2.5 : 1
Triplets	6919	487	14.2 : 1
Quadruplets	627	5	125.4 : 1
Quintuplets and higher multiples	79	0.06	1316.7 : 1

Total births in 1998 – 3 941 553

Despite the increase in the use of ART[5], however, the proportion of those cases that are badly hyperstimulated, resulting in quintuplets or more, has dramatically decreased to less than 10%. For those cases of ovulation stimulation, however, particularly those using Metrodin®, the proportion of cases that carry quintuplets or more has remained consistent over the past decade at about 30%. There has been no improvement over the past few years. Such data continue to speak very strongly for the need to have significant vigilance in the monitoring of infertility therapies. While the vast majority of cases appear to be occurring to physicians with the best of equipment and with the best of intentions, but who have an unfortunate and reasonably unpredictable or unpreventable maloccurrence, there clearly are some cases that might have been prevented if increased vigilance had been used.

Public fascination with multifetal pregnancies extends back to the 1930s, with the Dionne quintuplets in Ontario, Canada. The same fascination has existed in the 70 years since then[6]. In the 1980s, quintuplets would make the national news, but now the bar keeps getting set higher and higher for lay press interest. In the early 1990s, sextuplets, such as those of the Dilly family in Indiana, drew several rounds of national attention, and help from diaper companies, formula companies, crib companies, and the support of neighbors in their small town. The ultimate example of that was the MacCaughy septuplets in Iowa, where virtually the entire town of Carlyle, Iowa was marshaled to help the family deal with the rigors of so many children at once. The family was given a van by a local automotive dealer, and the state of Iowa contributed a house. Miraculously, that pregnancy lasted until about 31 weeks, and the national media reported that all was doing well. Closer inspection revealed that the presenting fetus was a transverse lie, which fundamentally blocked the cervix from opening, rather than acting as the usual wedge to cause dilatation. Media reports of the children at age 4 years reveal that two of them have been diagnosed with cerebral palsy, a fact that has been glossed over and ignored by the media, and a third has epilepsy. Three have required feeding tubes for nearly their entire life. The American octuplets in 1998 received much less attention. Whether this lack of attention was due to saturation of the concept of multifetal pregnancies or racism is open to speculation. One of these fetuses died very shortly after birth, and the other seven are said to be doing reasonably well at 3 years of age.

PROCEDURES

Multifetal pregnancy reduction (MFPR) is a clinical procedure that dates back to the mid-1980s when a small number of centers in both the United States and Europe began to try to ameliorate the usual, tremendously adverse sequelae of multifetal pregnancies by selectively terminating, or reducing, the number of fetuses to a more manageable number. The first European reports by Dumez[7], and the first American report by Evans et al.[8], followed by another report by Berkowitz et al.[9] and later Wapner et al.[10], laid out for physicians a possible dramatic surgical approach to improve the outcome in such cases. Even early reports, however, recognized the ethical conundrum faced by couples and physicians under such difficult circumstances[8]. In the mid-1980s despite relatively mediocre ultrasound visualization, needles were inserted transabdominally and maneuvered into the thorax of the fetus with either mechanical destruction, air embolization, or potassium chloride injections. Transcervical aspirations were also tried, without much success. Some centers have also used trans-vaginal mechanical disruption, but recent data suggest a significantly higher loss rate than with the transabdominal route[11].

Today virtually all experienced operators perform the procedure inserting needles transabdominally under ultrasound guidance. We find it best to line up the needle with the thorax first in the longitudinal plane. Under transverse visualization, the needle is carefully thrust into the thorax and a syringe attached to the needle. KCl is then injected slowly so as not to dislodge the needle tip. A pleural effusion should be seen, as well as asystole.

OUTCOMES

Several of the centers with the world's largest experience began collaborating to increase the power of their data. The first collaborative report, published in 1993, showed a 16% pregnancy loss rate up to 24 completed weeks[12]. This was already a large improvement as compared to expectations of higher-order multiple pregnancies, particularly of quadruplets and above. Further collaborative efforts were published in 1994, 1996 and 2001 and have shown continued dramatic improvements in the overall outcomes of such pregnancies (Table 3)[13–15]. The 2001 collaborative data show that the outcome of triplets reduced to twins, and quadruplets reduced to twins, now perform essentially as if they started as twins. Even with the tremendous advances in neonatal care, the 95% take-home-baby rate for triplets and the 92% take-home-baby rate for quadruplets are clearly dramatic improvements over natural statistics. Not only has the pregnancy loss rate been substantially reduced, but so has the rate of very early prematurity. Both the loss and the prematurity rates continue to be a function of the starting number, showing that there is still a real price to be paid for over-aggressive infertility therapies.

Finishing number data also showed lowest pregnancy loss rates for those cases reduced to twins, with increasing losses for singletons, followed by triplets. However, the rate of early premature delivery was, not surprisingly, highest with triplets followed by twins and lowest with singletons. Mean gestational age at delivery was also lower for higher-order cases.

Birth weights following MFPR decreased with starting and finishing numbers reflecting increased prematurity. However, analysis of birth weight centiles, particularly for singletons, reflects falling centiles with starting number, from 51.75 for 2→1, to 31.26 for 4→1. Furthermore, in remaining twins, the rate of birth weight centile discordancy among the twins increased from 0.57% for starting

triplets to 4.86% for starting 5 or more. For remaining triplets, the centile differences were even greater.

Analysis of the data suggests that the improvements in multifetal pregnancy reduction outcomes are a function of extensive operator experience combined with improved ultrasound.

Historically, most observers, except those completely opposed to intervention on religious grounds, have accepted MFPR with quadruplets or more, and saw no need with twins[16]. The debate was over triplets. While there are conflicting data in the literature, our experiences suggest that triplets reduced to twins do much better in terms of loss and prematurity than unreduced triplets. We believe that, if a patient's primary goal is to maximize the chances of healthy children, reduction of triplets to twins achieves the best results.

Several previous papers have argued about whether triplets have better outcomes 'reduced' or not. In a 1999 paper, Yaron et al.[17] looked at 3→2 and compared these data to unreduced triplets with two large cohorts of twins. The data show substantial improvement of reduced twins, as compared to triplets. The data from the most recent collaborative series suggest that pregnancy outcomes for cases starting at triplets or even quadruplets reduced to twins do fundamentally as well as starting as twins, and therefore support some cautious aggressiveness in infertility treatments to achieve pregnancy in tough situations. However, when higher numbers occur, good outcomes clearly diminish. A 2001 paper suggested that reduced triplets did worse than continuing ones. However, analysis of that

Table 3 *Multifetal pregnancy reduction: losses by years*

		Losses (weeks)		Deliveries (weeks)			
	Total	% <24	% >24	% 25–28	% 29–32	% 33–36	% 37+
1986–90	508	13.2	4.5	10.0	21.1	15.7	35.4
1991–94	724	9.4	0.3	2.8	5.4	21.1	61.0
1995–98	1356	6.4	0.2	4.3	10.2	31.5	47.4

From reference 15

series showed a loss rate following MFPR twice that seen in our collaborative series[14–17] and worse outcome data in every other category for remaining triplets. The point is that one must use extreme caution in choosing comparison groups.

Pregnancy loss is not the only poor outcome. Very early premature delivery correlates with the starting number. The data on diminishing birth weight centile in singletons, and discordancy in twins, are of concern, consistent with a belief that there is perhaps a fundamental 'imprinting' of the uterus early in pregnancy that is not completely undone by MFPR[15,18].

The subset of patients in the 2001 collaborative report reduced from two to one (not for fetal anomalies) included 154 patients. Nine lost their pregnancies before 24 weeks, and two delivered between 25 and 28 weeks. While the numbers, in absolute terms, are not large as compared the other categories, they suggest a loss rate comparable to 3→2. In an earlier series, in about one-third of the 2→1 cases, there was a medical indication for the procedure – e.g. maternal cardiac disease or prior twin pregnancy with severe prematurity, or uterine abnormality[14]. In recent years, however, the vast majority of such cases have been from women in their forties or even fifties who are using donor eggs and who, more for social reasons than medical, only want a singleton pregnancy[19]. The effect of maternal age *per se*, however, is negligible, only explaining 3.5% of the variance, suggesting that, with reduction, 'older' gravidas do nearly as well as their younger counterparts[14,19].

PATIENT ISSUES

The demographics of patients seeking multifetal pregnancy reduction have evolved over the past decade[19]. Particularly with the availability of donor eggs, the number of 'older women' seeking MFPR has increased dramatically. In several programs, over 10% of all patients seeking MFPR are over 40 years of age, and most are using donor eggs. As a consequence of the shift to older patients, many of whom already had previous relationships and children, there is an increased desire by these patients to have only one further child. The number of experienced centers willing to do 2→1 reductions is still limited, but we believe it can be justified in the appropriate circumstances.

Likewise, for patients who are older and using their own eggs, the issue of genetic diagnosis comes into play. In the 1980s and early 1990s, the most common approach was to offer amniocentesis at 16–17 weeks on the remaining twins. One report suggested an 11% loss rate in these cases, which caused considerable concern[20]. However, a much larger collaborative series then settled the question by showing that loss rates were no higher than comparable controls of MFPR patients who did not have amniocentesis[21]. The collaborative data shared a loss rate of 5%, which was certainly no higher than in the group of patients post-MFPR who did not have genetic studies.

Given that the centers with the most MFPR experience also happened to be the ones that also had the same accomplishments with chorionic villus sampling (CVS), combinations of the procedures were very logical.

There have been two principal schools of thought as to the best approach to first-trimester genetic diagnosis, i.e. should it be before or after the performance of MFPR? Published data in the early 1990s about doing the CVS first, followed by reduction, have suggested a 1–2% error rate as to identifying which fetus was which, particularly if the entire karyotype was obtained before the reduction[22]. Therefore, for the first 10–15 years, the approach that one of us used was to prefer generally to do the reduction first at approximately 10.5 weeks in patients reducing down to twins or triplets, followed by CVS approximately 1 week later. However, in patients reducing to a singleton pregnancy, therefore putting 'all of their eggs in one basket', we believed the best approach was to know what was in the 'basket' before reducing the other embryos[15,19]. In these cases we performed CVS on usually all the fetuses, or one more than the intended stopping number, and performed a fluorescent *in situ* hybridization (FISH) analysis with probes for chromosomes 13, 18, 21, X and Y. While we have published about 30% of anomalies seen on karyotype that would not be detectable by FISH with these probes[23], the absolute risk given a normal FISH and a normal ultrasound examination is about 1/500. We believe that risk is lower than the increased risk from the 2-week wait necessary to obtain the full karyotype. We have now commonly extended this approach to all patients who are appropriate candidates for prenatal diagnosis, regardless of the fetal number.

The other approach used by the Philadelphia group was to perform the CVS and complete karotype first, and have the patient come back for the reduction. While mistakes were common 10 years ago, the chance of error has been considerably reduced, and this group believed the benefits of the full karyotype justified the wait. The issue as to the better of these two approaches is currently unsettled.

SOCIETAL ISSUES

MFPR continues to be controversial. Feelings on MFPR have not, in our experience, ever followed the classic 'pro-choice/pro-life' dichotomy. As far back as the mid- to late 1980s, opinions about the subject were highly varied. Even then, when much less was known about the subject, opinions did not always parallel the usual pro-choice/theological boundaries. We believe that the real debate over the next 5–10 years will not be whether or not MFPR should be performed with triplets or more. The fact is that MFPR does clearly improve those outcomes. A serious debate will emerge over whether or not it will be appropriate to offer MFPR routinely for twins, even natural ones for whom the outcome is commonly considered 'good enough'. Our data suggest that reduction of twins to a singleton actually improves the outcome of the remaining

fetus. No consensus on appropriateness of routine 2→1 reductions, however, is ever likely to emerge.

The ethical issues surrounding MFPR will also always be controversial. Over the years, much has been written on the subject. Opinions will always vary substantially from outraged condemnation to complete acceptance. No short paragraph could do justice to the subject other than to state that most proponents do not believe that this is a frivolous procedure, but do believe in the principle of proportionality, i.e. therapy to achieve the most good for the least harm[8,24-26].

Over the past 15 years MFPR has become a well-established and integral part of infertility therapy, and attempts to deal with the sequelae of aggressive infertility management. In the mid-1980s, the risks and benefits of the procedure could only be guessed[8-10]. We now have very clear and precise data on the risks and benefits of the procedure and an understanding that the risks increase substantially with the starting and finishing number of fetuses in multifetal pregnancies. The collaborative loss rate, i.e. 4.5% for triplets, 8% for quadruplets, 11% for quintuplets and 15% for sextuplets or more, seems reasonable to present to patients for the procedure performed by an experienced operator. Our own experiences and anecdotal experiences from other groups suggest that less experienced operators have worse outcomes.

It is very clear that pregnancy loss is not the only poor outcome. The other main issue with which to be concerned is very early premature delivery. Here again there is an increasing rate of poor outcomes correlated with the starting number. The finishing numbers are also critical, with twins having the best outcomes for cases starting with three or more. Triplets and singletons do not do as well. We continue to hope, however, that MFPR will become obsolete as better control of ovulation agents and assisted reproductive technologies make multifetal pregnancies uncommon.

References

1. *National Vital Statistics Report*. 2000;48:17
2. Evans MI, Rodeck CH, Stewart KS, Yaron Y, Johnson MP. Multiple gestation: genetic issues, selective termination, and fetal reduction. In Gleisher N, Buttino L Jr, Elkayam U, Evans MI, Galbraith RM, Gall SA, Sibai BM, eds. *Principles and Practices of Medical Therapy in Pregnancy*, 3rd edn. Norwalk, CT: Appleton and Lange, 1998: 235–42
3. Baker C, Feldman B, Shalhoub AG, Ayoub MA, Evans MI. Demographic determinants on the utilization of invasive genetic testing after multi-fetal pregnancy reduction (MFPR). *Fetal Diagn Ther* 2002; in press
4. Evans MI, Dommergues M, Wapner RJ, *et al*. Efficacy of transabdominal multifetal pregnancy reduction: collaborative experience among the world's largest centers. *Obstet Gynecol* 1993;82:61–7
5. Evans MI, Littman L, St Louis L, *et al*. Evolving patterns of iatrogenic multifetal pregnancy generation: implications for aggressiveness of infertility treatments. *Am J Obstet Gynecol* 1995; 172:1750–3
6. Evans MI, Fletcher JC. Multifetal pregnancy reduction. In Reece EA, Hobbins JC, Mahoney MJ, Petrie R, eds. *Medicine of the Fetus and its Mother*. Philadelphia: Lippincott Harper, 1992:1345–62
7. Dumez Y, Oury JF. Method for first trimester selective abortion in multiple pregnancy. *Contrib Gynecol Obstet* 1986;15:50
8. Evans MI, Fletcher JC, Zador IE, Newton BW, Struyk CK, Quigg MH. Selective first trimester termination in octuplet and quadruplet preg-nancies: clinical and ethical issues. *Obstet Gynecol* 1988;71:289–96
9. Berkowitz RL, Lynch L, Chitkara U, *et al*. Selective reduction of multiple pregnancies in the first trimester. *N Engl J Med* 1988;318:1043
10. Wapner RJ, Davis GH, Johnson A. Selective reduction of multifetal pregnancies. *Lancet* 1990; 335:90–3
11. Timor-Tritsch IE, Peisner DB, Monteagudo A, Lerner JP, Sharma S. Multifetal pregnancy reduction by transvaginal puncture: evaluation of the technique used in 134 cases. *Am J Obstet Gynecol* 1993;168:799–804
12. Evans MI, Dommergues M, Wapner RJ, *et al*. Efficacy of transabdominal multifetal pregnancy reduction: collaborative experience among the world's largest centers. *Obstet Gynecol* 1993;82: 61–6
13. Evans MI, Dommergues M, Timor-Tritsch I, *et al*. Transabdominal versus transcervical and transvaginal multifetal pregnancy reduction: international collaborative experience of more than one thousand cases. *Am J Obstet Gynecol* 1994;170:902–9
14. Evans MI, Dommergues M, Wapner RJ, *et al*. International collaborative experience of 1789 patients having multifetal pregnancy reduction: a plateauing of risks and outcomes. *J Soc Gynecol Invest* 1996;3:23–6
15. Evans MI, Berkowitz R, Wapner R, *et al*. Multifetal pregnancy reduction (MFPR): Improved outcomes with increased experience. *Am J Obstet Gynecol*, 2001;184:97–103
16. Evans MI, Drugan A, Fletcher JC, *et al*. Attitudes on the ethics of abortion, sex selection & selective termination among health care professionals, ethicists & clergy likely to encounter such situations. *Am J Obstet Gynecol* 1991;164: 1092–9
17. Yaron Y, Bryant-Greenwood PK, Dave N, *et al*. Multifetal pregnancy reduction (MFPR) of triplets to twins: comparison with non-reduced triplets and twins. *Am J Obstet Gynecol* 1999:180: 1268–71
18. Torok O, Lapinski R, Salafia CM, Bernasko J, Berkowitz RL. Multifetal pregnancy reduction is not associated with an increased risk of intra-uterine growth restriction, except for very high order multiples. *Am J Obstet Gynecol* 1998;179: 221–5
19. Evans MI, Hume RF, Polak S, *et al*. The geriatric gravida: multifetal pregnancy reduction (MFPR) donor eggs and aggressive infertility treatments. *Am J Obstet Gynecol* 1997;177:875–8
20. Tabsh KM, Theroux NL. Genetic amniocentesis following multifetal pregnancy reduction twins: assessing the risk. *Prenat Diagn* 1995;15:221–3
21. McLean LK, Evans MI, Carpenter RJ, Johnson MP, Goldberg JD. Genetic amniocentesis (AMN) following multifetal pregnancy reduction (MFPR) does not increase the risk of pregnancy loss. *Prenat Diagn* 1998;18:186–8
22. Brambati B, Tului L, Baldi M, Guercilena S. Genetic analysis prior to selective termination in multiple pregnancy: technical aspects and clinical outcome. *Hum Reprod* 1995;10:818–25
23. Evans MI, Henry GP, Miller WA, *et al*. International, collaborative assessment of 146,000 prenatal karyotypes: expected limitations if only chromosome-specific probes and fluorescent *in situ* hybridization were used. *Hum Reprod* 1999;14:1213–16
24. Evans MI, Fletcher JC, Rodeck C. Ethical problems in multiple gestations: selective

termination. In Evans MI, Fletcher JC, Dixler AO, Schulman JD, eds. *Fetal Diagnosis and Therapy: Science, Ethics, and the Law*, Philadelphia: Lippincott Harper, 1989:266–76

25. The Committee on Ethics. *ACOG Ethics Statement: Multifetal Pregnancy Reduction and Selective Fetal Termination*. American College of Obstetricians and Gynecologists, 1990

26. Chervenak FA, McCullough LB, Wapner R. Three ethically justified indications for selective termination in multifetal pregnancy: a practical and comprehensive management strategy. *J Assist Repro Med* 1995;12:531–6

Evaluation of intrapartum long-term cardiotocography with artificial neural network analysis

18

K. Maeda, M. Utsu, Y. Noguchi and F. Matsumoto

INTRODUCTION

The usefulness of intrapartum cardiotocography (CTG) followed by interventional delivery was confirmed by the fact that perinatal mortality was reduced in the fetal monitoring group in the controlled study of Tottori University[1]. Perinatal mortality, neonatal asphyxia and cerebral palsy (CP) were reduced in Yohka hospital after full fetal monitoring was introduced[2], and CP was reduced after wide use of fetal monitoring in the Tottori area[3]. Beneficial improvements in the reports were obtained by continuous or very frequent observation and evaluation of the CTG during labor. However, the procedure is not easy for obstetric staff, and therefore we intended to introduce computerized analysis of the intrapartum fetal heart rate (FHR) by using an experts' knowledge system (EKS), where the computer evaluation was uniform and it worked without fatigue. Details of CTG are listed, and abnormal FHR signs and fetal distress are recognized by the EKS, with sound and red-color letters in the centralized monitoring of multiple fetuses.

Meanwhile, correct diagnosis has sometimes been difficult after long CTG recording for several hours, if the evaluation is conventional with visual observation. Empirically, we diagnosed late decelerations after recording the phenomena for 15 or more minutes. In this common computerized technique, each analysis time is usually fixed at 5–30 min, e.g. our FHR score is determined in 5 min and fetal distress (FD) index in 5–15 min. Usual analysis time is 15 min and processed every 5 min in our artificial neural network system. Very pathological or totally normal FHR is clearly diagnosed because of its clear trend toward abnormality or normality. The changes, however, usually show time-to-time variation, and therefore the impression from the trendgram of 15 min of analyzing time is unstable. Long analysis time is set at 50 min in our artificial neural network system[6], but we were unable to evaluate the change before the end of 50 min. We have to create new techniques to evaluate the total length of the past CTG at any moment in the course of labor. The purpose of this study was to assess the outcome after recording long-term CTG with a new computer processing technique.

MATERIALS AND METHODS

The experts' knowledge system (EKS) was programmed by Maeda in 1980[4] and was composed of two parts, repeated FHR analysis and its evaluation every 5 min. Basic jobs are determination of FHR parameters and its evaluation with FHR score and FD index. FHR miscounts and false decelerations due to transient tachycardia are eliminated. If detached the transducer is alarmed. FHR score is ten or more if the fetus deteriorates, and FD index is three or more if the umbilical pH is lower than 7.25[5].

Wireless telemetry transmits fetal heart beats and contractions to the central monitor which analyzes FHR by a conventional program[4]. Neither is the chart recorder incorporated, nor is the CTG chart recorded, in the monitor. FHR abnormalities are detected by the computer and alarmed by sound and red lettering on the monitor. Telemeter signals are stored in an MO disk and they are replayed after hearing the alarm sound, then the past CTG is evaluated. The fetus is diagnosed by CTG and automated analysis, both on the monitor screen. At most, 16 cases are simultaneously monitored by a single system. The CTG is printed by computer to a hard copy on ordinary paper.

The artificial neural network computer system has recently been developed[6], and the network is trained 10 000 times with eight FHR parameters of typical outcome cases before the diagnosis is made by the probability in percentage to be normal, pathological or suspicious. Input CTG parameters are baseline FHR, variability amplitude, presence of sinusoidal pattern, number of decelerations and four detailed components of deceleration, i.e. it is a hybrid neural network system. The same FHR parameters of patients are analyzed by the trained neural system. The system is composed of three layers, i.e. the first layer consists of 24 units in the case of 15 min of diagnosis, intermediate layer 30 units and output layer three units that output normal, pathological and suspicious probability percentages (Figure 1). Its diagnostic ability is maximized by the application of a back propagation system. Initially the network was trained for the diagnosis of 50 min of FHR, and the accuracy of its evaluation was 86.2%[6]. Analytic results of 15 min of data every 5 min form trendgrams (Figure 2). Apparently normal or pathological CTG is easily recognized in the trendgram, but the decision is vague in cases of intermediate changes in the long trendgram.

A combination of experts' and neural systems is intended to promote further FHR studies with the systems. Although the decision is easy in the analysis with the probability percentage obtained by neural network system, various CTG details are not demonstrated by the neural system. In addition, FHR parameters used in the neural network are supplied by an analytic part of a conventional experts' system. Accordingly, it is

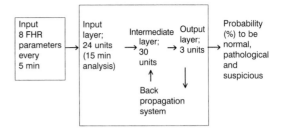

Figure 1 *Schematic illustration of the artificial neural network computer construction. It shows the setting in 15 min of analysis where eight fetal heart rate (FHR) parameters are input every 5 min, and therefore the input layer is composed of 24 units*

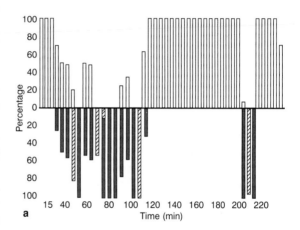

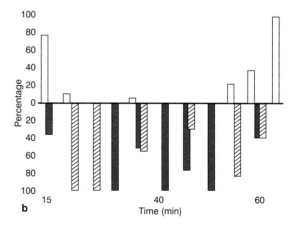

Figure 2 *Probability trendgrams from two cases obtained by the artificial neural network fetal heart rate (FHR) analysis. Upward hollow bars, probability to be normal; downward shaded bars, pathological; hatched bars, suspicious. (a) is a long-term CTG trendgram and (b) a shorter-term trendgram*

reasonable to combine conventional and artificial neural network systems. The conventional one detects CTG details and recognizes its abnormalities, and its analytic part outputs CTG parameters for the neural system every 5 min, then the neural system reports percentages of three outcome probabilities. Long-term FHR analyses are scheduled to be incorporated in the new system.

Long-term CTG is hardly evaluated at any requested time during labor in most manual as well as automatic techniques. At present, we intend to accumulate and average 15 min of normal and pathological probabilities obtained every 5 min by our artificial neural network system. The series of probabilities in the trendgrams[6] is manually processed by using a simple BASIC program incorporated in a pocket computer. It is a preliminary trial with the purpose of confirming the utility of the new method before constructing a complicated automatic system.

RESULTS

Ten cases were analyzed with probability trendgrams in the first report of the artificial neural network system[6]. The probabilities were totally pathological in a case of late

decelerations showing 100% pathological negative deflections, and a normal outcome case revealed 100% normal positive deflections. Therefore, no vague trendgram existed in totally pathological or normal cases. Most of the cases, however, showed a mixture of normal, pathological and suspicious probabilities, and the trendgrams were constructed of mixed deflections; therefore, a definitive decision was hard to make and the diagnosis was done by visual impression in most of the long-term analyses (Figure 2).

The long-term analysis of accumulated and averaged probabilities obtained by our neural network system in two cases are shown in Figures 3 and 4. The cases are not included in Figure 2. The technique is simple, but needs repeated calculations every 5 min, i.e. 42 accumulations and 42 averagings are done in pathological and normal probabilities from 15 min after initiation of 2 h monitoring. In the case of Figure 3, the accumulated and averaged curve of normal probability lies above the pathological probability curve, and the diagnosis is normal outcome. The neonatal condition is normal and coincides with antenatal diagnosis.

In the Figure 4 case, the probability curve is initially highly pathological, then gradually lowers, but pathological probability is

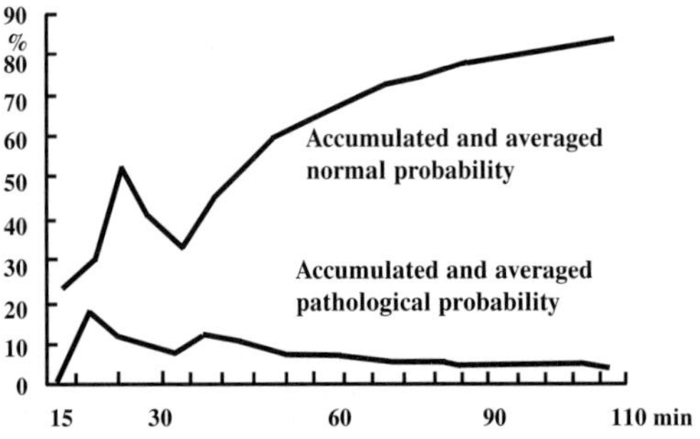

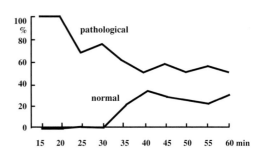

Figure 3 *Probabilities for normal and pathological outcomes are obtained by the artificial neural network in 15-min periods, and they are accumulated and averaged in the two curves every 5 min during fetal monitoring of about 2 h duration. As the normal probability curve consistently lies above the pathological one, prenatal diagnosis is normal. Actual outcome of normal neonate coincides with prenatal diagnosis*

Figure 4 *Methods are the same as in Figure 3. Pathological probability curve consistently lies above the normal probability curve. Therefore, prenatal diagnosis is abnormal, and actual outcome is neonatal depression which coincides with prenatal diagnosis. Final state of the relation of the two curves is important in predictive diagnosis for the outcome*

190

consistently higher than normal. The prenatal diagnosis is abnormal, and coincides with the clinical condition known as neonatal suppression.

Figure 2a case was expected to be normal by the trendgram, the decision of accumulation and average technique is normal and clinical outcome is normal. Figure 2b case was expected to be abnormal by the trendgram and outcome was neonatal suppression. Other long CTG cases showed clinical results coinciding with the prenatal decision made by the accumulation-average probability technique in the neural network analysis.

DISCUSSION

As the results of artificial neural network FHR analysis are shown by the percentage of outcome probabilities, the interpretation is usually easy, because it is unnecessary to study their meaning prior to FHR analysis, i.e. visual CTG diagnosis needs detailed knowledge of FHR parameters and patterns, several manual scoring methods need calculation techniques and criteria, and even in computerized diagnosis, FHR score or FD index needs particular knowledge to evaluate the index values. In our artificial neural network, the outcome is shown by probability percentage which is promptly understood without any preparatory knowledge.

Although there is a single pathological index for the CTG evaluation in other common techniques, two simultaneous normal and pathological probabilities are useful in long-term CTG analysis with the artificial neural network system. Two parameters offer more than double the information compared to a single index. Comparison of normal and pathological probabilities makes it possible to assess neonatal conditions from the CTG. Automated evaluation of long-term CTG at any time during labor has been present only

very rarely, and this is the first time we have achieved success by using the two probability techniques.

Whereas there are chronological variations of fetal condition in the accumulated and averaged curves of two outcome probabilities, the final values will show the state of the fetus immediately before the delivery. Therefore, we can take the final cutting edge of the two probabilities as the indices of fetal survival, i.e. we can decide neonatal condition by the last part of the accumulated and averaged probabilities.

It is natural to assess fetal injury during labor from the clear elevation of pathological probability that is higher than normal in the accumulated-averaged probability curves. Therefore, the method may also indicate neonatal morbidity. The possibility of assessing the morbidity will be further studied in the future.

SUMMARY

Wider and more intensive fetal surveillance in general delivery and improved perinatal outcome are the aims of our studies on computerized monitoring. The studies show improved results using the conventional computer, particularly in multiple simultaneous monitoring. The artificial neural network computer system is characterized by its output of three normal, pathological and suspicious probability percentages which are the most easily understood among visual CTG evaluation and computer processing. Although long-term CTG recorded in hours is hardly evaluated at any time during labor by conventional techniques, this is the first time we have succeeded in its evaluation with the comparison of normal and pathological probabilities after the accumulation and averaging of all past 15 min of values analyzed every 5 min.

References

1. Maeda K. Healthy baby and reduced fetal death by improved obstetric management. In Karim SMM, Tan KL, eds. *Problems in Perinatology.* Singapore: Singapore University, 1979:525–9
2. Maeda K, Tsuzaki T. Improved fetal outcome by fetal monitoring: 17 years' experience in Yohka hospital. In Chervenak FA, Kurjak A, eds. *Current Perspectives on the Fetus as a Patient.* Carnforth, UK: Parthenon Publishing, 1996:379–83
3. Takeshita K, *et al.* Cerebral palsy in Tottori, Japan. *Neuroepiemiology* 1989;4:184–92
4. Maeda K, *et al.* Computer-aided fetal heart rate analysis and automatic fetal distress diagnosis during labor and pregnancy utilizing external technique in fetal monitoring. In Lindberg DAB, Kaihara S, eds. *MEDINFO80.* Amsterdam: North-Holland, 1980:1214–18
5. Irie T. Automated fetal heart rate analysis and its trendgram in relation to the gas analysis and acid-base balance of umbilical cord arterial blood. *Acta Obstet Gynaecol Jpn* 1986;38:1623–31
6. Maeda K, Noguchi Y, *et al.* Neural network computer analysis of fetal heart rate. *J Matern Fetal Invest* 1998;8:163–71

Objective definition of intrauterine growth restriction and practical consequences

19

G. P. Mandruzzato, Y. J. Meir, G. Maso and L. Fischer

INTRODUCTION

For a long time it has been recognized that newborns presenting a birth weight lower than the 10th centile for gestational age carry an increased risk of poor perinatal outcome. These newborns are defined as small for dates (SFD) and it has been postulated that the reduced birth weight is the expression of a restriction of fetal growth (IUGR). As a consequence the two terms of SFD and IUGR became synonymous. Until about 20 years ago this concept was acceptable, owing to the fact that at that time an accurate prenatal assessment of the characteristics of fetal growth was not commonly available, and the diagnosis of IUGR remained a postnatal one solely based on the birth weight. After the introduction into clinical practice of ultrasound fetal biometry, it has become possible to evaluate with good accuracy the characteristics of growth. The results of a number of randomized studies regarding ultrasound screening in pregnancies after 24 weeks have been published[1,5] and have represented the basis of a Cochrane review[6] whose conclusion has been that routine late pregnancy ultrasound scanning in a low-risk or unselected population does not confer benefit to the mother or baby, or for the prenatal detection of IUGR. The weak point of all these studies and their conclusions is represented by the fact that they were all directed to the prediction of the birth of a SFD infant and not to monitoring growth failure.

In the past years the scenario regarding the definition of IUGR has changed. Evidence has been given of what was easy to believe, that by serially monitoring fetal growth, the first appearance of ultrasonic parameters, the biparietal diameter (BPD) and/or abdominal circumference (AC), indicating reduced growth was widely distributed among pregnancies. Taking into consideration the birth weight as an end-point, the sensitivity of this technique is strongly dependent on the time between the last measurement and the birth[7]. Moreover, it has been shown that taking the birth weight at the indicated threshold of the 10th centile is inadequate, because fetal mortality is excessively high in cases presenting a birth weight between the 10th and 15th centiles[8]. It has been also observed that signs of hypoxemia, the most important complication of IUGR fetuses, are present with the same frequency in cases presenting a birth weight over the 50th centile, but showing restriction of growth at ultrasound investigation, and among SFD fetuses[9].

As a consequence, it appeared clear that identifying IUGR cases on the basis of the birth weight induced possible overestimation or underestimation of this clinical problem. An approach to identify, after birth, the cases in which fetal growth restriction took place has been proposed by adding to the birth weight the evaluation of the ponderal index. As a consequence, the concept of 'normal weight growth restriction' has been introduced[10]. This more comprehensive definition, based on a postnatal assessment, is very useful for epidemiological studies and newborn management, but no useful information is offered to the gynecologist in charge of prenatal management.

More than 10 years ago it began to be evident that concepts and definitions of IUGR based on birth weight were inaccurate and of little use in obstetric practice. In 1989 Altman and Hytten pointed out that fetal size is confused with growth, and the assessment of growth rather than size is important[11]. Subsequently many other papers dealing with this problem have been published[12-16]. More recently an ACOG practice bulletin[17] has pointed out that the use of ambiguous terminology and lack of uniform diagnostic criteria can complicate diagnosis and management of this clinical condition, suggesting that the term IUGR should be used in reference to the fetus while the term SGA (small for gestational age) should refer to the newborn.

Summarizing their conclusions it is possible to express some basic concepts:

(1) Small for gestational age is not a diagnosis[18];
(2) SFD and IUGR are not synonymous[12];
(3) Prediction of IUGR should reflect function rather than size[14];
(4) Poor perinatal outcome is connected with restriction of growth and not with weight alone[16].

As a consequence, taking into consideration both prenatal and postnatal evaluation, it is possible to distinguish two groups: SGA-IUGR and AGA-IUGR (where AGA refers to appropriate for gestational age). This distinction has limited interest from a practical point of view, as the prevalence of hypoxemia is similar in both groups. In the postnatal period by coupling birth weight and the ponderal index it is possible to make such a distinction, while during pregnancy the assessment of the characteristics of individual fetal growth is crucial for the recognition of IUGR.

There are two practical consequences of this approach to the clinical problem of IUGR in order to improve the perinatal outcome. The first is represented by the necessity to recognize the restriction of growth prenatally; and the second is the distinction, possible by applying second-level tests, between the IUGR cases that are affected by hypoxemia from those that are simply small, in order to optimize the characteristics of clinical management.

IUGR RECOGNITION

After the acceptance of this more correct concept of IUGR, based on the characteristics of fetal growth and not on weight or size, it has been pointed out that there is a need for better screening techniques for a timely detection of intrauterine growth failures[19]. As far as ultrasound biometry is concerned, the disappointing results obtained to date are the consequence of many confounding factors. First, in all the studies, the considered end-point has been birth weight and not the restriction of growth. Second, no uniform definition of growth restriction at ultrasound examinations has been offered. Third, no uniform protocols of management have been indicated to be applied after IUGR suspicion. As a logical consequence, no evidence of benefit has been obtained in terms of possible improvement of the perinatal outcome.

It is therefore necessary to revise the possible screening policies for IUGR. The fundal-height measurement has been proposed as a screening technique[17]. Unfortunately, this very simple and inexpensive procedure has an unsatisfactory sensitivity and specificity and therefore it is questionable whether its use is advisable[20,21].

On the other hand, the accuracy of ultrasound fetal biometry is well established. The most commonly used parameters are represented by the biparietal diameter (BPD), the abdominal circumference (AC) and the femur length (FL). The abdominal circumference offers the best sensitivity and specificity and its reproducibility is good: the intraoperator and interoperator variability are within acceptable limits[22].

In normal conditions these measurements are easy to perform in less than 10 min. They do not cause discomfort to the patient and by using probes with frequencies and power within the recommended limits there is no evidence that they cause harm to the fetus. Therefore, ultrasound fetal biometry should be considered the technique of choice for the screening of IUGR if the aim of the procedure is to monitor the characteristics of growth and not to predict fetal or neonatal weight. Not only is reduced fetal or neonatal weight not synonymous with IUGR, but fetal weight estimation also carries a large margin of error. Many formulas have been proposed for fetal weight estimation[23,24], but the error is between 7.5% and 10% of the actual weight. Accepting these considerations, in order to obtain reliable results some prerequisites must be respected. The first is the availability of fetal biometry in early pregnancy and not later than 20 weeks in order to adjust the gestational age, if necessary. Thus, at subsequent scans it is possible to observe whether any significant deviation from the expected curve of growth is present. In order to confirm a suspicious finding, a second biometric evaluation is needed. In order to avoid an excessive rate of false-positive findings, the second one should be performed after no more than 2 weeks. If this procedure is followed, the single fetus becomes its own control and the patterns of its growth can be monitored by serial biometry. If a screening policy for IUGR is accepted, some basic aspects should be discussed.

(1) Should this screening be comprehensive or selective?
(2) How many scans must be offered in clinically normal pregnancies and when?
(3) What must be the definition of IUGR on the basis of ultrasound biometry?
(4) What is the end-point to be considered for assessing the efficacy of the procedure?
(5) Is it necessary to have uniform protocols of management of IUGR cases in order to draw possible conclusions on the perinatal outcome?

Many conditions (anamnestic or actual) represent an increased risk for inducing restriction of fetal growth; it is accepted that in those cases serial biometry should be offered. Unfortunately, more than 50% of IUGR cases are observed in pregnancies not presenting detectable risk conditions[25,26]. As a consequence, in order to detect these cases in a timely fashion, a general screening policy should be applied.

As already stated, in order to assess the characteristics of fetal growth adequately, the availability of an ultrasonic scan performed before 20 weeks of gestational age is fundamental. If the target of the procedure is to recognize any growth failure, a second scan should be offered at gestational age 28–30 and a third at 34–36 weeks. It has been shown that more than 50% of cases presenting defective growth of the AC are observed after 32–33 weeks[26]. Therefore, including the anomaly scan usually performed at 21 weeks, a four-scan policy seems to be advisable.

There is no uniformity in the medical literature regarding the criteria that should be used for defining IUGR on the basis of fetal biometry. The most commonly proposed indicator is represented by the finding of an AC below the 10th centile or the 2nd standard deviation of the expected curve of growth. This criterion has implicit limitations, because it does not recognize the IUGR fetuses that present significant deviation of the AC from the expected curve of growth, but do not fall below the 2nd SD, as can occur in the case of fetuses whose expected growth was larger than the normal.

Taking the birth weight as an end-point is no more acceptable. If the target of the screening is to recognize defective growth possibly associated with fetal hypoxemia, the recognition of this adverse condition, possible by applying second-level tests, should be at the end-point. As perinatal deaths, NICU admission and/or stay, seizures and late handicaps are strongly dependent on prematurity, common in IUGR, they seem not to be objective and useful indicators.

As already stated, many variables influence the perinatal outcome of IUGR fetuses. After exclusion of fetal abnormalities, the most relevant are the magnitude of hypoxemia and the gestational age at recognition and at birth. In order to make possible the evaluation of the efficacy of the screening and the comparison of the results it is clear that the management following IUGR recognition must be as uniform as possible. As a consequence, for assessing the validity of any proposed screening policy, at least as far as the possible improvement of the perinatal outcome is concerned, a uniform protocol of management should be adopted in the studies directed toward the investigation of these aspects.

It has been shown that, by applying a four-scan screening protocol (first trimester, 21–22, 28–30 and 34–36 weeks' gestation) in an unselected population, about 70% of fetuses showing restricted growth have been detected after 32 weeks, and 25% of them were affected by hypoxemia[26]. This observation seems to justify such a policy, but the cost/benefit ratio must be evaluated.

ASSESSMENT OF FETAL OXYGENATION

The most frequent complication affecting about 30% of IUGR fetuses is represented by hypoxemia, the consequence of obliterative vasculopathy of the placenta. This is the principal cause of the poor perinatal outcome that (according to the severity and duration of the reduced oxygen supply) can lead to intra-uterine death before labor, acute fetal distress in labor and increased neonatal mortality and morbidity (immediate or late). Therefore, in order to improve the clinical outcome, it is fundamental to exclude or recognize the presence of hypoxemia, distinguishing between fetuses that are growing poorly and those that are suffering from reduced maternal–fetal gas exchange.

As the hypoxemic fetus first adapts to the adverse condition by altering many vital functions, it is by investigating the characteristics of these changes that it is possible to make that distinction and also to assess the dimension of the fetal compromise. The first mechanism of adaptation is represented by blood flow redistribution. This induces hemodynamic changes at the level of fetal vessels (arterial and venous). Later, cardiac function shows modifications, the fetal movements can be reduced and reduction of fetal urine production induces oligohydramnios.

The method of choice for assessing hemodynamic changes is Doppler fluximetry. By spectral analysis it is possible to obtain and examine the Doppler velocity waveform (DVWF), whose shape is mainly dependent on the peripheral resistance below the explored segment of the arterial vessel, particularly altering the characteristic of the diastolic phase of the DVWF.

After the introduction of the angle-independent parameters, the pulsatility index (PI) being the most commonly used, and color flow mapping, it becomes possible to investigate very tiny fetal vessels, building a map of their patterns in normal pregnancies and in those complicated by hypoxemia. In normal conditions, the fetal vessels show a fairly constant PI throughout pregnancy. When hypoxemia occurs, the PI is increased at the level of the somatic vessels and can be decreased in the cerebral arteries. The changes are induced by peripheral somatic and splanchnic vasoconstriction and cerebral vasodilatation, and when both are present they represent the so-called 'brain-sparing effect'. By studying the fetal hemodynamic characteristics, it is possible to identify the cases in which growth failure is complicated by hypoxemia.

When Doppler investigation is applied on the umbilical arteries, it is possible to study the characteristics of the vascular bed of the placenta. When these are more or less obliterated, reduction of maternal–fetal exchange occurs, leading to fetal hypoxemia. The alterations of the DVWF and of the PI are proportional to this obliteration[27]. By exploring with Doppler technology the fetal and umbilical arteries, it is possible to observe both the effect and the cause of hypoxemia.

Taking into consideration the DVWF characteristics and the PI values observed in both vascular districts (fetal thoracic descending aorta and umbilical arteries) it is possible to divide IUGR into four groups[28]. In the first group are cases presenting absent or reverse diastolic flow (ARED); in the second group are cases presenting PI values above the 2nd standard deviation in both vessels; in the third group are cases in which PI values above the 2nd standard deviation have been observed only in the fetal aorta; in the fourth group are cases presenting restriction of growth but with PI values within the range of normality.

In a cohort of 588 IUGR fetuses divided according to this hemodynamic criterion, the prevalence of fetal distress (abnormal antepartal cardiotocography and/or late decelerations in labor and/or fetal acidemia) necessitating abdominal delivery was calculated in each group. In the first group it was 100%, in the second group 75.5%, in the third 38.6% and in the fourth 12.6%; the differences were statistically significant. In the other cases spontaneous vaginal delivery with favorable outcome occurred.

Perinatal mortality (fetal or neonatal) has been observed only in the cases presenting ARED flow. The efficacy of Doppler for predicting hypoxemia and/or fetal distress is different according to the investigated vascular district. Sensitivity is better for the aorta as compared to the umbilical artery, while specificity is better for umbilical arteries than for fetal vessels. The pathophysiological background explains the reason for the difference. Fetal vessel Doppler changes indicate adaptation to hypoxemia, while umbilical artery Doppler changes indicate vascular alteration at the level of the placental bed. Moreover, it is true that the DVWF alterations are proportional to the obliteration of the placental vascular bed, but it is necessary that more than 60% of that vascular bed is obliterated before changes are observable in the DVWF[29]. Therefore, it is possible to say that Doppler investigation of fetal and umbilical arteries is a useful second-level test after recognition of IUGR. According to this information it is possible to modulate the characteristics of the management. Evidence has been shown that the use of Doppler semeiology can improve the perinatal outcome of IUGR cases[30].

Hemodynamic changes are evident in the hypoxemic fetus in different venous districts (inferior vena cava, ductus venosus, umbilical vein) and in the fetal heart. Unfortunately, these are usually a late symptom of fetal deterioration and their use in clinical practice needs further investigation.

Cardiac function is also altered in the case of reduced oxygen supply. Of the many alterations observable in chronic hypoxemia, the reduction of the fetal heart variability seems to be the most accurate indicator. This reduction is well correlated with the level of fetal hypoxemia and acidemia[28–31]. The fetal heart rate variability is easily evaluated by using computer-assisted cardiotochography[32].

Serial investigation allows detection of even subtle changes in this heart function; observing the trend of the values it is possible to modulate the timing of delivery, when necessary. Practically, as far as short-term variability (STV) is concerned, fetal acidemia and/or demise can be expected in more than 70% of the cases if STV values below 3.6 are observed. The probability of having such an unfavorable outcome progressively decreases as STV increases. The Doppler findings, the STV values and the level of hypoxemia and/or acidemia show a good correlation. As a practical consequence, by using Doppler investigation and computer-assisted CTG, it is possible to monitor, with good accuracy, the level of fetal oxygenation and its evolution, optimizing the timing of delivery when indicated.

CONCLUSIONS

IUGR is one of the leading causes of perinatal mortality and morbidity. The principle cause of poor perinatal outcomes is fetal hypoxemia and/or acidemia, which are encountered in about 30% of the cases in which restriction of growth has been observed. For a long time IUGR and SFD have been considered as synonymous. After the introduction into clinical practice of ultrasonic fetal biometry, it became possible to monitor the characteristics of growth. It has been observed that a poor perinatal outcome is more dependent on the restriction of growth than solely on the weight. Hypoxemia is present in about 25% of cases presenting restriction of growth, but with birth weight within the range of normality.

It has also been shown that the clinical outcome can be improved by optimizing the management by applying a second-level test such as Doppler technology or computer-assisted cardiotochography. As a consequence, the recognition of IUGR during pregnancy is crucial in order to apply rational management.

Therefore, there is a need to investigate the utility of screening policies for IUGR and their characteristics. As at the moment there is no evidence of the efficacy of such policies, there is a need to address this problem by properly designed studies offering a clear definition of IUGR at fetal biometry, and not considering only the birth weight as an end-point, and proposing uniform protocols of clinical control and management.

It is likely that this will show whether screening for IUGR is advisable or not.

References

1. Eik-Nes SH, Okland O, Aure JC. Ultrasound screening in pregnancy: a randomised controlled trial. *Lancet* 1984;16:1347
2. Bakketeig LS, Eik-Nes SH, Jacobsen G, *et al*. Randomised controlled trial of ultrasonographic screening in pregnancy. *Lancet* 1984;28:207–11
3. Newnaham JP, Evans SF, Michael CA, *et al*. Effects of frequent ultrasound during pregnancy: a randomised controlled trial. *Lancet* 1994;342: 887–91
4. Ewigman BG, Crane JP, Frigoletto FD, *et al*. Radius Study Group. Effect of prenatal ultrasound screening on perinatal outcome. *N Engl J Med* 1993;329:821–7
5. Eik-Nes SH, Salesen KA, Okland O, *et al*. Routine ultrasound fetal examination: the 'Alesund' randomized controlled trial. *Ultrasound Obstet Gynecol* 2000;15:473–8
6. Bricker L, Neilson JP. Routine ultrasound in late pregnancy (after 24 weeks gestation). Cochrane Review. In *The Cochrane Library* 2000: Issue 3 (Oxford: Update Software)
7. Mandruzzato GP, D'Ottavio G, Rustico MA, *et al*. Management of intrauterine growth retardation: diagnostic and clinical aspects. *Fetal Ther* 1986;1: 126–8
8. Seeds JW, Peng T. Impaired growth and risks of fetal death: is the tenth percentile the appropriate standard? *Am J Obstet Gynecol* 1998;178:658–69
9. Danielian PJ, Allman ACJ, Steer PJ. Is obstetric and neonatal outcome worse in fetuses who fail to reach their own growth potential? *Br J Obstet Gynaecol* 1992;99:452–4
10. Chard T, Costeloe K, Leaf A. Evidence of growth retardation in neonates of apparently normal weight. *Eur J Obstet Gynaecol Reprod Biol* 1992;45:59–62
11. Altman DG, Hytten FE. Intrauterine growth restriction: let's be clear about it. *Br J Obstet Gynaecol* 1989;96:1127–32
12. Ott WJ. Intrauterine growth retardation: refining the definition. *J Matern Fetal Invest* 1992;2:101–4
13. Chard T, Yoong A, Macintosh M. The myth of fetal growth retardation at term. *Br J Obstet Gynaecol* 1993;100:1076–81
14. Mahadevan N, Pearce M, Steer P. The proper measure of intrauterine growth retardation is function, not size. *Br J Obstet Gynaecol* 1994;101: 1032–5
15. Steer P. Fetal growth. *Br J Obstet Gynaecol* 1998; 105:1133–5
16. de Jong CLD, Francis A, van Geijn HP, *et al*. Fetal growth and adverse perinatal events. *Ultrasound Obstet Gynecol* 1999;13:86–9
17. ACOG practice bulletin. Intrauterine growth restriction. *Int J Obstet Gynecol* 2001;72:85–6
18. Soothil PW, Bobrow CS, Holmes R. Small for gestational age is not a diagnosis. *Ultrasound Obstet Gynecol* 1999;13:225–8
19. Mongelli M, Gardosi J. Fetal growth. *Curr Opin Obstet Gynecol* 2000;12:111–15
20. Rosenberg K, Grant JM, Tweedie I, *et al*. Measurement of fundal height as a screening test for fetal growth retardation. *Br J Obstet Gynaecol* 1982;89:447–50
21. Lindhard A, Neilsen PV, Mouritsen LA, *et al*. The implications of introducing the symphyseal–fundal height-measurement. A prospective randomized controlled trial. *Br J Obstet Gynaecol* 1990;97:675–80
22. Deter RL, Harrist RB, Hadlock FP, *et al*. Fetal head and abdominal circumferences >1. Evaluation of measurement errors. *J Clin Ultrasound* 1982;10:357
23. Shepard MJ, Richards VA, Berkovitz RL. An evaluation of two equations for predicting fetal weight by ultrasound. *Am J Obstet Gynecol* 1982; 142:47
24. Hadlock FP, Harrist RB, Sharman RS, *et al*. Estimation of fetal weight with the use of head, body and femur measurements. A prospective study. *Am J Obstet Gynecol* 1985;151:333–7
25. Ott WJ. The ultrasonic diagnosis and evaluation of intrauterine growth restriction. *Ultrasound Rev Obstet Gynecol* 2001;1:205–15
26. Mandruzzato GP, Bogatti P, Fischer Tamaro L, *et al*. The clinical significance of absence of reverse end diastolic flow in the fetal aorta and umbilical artery. *Ultrasound Obstet Gynecol* 1991;1: 192

27. Trudinger B, Cook CM. Doppler umbilical and uterine flow waveforms in severe pregnancy hypertension. *Br J Obstet Gynaecol* 1990;97:142

28. Mandruzzato GP, Meir YJ, Natale R, *et al.* Antepartal assessment of IUGR fetuses. *J Perinat Med* 2001;29:222–9

29. Giles W, Trudinger B, Bailard P. Fetal umbilical artery flow velocity waveforms and placental resistance: pathological correlation. *Br J Obstet Gynaecol* 1985;92:31

30. Neilson JP, Alfirevic Z. Doppler ultrasound for fetal assessment in high risk pregnancies. Cochrane Review. In *The Cochrane Library* 1999; Issue 1 (Oxford: Update Software)

31. Mandruzzato GP, Meir YJ, Fischer Tamaro L. Monitoring fetal hypoxemia: Doppler flow measurement and computerized cardiotocography. In Chevernak FA, Kurjak A, eds. *Current Perspectives on The Fetus as a Patient*. Carnforth, UK: Parthenon Publishing, 1996:393–404

32. Dawes GS, Moulden M, Redman CWG. Short term fetal heart rate variation, decelerations, and umbilical flow velocity waveforms before labour. *Obstet Gynaecol* 1992;80:673

Fetal risks of macrosomia

20

V. Váradi

DEFINITION

Macrosomia is one of the terms used to categorize the large infant. It has several definition thresholds (4000 g, 4250 g and 4500 g). In 1991, the American College of Obstetricians and Gynecologists suggested that macrosomia be defined as a birth weight of 4500 g or more. Hungarian handbooks define macrosomia as a birth weight of 4000 g or more[1,2].

Within this category there is a heterogeneous group of fetuses and newborns with varying concerns, and it is difficult to ascertain the underlying cause[3]. Some macrosomic fetuses are at increased risk for certain perinatal complications such as hypoxia, birth injuries and impairment of neonatal adaptation. Recently, even long-term sequelae of macrosomia, e.g. higher incidence of certain congenital tumors, such as acute lymphatic leukemia, Wilms tumor and neuroblastoma, low blood pressure at 7 years of age, a higher incidence of diabetes mellitus and obesity in adolescence, have been recognized[4–6]. However, the majority of infants with macrosomia are normal, genetically driven, large infants.

Using this definition, a fetus weighing 3900 g on delivery at 36 weeks of gestation would not be classified as macrosomic, even though its weight would be greater than the 90th centile for its gestational age.

Another term for large fetuses and neonates is 'large for gestational age' (LGA). The classic definition of large for gestational age is: fetal/neonatal weight greater than or equal to the 90th centile for a given gestational age. Using this criterion, 70% of LGA infants will be determined by genetic factors and the remaining 30% can be considered 'abnormally' large for gestational age and will require special clinical attention.

In addition to weight, some have argued that neonatal body proportions have a role in defining macrosomia. Macrosomic fetuses of diabetic mothers have a greater shoulder circumference to head circumference ratio than fetuses of similar weight from non-diabetic women. Disproportionate macrosomia, as evidenced by a high ponderal index, has also been associated with an increased likelihood of neonatal complications among infants of diabetic mothers[2].

INCIDENCE

Using the 4000-g threshold, the incidence of newborn infants with macrosomia is 8–10%, while 0.1% of fetuses have a birth weight of 4500 g or more. In the Obstetrical Statistical Cooperative Study of more than 104 000 deliveries, macrosomic neonates resulted from 15.4% of postmature deliveries, 10% of morbidly obese mothers, 9.2% of diabetic mothers and 6.4% of mothers with gestational diabetes[2].

FACTORS AFFECTING FETAL GROWTH

In general, fetal growth differs from postnatal growth. Intrinsic fetal growth potential relies upon genetic material, sex and anatomy of the fetus, and the length of gestation. Race and ethnicity have been shown to be contributing factors, and several congenital disorders are associated with macrosomia[2]. Factors affecting fetal growth are fetal, placental and maternal in origin[7].

Fetal growth potential is determined by genetic factors, as studies performed in monozygotic and dizygotic twins have demonstrated[4]. However, genetic potential accounts for only about 35–40% of variations in fetal weight.

Apart from genetic factors, fetal hormones are also related to intrauterine growth. The most important fetal hormone affecting intrauterine growth is insulin, derived from the fetus itself. Insulin is already present at 8–10 weeks of gestation. However, it remains relatively inactive until the 20th week of gestation. Insulin-like growth factors (IGF-I and IGF-II) are proinsulin-like polypeptides that stimulate cell division and differentiation. IGF-I is strongly related to fetal growth and macrosomia in pregnant women without diabetes. Macrosomia was found to be associated with high levels of maternal IGF-I and II. The higher the birth weight, the higher the levels of IGF I and II[8]. Contrary opinions and evidence suggest that IGF II is not associated with fetal growth.

Other hormones, such as thyroid hormone and growth hormone, whose role in postnatal growth is well known, have no effect on prenatal growth.

Leptin has been discovered to be the protein product of the obese gene. It is synthesized in the adipose tissue and secreted into the circulation. There is a significant association between cord serum leptin and infant birth weight. Since maternal leptin does not cross the placenta, it is probably fetal in origin.

Placental dysfunction (toxema, infarct) constrains the development of genetic factors in fetuses. There is growing agreement that impaired uteroplacental and fetoplacental blood flow is an important factor in the pathophysiology of intrauterine fetal growth restriction. Severe maternal malnutrition is one of the main causes of intrauterine growth retardation. Deprivation of adequate fetal nutrition alters cellular homeostasis. Limited bioavailability of amino acids for protein synthesis is the origin of a series of modifications[9].

Maternal risk factors

Many authors describe their observations according to the association between maternal preconceptional weight, maternal height and weight gain during pregnancy and postmaturity[10].

In a series of 393 large-for-dates babies born during the 3 years from 1998 to 2000 at the St Margaret Hospital in Budapest, Hungary, we found a significant correlation between fetal macrosomia and maternal preconceptional weight, maternal height and weight gain during pregnancy. However, unlike most other authors[11,12], we found no association between macrosomia and postmaturity among our fetuses.

COMPLICATIONS OF FETAL MACROSOMIA

Some complications, such as protracted labor, perinatal asphyxia, skeletal injuries, shoulder dystocia and increased risk of Cesarean section, are more common among macrosomic fetuses than 'normal weight' fetuses, regardless of the exact cause of macrosomia.

Correlation between macrosomia and perinatal asphyxia is not obvious, not even among the fetuses of diabetic mothers[13]. In addition to that, a recent study even suggests that, in the fetuses of diabetic mothers, the insulin growth factor system may have a neuroprotective role against asphyxial brain injury[2].

Although there is a lot of ambiguity, there seems to be a correlation between increased fetal size and the risk of shoulder dystocia. In the general population, the risk of shoulder dystocia is approximately 1% in cases of cephalic vaginal delivery[13]. The incidence increases to 7.3% when birth weight is 4500 g. An additional risk for shoulder dystocia is the presence of maternal diabetes and vacuum or forceps delivery.

In 4–40% of shoulder dystocia cases, brachial plexus injury may occur. In the majority of cases, brachial plexus injury is transient and resolves without treatment, or with conservative treatment involving observation and physiotherapy during the first months of life. In serious, permanent cases it produces medicolegal concerns as well. Indications and timing for microsurgery and nerve grafting are still controversial.

A review of the literature shows that numerous risk factors can be identified for shoulder dystocia. Risk factors consistently identified in all studies include fetal macrosomia and maternal diabetes mellitus. Operative delivery also appears to be an important risk factor in many studies. Shoulder dystocia risk factors and shoulder dystocia are relatively common in the obstetric population, but the true concern, permanent plexus brachialis injury, is extremely rare. Risk factors associated with shoulder dystocia are identified quite frequently in the general obstetric population[15]. Besides maternal diabetes mellitus combined with expected birth weight of more than 4250 g and the combination of known macrosomia and second-stage labor arrest with mid-pelvic operative delivery, there is no single predictor of shoulder dystocia. Iffy and colleagues[16] have called attention to the physiology of the labor process and suggested that the rotation and passage of the shoulders through the pelvis at the peak of the next contraction is a physiological process that need not occur immediately after delivery of the head, but as much as 2–4 min later. They suggest that, if the shoulders are not delivered with the next uterine contraction, oxytocin should be administered to assist in delivery of the shoulders.

Among the numerous risk factors identified for shoulder dystocia, the following three have proved to be clinically significant:

(1) Fetal macrosomia;
(2) Maternal diabetes mellitus;
(3) Operative (forceps or vacuum) delivery.

A direct correlation was found in diabetic patients between the level of fetal truncal asymmetry measured sonographically and the incidence and severity of shoulder dystocia[17].

Despite the association between birth weight and shoulder dystocia, most authors do not advocate elective Cesarean section for macrosomia. The one exception is the judicious use of Cesarean delivery in diabetic mothers with an estimated fetal birth weight of more than 4250 g, which should reduce the risk of shoulder dystocia in this subgroup of patients[18,19].

Elective Cesarean section is not desirable, because it requires a great number of unnecessary procedures to avoid a single neonatal injury[20]. Furthermore, prediction of macrosomia by ultrasound examination is limited by substantial inherent false-positive and false-negative rates. Sensitivity of ultrasonography in estimating fetal weight is 60%, its specificity 90%. The incidence of macrosomia is 8.2% in > 4000 g and 1.6% in > 4500 g in infants born to mothers without diabetes, versus 17% and 6%, respectively, for infants born to diabetic mothers. Using these data in a hypothetical group of 100 pregnant women, 12% would have macrosomic infants weighing > 4000 g. Although ultrasound would identify 16 fetuses with macrosomia, only seven would actually be macrosomic. Conversely, five of the 12 fetuses with macrosomia would be incorrectly identified as having normal weight. Thus, any policy of prophylactic Cesarean delivery for suspected fetal macrosomia would result in unnecessary Cesarean deliveries of normal-weight fetuses and the trial of labor and vaginal delivery of infants with macrosomia whose weights were underestimated[21].

Sokol and colleagues[22] were able to improve the accuracy of identifying fetal macrosomia compared to the reliance on the equation by Hadlock et al.[23]. There was a chance for a fetus to have significantly increased risk for birth weight > 4000 g when the estimated fetal weight based on abdominal circumference was greater than that based on either head circumference or femur length. Taking into account maternal height, weight and the presence of maternal diabetes mellitus in addition to these ultrasonographic measurement protocols, accuracy in the prediction of macrosomia can improve. Intrapartum sonographic evaluation of abdominal circumference in suspected macrosomic fetuses during early labor is advised to help with decision making[24].

Sylvestre et al. found that in post-date patients routine glucose challenge testing performed early in pregnancy (24–28 weeks) can improve the test characteristics of sonography in predicting macrosomia. The value of sonographically suspected macrosomia increased from 60 to 71%, when the glucose level was ≥ 120 mg%[25].

Thus, indicating a prophylactic Cesarean section in cases of fetal macrosomia defined by ultrasound will lead to unnecessary Cesarean sections for fetuses of normal birth weight and advice for vaginal delivery for macrosomic fetuses with underestimated weight[26]. Others also found that a policy of elective Cesarean delivery in cases with fetal macrosomia had a non-significant effect on the incidence of brachial plexus injury and made only a small contribution to the rate of Cesarean deliveries[1].

Early induction of labor to limit fetal growth led to substantial increase in Cesarean section rate, because of failed induction. Induction at 38 weeks or before is associated with an increased rate of Cesarean delivery. A fetal weight of 4000 g or more is not an indication for induction of labor. Even post-date labor complicated by fetal macrosomia seems to be best managed expectantly[9,12,27]. The best policy seems to be spontaneous birth or induction only after the completion of 42 weeks. In cases complicated with diabetes mellitus, there are reasons for elective induction when macrosomia is suspected, and indication for Cesarean section if the calculated birth weight is greater than 4250–4500 g[19,28,29]. We agree with the opinion that physician factors have an important role in the risk for Cesarean delivery in diabetic patients[30].

Macrosomic infants have increased incidence of prolonged labor, operative vaginal delivery and emergency Cesarean section compared with normal-weight babies. These complications are more pronounced in primigravida than in multigravida. Shoulder dystocia seems to occur with equal frequency in primigravida and multigravida[31].

OUR EXPERIENCE

Between 1 January 1998 and 31 December 2000, we retrospectively reviewed the medical records of 392 mothers with macrosomic fetuses – 7.46% (392/5252) of all deliveries. Fourteen mothers had gestational diabetes and one mother had diabetes mellitus. We examined the mothers' weight, height and weight gain during pregnancy and compared the data with those of mothers with non-macrosomic fetuses. We found significant parallel correlation between the maternal height, preconceptional weight, weight gain during pregnancy and fetal macrosomia. The overall Cesarean section rate was 22.5% (1185/5252) during the examined 3 years, and 29.5% (116/392) in the macrosomic group. In 16 cases out of the 392, elective Cesarean section was carried out, owing to gestational diabetes and other associated conditions.

In 168 cases birth induction was chosen during the 40th and 41st gestational weeks, mostly because of fetal macrosomia. Out of these 168 cases, 63 Cesarean sections were carried out, mostly owing to prolonged second stage of labor and signs of intrauterine asphyxia. Therefore, 37.5% (63/168) of all induced labors ended in Cesarean sections.

Two-thirds of all labor (224/392) started spontaneously. From this group 23.5% (53/224) of Cesarean sections occurred later, owing to indications similar to those in the induced group. There was a significant difference between the Cesarean section rates for macrosomic fetuses of the spontaneous and induced labor groups (23.5% versus 37.5%). As far as the birth injury is concerned, there were two cases of transient plexus brachialis paresis in the spontaneously born group and none among the newborns born by Cesarean section. The mode of delivery did not influence the 1 and 5 min Apgar score, or the postnatal adaptation of macrosomic infants (V. Váradi, unpublished data).

References

1. Gonen O, Bader D, Ajami M. Effects of a policy of elective cesarean delivery in cases of suspected fetal macrosomia on the incidence of brachial plexus injury and the rate of cesarean delivery. *Am J Obstet Gynecol* 2000;183:1296–300

2. Grassi AE, Giuliano MA. The neonate with macrosomia. *Clin Obstet Gynecol* 2000;43:340–8

3. Divon MY. Fetal macrosomia. *Clin Obstet Gynecol* 2000;43:225–350

4. Mikulandra F, Gruric J, Banovic I, Perisa M, Zakanj Z. The effect of high birth weight (4000 g or more) on the weight and height of adult men and women. *Coll Anthropol* 2000;24:133–6

5. Yeazel MW, Ross JA, Buckley JD. High birth weight: a risk for childhood cancer: a report from the Children's Center Group. *J Pediatr* 1997;131:671–7

6. Yiu V, Buka S, Zurakowski D. Relationship between birth weight and blood pressure in childhood. *Am J Kidney Dis* 1999;33:253–60

7. Langer O. Fetal macrosomia: etiologic factors. *Clin Obstet Gynecol* 2000;43:283–97

8. Lauszus FF, Klebe JG, Flyvbjerg A. Macrosomia associated with maternal serum insulin-like growth hormone I and II in diabetic pregnancy. *Obstet Gynecol* 2001;97:734–41

9. Carrera JM, Devesa R, Salvador J. Etiology and pathogenesis of intrauterine growth retardation. In Kurjak A, ed. *Textbook of Perinatal Medicine*. Carnforth, UK: Parthenon Publishing, 1998:1171–91

10. Hardy DS. A multiethnic study of the predictors of macrosomia. *Diabetes Educ* 1999;25:925–33

11. Chervenak FA, Divon MY, Hirsch HJ, Girz B, Langer O. Macrosomia in the postdate pregnancy: is routine ultrasonographic screening indicated? *Am J Obstet Gynecol* 1989;161:753–6

12. Horrigan TJ. Physicians who induce labor for fetal macrosomia do not reduce cesarean delivery rates. *J Perinatol* 2001;21:93–6

13. Wollschlaeder K, Nieder J, Koppe I, Hartlein K. A study of fetal macrosomia. *Arch Gynecol Obstet* 1999;263:51–5

14. Dildy GA, Clark SL. Shoulder dystocia: risk identification. *Clin Obstet Gynecol* 2000;43:265–82

15. Iffy L, Váradi V, Jakobovits A. Common intrapartum denominators of shoulder dystocia related birth injuries. *Zentralbl Gynekol* 1994;116:133–7

16. Iffy L, Ganesh V, Gittens L. Obstetric maneuvers for shoulder dystocia. *Am J Obstet Gynecol* 1998;179:1379–80

17. Berkus MD, Conway D, Langer O. The large fetus. *Clin Obstet Gynecol* 1999;42:766–84

18. Larger O, Berkus MD, Huff RW, Samueloff A. Shoulder dystocia: should the fetus weighing > 4000 grams be delivered by cesarean section? *Am J Obstet Gynecol* 1991;165:831–7

19. Wagner RK, Nielsen PE, Gonik B. Shoulder dystocia. *Obstet Gynecol Clin North Am* 1999;26:371–83

20. Rouse DJ, Owen J. Prophylactic cesarean delivery for fetal macrosomia diagnosed by means of ultrasonography. A Faustian bargain? *Am J Obstet Gynecol* 1999;181:332–8

21. O'Reilly-Green C, Divon M. Sonographic and clinical methods in the diagnosis of macrosomia. *Clin Obstet Gynecol* 2000;43:319–20

22. Sokol RJ, Chik L, Dombrowski MP, Zador IE. Correctly identifying the macrosomic fetus: improving prediction. *Am J Obstet Gynecol* 2000;182:1489–95

23. Hadlock FP, Harrist RB, Sharman RS, Deter RL, Park SK. Estimation of fetal weight with the use of head, body and femur measurements – a prospective study. *Am J Obstet Gynecol* 1985;151:333–7

24. Al Inany H, Alaa N, Momtaz M, Abdel Badii M. Intrapartum prediction of macrosomia: accuracy of abdominal circumference estimation. *Gynecol Obstet Invest* 2001;51:116–19

25. Sylvestre G, Divon MY, Onyeije C, Fischer M. Diagnosis of macrosomia in the postdates population: combining sonographic estimates of fetal weight with glucose challenge testing. *J Matern Fetal Med* 2000;9:287–90

26. Parry S, Severs CP, Sehdev HM, Macones GA, White LM, Morgan MA. Ultrasonographic prediction of fetal macrosomia: association with cesarean delivery. *Reprod Med* 2000;45:17–22

27. Gonen O, Rosen DJ. Dolfin Z, Tepper R, Markov S, Fejgin MD. Induction of labor versus expectant management in macrosomia: a randomized study. *Obstet Gynecol* 1997;89:913–17

28. Conway DL, Langer O. Elective delivery of infants with macrosomia in diabetic women: reduced shoulder dystocia versus increased cesarean deliveries. *Am J Obstet Gynecol* 1998;178:922–6

29. Haram K, Bergsjo P, Pirhonen J. Suspected large fetus in the last period of pregnancy – a difficulty. *Tidsskr Nor Laegeforen* 2001;121:1369–73

30. Blackwell SC, Hassan SS, Wolfe HW, Michaelson J, Berry SM, Sorokin Y. What are cesarean delivery rates so high in diabetic pregnancies? *J Perinat Med* 200;28:316–20

31. Mocanu EV, Greene RA, Byrne BM, Turner MJ. Obstetric and neonatal outcome of babies weighing more than 4250 g: an analysis by parity. *Eur J Obstet Gynecol Reprod Biol* 2000;92:229–33

Normal and abnormal fetal growth in multiple pregnancies

21

I. Blickstein

INTRODUCTION

Animal and human models demonstrated that both birth weight and gestational age at birth bear a reciprocal relationship with litter size. In the human, the mean gestational age and birth weight were 39.0 weeks/3357 g, 35.8 weeks/2389 g and 32.5 weeks/1735 g for singletons, twins and triplets, respectively[1]. These relationships suggest that the uterine milieu, comprising uteroplacental as well as maternal and fetal components, clearly limits the growth potential of the individual fetus in a multiple pregnancy. This concept implies that, as a rule, all multiples are growth restricted, compared with singletons.

However, at the same time that the uterine milieu is overwhelmed by the multiple pregnancy, it exhibits remarkable adaptation. Consider the situation at 40 weeks' singleton gestation, in which the 50th birth weight centile is 3515 g. This birth weight is achieved in twins by 32 weeks, when the 50th centile of the total fetal birth weight is 3628 g[1]. It follows that after this gestational age, the total twin pregnancy is growth promoted, rather than restricted. In triplets, the 50th singleton birth weight centile is attained even earlier, at 29 weeks.

The extent of adaptation is best illustrated at the mean gestational age at birth for multiples. Consider the total twin birth weight at 36 weeks (2 × 2500 g = 5000 g) and the total triplet birth weight at 33 weeks (3 × 1701 g = 5103 g). Both total birth weights exceed by far the 90th centile of singletons at term.

This chapter does not discuss maternal morbidities that may affect fetal growth (i.e. diabetes, pre-eclamptic toxemia, etc.). However, the chapter focuses on several aspects of the unique and intriguing situation whereby the individual fetus is growth restricted at the same time that the entire pregnancy is growth promoted.

THE COMPLEX GROWTH PATTERNS OF MULTIPLES

It is clear that not all small for gestational age (SGA) fetuses are growth restricted. However, the SGA designation helps to identify those with a lower birth weight than most (usually 95–97%) of the infants of the same gestational age. Whether the SGA status results from true growth restriction (i.e. restricted by the uterine milieu) or from a constitutional background (i.e. part of the normal variability) is sometimes difficult to establish[2]. This difficulty, which leads frequently to confusion, is much more complex in multiple pregnancies for several reasons. First, a significant proportion of twins will be considered SGA by singleton standards, and therefore, it has been repeatedly argued that such a definition should be based only on twin standards[3]. Regrettably, there are few population-based data from which accurate statistical inference can be made.

Second, twins exhibit a paired situation and it is not infrequent to find that each member of a twin pair has a different definition. Table 1 shows the analysis of 7196 Swedish pairs born between 1991 and 1995. Each twin was defined as large (>95th centile), small (<5th centile) or appropriate (5th–95th centile) for gestational age (LGA, SGA and AGA, respectively), based on twin standards derived from the same population (Blickstein I, Goldman RD, Rydhstroem H, unpublished data) The incidence of a single

Table 1 *Frequencies (%) of size combinations among twins. Large for gestational age, LGA; appropriate for gestational age, AGA; small for gestational age, SGA. (Blickstein I, Goldman RD and Rydhstroem H, unpublished data)*

	Twin A		
Twin B	LGA	AGA	SGA
LGA	0.4	2.0	0.03
AGA	2.0	91.0	1.2
SGA	0.07	3.0	0.3

SGA twin was 4.3%, with an increased risk that twin B would be SGA (odds ratio (OR) 2.5; 95% confidence interval (95% CI) 1.9, 3.6). The incidence of both twins being SGA was 0.3%. Very large discordance (i.e. SGA/LGA and LGA/SGA) was rarely observed – 0.1% of all twins. Similarly, the incidence of one LGA twin was 4.1% and that of two LGA twins was 0.4%.

Another way to establish the risk of growth aberration is to look at deliveries of very low (<1500 g) and extremely low birth weight (<1000 g) (VLBW and ELBW, respectively) among multiples. This risk was determined in a cohort of 12 567 live-born twin pairs delivered from 1993 to 1998 in Israel[4]. The numbers of pairs with VLBW and low birth weight (LBW) (<2500 g) neonates were counted in three combinations: VLBW–VLBW, VLBW–LBW and VLBW–over 2500 g. Comparisons were made between the subsets of nulliparas and multiparas and like- versus unlike-sex pairs. The frequency of at least one VLBW twin was significantly higher among nulliparas than multiparas (OR 2.3; 95% CI 2.1, 2.6; $p < 0.001$). For pairs with VLBW–VLBW and VLBW–LBW combinations, a significantly higher frequency was found among nulliparas than multiparas (OR 2.0; 95% CI 1.7, 2.8; $p < 0.001$ and OR 2.6; 95% CI 2.2, 3.1; $p < 0.001$, respectively). The risk seemed to be accentuated in like-sex twins. Overall, the risk of having at least one VLBW infant was 1 : 5 among nulliparas and 1 : 12 among multiparas. The risk of having two VLBW twins among nulliparas (1 : 11) was double that of multiparas (1 : 22).

The same approach was used in a nation-wide perinatal database collected by Matria Healthcare, Inc. (Marietta, GA)[5]. The number of sets with one, two and three ELBW neonates was counted in a cohort of 3288 triplets sets. The odds of delivering at least one ELBW infant was significantly higher among nulliparas (1 : 7) than among multiparas (1 : 13), OR 1.9, 95% CI 1.9, 2.5. The odds of having at least two ELBW sibs in nulliparas (1 : 16) was twice higher than in multiparas (1 : 32), 95% CI 1.3, 2.9. Nulliparas and multiparas had similar odds of delivering three ELBW infants (1 : 28 vs. 1 : 39, OR 1.3, 95% CI 0.9, 2.1).

TRENDS OF FETAL GROWTH OF MULTIPLES RELATIVE TO SINGLETONS

The uterine milieu efficiently provides for fetal growth until a certain gestational age is reached. At that age, growth velocity of multiples decelerates as compared with singletons, exhibiting a growth restriction pattern. This pattern is observed before birth (by prenatal ultrasound) and by using birth weight by gestational age ('growth') curves. With ultrasound assessments of various fetal indices, this decelerating pattern starts sometime between 30 and 33 weeks' gestation[6,7]. Of importance was the observation that this pattern starts earlier in triplets[8] than in twins[7] and in twins earlier than in singletons.

The corresponding observation postpartum is found in large population-based growth curves. Alexander *et al.*[1] clearly show that until 27 weeks, there is no difference between birth weights of singletons, twins or triplets. At 28 weeks, birth weight of twins and triplets starts to lag after that of singletons, with little difference between twins and triplets until 32 weeks. Thereafter, a marked distinction between singleton, twins and triplets is evident.

To appreciate the adaptation of the uterine milieu to nurture multiples, the data presented by Alexander *et al.*[1] were re-assessed to compare the ratio between the median (50th) birth weight centile of twin/singleton and triplet/singleton (Figure 1). Figure 2 is a schematic

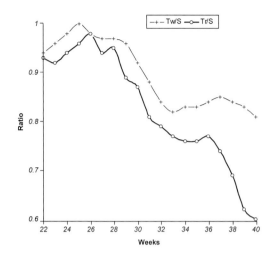

Figure 1 *Ratio between the median birth weight of twin/singleton (Tw/S) and triplet/singleton (Tr/S). Data adapted from reference 1*

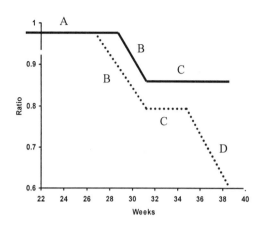

Figure 2 *Schematic presentation of the trend lines shown in Figure 1. Solid line, twins; dotted line, triplets. The four phases (A–D) are discussed in the text*

illustration of the trend lines shown in Figure 1. The pattern suggests four phases (A to D).

In phase A, a ratio of 0.9–1.0 (i.e. very similar birth weights to singletons) is maintained until 28 and 30 weeks' gestation in twins and triplets. This means that the uterine milieu is fully capable of providing for growth of the individual multiple fetuses to the same extent as for singletons, but for some reason (i.e. cervical incompetence) is unable to promote gestational age. Multiples delivered at this phase are not likely to demonstrate growth restriction albeit that they have VLBW and ELBW. Phase B starts at 30 weeks in twins and is characterized by a steady decrease in birth weight of the individual twins relative to singletons. In triplets the same pattern is observed, but phase B starts earlier than in twins. In this phase the uterine milieu is inadequate to provide fully for growth of the individual multiple fetuses, and individual twins and triplets may be smaller relative to singletons by as much as 15 and 20%, respectively. At the same time, the uterine environment promotes maturity. Phase C is characterized by a stabilized ratio, which does not change significantly over time. This phase, in which twin and triplet birth weights are

maintained at about 15% and 20% less than singletons, respectively, continues until 40 weeks in twins, but is of short duration – between 33 and 36 weeks – in triplets. The uterine environment during this phase exhibits an adaptation to the presence of twins; in triplets, however, this adaptation cannot be sustained for a long period. Phase C deliveries include growth restricted and gestational age promoted multiples. Phase D, which is seen in triplets only, represents the inability of the overwhelmed uterine milieu to adapt, leading to a marked decrease in triplet birth weight relative to singleton until 40 weeks. Phase D deliveries are purely gestational age promoted.

The different individual fetal growth of twins and triplets compared with singletons is based on cross-sectional rather on longitudinal data. At this time it cannot be postulated that a given uterine environment undergoes changes during a multiple pregnancy. It could be argued, however, that there are two different environments – promoting age and maintaining size (A and C), and promoting age and restricting size (B and D). It also can be argued that nature seems to favor advanced gestational age (i.e. maturity) at the expense of size.

SIZE DISCORDANCE: FACTS AND HYPOTHESES

The discussion about fetal size in multiple pregnancy should always include reference to divergent growth patterns of the multiples resulting in discordant birth weights.

There are several definitions of discordant birth weight. The most popular is the per cent definition whereby the intertwin difference is measured as a proportion of the larger twin[9]. Growth discordance is frequently associated with adverse perinatal outcome similar to that seen in growth restriction. It should be stressed, however, that discordant growth (relative growth restriction) does not necessarily mean absolute growth restriction: consider a 3500/2500 set, which is certainly discordant (1000/3500 g = 28.6%) but is obviously not growth restricted, even by singleton standards.

Incidence

The incidence of discordant pairs depends on the per cent definition used[10,11]. Figure 3 shows that the frequency of discordant pairs decreases with increasing discordance levels, satisfying an inversely logarithmic function (Pearson's R^2 = 0.988). This correlation means that the frequency of discordant pairs drops faster at the lower and slower at the upper range of discordance levels.

Birth order

For many years it was believed that the smaller twin is usually the second-born twin. While this was disproved on many occasions, it has been shown that the likelihood of the second-born twin being smaller increases with increasing discordance levels as a quadratic function (Pearson's R^2 = 0.946) (Figure 4)[10,11].

Fetal sex

It is well known that females have a lower birth weight than males, a phenomenon seen in singletons as well as in multiples. Thus, the possible effect of a male fetus on growth of the

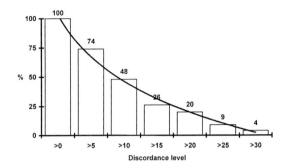

Figure 3 *Frequencies of discordant pairs by discordance level. Adapted from reference 11*

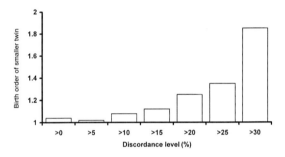

Figure 4 *Birth order of the smaller twin by level of discordance. Adapted from reference 11*

female co-twin is intriguing, although the growth promoting or growth restricting mechanisms are totally obscure.

A comparison of 71 male–female pairs with 82 female–male pairs showed similar mean twin birth weight and frequency of birth weight discordance. However, males were significantly heavier compared with females in the male-first but not in the female-first combination. The frequency of females being the smaller twins was significantly higher compared with males in both fetal sex combinations[12].

Orlebeke *et al.*[13] challenged this hypothesis in a study of 3069 twin pairs born in The Netherlands. Results show that among DZ twins, birth weight is not affected by the sex of the co-twin. Therefore, birth weight differences in unlike-sexed pairs have to be ascribed to the general effects of sex and birth order but not to a specific effect for unlike-sexed pairs only.

This debate is not settled yet. Glinianaia *et al.*[14] observed a tendency for female birth weight to be influenced by the presence of a male co-twin and concluded that this may have a biological significance and should lead to a close follow-up with respect to hormone-sensitive disorders and reproductive ability among the female twins. However, in a recent study conducted on a cohort of over 12 000 twin pairs, we could not substantiate the tendency described be Glinianaia and her co-workers (Bloomrozen-Avraham E and Blickstein I, unpublished data).

Fetal presentation

In accord with the concept that the uterine space is limited, it was postulated that twins may arrange in second-breech presentations as an adaptive measure to promote growth. Breech–breech pairs were delivered at a significantly earlier gestational age compared with vertex-second twins but attained similar or larger birth weights. Discordant-second twins were found five times more frequently in breech-second pairs when twin A was in the vertex presentation[15]. This hypothesis could be supported in part by sonographic measurements[16].

MATERNAL PARITY IN RELATION TO TWIN GROWTH

Maternal parity is perhaps the most consistent factor that influences growth in twins. It was known from singleton gestations that birth weight increases in successive deliveries with a clear disadvantage for the nullipara (primipara at twin birth). It was not until 1995 that the hypothesis regarding the association between increased twin birth weight and increased parity was tested[17]. In a retrospective evaluation of 430 twins, divided in five parity groups (para 1–4 and ≥ 5) the mean birth weight of twin A, B and both twins was significantly lower in primiparas compared to para 2–4, but not as compared to para ≥ 5 patients. These

observations were fully supported by a much larger population-based study[4]. Because multiparas are usually older than primiparas, the effect of maternal age could be a confounding variable. To assess this question, birth weight characteristics in mothers aged ≥ 40 years (n = 510) were compared with those of mothers aged 35–39 years (n = 2102) delivered during the late 1990s[18].

Interestingly, the incidence of twin mothers aged 40 years or more increased 50% during the study period, ten times more than mothers aged 35–39. The mean twin birth weight, total twin birth weight <3000 g, 3000–4999 g and ≥ 5000 g, and frequencies of VLBW twin neonates delivered to mothers aged ≥ 40 were not different from those delivered to 35–39-year-old mothers.

Because interest was focused on the adverse outcome of the primipara, a comparison was done between primiparas (n = 4793) of different age groups (<20 years, 20–24, 25–29, 30–34, 35–39 and ≥ 40 years)[19]. Interestingly, a highly significant inverse correlation between the proportion of nulliparas and maternal age group, decreasing from 71.8% at less than 20 years to 18.6% at age 35–39 years was found (Pearson $R^2 = 0.98$). Nevertheless, this trend changed abruptly to the observed figure of 25.9% nulliparas aged 40 years or more instead of the expected 2.8%. Nevertheless, maternal age of primiparas was not associated with different birth weight characteristics of their twins.

In summary, maternal parity and not maternal age is the key factor that influences growth, supporting the notion that the parous uterus is more capable of nurturing twins.

SIZE DISCORDANCE DURING THE FIRST HALF OF GESTATION

When discussing growth trends of multiples, it was repeatedly pointed out that differences are expected not earlier than the 27th week. However, early discordant growth is a well-known but poorly understood phenomenon.

According to famous Greek mythology, the twins Castor and Pollux were delivered to Leda following the bipaternal conceptions with Zeus

(King of Gods, disguised as a swan) and with her husband Tyndareus. Indeed, Aristotle suggested that twins are a result of super-fecundation, albeit he did not insist on heteropaternity as the etiology for twinning. Studies conducted 2500 years later found three cases of heteropaternal superfecundation in a parentage test database of 39 000 records[20]. James, however, estimated that at least one DZ twin maternity in twelve is produced by superfecundation[21]. He suggested that among DZ twins born to married white women in the USA, about one pair in 400 is bipaternal with substantially higher rates among selected groups of dizygotic twin maternities.

Superfecundation means that twins have different gestational ages. It is unknown, however, what is the possible maximal time interval between fertilizations. It is logical to assume that intervals of less than 1 week may not cause large birth weight differences. There are also documented cases of discordant embryonic growth when conception was not achieved by superfecundation. The first case[22] demonstrated persistent first-trimester growth disparity following *in vitro* fertilization (IVF). The crown–rump length of the two fetuses was substantially different at 7 and 11 weeks and from the 20th week onwards, intertwin dif-ferences in abdominal circumferences and estimated fetal weights were observed. Birth weight discordance was 26.6% (1600/2180 g).

The outlook of early discordance may not be bright at all. Tadmor and his co-workers described a twin pregnancy with abnormal sac size/crown–rump length ratio at 9 weeks[23]. By 14 weeks, discordant heart rates and umbilical artery flow velocities were detected, and progressively discordant size became apparent. At 30 weeks, the patient delivered a live 1350 g infant and a 400 g dead fetus.

Indeed, early discordance is an ominous sign: Weissman *et al.*[24] evaluated the clinical significance and the natural course of dis-cordant twin growth found during the first trimester of pregnancy defined as a difference in crown–rump length corresponding to 5 or more days in the estimated gestational age. Five cases with first-trimester discordant twin growth were identified and all had major congenital anomalies in the smaller twin, such as diaphragmatic hernia, ventriculomegaly, schizencephaly, critical aortic atresia and sacral agenesis. This observation certainly calls for a meticulous search for congenital anomalies in such cases.

Finally, it should be noted that many early discordant twins are actually not discordant. Sometimes, a wrong image plane depicts divergent crown–rump lengths. It is suggested that whenever such an image is found, a repeated scan should be done after 2–3 days to confirm the diagnosis. In addition, individual embryonic measurement rather than a dual presentation on the same image is recom-mended.

In summary, discordant growth starting at the first half of gestation is either very rare or associated with adverse outcome of the smaller twin.

IS SIZE DISCORDANCE A RISK FOR PRETERM BIRTH?

It is well known that the smaller twin of a discordant pair may not even be relatively growth restricted. On the contrary, the smaller twin may be appropriately grown, but the larger twin may be growth promoted. Such cases can only be found if twins are followed by sonographic biometry on a regular basis throughout gestation. It is unknown what are the factors that influence such a growth pattern.

In a study comparing perinatal variables of twin pregnancies comprising the tenth decile of the mean twin birth weight distribution with pregnancies in the ninth decile, no significant difference was found[25]. However, the incidence of growth discordant pairs was significantly higher in the heavier group as compared with the general twin population, and as expected, the tenth-decile group contained significantly fewer primiparas. Maternal obesity and diabetes were infrequent and could not explain the increased birth weight. The neonatal outcome was excellent. Although the comparison revealed insignificant differences, higher parity may be operative in the genesis of large twins.

This study led to the idea that growth discordance is not clinically significant after a certain gestational age and birth weight. To test this hypothesis, a cohort of 14 pairs delivered at ≥ 37 weeks, of at least 15% discordance, but weighing at least 2500 g were compared with 28 randomly selected term and appropriate for gestational age twin pairs without discordance[26]. The comparison showed no significant difference in maternal age, parity, gestational age, incidence of maternal hypertension or perinatal outcome. This study suggested that discordant growth is not a risk factor when the twin pair has reached term and the lighter twin weighs at least 2500 g. The other side of the coin would mean that discordant growth is clinically significant if present before that gestational age or at a lower birth weight.

The clinical significance of gestational age and birth weight has important clinical implications. In one study[27] the authors found that greater birth weight discordance was significantly associated with preterm delivery due to intervention and consequential neonatal morbidity due to prematurity. This intriguing view was examined in another study[28]. The authors found that the level of >30% discordance correlated strongly with risk for live preterm (<32 weeks) birth. Interestingly, of the 42 preterm twin births at <32 weeks' gestation with discordances ≥ 40%, 51% were attributable to fetal growth restriction and 16% to large size for gestational age in one infant. Thus, by contrast to Hollier et al.[27] who suggested the iatrogenic nature of preterm birth of discordant twins, Cooperstock et al.[28] proposed that discordant growth is itself a risk factor for preterm birth. Based on the study of Talbot et al.[29] and a census study published more than a decade ago[30], it is my view that size discordance alone does not appear to be an indication for preterm delivery of twins. When results of antenatal testing are normal and growth restriction is absent, attempts should be made to achieve a gestational age >32 weeks and weight >2000 g before delivery is

considered[29]. Also, in the subset of preterm twin gestations, the cut-off level of 30% birth weight difference seems most clinically relevant in identifying those infants at risk for adverse perinatal outcome[31].

In summary, twins may be growth promoted in general, adding up to over 6000 g. Moreover, one of the twins may exhibit better growth than its normally growing co-twin and the pair, albeit discordant, is perfectly normal. On the other side of the scale, opinions differ whether preterm birth results from or is induced because of discordant growth.

THE EFFECT OF ZYGOSITY AND CHORIONICITY ON TWIN GROWTH

The influence of zygosity on outcome is well established. Monozygotic (MZ) twins are associated with increased risk of fetal malformations and with adverse outcome related mainly to the subset of monochorionic (MC) placentas. Zygosity is perhaps the least available information in twin studies. By and large, MZ twinning is inferred when a MC placenta is found or when early sonography is highly suggestive of a MC pregnancy. It follows that all MZ twins with a dichorionic (DC) placenta cannot be differentiated from like-sex dizygotic (DZ) who have always a DC placenta. Based on the proportions of 50% like-sex DZ, 2/3 DZ:1/3 MZ, and the proportion of 2/3 MC:1/3 DC placentas among the MZ twins, one can safely assume that 11% of the twins (MZ twins with DC placentas) cannot be differentiated from 33% of the twins (like-sex DZ twins). Thus, uncertainty about zygosity is encountered in as many as 44% of the twins. To bypass this deficiency, researchers either used MC twins to represent the MZ twins (failing to include one-third of the MZ twins), or compared like-versus unlike-sexed twins (failing to exclude half of the DZ twins).

Irrespective of the mode of zygosity ascertainment, it is expected that MZ and like-sexed twins will be more similar than DZ and unlike-sexed twins, respectively. This similarity is expected in cases without overt growth discrepancies resulting from anomalies or twin–twin transfusion[32]. Indeed, divergent growth has always been a part of twin–twin transfusion syndrome, albeit it is currently not essential for the diagnosis. It should be stressed that substantial twin–twin transfusion affects about 10% of all MC twins (<3% of all twins) and can account for birth weight discordance in only a small fraction of the cases. Growth abnormalities in twin–twin transfusion will be discussed separately in this chapter.

To establish fetal growth nomograms for twin gestations by placental chorionicity, Ananth *et al.*[33] produced birth weight curves derived separately for MC and DC twins. Twins from MC gestations weighed, on average, 66.1 g less than twins from DC gestations after correcting for gestational age. Analyses indicate that singleton nomograms approximate twin growth reasonably well between 32 and 34 weeks, but they underestimate twin growth at earlier gestational ages (between 25 and 32 weeks) and overestimate twin growth beyond 34 weeks' gestation. Senoo *et al.*[34] measured longitudinally by ultrasound biometry 70 cases of concordant twins (24 MC, 46 DC) and 45 cases of discordant twins (25 MC, 20 DC). There were no differences in incremental growth between concordant MC and DC twins. However, in the discordant twins, the growth of the larger twin matched the growth curve of a singleton or concordant twin, but the growth of the smaller twin gradually decreased to the range of growth restriction. Victoria *et al.*[35] evaluated differences in pregnancy outcomes and placental findings among severely discordant MC and DC twins. Severe discordance (>25%) occurred significantly more often in MC than in DC twins and was associated with significantly more deliveries before 36 weeks and more newborns remaining more than 10 days in the neonatal intensive care unit. Severely discordant MC and DC twins had significantly worse perinatal mortality and morbidity than mildly discordant (5–25%) and concordant twins. The most frequent findings in the placentas of severely discordant twins were small placental weight and umbilical cord abnormalities.

In summary, growth patterns of MC and DC twins are different. Some of the differences may result from different fetal sex in the DC group. Regardless, all authors point to the need of sonographic chorionicity assessment early in pregnancy.

PLACENTAL ETIOLOGY FOR DISCORDANCE

When fetal (intrinsic and constitutional) causes of growth aberration are excluded, most of the other reasons have a common pathway – the uterine milieu. It has been proposed that different implantation sites and/or placental aging are responsible for divergent supply to the growing fetuses. However, a complete explanation for why one of the placentas is less efficient than the other to nurture twins is still needed.

There have been several attempts to evaluate this issue. Bleker *et al.*[36] studied the birth weights and placental weights of 3000 singletons, 1500 twin pairs and 67 triplets in relation to the gestational age. These authors found that placental indices (placental weights related to birth weights) are similar in singletons, twins and triplets. However, starting at 24 weeks, placental weights of twins and triplets were smaller than those of singletons. The authors used the term 'placental crowding' to denote poor early placental development that preceded growth restriction in multiples. This concept was re-emphasized by the same group in a later study on 487 DC twin pairs with separate placentas[37]. Not everyone supports the view that placental size alone is related to aberrant twin growth. Eberle and co-workers studied 99 DC and 48 MC structurally normal twin pairs and found that in DC, but not in MC twins, birth weight discordance >20% was not attributable to differences in placental weight but to a significantly greater number of placental lesions in the lighter twin than in the heavier twin[38]. In the Scottish Grampian population, Campbell and MacGillivray[39] observed, in the subset of pregnancies who developed hypertensive disease, that birth weight was lower and placental weight greater in MC compared to either MZ or DZ twins with a DC placenta. Hence, a higher placental index is expected in such cases. Victoria *et al.*[40] evaluated differences in pregnancy outcomes and placental findings among severely discordant MC and DC twins. Severe discordance (>25%) occurred significantly more often in MC than in DC twins. Placental weight of the smaller fetus in severely discordant DC twins with separate placentas and the total placental weight in severely discordant MC twins were significantly smaller than the weights of the placentas in their concordant (<5%) and mildly discordant (5–25%) counterparts.

It seems that size alone is not the only way that the placenta might influence growth. Victoria *et al.*[40] noticed that the umbilical cords of the smaller fetuses in both DC and MC pregnancies inserted significantly more often as velamentous and had single umbilical arteries more often than in concordant or mildly discordant twins of similar chorionicity. This observation supports the view of Machin who analyzed 60 consecutive MC placentas by cord insertion patterns. The group with one velamentous/marginal cord (53% of the cases) had the highest rates of growth discordance >20%, unequal placental parenchymal sharing, uncompensated anastomoses and perinatal demise[41].

Finally, in order to determine whether fetal growth is regulated by placental and/or fetal factors, the Manchester group recently measured maternal and fetal concentrations of insulin-like growth factor-I (IGF-I), IGF-II and insulin-like growth factor binding protein-1 in DC and MC twins with or without discordant birth weight[42]. The data suggest that growth discordance of twins exposed to the same maternal environment may be due to variations in either IGF-I or IGF-II/IGFBP-1, depending upon the functioning of the placenta.

In summary, although views may differ, there is little doubt that placental type, size, morphology and pathology significantly influence fetal growth. The molecular level of analysis may further clarify the interplay between the uterine milieu and fetal growth.

TO WHAT EXTENT IS BIRTH WEIGHT DISCORDANCE A NORMAL VARIATION?

There is a clinical ambiguity towards birth weight discordance that originates from cases of discordant pairs that have normal outcomes. It follows that there is a level of discordance below which the difference in size might be a consequence of the biological variation between sibs. At the same time, this view suggests that differences above this cut-off level are more likely to be associated with abnormal growth. If the total twin birth weight represents the capacity of the uterine milieu to nurture twins at any given time, then the frequencies of discordant pairs should be comparable across gestational ages and total twin birth weights.

This concept was studied in two steps. The first was counting and comparing the frequencies of birth weight discordance of more than 25% in an unlike-sexed twin cohort (*n* = 1244 pairs) and in a population-based twin cohort (*n* = 7570 pairs) across the deciles of the total twin birth weight (twin A + twin B) distribution[43]. Similar frequencies of discordant pairs were found in both cohorts (11% and 12%, respectively). In the discordant pairs, the presenting twin was much more often the heavier twin in all birth weight deciles and in both cohorts (OR 5.9 to 3.1). Both cohorts showed a similar non-linear, inversely logarithmic, trend (Figure 5). This observation suggested

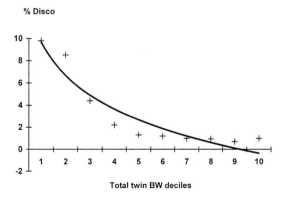

Figure 5 *Frequency of >25% discordant pairs (Disco) by total birth weight (BW) deciles. Adapted from reference 43*

that the more favorable the uterine milieu for carrying twins, the smaller the likelihood of discordant twin growth, a conclusion valid for both like and unlike-sexed twins.

At the next step, our group analyzed a cohort of 12 565 Israeli live-born twin pairs[44]. We found a marked change in the best-fit correlation function with increased discordance. At a level of 15–24.9%, the function was inversely linear, supporting the hypothesis that with being a normal variation, the frequencies of discordant pairs should be quite similar at any total twin birth weight. However, at levels 25–34.9% and over 34.9%, the observed patterns of birth weight discordance did not substantiate a normal variation, as both functions were inversely logarithmic with a much steeper decrease at the ≥ 35% level (Figure 6).

Our explanation for this pattern is that the uterine environment limits discordant growth up to about the median total birth weight. Thereafter, with increasing gestational age at a given uterine 'size', discordant growth may be induced as an adaptation to promote maturity. Adverse outcome of discordant pairs may occur if adaptation fails, as was shown by Hollier et al.[27], who found that greater birth weight discordance was associated with various signs of uterine maladjustment. This model also fits with the observation that when twins overcome the risks of prematurity and low birth weight, there was no excess risk of adverse outcome for discordant pairs[26].

In summary, it was proposed that significant birth weight discordance is a result of the uterine inability to nurture twins equally. In order to promote gestational age, mild compensating events begin at a relatively early phase. Those pairs who exhibit marked differences early in pregnancy predispose to adverse outcome. Conversely, the uterine milieu that competently nurtures twins is associated with increased total birth weight and decreased discordance frequencies. Effective adaptation results in discordant pairs delivered at an advanced gestational age that fare as well as growth concordant pairs. On the other hand, failure to adapt may cause adverse outcomes among discordant pairs.

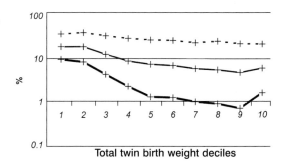

Figure 6 *Frequency of 15–24.9% (upper curve), 25–34.9% (middle curve) and ≥ 35% (lower curve) discordant pairs by total birth weight deciles. Logarithmic scale. Adapted from reference 44*

FETAL GROWTH OF TRIPLETS

The small size of reported triplet series has resulted in conflicting views regarding triplet birth weight[45]. In a study of 196 triplet pregnancies, Newman et al.[46] found that birth weight appeared to be higher in males and when delivered to mothers of higher parity. This relationship was independent of gestational age, pre-eclampsia, maternal race and zygosity, as well as of the mode of conception. As with twins, the heaviest triplet did present first more often than would be expected by chance alone.

The relation of birth weight of infants registered as twins or triplets and gestational age demonstrated a linear growth phase followed by a plateau after 38 and 37 weeks for twins and triplets, respectively[1]. Jones et al.[47] found that triplets exhibit linear growth that lacks the accelerated growth pattern seen in singletons and speculated that the failure to identify such an acceleration in triplet pregnancies may be the result of suboptimal transfer of nutrients by the uteroplacental unit, representing a pattern of growth restriction compared to singletons. We have analyzed a 1988–2000 prospective cohort of 3238 United States live-born triplets and correlated the mean individual (heaviest, middle and lightest) and total triplet birth weight with gestational age in nulliparous and multiparous patients[48]. The mean total triplet birth weights significantly correlated, in an almost perfect linear pattern, with gestational ages between 26 and 37 weeks, for both nulliparas and multiparas, but the respective regression lines were significantly different. The respective regression lines for individual triplets also showed a highly significant linear correlation. Our observation of the linear but diverging slopes for all sibs complements the findings of Jones et al.[47] and seems to provide the explanation for the lack of accelerated growth based on the individual triplet growth pattern.

Although it could be expected that each member of a triplet set would have a different growth pattern included within the overall mean ± standard deviation, neither the type (linear or non-linear) nor the slope were known. Moreover, it was unknown if the slopes were similar (parallel) or diverging. The findings clearly demonstrate the diverging nature of the slope for both nulli- and multiparas, suggesting that each fetus has its own linear growth pattern, with a significantly different inclination to that of its sibs. The resultant discordant growth is proposed to be a physiological, differential and gestational age-dependent event in triplets. Finally, the linear pattern for all sibs suggests that although the lightest triplets seem to be growth-restricted relative to the heaviest, their growth pattern is not similar to the flattening curves seen in growth-restricted singletons.

The data indicate that the uteroplacental unit is not overwhelmed until 33 weeks of a triplet gestation, leading to the distinct periods discussed above (Figure 2).

In summary, the data point to a physiological differential growth restriction that characterizes advanced gestational age in triplets. As in twins, this phenomenon may suggest that nature favors advanced gestational age over fetal size and also that differential growth restriction may be an adaptive measure to promote gestational age.

BIRTH WEIGHT DISCORDANCE IN TRIPLETS

The inadequate definition of birth discordance in twins is even more complex in triplets. Authors usually used the per cent definition of twins and used the difference between the largest and smallest triplet of each set[47,49,50]. By this definition, Jones et al.[47] found that 30.4% of 196 sets exhibited at least 25% discordance, a figure similar to the nearly 25% found by Mordel et al.[49] and 34.2% found by Fountain et al.[50]. Extreme discordance over 40% was found in 7[47] to 11.8%[50] of the cases. These percentages are much larger than those reported in twins.

The difference between the heaviest and the lightest triplets used for the per cent definition ignores the middle one – and as a result the true inter-triplet relationship. We therefore proposed a new description in which the relative birth weight of the middle triplet was defined[51]. First, we used the per cent definition to define concordant sets as those with a difference between the largest and smallest triplet of less than 25% of the largest triplet birth weight. Differences of 25.1–35% and more than 35% were defined as moderate and severe discordance, respectively. Next, we calculated the relative birth weight of the middle triplet by dividing the difference between the middle and the smallest triplets by the difference between the largest and the smallest triplets. The middle triplet was defined as symmetrical when the ratio was between 0.25 and 0.75 (i.e. within ±25% of the average birth weight between the larger and smaller triplet), as low-skew when the ratio was less than 0.25 (i.e. a set comprising one large and two small triplets) and defined as high-skew if the ratio was more than 0.75 (i.e. a set comprising two large and one small triplets) (Figure 7). We found discordance of 25.1–35% and >35% in 19.4% and 9.5% of the 2804 triplets analyzed, respectively, three times higher than the 3.1% found in twins[44]. Nulliparas had significantly fewer concordant sets as a result of less moderately discordant sets (OR 0.7; 95% CI 0.6, 0.9) and more symmetrically discordant sets (OR 1.5; 95% CI 1.1, 1.9).

The high rate of severe discordance may imply a physiological phenomenon and pertain to the different individual growth patterns of the triplets[48]. On the other hand, the large difference may indicate genuine growth restriction of the smaller triplet. Regardless, the obvious

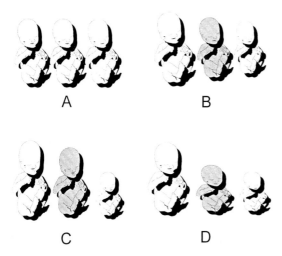

A

B

C

D

Figure 7 *Proposed definition of discordant growth in triplets. A, Concordant sets; B, discordant sets, symmetrical; C, discordant sets, high skew; D, discordant sets, low skew*

dissimilarity between twins and triplets indicates a special conceptual approach to birth weight discordance in triplets. Discordance >25% in triplets is a gestational age dependent event, following a best-fit polynomial function, with a moderate increase until 31 weeks' gestation and a steeper decrease thereafter. The polynomial function between frequencies of >25% discordant sets and birth weight deciles is also different from the inverse logarithmic relationship found in twins[44]. From a clinical perspective, the difference between the two functions seems to be consistent with the difference between the uterine capacities; whereas in twins 'capacity' is associated with an inversely logarithmic decline of the frequencies of discordant pairs, the uterine environment in triplets is unable to limit the frequencies of discordant sets as the uterine size increases. Nonetheless, in triplets as in twins, the more favorable the uterine milieu for carrying multiples, the smaller the likelihood that these multiples will exhibit discordant growth.

The designation of sets as symmetrical, high- and low-skew sets may denote different severity. Of importance, the frequencies of different types of triplet discordance did not change with gestational age. This observation may

suggest three distinct, gestational-age independent, types of discordant growth in triplets (average values: symmetrical 57%, high-skew 30% and low-skew 13%). The data indicate that symmetrically discordant sets are probably the standard arrangement favored by the uterine environment. Also, among discordant sets, one rather than two of the triplets was more often smaller.

Parity seems to protect against discordance only at moderate levels and for the symmetrical type, supporting the view that even parity is of less effect in triplets.

In summary, the observations suggest that the higher frequency, severity and the special relationships of birth weight discordance in triplets are the result of an exhausted uterine milieu.

DIAGNOSIS OF DISCORDANT GROWTH

The diagnosis of discordant fetal growth involves two steps: estimation of each twin's weight and calculating the difference. The first step involves an error of around 10% in the estimated fetal weight (as in singletons) and therefore the literature demonstrated adequate estimations of the individual twin birth weight. However, in a paired construct of discordance estimation, rather low predictive values are to be expected[52,53]. Consider the case of a 2000/2000 g pair in which the first of these absolutely birth weight concordant twins is overestimated by 10% and the second twin is underestimated by 10%. While the actual birth weights are within a satisfactory error range (i.e. ±10%), the estimation for this pair will result in a 2200/1800 g discordance, or 18.2%. If a pair is only mildly (10%) discordant, say 2200/2000 g, the same diverging estimations will show a 2420/1800 g or 25.6% discordance. Thus diverging estimations are expected to increase the negative predictive value of the test. By contrast, converging estimations will reduce the positive predictive value. For example, in a 2400/1800 g pair (25% discordance), if the larger twin is underestimated by 10% and the smaller is overestimated by 10%, the converging estimations will show a 2160/1980 g or only 8.3% discordance[52]. For the time being, it is unknown which cases are more prone to either type of error in estimating discordant growth.

One way to circumvent the inherent error in estimating birth weight discordance was to compare individual biometric measures. Indeed, comparison of biparietal diameters was suggested during the early days of ultrasonography. Values of >5 mm difference were considered suggestive of birth weight discordance[54]. However, because of skull changes due to intrauterine crowding, these measurements proved to be unreliable[55] and other parameters such as differences between femur lengths and abdominal circumferences were introduced[56,57]. In the final stage, comparisons were done between various formulas to estimate fetal weight[58].

The increased interest in the sonographic prediction of birth weight discordance produced initially optimistic results[59,60]; however, the optimism changed when more data and experience were accumulated[52,53]. We, for example, examined 90 pairs within 2 weeks before delivery[52]. We used Bayes' theorem to compare the rates of false-positive and false-negative prediction of the cut-off values of 15, 20 and 25% intertwin birth weight discordance by the intertwin estimated birth weight difference and by an intertwin abdominal circumference difference of ≥ 18 mm. Both methods had similar negative predictive values and the same efficacy to exclude discordant growth and, of notice, similar relatively low positive predictive values.

Recently, Gernt et al.[61] reported on somewhat better sonographic prediction. They found sensitivity of 55%, specificity of 97%, positive predictive value of 82% and negative predictive value of 91% in predicting actual intertwin birth weight discordance $\geq 25\%$. On the other hand, Caravello and co-workers[62] examined the receiver-operating characteristic curves of the current methods (differences in abdominal circumference ≥ 20 mm or in estimated fetal weight of $\geq 25\%$). They showed that both diagnostic tests yielded areas under the two curves not significantly different from the area under the non-diagnostic line. Prediction limit calculations indicated that a 90% certainty that an actual birth weight discordance of at least 25% was achievable only if the difference in abdominal circumference was ≥ 172 mm or the difference in estimated weights was 112% or more. They concluded that current methods for predicting discordant twin growth have limited accuracy. Also, the fetal ponderal index (estimated fetal weight divided by femur length[3]) poorly correlated with birth weight discordance and thus was a poor predictor of discordant growth[63].

Another way to improve the prediction of growth disparity was to look for discordant umbilical Doppler velocimetry. The initial attempts were reported by Gerson et al.[64] who used traditional ultrasonic methods and duplex Doppler ultrasound. Duplex Doppler ultrasound predicted normal growth in 98% normal sets of fetuses, and correctly predicted discordant growth in 82% discordant sets of twins. Additional observations from umbilcal cord Doppler velocimetry alone[65,66] or in combination with sonography[67] yielded promising results. It should be stressed that because of their small sample size, the results should be interpreted with caution.

In summary, the ability of ultrasonography accurately to assess estimated weight of the individual fetuses in twin gestations is not much different from that in singletons, but there are conflicting results regarding the detection of discordant growth.

GROWTH IN THE TWIN–TWIN TRANSFUSION SYNDROME

As mentioned above, twin–twin transfusion is frequently associated with abnormal growth[32]. However, fetal growth abnormalities are quite distinct from the causes in other multiple pregnancies and are briefly discussed here.

In the mechanistic explanation of the syndrome, which exclusively occurs in MC twins, blood (and nutrients) is transfused from the donor to the recipient twin via an open artery-to-vein transplacental anastomosis. The diagnosis prior to the 1990s was therefore based on the occurrence of intertwin hemoglobin and birth weight discordance. However, Wenstrom et al.[68] evaluated the frequency, distribution and most likely etiology of weight discordance in pathologically proven MC twins. Thirty-four twin pairs (35%) were discordant for weight. In half of these (17 of 34), the hemoglobin levels were concordant. In 18% (six of 34), the smaller twin had the higher hemoglobin. On the other hand, 23 of 63 size-concordant pairs (36%) were discordant for hemoglobin. The authors concluded that weight and/or hemoglobin discordance is relatively common in MC twins and in itself is not sufficient to diagnose twin–twin transfusion. The antenatal diagnosis, based on sonographic criteria, soon prevailed.

Although the unbalanced nutrition of the twins is a good explanation, it is not the only one. Divergent size may also result from fetal hydrops in the recipient as a consequence of cardiac overload and decompensation. However, this situation should be rare when the diagnosis is made and treatment is implemented at the early stages of the syndrome.

Recently, Denbow and co-workers[69] correlated placental vasculature with fetal growth and outcome in MC twins. Pregnancies affected by twin–twin transfusion syndrome had numbers of arteriovenous and venovenous anastomoses that were similar to those in pregnancies without the syndrome but fewer arterioarterial anastomoses. The syndrome occurred in 78% of pregnancies with at least one arteriovenous and no arterioarterial anastomoses. Birth weight discordancy correlated with placental territory discordancy and the degree of balance in arteriovenous anastomoses. The larger placental share twin had a greater growth velocity than its smaller placental share co-twin in most anastomotic patterns. Where arteriovenous anastomoses were aligned with the net venous outflow to the fetus with the smaller territory, co-twins had similar birth weights and growth velocities irrespective of placental share. Survival of both fetuses was inversely associated with birth weight discordancy.

In conclusion, the unequal share of nutrients complement the unequal sharing of the placental territory and the pattern of anastomoses that influence fetal growth in twin–twin transfusion.

CLINICAL CONSIDERATIONS

Early chorionicity assessment is the first step in managing multifetal pregnancies. Once chorionicity is established, the appropriate management of aberrant fetal growth starts with an antenatal suspicion of absolute or relative growth restriction. Early discordance should lead to an extensive anatomical survey, and to exclude signs of twin–twin transfusion when a monochorionic gestation is diagnosed. Once twin–twin transfusion and fetal anomaly are excluded, the degree of discordance should be established.

In order to establish a protocol that considers the definition, diagnosis and management of growth-discordant twin gestations, an international census survey was carried out[30]. Although this survey was conducted more than a decade ago, the compiled views generally conform with current practice. First, because of the low predictivity of sonography, a graded definition of discordance was suggested. Currently, this implies a cut-off level of 25% between mild and severe discordance, to identify those who need further (second or third level) evaluation. Expectant management was advocated by the majority of participants with out-patient follow-up for mild discordants. When a severely discordant pair is diagnosed, a much closer surveillance is recommended, just as for every suspected fetal growth restiction case. Follow-up should be done by non-stress testing (daily to twice weekly), sonographic biophysical profile assessment (daily to twice weekly) and sonographic biometry (bi-weekly). Doppler velocimetry (once weekly) may be added to the follow-up. Grobman and Parilla[70] examined ultrasonographic surveillance for growth abnormalities in twin gestations as a function of gestational age. The positive predictive value for the occurrence of a growth abnormality at birth, after an abnormal growth finding on ultrasonography at any time during gestation was, as expected, low (47.7%), but greatest (85%) when suspected growth restriction was first documented at 20–24 weeks of gestation. An interval 10.3 ± 3.9 weeks was needed until a growth abnormality was subsequently detected in normally growing twins at 20–24 weeks, calling for a routine 2- to 4-week interval between sonograms for all twin gestations.

Opinions about intertwin growth discordance as an indication for termination of pregnancy were divided in the 1991 study, as they are today. Based on the concepts discussed in this volume, it seems that the key might be the ability to identify the transition from the physiological adaptation into the pathological process of growth restriction. In this respect, a clinical correlate between outcome of 'adapted' and 'non-adapted' multiple pregnancies is necessary. Regrettably, there are no randomized controlled trials on the management of discordant twins and triplets. For the time being it seems prudent to intervene when

arrest of growth, but not decelerated growth, is documented. In addition, intervention may be indicated when the close follow-up identifies fetuses with growth restriction associated signs of distress, such as an abnormal amount of amniotic fluid and abnormal Doppler, biophysical and cardiotocographic findings.

Finally, discordant growth in a twin pregnancy may set the stage for interfetal conflicts[71]. With lesser degrees of discordance, little controversy is present about the role of conservative management, as is the case in moderately growth-restricted singletons. However, in a remote-from-term severely growth discordant pair, when the smaller twin has sonographic features of severe growth restriction and Doppler studies show impending demise, the option for rescue by delivering the affected fetus concomitantly puts the normally growing fetus at increased risks of severe prematurity. Currently, there are no guidelines for the clinician to solve such conflicts.

References

1. Alexander GR, Kogan M, Martin J, Papiernik E. What are the fetal growth patterns of singletons, twins, and triplets in the United States? *Clin Obstet Gynecol* 1998;41:114–25

2. Ott WJ. Current perspective on the evaluation of suspected intrauterine growth retardation. In Chervenak FA, Kurjak A, eds. *Current Perspectives on the Fetus as a Patient*. Carnforth, UK: Parthenon Publishing, 1996:49–73

3. Leroy B, Lefort F, Neveu P, Risse RJ, Trevise P, Jeny R. Intrauterine growth charts for twin fetuses. *Acta Genet Med Gemellol* 1982;31:199–206

4. Blickstein I, Goldman RD, Mazkereth R. Risk for one or two very low birth weight twins: a population study. *Obstet Gynecol* 2000;96:400–2

5. Blickstein I, Jacques D, Keith LG. The odds of delivering one, two or three extremely low birth weight (<1000 g) triplet infants: a study of 3288 sets. 2001;submitted

6. Grumbach K, Coleman BG, Arger PH, Mintz MC, Gabbe SV, Mennuti MT. Twin and singleton growth patterns compared using US. *Radiology* 1986;158:237–41

7. Taylor GM, Owen P, Mires GJ. Foetal growth velocities in twin pregnancies. *Twin Res* 1998;1:9–14

8. Mordel N, Laufer N, Zajicek G, Shalev Z, Lewin A, Schenker JG, Sadovsky E. Sonographic growth curves of triplet conceptions. *Am J Perinatol* 1993;10:239–42

9. Blickstein I, Lancet M. The growth discordant twin. *Obstet Gynecol Surv* 1988;43:509–15

10. Blickstein I, Shoham-Schwartz Z, Lancet M, Borenstein R. Characterization of the growth-discordant twin. *Obstet Gynecol* 1987;70:11–15

11. Blickstein I, Smith-Levitin M. Twinning and twins. In Chervenak FA, Kurjak A, eds. *Current Perspectives on the Fetus as a Patient*. Carnforth, UK: Parthenon Publishing, 1996:507–25

12. Blickstein I, Weissman A. Birth weight discordancy in male-first and female-first pairs of unlike-sexed twins. *Am J Obstet Gynecol* 1990;162:661–3

13. Orlebeke JF, van Baal GC, Boomsma DI, Neeleman D. Birth weight in opposite sex twins as compared to same sex dizygotic twins. *Eur J Obstet Gynecol Reprod Biol* 1993;50:95–8

14. Glinianaia SV, Magnus P, Harris JR, Tambs K. Is there a consequence for fetal growth of having an unlike-sexed cohabitant *in utero*? *Int J Epidemiol* 1998;27(4):657–9

15. Blickstein I, Lancet M. Second-breech presentation in twins – a possible adaptive measure to promote fetal growth. *Obstet Gynecol* 1989;73:700–2

16. Blickstein I, Namir R, Weissman A, Diamant Y. The influence of birth order and presentation on intrauterine growth of twins. *Acta Genet Med Gemellol* 1993;42:151–8

17. Blickstein I, Zalel Y, Weissman A. Pregnancy order. A factor influencing birth weight in twin gestations. *J Reprod Med* 1995;40:443–6

18. Blickstein I, Goldman RD, Mazkereth R. Incidence and birth weight characteristics of twins born to mothers aged 40 years or more compared with 35–39 years old mothers: a population study. *J Perinat Med* 2001;29:128–32

19. Blickstein I, Goldman RD, Mazkereth R. Maternal age and birth weight characteristics of twins born to nulliparous mothers: a population study. *Twin Res* 2001;4:1–3

20. Wenk RE, Houtz T, Brooks M, Chiafari FA. How frequent is heteropaternal superfecundation? *Acta Genet Med Gemellol* 1992;41:43–7

21. James WH. The incidence of superfecundation and of double paternity in the general population. *Acta Genet Med Gemellol* 1993;42:257–62

22. Ahiron R, Blickstein I. Persistent discordant twin growth following IVF-ET. *Acta Genet Med Gemellol* 1993;42:41–4

23. Tadmor O, Nitzan M, Rabinowitz R, Skomorovsky Y, Aboulafia Y, Diamant YZ. Prediction of second trimester intrauterine growth retardation and fetal death in a discordant twin by first trimester measurements. Case report and review of the literature. *Fetal Diagn Ther* 1995;10:17–21

24. Weissman A, Achiron R, Lipitz S, Blickstein I, Mashiach S. The first-trimester growth-discordant twin: an ominous prenatal finding. *Obstet Gynecol* 1994;84:110–14

25. Blickstein I, Weissman A. 'Macrosomic' twinning: a study of growth promoted twins. *Obstet Gynecol* 1990;76:822–4

26. Blickstein I, Shoham-Schwartz Z, Lancet M. Growth discordancy in appropriate for gestational age, term twins. *Obstet Gynecol* 1988;72:582–4

27. Hollier LM, McIntire DD, Leveno KJ. Outcome of twin pregnancies according to intrapair birth weight differences. *Obstet Gynecol* 1999;94:1006–10

28. Cooperstock MS, Tummaru R, Bakewell J, Schramm W. Twin birth weight discordance and risk of preterm birth. *Am J Obstet Gynecol* 2000;183:63–7

29. Talbot GT, Goldstein RF, Nesbitt T, Johnson JL, Kay HH. Is size discordancy an indication for delivery of preterm twins? *Am J Obstet Gynecol* 1997;177:1050–4

30. Blickstein I. The definition, diagnosis, and management of growth-discordant twins: an international census survey. *Acta Genet Med Gemellol* 1991;40:345–51

31. Cheung VY, Bocking AD, Dasilva OP. Preterm discordant twins: what birth weight difference is significant? *Am J Obstet Gynecol* 1995;172:955–9

32. Blickstein I. The twin–twin transfusion syndrome. *Obstet Gynecol* 1990;76:714–22

33. Ananth CV, Vintzileos AM, Shen-Schwarz S, Smulian JC, Lai YL. Standards of birth weight in twin gestations stratified by placental chorionicity. *Obstet Gynecol* 1998;91:917–24

34. Senoo M, Okamura K, Murotsuki J, Yaegashi N, Uehara S, Yajima A. Growth pattern of twins of different chorionicity evaluated by sonographic biometry. *Obstet Gynecol* 2000;95:656–61

35. Victoria A, Mora G, Arias F. Perinatal outcome, placental pathology, and severity of discordance in monochorionic and dichorionic twins. *Obstet Gynecol* 2001;97:310–15

36. Bleker OP, Oosting J, Hemrika DJ. On the cause of the retardation of fetal growth in multiple gestations. *Acta Genet Med Gemellol* 1988;37:41–6

37. Bleker OP, Wolf H, Oosting J. The placental cause of fetal growth retardation in twin gestations. *Acta Genet Med Gemellol* 1995;44:103–6

38. Eberle AM, Levesque D, Vintzileos AM, Egan JF, Tsapanos V, Salafia CM. Placental pathology in discordant twins. *Am J Obstet Gynecol* 1993;169:931–5

39. Campbell DM, MacGillivray I. Preeclampsia in twin pregnancies: incidence and outcome. *Hypertens Pregnancy* 1999;18:197–207

40. Victoria A, Mora G, Arias F. Perinatal outcome, placental pathology, and severity of discordance in monochorionic and dichorionic twins. *Obstet Gynecol* 2001;97:310–15

41. Machin GA. Velamentous cord insertion in monochorionic twin gestation. An added risk factor. *J Reprod Med* 1997;42:785–9

42. Westwood M, Gibson JM, Sooranna SR, Ward S, Neilson JP, Bajoria R. Genes or placenta as modulator of fetal growth: evidence from the insulin-like growth factor axis in twins with discordant growth. *Mol Hum Reprod* 2001;7:387–95

43. Blickstein I, Goldman RD, Smith-Levitin M, Greenberg M, Sherman D, Rydhstroem H. The relation between inter-twin birth weight discordance and total twin birth weight. *Obstet Gynecol* 1999;93:113–16

44. Blickstein I, Goldman RD, Mazkereth R. Adaptive growth restriction as a pattern of birth weight discordance in twin gestations. *Obstet Gynecol* 2000;96:986–90

45. Elster AD, Bleyl JL, Craven TE. Birth weight standards for triplets under modern obstetric care in the United States, 1984–1989. *Obstet Gynecol* 1991;77:387–93

46. Newman RB, Jones JS, Miller MC. Influence of clinical variables on triplet birth weight. *Acta Genet Med Gemellol* 1991;40:173–9

47. Jones JS, Newman RB, Miller MC. Cross-sectional analysis of triplet birth weight. *Am J Obstet Gynecol* 1991;164:135–40

48. Blickstein I, Jacques DL, Keith LG. Total and individual triplet birth weight as a function of gestational age. *Am J Obstet Gynecol* 2002; in press

49. Mordel N, Benshushan A, Zajicek G, Laufer N, Schenker JG, Sadovsky E. Discordancy in triplets. *Am J Perinatol* 1993;10:224–5

50. Fountain SA, Morrison JJ, Smith SK, Winston RM. Ultrasonographic growth measurements in triplet pregnancies. *J Perinat Med* 1995;23:257–63

51. Blickstein I, Jacques DL, Keith LG. Intertriplet birth weight discordance. 2002;submitted

52. Blickstein I, Manor M, Levi R, Goldchmit R. Is intertwin birth weight discordance predictable? *Gynecol Obstet Invest* 1996;42:105–8

53. Jensen OH, Jenssen H. Prediction of fetal weights in twins. *Acta Obstet Gynecol Scand* 1995;74:177–80

54. Chitkara U, Berkowitz GS, Levine R, Riden DJ, Fagerstrom RM Jr, Chervenak FA, Berkowitz RL. Twin pregnancy: routine use of ultrasound examinations in the prenatal diagnosis of intrauterine growth retardation and discordant growth. *Am J Perinatol* 1985;2:49–54

55. Brown CE, Guzick DS, Leveno KJ, Santos-Ramos R, Whalley PJ. Prediction of discordant twins using ultrasound measurement of biparietal diameter and abdominal perimeter. *Obstet Gynecol* 1987;70:677–81

56. Storlazzi E, Vintzileos AM, Campbell WA, Nochimson DJ, Weinbaum PJ. Ultrasonic diagnosis of discordant fetal growth in twin gestations. *Obstet Gynecol* 1987;69:363–7

57. Blickstein I, Friedman A, Caspi B, Lancet M. Ultrasonic prediction of growth discordancy by intertwin difference in abdominal circumference. *Int J Gynaecol Obstet* 1989;29:121–4

58. Rodis JF, Vintzileos AM, Campbell WA, Nochimson DJ. Intrauterine fetal growth in discordant twin gestations. *J Ultrasound Med* 1990;9:443–8

59. Watson WJ, Valea FA, Seeds JW. Sonographic evaluation of growth discordance and chorionicity in twin gestation. *Am J Perinatol* 1991;8:342–4

60. Chauhan SP, Washburne JF, Martin JN Jr, Roberts WE, Roach H, Morrison JC. Intrapartum assessment by house staff of birth weight among twins. *Obstet Gynecol* 1993;82:523–6

61. Gernt PR, Mauldin JG, Newman RB, Durkalski VL. Sonographic prediction of twin birth weight discordance. *Obstet Gynecol* 2001;97:53–6

62. Caravello JW, Chauhan SP, Morrison JC, Magann EF, Martin JN Jr, Devoe LD. Sonographic examination does not predict twin growth discordance accurately. *Obstet Gynecol* 1997;89:529–33

63. Blickstein I, Manor M, Levi R, Goldchmit R, Weissman A. The intrauterine ponderal index in relation to birth weight discordance in twin gestations. *Int J Gynaecol Obstet* 1995;50:253–5

64. Gerson AG, Wallace DM, Bridgens NK, Ashmead GG, Weiner S, Bolognese RJ. Duplex Doppler ultrasound in the evaluation of growth in twin pregnancies. *Obstet Gynecol* 1987;70:419–23

65. Shah YG, Gragg LA, Moodley S, Williams GW. Doppler velocimetry in concordant and discordant twin gestations. *Obstet Gynecol* 1992;80:272–6

66. Chittacharoen A, Leelapattana P, Phuapradit W. Umbilical Doppler velocimetry prediction of discordant twins. *J Obstet Gynaecol Res* 1999;25:95–8

67. Chittacharoen A, Leelapattana P, Rangsiprakarn R. Prediction of discordant twins by real-time ultrasonography combined with umbilical artery velocimetry. *Ultrasound Obstet Gynecol* 2000;15:118–21

68. Wenstrom KD, Tessen JA, Zlatnik FJ, Sipes SL. Frequency, distribution, and theoretical mechanisms of hematologic and weight discordance in monochorionic twins. *Obstet Gynecol* 1992;80:257–61

69. Denbow ML, Cox P, Taylor M, Hammal DM, Fisk NM. Placental angioarchitecture in monochorionic twin pregnancies: relationship to fetal growth, fetofetal transfusion syndrome, and pregnancy outcome. *Am J Obstet Gynecol* 2000;182:417–26

70. Grobman WA, Parilla BV. Positive predictive value of suspected growth aberration in twin gestations. *Am J Obstet Gynecol* 1999;181:1139–41

71. Blickstein I. Controversial issues in the management of multiple pregnancies. *Twin Res* 2001;4:165–7

Twin–twin transfusion syndrome

22

R. A. Quintero

DEFINITION

Twin–twin transfusion syndrome (TTTS) is a complication of monochorionic multiple pregnancies defined sonographically as the combined presence of polyhydramnios in one sac and oligohydramnios in the other sac in a monochorionic–diamniotic twin gestation. Polyhydramnios is defined as a maximum vertical pocket (MVP) of >8 cm, and oligohydramnios as a MVP of <2 cm ('poly8–oligo2'). Monochorionicity is established by the presence of a single placenta, absence of a twin-peak sign, thin dividing membrane and same gender.

Variations in the definition

Although the condition affects mostly twin pregnancies, it can also occur in triplet or higher-order multiple gestations provided at least two fetuses are monochorionic. In monoamniotic twins, the lack of a dividing membrane precludes the combined presence of polyhydramnios and oligohydramnios. In these patients, the syndrome can be suspected by the presence of polyhydramnios and differences in bladder filling of the two fetuses. In monochorionic triplet pregnancies, two or all three fetuses may be involved.

Definitions no longer used

Until a few years ago, TTTS was diagnosed postnatally if an intertwin hemoglobin difference of >5 g/dl[1] and a birth weight difference of >20%[2] existed. However, in a study by Danskin and Neilson[3] in 178 twin pairs, only four pairs had a hemoglobin difference of >5 g/dl and a weight difference of >20%; none of these pregnancies showed evidence of polyhydramnios or oligohydramnios. Similarly,

percutaneous umbilical blood sampling in six TTTS patients failed to show hemoglobin differences of >5 g/dl except in one pregnancy[4]. A difference of only 1.7 g/dl was found in four patients by Saunders and collaborators[5]. Therefore, the previous pediatric criteria are no longer applicable.

Older sonographic criteria are also no longer applicable. Wittmann *et al.* suggested that the diagnosis be based on a discrepancy greater than 10 mm of either the biparietal diameter or the transverse diameter of the trunk between the twins, and on the hydramnios surrounding the larger twin[6]. Brennan *et al.* suggested that the presence of same sex, a disparity in size or in the number of vessels in the umbilical cords, a single placenta with different echogenicity of the cotyledons supplying the two cords, and evidence of hydrops in either twin or congestive heart failure in the recipient be added to the criteria[7]. The definition used today of poly8–oligo2 simplifies and standardizes the diagnosis of TTTS.

INCIDENCE

TTTS occurs in approximately 5.5–17.5%[2,7–10] of all monochorionic pregnancies. Variations in the reported incidences may reflect variations in the definitions used, as standard sonographic criteria did not exist at the time.

ETIOLOGY

The syndrome appears to result from a net unbalanced flow of blood between two monochorionic fetuses through placental vascular communications. This results in a donor twin and a recipient twin. Although documentation of the unbalanced blood flow remains elusive, it is apparent from our endoscopic observations[11].

The first description of the syndrome was given in 1882 by Schatz who noted that certain placental cotyledons could be perfused by an artery from one twin and a vein to the other[12]. Placental injection studies showed that anastomoses are almost universally present in monochorionic placentas[10]. Two general types of anastomosis may be present: superficial or deep. Superficial anastomoses include arterioarterial and venovenous anastomoses. Deep anastomoses correspond to shared cotyledons, perfused by an artery and a vein from each twin[13]. Both deep and superficial communications may be single or multiple and result in a net transfer of blood from one twin to the other. An average of 3.1 anastomoses per placenta are present in each twin pair. In addition to vascular anastomoses, monochorionic placentas have individually perfused cotyledons, within which exchange of blood between the fetuses does not take place. The mechanisms responsible for the particular vascular design of monochorionic placentas are unknown.

Vascular anastomoses may be responsible *per se* for the development of TTTS if the vascular design is such that it forces a net flow from donor to recipient[11]. Alternatively, the vascular anastomoses may play a passive role in the development of the syndrome but nonetheless allow its development. This is the case of monochorionic twins discordant for congenital heart disease, cardiomyopathies, cord anomalies or other conditions associated with uneven hemodynamic competence.

DIAGNOSIS

The diagnosis of TTTS is made by ultrasound by noting the presence of combined polyhydramnios and oligohydramnios in a monochorionic–diamniotic twin pregnancy. Polyhydramnios is defined as a MVP of >8 cm, and oligohydramnios as a MVP of <2 cm. Differences in estimated fetal weight are no longer used to define the syndrome. Adherence to these criteria is important to distinguish TTTS from other entities.

The use of Doppler to define the syndrome is also unwarranted, as evidenced by conflicting reports from several authors[9,14–17].

Differential diagnosis

(1) *Simple amniotic fluid volume discordance* Differences in amniotic fluid volume not meeting the above criteria can be present in up to 26% of all monochorionic twins (Nicolaides, personal communication).

(2) *Isolated polyhydramnios* Discordance may include a MVP of >8 cm in one sac, but a MVP of >2 cm in the other (isolated polyhydramnios). Occasionally, isolated polyhydramnios may be significant enough to warrant therapy (MVP >10 cm). We have treated one such case with a single therapeutic amniocentesis without recurrence of the polyhydramnios and delivery of two healthy fetuses at 35 weeks.

(3) *Isolated oligohydramnios* Alternatively, the MVP in one sac may be <2 cm, but the MVP in the other sac be <8 cm (isolated oligohydramnios). This may occur in cases of bilateral renal agenesis or other urinary tract abnormalities of one fetus, undiagnosed premature rupture of membranes, or in selective intrauterine growth retardation.

STAGING

Aside from the common standard sonographic criteria of polyhydramnios of >8 cm and oligohydramnios of <2 cm, the sonographic presentation of TTTS is not homogeneous. In this sense, and based on our own observational data, we believe the disease may follow a certain time course characterized by progressive development of renal failure in the donor twin, abnormal Doppler studies, congestive heart failure with hydrops and fetal demise. To this extent, we have proposed a staging system as follows[18]:

(1) Stage I: The bladder of the donor twin is still visible.

(2) Stage II: The bladder of the donor twin is no longer visible. This fetus is in renal failure.

(3) Stage III: Critically abnormal Doppler studies: absent or reverse end-diastolic velocity in the umbilical artery, or pulsatile umbilical venous flow, or reverse flow in the ductus venosus.

(4) Stage IV: Hydrops of one or both fetuses.

(5) Stage V: Demise of one or both fetuses.

Expectant management of patients may show no progression from one stage to the next, or sequential or non-sequential progressive disease. Regardless of whether the disease follows an orderly pattern, the proposed staging system has prognostic value, as will be discussed below.

TREATMENT

Undoubtedly, the most controversial aspect of TTTS is with respect to treatment. Interpretation of published therapeutic results must be done with caution, as not all investigators have adhered to standard diagnostic sonographic criteria. Expectant management of TTTS has been associated with almost 100% perinatal mortality[19]. In a collective series reported by Nicolaides' group, only five of 106 pregnancies had a successful outcome[20]. Medical treatment either with digoxin[21], or indomethacin[22] has no role. Having said this, it is possible to follow stage I patients expectantly, provided the degree of polyhydramnios is not large (MVP 8–9 cm) and the cervical length is adequate (> 2.5 cm), particularly if disease is diagnosed after 22–24 weeks of gestation. Such pregnancies may remain stable and not require invasive therapy. Invasive therapeutic alternatives include serial amniocentesis, laser therapy and umbilical-cord occlusion. Other options proposed include purposeful disruption of the dividing membrane (so-called 'septostomy'), and purposeful injection of fluid in the sac of the donor, neither of which can be recommended today.

Serial amniocentesis

The goal of this therapy is to decrease the likelihood of miscarriage or preterm labor by reducing the amniotic fluid volume in the sac of the recipient twin[7,23–38]. The procedure is repeated as often as necessary, depending on the rate of reaccumulation of fluid in the sac of the recipient twin. Occasionally, no further reaccumulation of fluid occurs, and a single procedure is all that is necessary. Although therapy can be started at any level of polyhydramnios, we normally do not start treatment until a MVP of 9–10 cm is reached. Serial amniocentesis is associated with an overall success rate of 66% (likelihood of at least one twin surviving), with an average risk of cerebral palsy of 15%.

There is no standard technique for the performance of serial amniocentesis. How much fluid should be removed, at what rate, what needle or what type of anesthesia should be used are among the issues that could benefit from standardization. Our technique involves the use of an 18-gauge Echotip® needle (Cook Ob/Gyn, Spencer, IN) under local anesthesia. The needle is inserted in a placenta-free area, with care not to disrupt the dividing membrane. Extension tubing is attached to the needle with a luer-lock adaptor, connected to wall suction (maximum vacuum pressure 200 mmHg). The patient and the fetuses are previously sedated with 5–10 mg of intravenous (IV) morphine sulfate and 5–10 mg of IV diazepam. Fluid is removed until a MVP of approximately 6–7 cm is reached. We do not attempt to reach a particular level of MVP, but rather limit the amount of fluid extracted by the amount of space surrounding the donor twin. Indeed, if too much fluid is removed, the donor twin may become compromised from cord compression and die, as it is unable to change its position within the uterine cavity.

Laser therapy

The goal of this approach is to eliminate all and any blood exchange between the fetuses[39–47]. This halts the disease process altogether, allowing each fetus to continue the pregnancy on its own. For many years, endoscopic identification of the communicating vessels remained an unresolved issue. The original technique, while fundamentally correct, did not specify how the vessels could be identified[39,40]. The next step in the evolution of the technique involved targeting vessels that crossed the dividing membrane[41–43,45]. Although this effectively interrupted the vascular communications between the twins, it could also target incorrectly many non-communicating vessels, owing to the lack of correlation between the vascular equator and the location of the dividing membrane. In 1998, we described a precise, reproducible technique capable of distinguishing communicating vessels from normal individually perfused areas of the placenta. We called this technique selective laser photocoagulation of communicating vessels, or SLPCV[44]. Basically, each placental artery is followed to its terminal end in the placenta (arteries cross over veins). A returning vein from that cotyledon should normally drain back to the same twin. If blood is drained to the other twin, a deep arteriovenous anastomosis (AV) is present. Arterioarterial or venovenous anastomoses are easily identified by noting the lack of a terminal end for an artery or a vein, respectively. We also developed reliable techniques to treat patients with anterior placentas[48]. SLPCV is associated with an 85% success rate (likelihood that at least one fetus survives), and a 3–5% risk of cerebral palsy. SLPCV compares favorably with the previous non-selective technique, resulting in a lower rate of dual fetal demise (5.6% vs. 22%, respectively)[47].

Umbilical-cord occlusion

The goal of this technique is to stop blood exchange between the fetuses at the level of the umbilical cord of one of the twins. This can be accomplished by ligating the umbilical cord either endoscopically or under ultrasound guidance[49,50], or by using bipolar electrocautery under ultrasound[51]. The procedure is reserved for severe cases where spontaneous fetal death of one of the twins is likely to occur, particularly with the presence of hydrops. We currently have a 76% successful pregnancy rate, with no quotable risk of cerebral palsy in patients treated with umbilical-cord ligation.

Iatrogenic disruption of the dividing membrane, or 'septostomy'

The goal of this procedure is to 'equilibrate' the pressures between the two amniotic cavities[52]. Under ultrasound guidance, the dividing membrane is pierced repeatedly with a needle, allowing fluid from the recipient twin's sac to enter the donor twin's sac. Proponents of this technique have not shown that different amniotic fluid pressures exist between the two cavities. Instead, we have shown in fact that the amniotic fluid pressures are similar, despite large differences in amniotic fluid volumes[53]. Iatrogenic membrane disruption may result in a pseudo-monoamniotic twin pregnancy, with cord entanglement and fetal demise[54]. In addition, the resulting artificial improvement in the amniotic fluid volume of the donor twin's sac no longer reflects the urinary function of this fetus (this also applies to cases where purposeful amnioinfusion of the donor twin is performed), which precludes adequate monitoring of the disease status of this twin. Lastly, disruption of the dividing membrane significantly hampers the performance of laser therapy, should this option be subsequently considered, as the floating dividing membrane hampers adequate visualization and location of the communicating vessels. Because the procedure is ill-based, does not result in improvement of the disease and may actually harm the pregnancy, we strongly discourage this practice.

Amniocentesis vs. laser

The controversy regarding the optimal treatment of TTTS has centered on the use of amniocentesis or laser. Unfortunately, lack of sonographic diagnostic standards, different inclusion criteria for gestational age, dogmatic views about the merits of each technique and the shortcomings of a surgical technique in development led to almost irreconcilable positions between the proponents of each approach. Risk factors for a poor pregnancy outcome with serial amniocentesis have been identified. Those include gestational age at diagnosis of <22 weeks, absent or reverse end-diastolic velocity in the umbilical artery, removal of > 1100 ml of amniotic fluid per week or fetal hydrops[55]. Despite limitations, two prospective non-randomized clinical studies have shown laser therapy to be superior to amniocentesis[41,46]. A randomized clinical trial is under way to address these concerns.

Outcome analysis in patients treated with either amniocentesis or laser has not been stratified by severity of the disease at presentation. Unfortunately, sub-analysis of trials by risk factors may yield insufficient power to find statistical differences. Our preliminary data comparing 79 patients treated with serial amniocentesis and 84 patients treated with SLPCV shows an inverse relationship between fetal survival rates and stage in the amniocentesis group ($p < 0.001$), but not with SLPCV. A direct relationship between fetal neurological morbidity and stage was also seen in the amniocentesis but not in the laser group (Quintero, in preparation). These findings suggest that the optimal teatment of TTTS may be tailored by stage: stage I and possibly II patients could fare well with serial amniocentesis, depending on the gestational age at diagnosis, whereas stage III and IV patients are best treated with SLPCV. A prospective clinical trial to address this hypothesis is in preparation by us.

SINGLE INTRAUTERINE FETAL DEMISE

Death of one of the twins is not an infrequent finding during the management of twin–twin transfusion patients. This complication has been associated with death or significant morbidity of the co-twin. The morbidity includes the development of porencephalic cysts and other major neurological complications[56–59]. Originally, these complications were thought to result from the release of thromboplastic substances from the dead twin into the surviving twin. More recently, however, an alternative mechanism has been proposed. Fetal blood sampling in one of the twins before and after the demise of its co-twin has shown the development of acute anemia in the surviving twin within a few hours. This suggests that post-mortem fetofetal hemorrhage may be responsible for the development of acute hypotension and thus may be responsible for the observed complications[60,61]. Since this complication can occur only if the vascular communications between the twins are patent, only through occlusion of these vessels can this event be avoided.

CONCLUSIONS

The understanding and management of twin–twin transfusion syndrome has evolved significantly in the past few years. Improved diagnostic criteria, understanding of the heterogeneic nature of the syndrome, development of a reproducible surgical technique for the identification of the vascular anastomoses, and technological advances and developments allow us to view the disease as a more readily understandable and treatable condition. Still, many tasks remain, including education of peers, better screening and diagnosis and further development of surgical instruments. Generalization of treatment outcomes should no longer apply, given the known varied results with disease stage. Confirmation of our tailored approach to the management of the disease according to stage should soon be possible with an appropriate clinical trial.

References

1. Rausen A, Seki M, Strauss L. Twin transfusion syndrome. *J Pediatr* 1965;66:613–28
2. Tan K, Tan R, Tan A. The twin transfusion syndrome. *Clin Pediatr* 1979;18:111–14
3. Danskin FH, Neilson JP. Twin-to-twin transfusion syndrome: what are appropriate diagnostic criteria? *Am J Obstet Gynecol* 1989;161:365–9
4. Fisk NM, Borrell A, Hubinont C, Tannirandorn Y, Nicolini U, Rodeck CH. Fetofetal transfusion syndrome: do the neonatal criteria apply *in utero*? *Arch Dis Child* 1990;65:657–61
5. Saunders N, Snijders R, Nicolaides K. Twin–twin transfusion syndrome during the 2nd trimester is associated with small intertwin hemoglobin differences. *Fetal Diagn Ther* 1991;6:34–6
6. Wittmann B, Baldwin V, Nichol B. Antenatal diagnosis of twin transfusion syndrome by ultrasound. *Obstet Gynecol* 1981;58:123–7
7. Brennan JN, Diwan RV, Rosen MG, Bellon EM. Fetofetal transfusion syndrome: prenatal ultrasonographic diagnosis. *Radiology* 1982;143:535–6
8. Benirschke K. Twin placenta in perinatal mortality. *NY State J Med* 1961;61:1499–508
9. Farmakides G, Schulman H, Saldana L, *et al.* Surveillance of twin pregnancy with umbilical arterial velocimetry. *Am J Obstet Gynecol* 1985;153:789
10. Robertson E, Neer K. Placental injection studies in twin gestation. *Am J Obstet Gynecol* 1983;147:170–3
11. Quintero R, Quintero L, Bornick P, Allen M, Johnson P. The donor–recipient (D–R) score: *in vivo* endoscopic evidence to support the hypothesis of a net transfer of blood from donor to recipient in twin–twin transfusion syndrome. *Prenat Neonat Med* 2000;5:84–91
12. Schatz F. Eine besondere Art von einseitiger Polyhydramnie mit anderseitiger Oligohydramnie bei einaugen Zwillingen. *Arch Gynaekol* 1882;19:329
13. Benirschke K, Driscoll S. *The Pathology of the Human Placenta.* New York: Springer-Verlag, 1967
14. Giles WB, Trudinger BJ, Cook CM, Connelly AJ. Doppler umbilical artery studies in the twin–twin transfusion syndrome. *Obstet Gynecol* 1990;76:1097
15. Ishimatsu J, Yoshimura O, Manabe A, Matsuzaki T, Tanabe R, Hamada T. Ultrasonography and Doppler studies in twin-to-twin transfusion syndrome. *Asia Oceania J Obstet Gynaecol* 1992;18:325–31
16. Pretorius D, Manchester D, Barkin S, *et al.* Doppler ultrasound of twin transfusion syndrome at 18 weeks of gestation. *JCV* 1983;11:442
17. Yamada A, Kasugai M, Ohno Y, Ishizuka T, Mizutani S, Tomoda Y. Antenatal diagnosis of twin–twin transfusion syndrome by Doppler ultrasound. *Obstet Gynecol* 1991;78:1058
18. Quintero R, Morales W, Allen M, Bornick P, Johnson P, Krueger M. Staging of twin–twin transfusion syndrome. *J Perinatol* 1999;19:550–5
19. Weir P, Ratten G, Beischner N. Acute polyhydramnios: a complication of monozygous twin pregnancy. *Br J Obstet Gynaecol* 1979;86:849–53
20. Saunders NJ, Snijders RJ, Nicolaides KH. Therapeutic amniocentesis in twin–twin transfusion syndrome appearing in the second trimester of pregnancy. *Am J Obstet Gynecol* 1992;166:820–4
21. De Lia J, Emery M, Sheafor S, *et al.* Twin transfusion syndrome: successful *in utero* treatment with digoxin. *Int J Gynecol Obstet* 1985;23:197
22. Jones J, Sbarra A, Dilillo L, *et al.* Indomethacin in severe twin-to-twin transfusion syndrome. *Am J Perinatol* 1993;10:24
23. Erskine JP. A case of acute hydramnios successfully treated by abdominal paracentesis. *Obstet Gynaecol Br Emp* 1944;51:549–51
24. Danziger RW, Chir B. Twin pregnancy with acute hydramnios treated by paracentesis uteri. *Br Med J* 1948;2:205–6
25. Brown GR. Acute hydramnios treated by abdominal paracentesis. *J Obstet Gynaecol Br Emp* 1958;65:61–3
26. Brown G, Macaskill S. Acute hydramnios, with twins, successfully treated by abdominal paracentesis. *Br Med J* 1961;1:1739–40
27. Mills W. Letter. *Br J Obstet Gynaecol* 1980;87:256
28. Brown G. Letter. *Br J Obstet Gynaecol* 1980;87:255
29. Montan S, Jorgensen C, Sjoberg N. Amniocentesis in treatment of acute polyhydramnios in twin pregnancies. *Acta Obstet Gynecol Scand* 1985;64:537–9
30. Schneider KTM, Vetter K, Huch R, Huch A. Acute polyhydramnios complicating twin pregnancies. *Acta Genet Med Gemellol* 1985;34:179–84
31. Feingold M, Centrulo CL, Newton ER, Weiss J, Shakr C, Shmoys S. Serial amniocentesis in the treatment of twin to twin transfusion complicated with acute polyhydramnios. *Acta Genet Med Germellol* 1986;35:107–13
32. Chescheir NC, Seeds JW. Polyhydramnios and oligohydramnios in twin gestations. *Obstet Gynecol* 1988;71:882–4
33. Bebbington MW, Wittmann BK. Fetal transfusion syndrome: antenatal factors predicting outcome. *Am J Obstet Gynecol* 1989;160:913–15
34. Nageotte M, Hurwitz S, Kaupke C, Vaziri N, Pandian M. Atriopeptin in the twin transfusion syndrome. *Obstet Gynecol* 1989;73:867–70
35. Urig M, Clevell W, Elliot J. Twin–twin transfusion syndrome. *Am J Obstet Gynecol* 1990;163:1522–6

36. Gonsoulin W, Moise KJ, Kirshon B, Cotton DB, Wheeler JW, Carpenter RJ. Outcome of twin–twin transfusion diagnosed before 28 weeks of gestation. *Obstet Gynecol* 1990;75:214–16

37. Elliott JP, Urig MA, Clewell WH. Aggressive therapeutic amniocentesis for treatment of twin–twin transfusion syndrome. *Obstet Gynecol* 1991;77:537–40

38. Elliott JP, Sawyer AT, Radin TG, Strong RE. Large-volume therapeutic amniocentesis in the treatment of hydramnios. *Obstet Gynecol* 1994;84: 1025–7

39. De Lia J, Cruiskshank D, Keye W. Fetoscopic neodymium : yttrium–aluminium–garnet laser occlusion of placental vessels in severe twin–twin transfusion syndrome. *Obstet Gynecol* 1990;75: 1046–53

40. De Lia J, Kuhlman R, Harstad T, *et al*. Twin–twin transfusion syndrome treated by fetoscopic neodymium : YAG laser occlusion of chorioangiopagus. *Am J Obstet Gynecol* 1993;168:308

41. Ville Y, Hyett J, Hecher K, Nicolaides K. Management of severe twin–twin transfusion: amniodrainage compared to endoscopic surgery [Abstract]. *Ultrasound Obstet Gynecol* 1994;4(Suppl 1):130

42. Ville Y, Hyett J, Hecher K, Nicolaides K. Preliminary experience with endoscopic laser surgery for severe twin–twin transfusion syndrome. *N Engl J Med* 1995;332:224–7

43. Ville Y, Van Peborgh P, Gagnon A, Frydman R, Fernandez H. [Surgical treatment of twin-to-twin transfusion syndrome: coagulation of anastomoses with a Nd : YAG laser, under endosonographic control. Forty four cases]. *J Gynecol Obstet Biol Reprod* 1997;26:175–81

44. Quintero R, Morales W, Mendoza G, *et al*. Selective photocoagulation of placental vessels in twin–twin transfusion syndrome: evolution of a surgical technique. *Obstet Gynecol Surv* 1998;53: s97–s103

45. Ville Y, Hecher K, Gagnon A, Sebire N, Hyett J, Nicolaides K. Endoscopic laser coagulation in the management of severe twin-to-twin transfusion syndrome. *Br J Obstet Gynaecol* 1998;105:446–53

46. Hecher K, Plath H, Bregenzer R, Hansmann M, Hackeloer BJ. Endoscopic laser surgery versus serial amniocentesis in the treatment of severe twin–twin transfusion syndrome. *Am J Obstet Gynecol* 1999;180:717–24

47. Quintero RA, Comas C, Bornick PW, Allen MH, Kruger M. Selective versus non-selective laser photocoagulation of placental vessels in twin–twin transfusion syndrome. *Ultrasound Obstet Gynecol* 2000;16:230–6

48. Quintero RA, Bornick PW, Allen MH, Johnson PK. Selective laser photocoagulation of communicating vessels in severe twin–twin transfusion syndrome in women with an anterior placenta. *Obstet Gynecol* 2001;97:477–81

49. Lemery D, Vanlieferinghen P, Gasq M, Finkeltin F, Beaufrere M, Beytout M. Fetal umbilical cord ligation under ultrasound guidance. *Ultrasound Obstet Gynecol* 1994;4:399–401

50. Quintero R, Romero R, Reich H, *et al*. In utero percutaneous umbilical cord ligation in the management of complicated monochorionic multiple gestations. *Ultrasound Obstet Gynecol* 1996;8:16–22

51. Deprest JA, Audibert F, Van Schoubroeck D, Hecher K, Mahieu-Caputo D. Bipolar coagulation of the umbilical cord in complicated monochorionic twin pregnancy. *Am J Obstet Gynecol* 2000;182: 240–5

52. Saade GR, Belfort MA, Berry DL, *et al*. Amniotic septostomy for the treatment of oligohydramnios–polyhydramnios sequence. *Fetal Diagn Ther* 1998; 13:86–93

53. Quintero R, Quintero L, Morales W, Allen M, Bornick P. Amniotic fluid pressures in severe twin–twin transfusion syndrome. *Prenat Neonat Med* 1998;3:607–10

54. Gilbert W, Davis S, Kaplan C, Pretorius D, Merrit T, Benirschke K. Morbidity associated with prenatal disruption of the dividing membrane in twin gestations. *Obstet Gynecol* 1991;78:623–30

55. Mari G. International TTTS registry group. *Am J Obstet Gynecol* 1998:s28

56. Bejar R, Vigliocco G, Gramajo H, *et al*. Antenatal origin of neurologic damage in newborn infants. Part II. Multiple gestations. *Am J Obstet Gynecol* 1990;162:1230

57. Melnick M. Brain damage in survivor after *in utero* death in monozygous co-twin [Letter]. *Lancet* 1977;2:1287

58. Schinzel A, Smith D, Miller J. Monozygotic twinning and structural defects. *J Pediatr* 1979;95: 921–30

59. Yoshioka H, Kadomoto Y, Mino M, *et al*. Multicystic encephalomalacia in liveborn twin with a stillborn macerated co-twin. *J Pediatr* 1979;95:798

60. Dudley D, D'Alton M. Single fetal death in twin gestation. *Semin Perinatol* 1986;10:65–72

61. Okamura K, Murotsuki J, Tanigawara S, Uehara S, Yahima A. Funipuncture for evaluation of hematologic and coagulation indices in the surviving twin following co-twin's death. *Obstet Gynecol* 1994;83:975–8

Non-immune fetal hydrops

H. N. Winn

23

Fetal hydrops is a condition of excessive accumulation of extracellular fluid in the forms of skin edema, ascites, pleural effusion and/or pericardial effusion that can be diagnosed by ultrasonography. In the early second trimester (<20 weeks of gestation) increased nuchal translucency may represent the earliest sign of fetal hydrops[1]. When the excessive fluid is limited to one of the body compartments, the condition may be classified as an isolated finding such as isolated ascites[2]. Commonly associated ultrasonographic findings include polyhydramnios and increased placental thickness.

Fetal hydrops may be secondary to maternal alloimmunization against fetal red blood cell (RBC) antigens. Non-immune fetal hydrops (NIH) is distinguished by the absence of maternal IgG antibodies against fetal RBC antigens. The incidence of NIH is about 1 in 3000 deliveries[3]. The main categories of fetal disorders that are associated with NIH are infection, chromosomal abnormalities, structural anomalies, hematological diseases, metabolic diseases and tumors. The list of conditions associated with NIH is extensive[4,5]; however, the following discussion will focus on the common ones.

INFECTION

Common infectious agents associated with NIH include *Toxoplasma gondii*, *Treponema pallidum*, parvovirus (B19), cytomegalovirus (CMV) and adenovirus[4,6]. Adenovirus is probably the most common viral infection in NIH[6]. Maternal infection with these agents tends to be asymptomatic.

Diagnosis of maternal infection with *T. gondii*, parvovirus or CMV is made by the presence of organism-specific IgG and IgM in the maternal serum using the enzyme-linked immunosorbent assay (ELISA).

Diagnosis of fetal infection with parvovirus, *T. gondii*, CMV or adenovirus can be made by demonstrating the presence of: (1) the organism in the amniotic fluid using the polymerase chain reaction (PCR)[6–8]; (2) detection of B19 capsid antigens (VP1 and VP2) in the amniotic fluid using monoclonal antibodies for parvovirus[9]; (3) the organism-specific IgM antibody in the fetal blood; or (4) positive culture of the virus from the fetal blood. *T. gondii* cysts may be found in the placenta fixed in formalin prior to freezing.

The pathogenesis of fetal hydrops in fetal infection includes severe fetal anemia from destruction of fetal erythroid precursors in the case of parvovirus infection and possible hepatic failure and excessive extramedullary hematopoiesis in other cases.

Toxoplasma gondii

The presence of *T. gondii*-specific IgG in the maternal serum prior to pregnancy confers protection on the fetus. Maternal serum *T. gondii*-specific IgM indicates a recent infection within 8 months of the test date[10].

Maternal administration of either a combination of pyrimethamine and sulfadiazine or Spiramycin® for *T. gondii* fetal infection may reduce the severity of the neonatal sequelae. Pyrimethamine and sulfadiazine are commonly used in the United States while Spiramycin is widely used in Europe and is available in the United States through the Centers for Disease Control. Pyrimethamine (a dihydrofolic acid reductase inhibitor) and sulfadiazine (a dihydrofolic acid synthetase inhibitor) block folic acid synthesis sequentially and produce synergistic activity against *T. gondii*. Pyrimethamine should not be used during the period of embryonic organogenesis since it is teratogenic in animals. In patients who are allergic to sulfonamides, clindamycin can be substituted for sulfadiazine. One of the recommended regimens includes pyrimethamine (50 mg/day) and sulfadiazine (3 g/day) continuously until delivery. Since both pyrimethamine and sulfadiazine may cause bone marrow suppression, folinic acid (calcium leucovorin) at the dosage of 5–10 mg/day or 50 mg weekly should be added to the regimen.

Parvovirus

In the case of B19 infection, severe fetal anemia plays an important role in the pathogenesis of NIH. Immune factors can also contribute to the development of fetal hydrops. In fact, the placentas of patients with non-immune hydrops, fetal death or spontaneous abortion in association with maternal parvovirus infection contain interleukin 2 (IL-2), and have an increased number of CD3-positive cells, compared to those of patients with non-infectious NIH or normal pregnancies[11]. Fetal transfusion of packed RBCs alleviates or corrects fetal hydrops, thus improving perinatal outcomes.

Syphilis

Maternal infection with syphilis is screened by serum Venereal Disease Research Laboratory (VDRL) or rapid plasma reagin (RPR) tests and confirmed by the microhemagglutination assay–*Treponema pallidum* (MHA-TP) or fluorescent treponemal antibody absorption (FTA-ABS) test. Fetal infection can be diagnosed by demonstrating *T. pallidum* IgM antibody in the fetal serum, the latter obtained by funicentesis. The treatment of choice for maternal syphilis is penicillin as the following: benzathine penicillin G 2.4 million units IM in a single dose for primary and secondary syphilis or latent syphilis of <1 year's duration; benzathine penicillin G 2.4 million units weekly for 3 weeks for latent syphilis of more than 1 year's duration or tertiary syphilis; aqueous crystalline penicillin G 3–4 million units IV every 4 h for 10–14 days for neurosyphilis. Pregnant patients who are allergic to penicillin should undergo desensitization prior to receiving penicillin.

CHROMOSOMAL ABNORMALITIES

Chromosomal abnormalities constitute a major cause of NIH and include Turner syndrome (45,X), trisomy 21, trisomy 18, trisomy 16, trisomy 13, triploidy and unbalanced translocations. Turner syndrome is one of the most common chromosomal abnormalities associated with NIH, especially cystic hygroma.

FETAL STRUCTURAL ANOMALIES

Fetal anomalies which may be associated with NIH include: cystic hygroma; pulmonary abnormalities; cardiovascular abnormalities and cardiac arrhythmia; gastrointestinal disorders such as meconium peritonitis and intestinal obstruction; and severe skeletal dysplasia such as thanatophoric skeletal dysplasia, achondroplasia, asphyxiating thoracic dysplasia and osteogenenesis imperfecta.

Cystic hygroma

Cystic hygroma is characterized by the presence of a single or multiloculated cyst in the paracervical area and is commonly accompanied by other features of fetal hydrops. Septated cyst is associated with a high incidence of NIH, aneuploidy and fetal demise, while non-septated cyst is more likely to resolve spontaneously with normal outcomes[12]. Cystic hygroma presumably develops from the lack or maldevelopment of the communication between the vascular and lymphatic systems[13]. The incidence of abnormal chromosomes in patients with first-trimester nuchal cystic hygroma in larger series, each containing at least 29 patients, ranges from 35 to 60%[14]. Cystic hygroma may also be transmitted as an autosomal recessive disorder[15]. Perinatal mortality is at least 90% in fetuses having cystic hygroma and other signs of fetal hydrops or abnormal chromosomes[13], but drops to about 10% in fetuses having first-trimester nuchal cystic hygroma and normal chromosomes[14].

Cardiovascular conditions

Fetal structural cardiac anomalies and fetal arrhythmia represent 17–35% of cases of NIH[16]. Fetal hydrops develops probably as a result of congestive heart failure as evidenced by a reduced cardiac output and/or right heart overload[16]. Cardiac anomalies associated with NIH include atrioventricular defect, hypoplastic left ventricle, subaortic stenosis, pulmonary atresia, Ebstein's anomaly, ectopia cordis, cardiomyopathy, rhabdomyoma and premature closure of the ductus arteriosus[17,18]. Severe fetal bradycardia, persistent supraventricular tachycardia (SVT), atrial flutter and atrial fibrillation can cause NIH. Severe fetal bradycardia can occur as part of either complex cardiac structural defects or an isolated congenital heart block[19]. Perinatal mortality of a congenital heart block associated with other cardiac structural anomalies is extremely high. The isolated congenital heart block tends to have good outcomes, uncommonly develops fetal hydrops, and is associated with maternal antinuclear antibodies (ANA), anti-SSA (Ro) antibodies and anti-SSB (La) antibodies[19].

Pulmonary conditions

Pleural effusion may occur as an isolated chylothorax or as a part of NIH. Congenital cystic adenomatoid malformation (CCAM), extralobar pulmonary sequestration, mediastinal teratoma and diaphragmatic hernia are the major pulmonary causes of NIH. The possible mechanism for NIH is impaired venous return or cardiac contractility from mediastinal shift and/or direct compression from the mass[20].

Congenital cystic adenomatoid malformation occurs when there is an abnormal overgrowth of terminal respiratory bronchioles prior to 7 weeks of gestation[21]. Adzick et al. divided CCAM into two groups: macrocystic tumors containing cysts of at least 5 mm in diameter, appearing ultrasonographically cystic, not usually associated with NIH and having favorable prognosis; and microcystic tumors containing cysts less than 5 mm, appearing ultrasonographically solid and being commonly

associated with NIH[22]. The perinatal survival rate of CCAM without fetal hydrops approaches 100%, while the combination of CCAM, NIH and no fetal therapy is almost invariably fatal[22–24].

Pulmonary sequestration (PS) is a mass of non-aerated lung tissues that receives its systemic circulation from the aorta. Pulmonary sequestration is located either within (lobar) or outside (extralobar) the pleura of the normal lungs, depending on the timing of its separation from the normal lungs. Adzick et al.[24] reported that 71% (27/38) of fetuses with extralobar PS and without NIH regressed spontaneously prior to birth. Among five fetuses with PS and NIH: the hydrops resolved spontaneously in one, after weekly fetal thoracocentesis in one and after placement of a thoracoamniotic shunt in two; and persisted without fetal intervention in one. The perinatal survival rate in purely PS with or without NIH is 80% or 100%, respectively, and is significantly reduced by the presence of other anomalies[25]. Postnatal treatment of persistent PS may include resection of the PS and/or extracorporeal membrane oxygenation.

NEOPLASM

Fetal or placental tumors such as teratoma, neuroblastomas, tuberous sclerosis and placental chorioangiomas have been associated with fetal hydrops. Fetal hyperthyroidism due to maternal Grave's disease has also been associated with NIH[26,27].

Teratomas contain tissues derived from the three germ cell layers and are usually located in the presacral-coccygeal area or the neck[28]. The American Academy of Pediatrics Surgical Section (AAPSS) classified the teratomas as the following: type I is primarily external and has only a small presacral component; type II is predominantly external but has a significant intrapelvic portion; type III is partially external but is predominantly intrapelvic with an abdominal extension; and type IV is located entirely within the pelvis and the abdomen[29]. The perinatal prognosis is dismal if NIH, which occurs in about 30–40% of fetal teratomas, exists. Non-immune fetal hydrops may develop as a result of high cardiac output failure from arteriovenous shunting, hypoxia and anemia. The latter may be due to hemorrhage into the tumor.

Neuroblastomas arise from the autonomic nervous system or the adrenal medulla and can be associated with NIH[30]. The tumor may cause either fetal anemia, by invading the bone marrow, or hypoproteinemia and increased hepatic vascular resistance, by invading the liver.

Tuberous sclerosis is an autosomal dominant disorder that manifests as fibroangiomatous tumors affecting many organs. Tuberous sclerosis may cause fetal heart failure or portal hypertension and hepatic failure if the tumors affect the fetal heart or the fetal liver, respectively.

Placental chorioangiomas occur in about 1% of pregnancies[31]. These tumors, especially those with diameters of more than 5 cm, function as high-volume arteriovenous shunts which predispose the fetus to heart failure and/or microangiopathic hemolytic anemia[32,33]. Pulse Doppler blood flow and color flow mapping can reveal arterial blood flow through the mass[32]. Fetal transfusion of red blood cells for anemia can reduce fetal hydrops and improve perinatal outcomes.

HEMATOLOGICAL DISORDERS

Fetal hemorrhage, hemoglobinopathies and hemolysis are the most common fetal hematological disorders that produce fetal hydrops from severe fetal anemia and fetal hypoxia. Fetal hemorrhage can occur spontaneously or in the setting of abruptio placentae, placenta previa, trauma or twin transfusion. The amount of fetomaternal hemorrhage can be estimated from the Kleihauer–Betke test. Fetal anemia can be confirmed by funicentesis, and severe fetal anemia can be treated with fetal transfusion of red blood cells.

α-Thalassemia is an autosomal recessive hemoglobinopathy that occurs mainly in descendants of those from Southeast Asia and the Mediterranean. Normal fetal hemoglobin (HbF) has a tetramer consisting of two α-chains

and two γ-chains. A patient with α-thalassemia has reduced or absent synthesis of the α-chains due to deletion of one or more genes and increased production of tetramers of γ-chains also known as Bart's hemoglobins. Fetal hydrops develops secondary to fetal hypoxia because Bart's hemoglobins do not release oxygen to the tissue effectively, owing to their high affinity to oxygen. The α-globin gene is duplicated, and deletion of all four α-globin genes is lethal. The adult carriers of hemoglobinopathy such as α-thalassemia or β-thalassemia have red blood cell mean corpuscular volume (MCV) less than 80. Diagnosis of fetal α-thalassemia can be made with DNA analysis of fetal chromosomes; the genes for the α-globins are located on chromosome 16.

Glucose-6-phosphate dehydrogenase (G-6PD) deficiency may subject the fetus to hemolysis of red blood cells upon exposure to oxidative agents such as fava beans, sulfasoxazole and methylene blue. This disorder is transmitted as an X-linked recessive pattern and occurs more commonly among African and Greek descendants. Fetal hydrops develops from severe fetal anemia that can be corrected by fetal transfusion of red blood cells.

CLINICAL MANAGEMENT

Perinatal morbidity and mortality are high and depend on the etiology and the severity of the fetal hydrops. Isolated fetal conditions such as chylous ascites without an identifiable cause have better outcomes[2].

Initial maternal screening tests include: indirect Coomb's test for red blood cell isoimmunization; a complete blood count (CBC) with differential and indices for infection and thalassemia; Kleihauer–Betke test for fetomaternal hemorrhage; serum IgG and IgM antibody titers to *Toxoplasma gondii*, parvovirus B19 and cytomegalovirus; and RPR or VDRL titers for *Treponema pallidum*.

A detailed ultrasound examination of the fetal anatomy, amniotic fluid and placenta is essential to determine coexisting major structural anomalies and signs of fetal infection such as calcifications and hepatosplenomegaly. Amniocentesis may be performed to obtain amniotic fluid for analyzing fetal chromosomes and DNA, identifying antigens of the involved organisms using PCR or monoclonal antibodies, or assessing fetal lung maturity. Funicentesis may be done to obtain fetal blood for determining the fetal hemoglobin, complete blood count, organism-specific antibodies or infectious organisms.

Fetal therapy may include maternal administration of medications for selected fetal infectious diseases and fetal arrhythmia. Fetal invasive procedures may include: thoraco-centesis for isolated fetal hydrothorax or chylothorax to alleviate compression of fetal lungs; surgical resection of the abnormal lung tissue or tumor for microcystic CCAM; fetal intravascular or intraperitoneal administration of red blood cells for fetal anemia; and fetal intravascular or intramuscular injection of medications for fetal arrhythmia. Close fetal monitoring of fetal well-being is indicated, since there is a high incidence of fetal demise.

The timing of delivery depends on the associated condition, gestational age, fetal growth, the potential success of fetal therapies, the status of fetal well-being and fetal lung maturity. The mode of delivery depends on the maternal condition, fetal size and fetal tolerance to labor. Paracentesis may be performed prior to labor and delivery to reduce the risk of abdominal dystocia, if fetal ascites is excessive. The presence of an attending neonatologist at the time of delivery for neonatal resuscitation and evaluation is recommended. Fetuses with NIH may benefit from a multidisciplinary approach, consisting of maternal–fetal medicine physicians, neonatologists, geneticists and appropriate pediatric medical or surgical subspecialists.

References

1. Jauniaux E. Diagnosis and management of early non-immune hydrops fetalis. *Prenat Diagn* 1997; 17:1261–8
2. Winn HN, Stiller R, Grannum PAT, Crane JC, Coster B, Romero R. Isolated fetal ascites: prenatal diagnosis and management. *Am J Perinatol* 1990;7:370–3
3. Machin GA. Hydrops revisited: literature review of 1414 cases published in 1980s. *Am J Med Genet* 1989;34:366–90
4. Norton MA. Nonimmune hydrops fetalis. *Semin Perinatol* 1994;18:321–32
5. Jones DC. Nonimmune fetal hydrops: diagnosis and obstetrical management. *Semin Perinatol* 1995;19:447–61
6. Van den Veyver IB, Ni J, Bowles N, *et al*. Detection of intrauterine infection using polymerase chain reaction. *Mol Genet Metab* 1998;63: 85–95
7. Kovacs BW, Carlson DE, Shahbahrami B, Platt LD. Prenatal diagnosis of human parvovirus B19 in nonimmune hydrops fetalis by polymerase chain reaction. *Am J Obstet Gynecol* 1992;167:461–6
8. Tobin JA, Griffin LD, Martin AB, *et al*. Intrauterine adenoviral myocarditis presenting as nonimmune hydrops fetalis: diagnosis by polymerase chain reaction. *Pediatr Infect Dis J* 1994; 13:144–50
9. Gentilomi G, Zerbini M, Gallinella G, *et al*. B19 parvovirus induced fetal hydrops: rapid and simple diagnosis by detection of B19 antigens in amniotic fluids. *Prenat Diagn* 1998;18:363–8
10. Sever JL. TORCH tests and what they mean. *Am J Obstet Gynecol* 1985;152:495
11. Jordan JA, Huff D, DeLoia JA. Placental cellular immune response in women infected with human parvovirus B19 during pregnancy. *Clin Diagn Lab Immunol* 2001;8:288–92
12. Bronstein M, Rottem S, Yoffe N, Blumenfeld Z. First-trimester and early second-trimester diagnosis of nuchal cystic hygroma by transvaginal sonography: diverse prognosis of septated from nonseptated lesion. *Am J Obstet Gynecol* 1989;161: 78–82
13. Chervenak FA, Isacson MD, Blakemore KJ, *et al*. Fetal cystic hygroma. *N Engl J Med* 1983;309:822–5
14. Trauffer PML, Anderson CE, Johnson A, Heeger S, Morgan P, Wapner RJ. The natural history of euploid pregnancies with first-trimester cystic hygromas. *Am J Obstet Gynecol* 1994;170:1279–84

15. Tricoire J, Sarramon MF, Rolland M, Lefort G. Familial cystic hygroma. Report of 8 cases in 3 families. *Genetic Counsel* 1993;4:265–9

16. Kleinman CS, Donnerstein RL, DeVore GR, *et al.* Fetal echocardiography for evaluation of *in utero* congestive heart failure: a technique for study of nonimmune fetal hydrops. *N Engl J Med* 1982; 306:568

17. Allan LD, Crawford DC, Sheridan R, *et al.* Aetiology of non-immune hydrops: the value of echocardiography. *Br J Obstet Gynaecol* 1986;93:223

18. Harlass FE, Duff P, Brady K, Read J. Hydrops fetalis and premature closure of the ductus arteriosus: a review. *Obstet Gynecol Surv* 1989;44: 541–3

19. Schmidt KG, Ulmer HE, Silverman NH, *et al.* Perinatal outcome of fetal complete atrio-ventricular block: a multicenter experience. *J Am Coll Cardiol* 1991;17:1360–6

20. Chin KY, Tang MY. Congenital adenomatoid malformation of one lobe of a lung with general anasarca. *Arch Pathol* 1949;49:221

21. Stocker TJ, Manewell JE, Drake RM. Congenital cystic adenomatoid malformation of the lung: classification and morphologic spectrum. *Hum Pathol* 1977;8:155

22. Adzick NS, Harrison MR, Glick PL, *et al.* Fetal cystic adenomatoid malformation: prenatal diagnosis and natural history. *J Pediatr Surg* 1985; 20:483

23. De Santis M, Masini L, Noia G, Cavaliere AF, Oliva N, Caruso A. Congenital cystic adenomatoid malformation of the lung: antenatal ultrasound findings and fetal–neonatal outcome. *Fetal Diagn Ther* 2000;15:246–50

24. Adzick NS, Harrison MR, Crombleholme TM, Flake AW, Howell LJ. Fetal lung lesions: management and outcome. *Am J Obstet Gynecol* 1998;179:884–9

25. Savic B, Birtel FJ, Tholen W, *et al.* Lung sequestration: report of seven cases and review of 540 published cases. *Thorax* 1979;34:96

26. Watson WJ, Fiegen MM. Fetal thyrotoxicosis associated with nonimmune hydrops. *Am J Obstet Gynecol* 1995;172:1039–40

27. Stulberg RA, Davies GAL. Maternal thyrotoxicosis and fetal nonimmune hydrops. *Obstet Gynecol* 2000;95:1036

28. Billmire DF, Grosfeld JL. Teratomas in childhood: analysis of 142 cases. *J Pediatr Surg* 1986;21: 548–51

29. Altman RP, Randolph JG, Lilly JR. Sacrococcygeal teratoma: American Academy of Pediatrics Surgical Section Survey 1973. *J Pediatr Surg* 1974;9:389

30. Moss TJ, Kaplan L. Association of hydrops fetalis with congenital neuroblastoma. *Am J Obstet Gynecol* 1978;132:905

31. Wentforth P. The incidence and significance of hemangioma of the placenta. *J Obstet Gynaecol Br Commonw* 1965;77:81–8

32. Hirata GI, Masaki DI, O'Toole M, Medearis AL, Platt LD. Color flow mapping and Doppler velocimetry in the diagnosis and management of a placental chorioangioma associated with non-immune fetal hydrops. *Obstet Gynecol* 1993;81: 850–2

33. Bauer CR, Fojaco RM, Bancalari E, Fernandez-Rocha L. Microangiopathic hemolytic anemia and thrombocytopenia in a neonate associated with a large placental chorioangioma. *Pediatrics* 1978;62: 574–7

Advances in the diagnosis of intrapartum asphyxia

24

R. Luzietti, G. Clerici, K. G. Rosén and G. C. Di Renzo

The aim of intrapartum fetal monitoring is to identify fetuses at risk of an adverse outcome, based on our understanding of the pathophysiology involved. What, therefore, is the information we are looking for? We know that intrapartum asphyxia is one reason why babies get damaged. How can we learn when a fetus is at risk and how can we separate those at risk from those who are coping? For the purposes of intrapartum monitoring there are three groups of fetuses that we should be able to identify:

(1) The fetus that is untroubled by the events of labor;
(2) The fetus that is troubled but able to compensate fully and is in no immediate danger;
(3) The fetus that is troubled and is utilizing key resources in an attempt to compensate, or is unable to compensate fully. This is the group that may benefit from appropriately timed intervention.

MULTIPLE DEFENSE MECHANISMS

The fetal ability to adapt to hypoxemia involves multiple defense mechanisms (Table 1). These consist primarily of cardiovascular compensation that increases blood flow to the most important organs – the brain, the heart and the adrenals – thereby counteracting the decreasing oxygen content. A second line of defense is the metabolic compensatory mechanisms. It is only when these compensatory mechanisms are insufficient that asphyxia will develop and along with it the possibility of central nervous system damage and handicap (for review, see Greene and Rosén, 1995).

The capacity of fetuses to handle hypoxemia may differ greatly, depending not only on the condition prior to labor but also on events during labor, which may affect the ability to mobilize these defense systems. Therefore, it may be difficult to rely on only the level of oxygenation. Instead, it could be more rewarding to try to interpret the reactions taking place in a high-priority organ like the heart or the brain.

CARDIOTOCOGRAPHY

Continuous fetal heart rate (FHR) and uterine contraction recording (cardiotocography; CTG) is widely used to assess fetal well-being during labor. This method has limitations, however. A normal CTG trace reflects optimal fetal oxygenation and is of reassurance regarding fetal conditions. The significance of FHR changes is often unclear and therefore difficult to interpret. In the clinical scenario this can result in unnecessary interventions for suspected fetal hypoxia or inappropriate delay in action, with potentially disastrous consequences for the fetus. A better training of medical and midwifery staff can overcome some of these difficulties. Evidence also suggests that the use of expert systems for decision support would provide a valuable contribution in improving the detection and clinical management of cases with abnormal CTG patterns. However, it is also evident that there are situations where the CTG changes are not specific enough for the presence of fetal hypoxia, and additional information is necessary for appropriate decision making.

Table 1 *The relationship between different fetal physiological and clinical patterns during labor. From Greene and Rosén, 1995*

Defense mechanisms		
• Increased tissue oxygen extraction • Increased sympathetic activity • Anaerobic metabolism		• Decreased non-essential activity • Redistribution of blood flow
Intact	**Reduced**	**Lacking**
• Healthy fetus responding to acute hypoxia during labor	• Previously healthy fetus exposed to repeated episodes of hypoxia with progressively diminishing reserves The post-term fetus	• Antenatal problems with chronic distress Potential defense utilized or not available Growth-restricted fetus
• Optimum reaction to hypoxia • Full compensation	• Blunted reaction to hypoxia • Reduced compensation	• Minimal or no reaction to hypoxia • Decompensation
• Characteristic signs of fetal distress • Low risk of asphyxial damage	• Variable signs of fetal distress • Risk of asphyxial damage	• Uncharacteristic signs of distress • High risk of asphyxial damage

FETAL BLOOD SAMPLING

Fetal blood sampling (FBS) can be used along with CTG monitoring to assess fetal acid–base status during labor and can reduce operative intervention, but it requires additional expertise, is time consuming, gives only intermittent information and is therefore not widely used.

Considering the need to improve our understanding of the process of intrapartum hypoxia, very little has emerged with regard to the analysis of scalp pH since the early work by Saling. At the same time as EFM + FBS has been shown to improve outcome, the use of FBS has also been questioned by analyzing outcome measures in a large clinical service where the rate of FBS decreased from 1.76% to 0.03% without any change in the Cesarean rate or an increase in indicators of perinatal asphyxia. Thus, the attitude towards the clinical usefulness of FBS and scalp pH, after 30 years, is still unclear.

To what extent should scalp pH add to our ability to identify fetuses at risk of intrapartum hypoxia? The limitation of scalp pH is that it will always reflect the status of the peripheral blood, where acidosis is inherent, due to the accumulation of CO_2. Respiratory acidemia is generated in the blood, whereas metabolic acidemia is generated in the tissues. This means that a scalp sample *per se* will not always reflect the state of the tissues. If the aim is to identify those fetuses suffering from metabolic acidosis, a scalp blood pH measurement may provide limited information, as the rise in P_{CO_2} will always dominate as the cause behind a decrease in pH. The rise in P_{CO_2} is part of normal labor and should not be regarded as a specific sign of intrapartum hypoxia.

Furthermore, the effectiveness of FBS in clinical practice is another problem. In the Plymouth trial, despite the use of a strict protocol, 39% of cases had FBS performed unnecessarily, and 33% of cases did not have it performed when it was indicated. The decision to obtain an FBS depends on the interpretation of the CTG. If the level of CTG interpretation is suboptimal, the value by monitoring with FBS is limited.

PULSE OXIMETRY

Fetal pulse oximetry monitoring provides a quantitative, direct and real-time measurement of fetal arterial oxygen saturation (Sp_{O_2}). The term oxyhemoglobin describes hemoglobin when all of the available binding sites of hemoglobin are fully bound with oxygen.

Hemoglobin molecules not carrying oxygen are referred to as deoxyhemoglobin. Oxygen saturation monitors measure the ratio of hemoglobin molecules bound with oxygen (oxyhemoglobin) to the total amount of hemoglobin molecules available to bind with oxygen (oxyhemoglobin plus deoxyhemoglobin). Oxyhemoglobin and deoxyhemoglobin differ in their absorption of red and infrared light. The pulsatile changes in absorption of red and infrared light are used to determine the SpO_2 of fetal blood.

The oximeter sensors used in the fetus (reflectance pulse oximetry) have light-emitting diodes and photo-detectors that are adjacent to one another on a flexible probe, and absorption of light is determined from the light that scatters back to the tissue surface. The probe is placed, when membranes have been ruptured and cervical dilatation is more than 2 cm, between the fetal cheek and the uterine wall. The per cent oxygen saturation values are printed continuously on the CTG paper.

A recent US multicenter randomized trial of 1010 laboring women with a non-reassuring fetal heart rate tracing showed a reduction in emergency Cesarean sections from 10% to 5% with the use of CTG plus pulse oximetry. However, unexpectedly, the study also showed an increase in the section rate for failure to progress in the test group (19% versus 9%), and the overall section rates were not different between the test and control groups.

Pulse oximetry appears to be a screening technique that can help in discriminating a non-reassuring fetal heart rate tracing. However, the issue still to be resolved is the ability of CTG plus pulse oximetry to provide diagnostic capacity on fetal metabolic acidosis. Thus, we may have a situation where the two parameters in combination may not be specific enough to enable the obstetrician to grade the impact of hypoxemia on fetal organ function.

Therefore, it may be difficult to rely on only the level of oxygenation. Instead it could be more rewarding to try to interpret the reactions taking place in a high-priority organ such as the heart or the brain.

FETAL ELECTROCARDIOGRAM

The PR–RR interval analysis

The P wave configuration and time constants are affected by changes in the autonomic nervous system controlling the heart pump function. Hypoxia may cause an alteration in the PR time constant with a PR shortening in spite of an RR lengthening. However, Luzietti *et al.* showed that *all* substantial decelerations occurring during labor would cause the hypoxic response of a PR shortening with an RR lengthening. Thus, the physiology behind these changes is not specific for hypoxemia but is more related to an attempt by the fetal heart to preserve an optimal diastolic filling of the atrium in situations of a decrease in blood returning to the heart.

Recently, the results of a multicenter randomized trial comparing PR-RR relationship analysis plus CTG with CTG alone have been published. This trial was set up to test the hypothesis that the use of PR–RR relationship analysis during labor could reduce the incidence of acidemia at birth. The analysis of the first 1038 cases, however, failed to confirm this hypothesis, as there was no change in the incidence of acidemia at birth between the two arms of the trial and only a trend towards a reduction in operative delivery for fetal distress with the use of time interval analysis. The trial has therefore been interrupted.

The ST waveform analysis

ST analysis of the electrocardiogram during exercise testing is a well proven technology to assess myocardial function in the adult. Similar to the adult stress test, ST waveform analysis of the fetal ECG, affected by the stress of labor, should provide key information about the ability of the high-priority organ, the fetal heart, to respond. This assumption seems to hold true, and ST analysis has emerged not as an alternative to cardiotocography but as a support tool to allow more accurate interpretation of intrapartum events, along the lines depicted in Figure 1. Furthermore, the fetal ECG is readily obtainable during labor from the same scalp electrode used to obtain the fetal heart rate.

Figure 1 indicates those parts of the ECG that have provided specific information on the fetal response to hypoxemia. The waveform marked P corresponds to the contraction of the atrium. The next sequence is the contraction of the ventricles, which is illustrated by the waveforms Q, R and S. The generation of these waveforms is a passive event and thus very stable and easily detected, which makes it well suited for fetal heart rate recording.

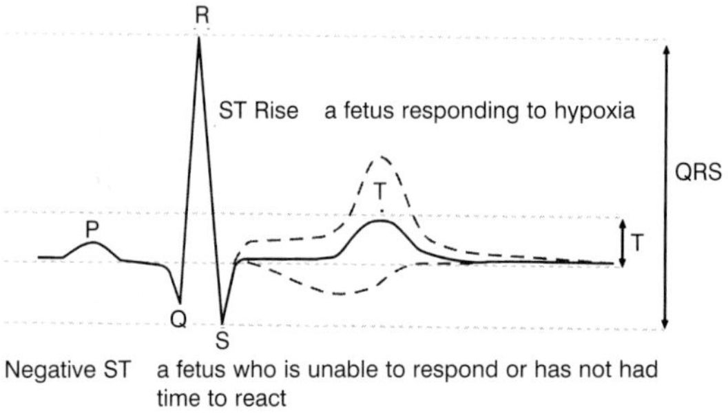

Figure 1 *The electrocardiogram with a schematic presentation of hypoxia-related changes. The T/QRS measurement is also indicated*

Physiology of ST waveform changes

The ST segment and T wave relate to the re-polarization of myocardial cells in preparation for the next contraction. This repolarization process is energy consuming. An increase in T wave height, quantified by the ratio between T and QRS amplitudes, the T/QRS ratio (Figure 1) occurs when the energy balance within the myocardial cells threatens to become negative. A negative energy balance means a situation when the amount of oxygen supplied to the cells no longer covers the energy required for metabolic activity. During hypoxia this balance becomes negative and the cells produce energy by the β-adrenoceptor-mediated anaerobic breakdown of glycogen reserves. The ability of these cells to produce energy in this manner and thereby maintain myocardial function is a vital compensatory defense mechanism. This process not only produces lactic acid but also potassium ions (K^+) that affect myocardial cell membrane potential and cause a rise of the ST waveform.

Hypoxemia is one way by which this myo-cardial energy balance situation can change, producing ST waveform changes. Another mechanism by which these ST changes may occur is the general surge of stress hormones (adrenaline, epinephrine) occurring in response to the squeezing and squashing of labor. This will stimulate the heart to increase its pumping activity but at the same time induce glyco-genolysis and high T waves. This general arousal is part of normal labor and in these cases the healthy fetus will display a reactive CTG, ensuring normality.

ST depression with negative T waves has been observed during hypoxia experiments in experimentally growth-retarded guinea pigs. Clinically, these changes have emerged as a specific sign of myocardial hypoxic stress. They reflect a myocardium that is not able or has not had the time to mobilize its defense to hypoxemia. The result is a decrease in myo-cardial activity and a risk of cardiovascular failure.

ST depression with T wave elevation (a biphasic ST waveform) is also seen when myo-cardial ischemia occurs in adults, and may represent an earlier stage in the development of myocardial ischemic hypoxia, when the action potential change is not uniform throughout the myocardium. The physiology behind biphasic ST events is related to the mechanical performance of the myocardium and the relationship between the inner (endocardium) and outer (epicardium) layers of the walls of the ventricles in particular. As we know it, biphasic ST illustrates an imbalance between these two layers, the reason being that the perfusion pressure of the endocardium is always lower at the same time as the mechanical strain is always larger. This means that unless the myocardium is generally activated (β receptor activation and enhanced Frank–Starling relationship, i.e. the ability of the myocardium to respond to volume load), any decrease in performance will cause biphasic ST. Thus, not only may hypoxia *per se* cause biphasic ST as a sign of maladaptation, but also basically all factors substantially altering the balance and the performance characteristics within the myocardial wall may institute these events.

To illustrate this one may list the following:

- Prematurity with less contractile elements making the heart less capable of responding to shifts in volume load and decreased ability to respond with glycogenolysis.
- Infections that may extend from general septicemia to non-specific inflammatory reactions altering membrane pumping mechanisms and reducing myocardial performance.
- Increased demand on the cardiovascular system, as may be seen with an increase in temperature or simply by marked tachycardia by itself. These situations may not be specific enough to cause an alarm reaction, but a slight ST depression may just inform that the myocardium is required to enhance its pumping performance somewhat beyond its optimum.
- Myocardial dystrophy. Unclear condition of poor performance *in utero*, recovering spontaneously after birth.
- Cardiac malformations.
- Long-term stress with an inability of the myocardium to adapt to emerging hypoxia.
- In the acute hypoxic phase, before adrenaline activation of β-adrenoceptors.

Basically, biphasic ST is the pattern to be expected whenever the myocardium is exposed to factors that may decrease its ability to respond.

Probably the most clinically important aspect of biphasic ST is once they have been flagged – a situation of potentially reduced myocardial performance has been identified and we should not expect 'classical' signs of fetal reactions to an emerging hypoxia. From what is stated above, it should be noted that a fetus displaying biphasic ST events is not usually in a situation of immediate hypoxia and metabolic acidosis. However, with further progress of labor and during the second stage in particular, these fetuses will suffer.

In conclusion, the evidence from experimental work indicates that ST waveform elevation reflects compensated myocardial stress and a switch to anaerobic myocardial metabolism. A progressive rise in the T/QRS ratio represents continuing anaerobic metabolism with a risk of eventual decompensation due to depletion of myocardial glycogen stores and a progressive metabolic acidosis. Persistently biphasic and negative waveform changes indicate myocardial decompensation as a result of direct myocardial ischemic hypoxia; other possibilities are myocarditis and non-specific myocardial dystrophy.

A unipolar fetal ECG lead is required to identify changes in ST configuration. Apart from a single spiral scalp electrode, this lead also requires an active skin electrode placed on the maternal thigh generating predominantly low-frequency signal noise. In the new STAN® recorder (STAN® S 21, Neoventa Medical, Gothenburg, Sweden) analog signal filters were replaced by digital signal processing techniques, which resulted in significant enhancement of signal quality, and automatic assessment of ST changes by means of an Expert System (ST log®) was introduced. The new system was tested extensively in observational studies prior to the second randomized trial of CTG versus CTG + ST.

The Plymouth randomized controlled trial

This was the first randomized controlled trial, where 2400 high-risk, term deliveries were studied comparing CTG + ST waveform analysis with standard CTG monitoring. The trial tested the hypothesis that the *combination* of ST waveform and CTG analysis would reduce operative interventions for fetal distress without placing the fetus at a risk.

There was a 46% reduction ($p < 0.001$) in operative deliveries for fetal distress in the ST + CTG arm with no difference in operative deliveries for other reasons. A retrospective analysis of the CTG showed operative deliveries for fetal distress in 2.7% of cases with normal CTG in the CTG only group, as compared with

0.3% in the STAN group. Thus, members of staff improved in their capacity correctly to identify a normal CTG in case they obtained support from a likewise normal ST waveform. Reductions in operative interventions were also noted with intermediate and abnormal CTG patterns of 19.5% vs. 9.6% and 44.4% vs. 35.3%, respectively. The overall effect was that 43% of operative interventions retrospectively were judged unnecessary in the CTG arm as compared with 5% in the STAN arm of the trial.

There were no significant differences in the measures of neonatal outcome, but fewer low 5-min Apgar scores (20 vs. 32, $p = 0.12$) and less metabolic acidosis (5 vs. 13, $p = 0.09$) in the ST + CTG arm were apparent. There was also a significant reduction in the use of fetal blood sampling. However, three babies in the ST arm showed evidence of perinatal asphyxia with ST events not being recognized. Two of these cases displayed biphasic ST events and the third a marked rise in T/QRS ratio.

These cases illustrated the need to improve data presentation, preferably by providing continuous assessment of significant ST events.

The ST log

The aim with this new feature is to provide a continuous support for the interpretation of ST waveform changes during labor. The following events are identified:

(1) Episodic rise in T/QRS ratio, i.e. an increase in the median filtered T/QRS values of >0.10 units for <10 min.

(2) Baseline rise in T/QRS ratio, i.e. consistent changes of more than 10 min in duration. The baseline T/QRS was calculated as the median value of data recorded for a 10-min époque, which was continuously updated on a minute-by-minute basis. A significant event was identified when the baseline T/QRS increased for >0.05 units.

(3) The appearance of repeated episodes of depression/negative slope of the ST segment. These changes are quantified by a scoring system where:

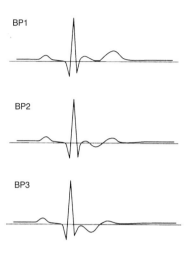

Figure 2 *Illustration of grading of biphasic ST*

Biphasic ST grade 1 (BP1) means a negative ST segment slope above baseline;
Biphasic ST grade 2 (BP2) means a negative ST segment slope cutting the baseline;
Biphasic ST grade 3 (BP3) means a negative/depressed ST segment below the baseline of the ECG (Figure 2).

(4) The appearance of repeatedly negative T waves with ST depression and negative T/QRS ratios.

Basically, the ST log automatically identifies and presents on screen and paper those changes that are significant in association with an abnormal CTG, i.e. an episodic rise in T/QRS of >0.10, an increase in baseline T/QRS of >0.05 and repeated episodes of biphasic ST grade 2 and 3 and negative T/QRS ratios.

The patterns identified as significant with regard to an intermediate CTG were an episodic T/QRS rise of >0.15 and a baseline rise of >0.10. Cases with episodes of BP2 and 3 for >5 min were also regarded as significant events.

Together with any ST log statement, signal quality is also assessed as the percentage of available ECG complexes used for fetal heart rate and ST waveform analysis. The ST log is restricted to situations where >75% of the ECG complexes are accepted. In situations with a risk of an inferior signal quality, the operator is notified and asked to check the ECG electrodes. A loosening scalp electrode will cause a gradual deterioration of the ECG signal quality. Furthermore, the scalp electrode may be inserted through the fetal membranes, in which case the ECG is distorted.

Episodic T/QRS

An episodic increase is defined as a rise in T/QRS ratio lasting less than 10 min. The ST log identifies all episodic changes exceeding 0.10, i.e. an increase from 0.07 to 0.18 will be recorded as a significant event. Clinical action depends on the corresponding CTG pattern according to the guidelines. In the majority of cases episodic ST changes appear in conjunction with a significant CTG event and action is required.

An episodic rise in T/QRS corresponds to an acute hypoxic event causing a negative myocardial energy balance. The fetus reacts by utilizing its myocardial glycogen stores, thus supplementing the failing aerobic metabolism with anaerobic metabolism. When the rise in the T/QRS ratio reaches a level as indicated in the guidelines, the event has become significant and action should follow.

Episodic ST changes usually appear in parallel with an abnormal CTG pattern, and a scalp pH will not add significant information but may delay intervention.

Figure 3. Observations

The CTG shows a baseline of 150 bpm, decreased variability and variable decelerations, occasionally with a slow return. The ST analysis shows a rise in the T/QRS ratio with each contraction. A significant episodic T/QRS increase from 0.08 to 0.24 occurred at 23:44. The recording continued for another 6 h with repeated significant episodic and baseline increase in the T/QRS ratio. Vaginal delivery at 05:35. Female 2510 g, Apgar scores 7–8–8, cord artery pH 6.92, BD_{ecf} 12.4 mmol/l, cord vein pH 7.22, BD_{ecf} 11.1 mmol/l. Neonatal seizures.

Figure 3. Comments

A case with marked ST changes indicating a significant hypoxic event at start of recording. The uncertainty about the previous history of this case together with significant ST changes and some CTG abnormality would indicate operative delivery at the time of the episodic increase in the T/QRS ratio at 23:44. The information from the STAN recorder showed a situation where significant resources (myocardial glycogen) had to be used to handle the contractions. Thus, the fetal/placental reserve was reduced and the ability to handle further stress would, if anything, be less and the fetus at risk of asphyxia.

Increase in baseline T/QRS

An increase in baseline T/QRS is defined as a change in the T/QRS ratio occurring for more than 10 min. The ST log is continuously recording baseline T/QRS and if a change of more than 0.05 has been found it will be indicated as a significant event. As could be seen from the clinical guidelines, such a change forms the grounds for an operative intervention in case of an abnormal CTG pattern. If the baseline T/QRS increases more than 0.10, a chronic hypoxic event should be suspected. The CTG may then provide uncharacteristic signs.

An increase in baseline T/QRS identifies a situation of more long-lasting hypoxia which tends to become permanent. Such a development may take hours and we may not be able to follow the development from the start. This means that when a recording starts one should be aware of the possibility of an ongoing hypoxic event and pay special attention to the CTG + ST pattern and any evidence of abnormality.

Baseline T/QRS

The actual T/QRS level is of importance in one situation. This is when the recording starts and hypoxia may already be present. After 20 min from the start, the ST log will have identified a

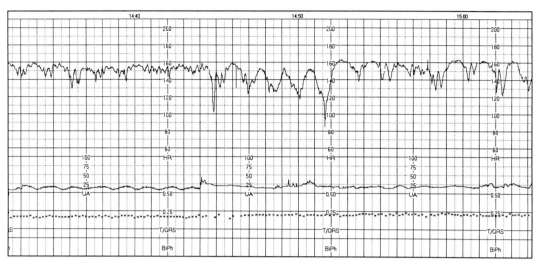

Figure 3 *Para 1, 40 + 1 weeks. Maternal hypertonia, treated with β-blockade. Induction because of decreased fetal movements, recording in early labor*

baseline T/QRS. In case this value is >0.25 and the CTG pattern is abnormal, clinical action is recommended. One must always be aware that sometimes a recording may start when there already is an ongoing hypoxic process. Under such circumstances, the fetus may already have utilized major resources and adapted to the hypoxia by decreasing its activity both neurologically and metabolically. From our experience, these cases are rare and a non-reactive FHR pattern with reduced variability at onset should always be regarded as a possible sign of ongoing hypoxia with need for intervention.

Figure 4. Observations

Baseline tachycardia, 160 bpm. Decelerations which gradually became more marked with a decrease in short-time variability. The baseline T/QRS ratio showed an increase from 0.11 at the start of the recording in the first stage of labour to 0.22, i.e. >0.10. Vacuum extraction due to threatening asphyxia at 15:30. Male baby 4730 g. Apgar scores 1–5–5. Cord artery pH 6.82. BD_{ecf} 17 mmol/l. Cord vein pH 6.89, BD_{ecf} 16 mmol/l. The baby developed neonatal seizures.

Figure 4. Comments

An illustration of progressive hypoxia developing into asphyxia. An uncharacteristic CTG pattern, which does not show marked changes until the last 30 min. During the last 2 h there is a gradual increase in T wave amplitude with a baseline T/QRS rise exceeding 0.10 at 14:48. According to the STAN clinical guidelines an operative delivery should be done at that point in time. These slow but persistently developing ST changes are sometimes difficult to identify without the support of the ST log. Furthermore, the combination of some CTG abnormality with a significant increase in baseline T/QRS is always related to significant hypoxic events.

Figure 5. Observations

Borderline tachycardia with onset of decelerations. Frequent contractions. The ST log shows onset of biphasic events at 17:13. A baseline T/QRS event occurred at 17:54 with a rise from 0.03 to 0.10 and with a further progress to 0.18 at the end of recording at 18:43. A FBS at 18:40 showed a pH of 7.13, and an outlet vacuum extraction was undertaken. Apgar scores 1–6–7. Cord arterial pH 7.07, BD_{ecf} 13.5 mmol/l.

Figure 5. Comments

A fetus displaying ST abnormalities consisting of biphasic ST, as illustrated by the three ECG averages, followed by a progressive rise in T amplitude. The biphasic ST, by themselves plus intermediary CTG would have indicated an abnormality and no further information is needed to tell that this fetus is unable to handle the stress of labor.

Observational data: the EC multicenter trial

In this descriptive study of 320 cases with the ST blinded to the clinician, the CTG was abnormal in 55 cases at retrospective analysis. Twenty-seven cases showed changes in ST waveform. In 21 cases these changes were represented by an increase in the T/QRS ratio. In six cases the changes were represented by a biphasic or negative ST waveform.

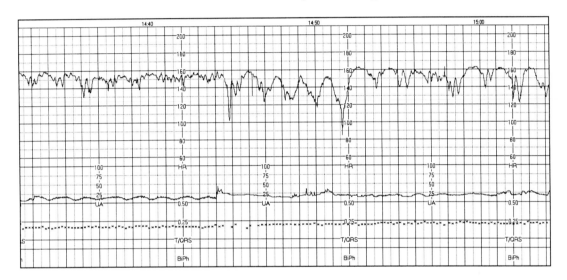

Figure 4 *Para 1, 42 + 1 weeks' gestation. Spontaneous start of labor. Recording during second stage*

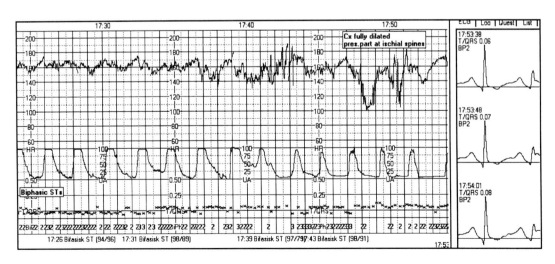

Figure 5 *Para 0, essential hypertension, no medication, 41 weeks, spontaneous onset of labor, clear amniotic fluid, epidural + oxytocin infusion*

Baseline rise in T/QRS

An increase in the T/QRS ratio lasting more than 10 min (baseline T/QRS increase) occurred in five cases. All these cases were associated with an abnormal CTG.

They all showed a low 1-min Apgar score (range 0–5) and evidence of cord artery acidemia (pH ≤ 7.10). This group included one case of intrapartum death, one case with neonatal seizures, and in two cases the neonates required assisted ventilation.

Episodic rise in T/QRS ratio

Episodic ST changes occurred in 16 of the 21 cases that showed an increase in T/QRS ratio during labor. An increase in T/QRS ratio of >0.10 for less than 10 min appeared in association with an abnormal CTG in all cases but one. The case with a rise in T/QRS ratio and normal CTG showed an episodic ST event lasting 2 min.

No baby required assisted ventilation. The lowest 5-min Apgar score was 7, and they all had an uneventful neonatal period.

Biphasic/negative ST

There were six cases that showed biphasic or negative ST changes. In five, these changes were intermittent, short lasting and associated with a normal CTG. All these cases had a normal outcome. One case showed a persistently biphasic ST with negative T waves associated with an abnormal CTG. This was an IUGR fetus (birth weight 2310 g at term). At birth this baby showed a low Apgar score (4 at 1 min) and cord artery acidemia (pH 7.05).

The EC descriptive multicenter trial used the STAN 8801 model linked to a PC for data acquisition. As considerable improvements in signal processing occurred after the study was completed with the introduction of digital signal processing, it was decided to conduct another descriptive study in Norway and Sweden using the prototype STAN S 21 fetal heart function monitor. In the four Swedish labor wards this also became part of the pilot phase of the large randomized controlled multicenter trial.

Nordic observational data

These data included CTG + ST recordings from 2694 term deliveries contained in the STAN database. Intrapartum hypoxia was assessed from cord acid–base status (cord artery pH <7.05, BD_{ecf} >12 mmol/l), Apgar scores and neonatal outcome. The ST log provided automatic statements on significant ST events. The results of this study are summarized in Table 2.

On the basis of observational data such as these, clinical guidelines have been formed to include both the ST and the CTG. The CTG + ST clinical guidelines recommend intervention, not only when there are ST + CTG changes but also when a preterminal CTG trace is recorded.

The high sensitivity of CTG + ST to predict fetal acidosis was associated with a significant increase in positive predictive values as compared with CTG only. Positive predictive values were calculated in a subset of 574 cases; 51% of cases with CTG + ST changes had a cord artery pH of <7.05 and 79% had a pH of <7.15. The corresponding figures for CTG only were 15 and 44%.

Table 2 *Distribution of cases related to cord artery metabolic acidosis, neonatal outcome and ST changes. The duration of ST events, i.e. time between an event indicated in the ST log and end of recording, is also shown*

	ST changes (n)	No ST changes (n)
Metabolic acidosis and neonatal symptoms (death or seizures)	4 (baseline T/QRS increase)	1 (preterminal CTG)
Onset ST changes – end recording (mean + range)	52 min (15–20 min)	
Metabolic acidosis and normal neonatal outcome	20	0
Onset ST changes – end recording (mean + range)	44 min (10–180 min)	

The Swedish multicenter randomized controlled trial

The aim of this large trial was to test the hypothesis that intrapartum monitoring of term fetuses with CTG and automatic ST waveform analysis results in a reduced rate of both operative deliveries for fetal distress (ODFD) and newborns with metabolic acidosis, as compared with CTG alone.

Four Swedish labor wards were equipped with the new STAN system. Term pregnancies in cephalic presentation were enrolled after a decision had been made to apply a single spiral scalp electrode. They were randomized to monitoring with CTG plus ST analysis or CTG only. Clinical action was guided by the study protocol. All ECG data were stored in both arms of the trial; 4421 cases were enrolled during the study period (December 1998 to June 2000).

The main outcome of the trial is given in Table 3. The CTG plus ST arm showed a 60% reduction in the number of cases with metabolic acidosis (cord artery pH<7.05 and base deficit >12 mmol/l) and there were 25% fewer

operative interventions for fetal distress as compared with the CTG arm, with no increase in operative deliveries for other reasons. The trial protocol allowed for an interim analysis after 1600 cases.

This analysis showed frequent breaches of protocol, as clinical management in the CTG + ST arm was conducted according to the 'old' CTG information. The result of this lack of compliance was not only more operative interventions but also babies being exposed to unnecessary intrauterine hypoxia. After retraining and enhanced experience with ST analysis during the second half of the trial, no baby in the CTG + ST arm was admitted to the NICU and a still more pronounced reduction in metabolic acidosis (–75%) and operative deliveries for fetal distress (–44%) was reported.

CONCLUSIONS

The prime aim of intrapartum fetal surveillance is to identify the fetuses forced to respond significantly to the stress of labor. The STAN concept of intrapartum fetal surveillance

Table 3 *Operative interventions and neonatal outcome. Analysis after exclusions of inadequate recordings and fetal malformations according to the protocol*

	CTG group (n (%))	CTG + ST group (n (%))	Odds ratio	95% CI	p Value
Total	2164	2228	—	—	—
Operative delivery for fetal distress	173 (8.0)	132 (5.9)	0.72	0.57–0.92	0.009
Cesarean section for fetal distress	63 (2.9)	43 (1.9)	0.66	0.44–0.97	0.04
Ventouse or forceps for fetal distress	110 (5.1)	89 (4.0)	0.78	0.58–1.03	0.10
Operative delivery for other indications	242 (11.2)	227 (10.2)	0.90	0.74–1.11	0.31
Cesarean section for other indications	110 (5.1)	103 (4.6)	0.91	0.68–1.20	0.52
Ventouse or forceps for other indications	132 (6.1)	124 (5.6)	0.91	0.70–1.17	0.49
Neonatal outcome					
Apgar score 1 min < 4	38 (1.8)	23 (1.0)	0.58	0.35–0.98	0.05
Apgar score 5 min < 7	21 (1.0)	17 (0.8)	0.78	0.39–1.55	0.56
Admission to NICU	151 (7.0)	132 (5.9)	0.84	0.66–1.07	0.18
Neonatal encephalopathy	6 (0.3)	0	—	—	0.01
Perinatal death	0	0			
Acid–base data, total	1871	1926	—	—	—
Cord artery metabolic acidosis	27 (1.4)	11 (0.6)	0.39	0.19–0.79	0.01

provides a unique opportunity to obtain online information related to the condition of a high-priority organ – the fetal heart. The data presented during the past year have documented the ability of ST waveform analysis together with the CTG to provide diagnostic information on intrapartum hypoxia. The outcome of the Swedish trial shows that, for term pregnancies, the STAN methodology of CTG with automatic ST waveform analysis substantially increases our ability to detect and more appropriately intervene in cases of a non-reassuring fetal status during labor. The trial also documented the need for educational efforts and local experience.

To guarantee the safe dissemination of the ST concept, an EU project was started in April 2000 and is still in progress with the following aims:

(1) Ten academic centers of excellence are established across Europe to become the regional hub of experience stimulating other units to follow in a structured fashion.

(2) Assisted learning on physiological and clinical aspects together with user certification will be validated through a system of continuous technology surveillance targeting a continuing reduction in the number of:

   (a) babies born at risk of intrapartum hypoxia;

   (b) operative intervention for threatening fetal oxygen deficiency.

The interim results of this project have confirmed the outcome of the Swedish RCT in that intrapartum monitoring with CTG combined with automatic ST waveform analysis increases the ability of obstetricians to identify fetal hypoxia and to intervene more appropriately, resulting in an improved perinatal outcome.

Bibliography

Amer-Wåhlin I, Hellsten C, Norén H, et al. Intrapartum fetal monitoring: cardiotocography versus cardiotocography plus ST analysis of the fetal ECG. A Swedish randomized controlled trial. Lancet 2001;358:534–8

Arulkumaran S, Lilja H, Lindecrantz K, Ratnam SS, Thavarasah AS, Rosén KG. Fetal ECG waveform analysis should improve fetal surveillance in labour. J Perinat Med 1990;18:13–22

Capstick JB, Edwards PJ. Medicine and the law. Lancet 1990;336:931–2

Dawes GS, Mott JC, Shelley HJ. The importance of cardiac glycogen for the maintenance of life in fetal lambs and newborn animals during anoxia. J Physiol 1959;146:516–38

Goodwin TM, Milner-Masterson L, Paul RH. Elimination of fetal scalp blood sampling on a large clinical service. Obstet Gynecol 1994;83:971–4

Greene KR, Rosén KG. Intrapartum asphyxia. In Levene MI, Bennett MJ, Punt J, eds. Fetal and Neonatal Neurology and Neurosurgery. Edinburgh: Churchill Livingstone, 1995:265–72

Greene KR. Intelligent fetal heart rate computer systems in intrapartum surveillance. Curr Opin Obstet Gynaecol 1996;8:123–7

Greene KR. Scalp blood gas analysis. In antepartum and intrapartum fetal assessment. Obstet Gynecol Clin North Am 1999;26:641–56

Hökegård KH, Eriksson BO, Kjellmer I, Magno R, Rosén KG. Myocardial metabolism in relation to electrocardiographic changes and cardiac function during graded hypoxia in the fetal lamb. Acta Physiol Scand 1981;113:1–7

Lilja H, Greene KR, Karlsson K, Rosén KG. ST waveform changes of the fetal electrocardiogram during labour – a clinical study. Br J Obstet Gynaecol 1985;92:611–17

Lindecrantz K, Lilja H, Widmark C, Rosén KG. The fetal ECG during labour. A suggested standard. J Biomed Eng 1988;10:351–3

Low JA. The relationship of asphyxia in the mature fetus to long-term neurologic function. Clin Obstet Gynecol 1993;36:82–90

Luzietti R, Erkkola R, Hasbargen U, Mattson LÅ, Thoulon JM, Rosén KG. European Community Multicentre Trial 'Fetal ECG analysis during labour': the P-R interval. J Perinat Med 1997;25:27–34

Luzietti R, Erkkola R, Hasbargen U, Mattsson L, Thoulon J-M, Rosén KG. European Community Multi-center Trial 'Fetal ECG analysis during labour': ST plus CTG analysis. *J Perinat Med* 1999; 27:431–40

Luzietti R, Rosén KG. ST waveform analysis of the fetal ECG and intrapartum hypoxia. XVII European Congress of Perinatal Medicine. *Prenat Neonat Med* 2000;5:30

MacLennan A. A template for defining a causal relation between acute intrapartum events and cerebral palsy: international consensus statement. *Br Med J* 1999;319:1054–9

Rosén KG, Isaksson O. Alterations in fetal heart rate and ECG correlated to glycogen, creatine phosphate and ATP levels during graded hypoxia. *Biol Neonate* 1976;30:17–24

Rosén KG, Dagbjartsson A, Henriksson BA, Lagercrantz H, Kjellmer I. The relationship between circulating catecholamines and ST waveform in the fetal lamb electrocardiogram during hypoxia. *Am J Obstet Gynecol* 1984;149:190–5

Rosén KG, Arulkumaran S, Greene KR, *et al.* Clinical validity of fetal ECG waveform analysis. In Sahling E, ed. *Perinatology*. New York: Raven Press, 1992: 95–110

Rosén KG, Lindecrantz A. STAN: the Gothenburg model for fetal surveillance during labour by ST analysis of the fetal electrocardiogram. *Clin Phys Physiol Meas* 1989;10:51–6

Rosén KG, Luzietti R. The fetal electrocardiogram: ST waveform analysis during labour. *J Perinat Med* 1994;22:502–12

Rosén KG, Murphy K How to assess fetal metabolic acidosis from cord samples. *J Perinat Med* 1991;19: 221–6

Rosén KG, Luzietti R. Intrapartum fetal monitoring: its basis and current developments. *Prenat Neonat Med* 2000;5:1–14

Rosén KG, Amer-Walin I, Bretones S, Luzietti R, Noren H, Pollanen P. Detection of intrapartum hypoxia. *Proceedings of the 5th World Congress of Perinatal Medicine*, Barcelona, 2001

Saling E. Neues vorgehen zur untersuchung des kindes unter der geburt-einführung, Technik, Grundlagen. *Arch Gynak* 1962;197:108–22

Siggaard-Andersen O. An acid base chart for arterial blood with normal and pathophysiological reference areas. *Scand J Clin Lab Invest* 1971;27:239–245

van Wijngaarden WJ. The fetal electrocardiogram: the PR-FHR relationship. *Proceedings of the 5th International Symposium on Intrapartum Fetal Surveillance*, Stockholm, 1999

Westgate J, Greene KR. How well is fetal blood sampling used in clinical practice? *Br J Obstet Gynaecol* 1994;101:250–1

Westgate J, Keith RD, Curnow JS, Ifeachor EC, Greene KR. Suitability of scalp electrodes for monitoring the fetal electrocardiogram during labour. *Clin Phys Physiol Meas* 1990;11:297–306

Westgate J, Harris M, Curnow JSH, Greene KR. Plymouth randomised trial of cardiotocogram only versus ST waveform plus cardiotocogram for intrapartum monitoring: 2400 cases. *Am J Obstet Gynecol* 1993;169:1151–60

Widmark C, Lindecrantz K, Murray H, Rosén KG. Changes in the PR, RR and ST waveform of the fetal lamb electrocardiogram with acute hypoxemia. *J Dev Physiol* 1992;18:99–103

Widmark C, Jansson T, Lindecrantz K, Rosén KG. ECG waveform, short term heart rate variability and plasma cathecholamine concentrations in response to hypoxia in intrauterine growth retarded guinea pig fetuses. *J Dev Physiol* 1991;15:161–8

The role of nucleated red blood cells in obstetrics

25

M. Y. Divon and A. Ferber

BACKGROUND

Nucleated red blood cells (NRBCs) are immature erythrocytes commonly found in the peripheral blood of healthy newborns[1,2]. It is believed that the presence of NRBCs reflects the relatively hypoxic nature of the fetal environment. A rapid decline in the number of hematopoietic progenitor cells is commonly observed after birth[3,4]. However, an elevated NRBC count has been described in association with various intrapartum pathological conditions.

One of the earliest descriptions of NRBCs was by Geissler and Japha[5] in 1901. The authors' impression was that the presence of NRBCs should be viewed as 'showing disease'. Similarly, in 1924, Lippman[6] stated that normoblasts in the peripheral blood of a newborn must be considered a pathological finding. The author reported that term neonates have an average of 3.2 NRBCs/100 white blood cells (WBCs) and that the number of NRBCs falls rapidly after birth. In 1941, Anderson[7] reported that the average count of NRBCs in cord blood smears of 200 infants was 7.3/100 WBCs for term deliveries and 11/100 WBCs for premature infants. His series included five peripartum deaths, all of which had elevated NRBC counts. Fox[8] was the first to relate the presence of NRBCs to fetal hypoxic events. He reported a very high incidence of asphyxial-type fetal distress accompanying placentas that had a high population of NRBCs[8]. Later, Dorros et al.[9] documented significantly higher NRBC counts in neonates who experienced 'distress during delivery' or were born with low Apgar scores when compared to healthy newborns (14.1/100 WBCs and 21.1/100 WBCs vs. 5.8/100 WBCs, respectively). A similar conclusion was reached by Merenstein et al.[10] who reported on the association between acute and chronic antenatal hypoxia, and lower Apgar scores with elevated NRBC counts.

PATHOPHYSIOLOGY

Several investigators have shown that the fetal hematopoietic system responds to hypoxia by elevating the level of erythropoietin (EPO)[11,12]. In turn, an elevated EPO results in an increase of erythroid production and in the release of immature forms of erythrocytes into the peripheral circulation. Georgieff et al.[13] used a fetal sheep model to document a significant reticulocytosis following either acute or chronic hypoxia. They observed a similar response following the administration of EPO. D'Souza et al.[14] studied 458 human, term newborns and reached the same conclusion. Fetal hypoxia was associated with increases in hemoglobin, red blood cell count, white blood cell count and hematocrit. Furthermore, the increase in the mean corpuscular volume combined with the decrease in mean corpuscular hemoglobin concentration was explained by a net influx of immature red blood cells into the peripheral circulation. Thus, the authors suggested that intrapartum fetal hypoxia stimulates erythropoiesis and results in mobilization of both immature erythrocytes and white blood cells into the peripheral circulation[14]. Snijders et al.[15] demonstrated that fetal EPO production and erythropoiesis increased in response to tissue hypoxia as early as 26 weeks' gestation. Moreover, these authors suggested that an abnormal elevated erythroblast count was a better measure of tissue hypoxia than blood pH levels. Maier et al.[11] argued that the presence of increased levels of EPO in umbilical cord blood samples indicated prolonged fetal hypoxia, and suggested that the determination of EPO levels in the umbilical cord would indicate the severity and timing of the asphyxial event. The EPO levels did not correlate with gestational age, meconium staining or Apgar scores, but they were related to umbilical artery pH and were elevated in growth-restricted fetuses.

Fetal animal studies indicate that several hours of hypoxemia are necessary before a rise in plasma EPO levels can be demonstrated[16,17]. This period is similar to that observed in both *in vivo* experiments in adult rats and *in vitro* kidney perfusion studies in adult dogs[18,19]. In these studies, the increase in EPO was found to be secondary to the synthesis of new hormone rather than the release of previously produced hormone. Widness et al.[20] studied the correlation between intrapartum fetal heart rate (FHR) patterns and umbilical cord EPO in 41 human fetuses. The authors reported that the highest level of EPO was observed in fetuses with the most abnormal FHR patterns. In addition, they concluded that a significant increase in EPO levels could be documented after only 3 h of hypoxia-related FHR abnormalities[20]. Thus, it is reasonable to conclude that prolonged rather than acute hypoxia results in a measurable EPO response.

Despite the lack of evidence supporting an EPO response to acute hypoxia, recent studies have shown that acute hypoxia is associated with elevated NRBC counts. Altshuler and Hyder[21] found that NRBC counts increased within 2 h of acute blood loss in healthy term fetuses. Benirschke[22] reported elevated NRBC counts within 1 h of an acute intrapartum fetal bleeding from disrupted velamentous vessels. Recently, Donaldson et al.[23] studied the impact of obstetric factors on umbilical cord blood composition and concluded that the overall number of nucleated cells is influenced by acute intrapartum events. Similarly, Lim et al.[24] demonstrated that 'stress during delivery' acutely increased the number of granulocytes, CD34+ cells and hematopoietic progenitor cells (i.e. NRBCs) possibly by acute-phase proteins

causing mobilization of stem cell line populations. They also showed that the longer the duration of 'stress', the higher the number of nucleated cells in the peripheral blood[24].

It is thus reasonable to conclude that both chronic and acute intrauterine hypoxic events elevate NRBC counts. Clearly, chronic hypoxia results in elevated EPO. However, the exact pathophysiology of an acute rise in NRBCs is yet to be determined.

PATHOLOGY

In order to establish normal values for NRBC counts in term singleton pregnancies, Hanon-Lundberg et al.[25] analyzed umbilical cord blood from 1112 such pregnancies. The mean number of NRBCs per 100 white blood cells was 8.6, with a standard deviation of 10.3, a median of 5, and a range of 0–89.

Fetal acidemia

In 1999, Hanlon-Lundberg and Kirby[26] prospectively collected umbilical blood from 1561 term live-born neonates. Arterial blood was analyzed for pH and blood gas values. Venous blood was analyzed for NRBC counts. Infants with arterial cord pH of < 7.2 demonstrated elevated NRBC counts when compared to infants with normal acid–base balance (18.5 ± 32.4 vs. 8.5 ± 16.2, respectively; $p = 0.001$). Infants with either respiratory acidemia or non-compensated metabolic acidemia had significantly elevated NRBC counts. More recently, Blackwell et al.[27] reported similar results in term neonates with umbilical artery pH ≤ 7.00.

Fetal growth restriction

In 1987, Soothill et al.[28] measured umbilical venous oxygen and carbon dioxide tensions, pH, lactate and glucose concentrations in fetal blood samples obtained by cordocentesis in 38 growth-restricted fetuses. The oxygen tension was below the normal mean for gestational age in 33 cases, and in 14 cases it was at least 2 standard deviations below the mean for normal pregnancy. The severity of fetal hypoxia significantly correlated with fetal hypercapnia, acidosis, hyperlacticemia, hypoglycemia and erythroblastosis (i.e. NRBCs).

The association between fetal circulatory abnormalities and elevated NRBC counts has received increased attention in recent years. Bernstein et al.[29] compared umbilical cord NRBC counts obtained from small-for-gestational age (SGA) neonates in whom umbilical artery end-diastolic velocity was present ($n = 33$) to SGA neonates with absent or reversed end-diastolic velocities ($n = 19$). Those with absent or reversed end diastolic velocities had significantly elevated NRBC counts (135.5 ± 138 vs. 17.4 ± 23.7, $p < 0.0001$). Infants with absent or reversed end-diastolic velocities exhibited lower birth weights, lower initial platelet counts, lower arterial pH, higher cord blood base excess and an increased likelihood of Cesarean delivery for 'fetal distress'. They also exhibited significantly longer time intervals for clearance of NRBCs from their circulation. A multivariate analysis revealed that absent or reversed end diastolic velocities and birth weight contributed independently to the elevation of NRBC counts (with a combined R^2 of 0.59).

In 1999, Baschat et al.[30] sought to determine the relationship between NRBC counts at birth and the circulatory status of growth-restricted fetuses. The authors evaluated 84 growth-restricted fetuses, which were divided into three subgroups according to their circulatory abnormality: (1) elevated umbilical artery pulsatility index (i.e. > 2 standard deviations above the mean for gestational age); (2) in addition, middle cerebral artery pulsatility index > 2 standard deviations above the mean for gestational age; (3) either peak velocity index > 2 standard deviations above the mean for gestational age in the inferior vena cava and ductus venosus or pulsatile flow in the umbilical vein, or both. Groups 2 and 3 had significantly higher NRBC counts relative to group 1, with a longer persistence of NRBCs in the neonates' circulation. The umbilical artery bicarbonate level was the strongest independent determinant of the peak NRBC count and

persistence of NRBCs in the neonatal circulation ($R^2 = 0.27$, $p < 0.001$ and $R^2 = 0.47$, $p < 0.0001$, respectively). The authors concluded that increasing abnormality of arterial and venous blood flows in growth-restricted fetuses was associated with increasing NRBC counts at birth[30]. Axt-Fliedner et al.[31] also sought to determine the effect of increasing circulatory impairment in fetuses on the neonatal NRBC counts. One hundred and thirty-four singleton pregnancies were included in the study and were allocated to four study groups according to Doppler findings. The systolic-to-diastolic (S/D) ratios of the umbilical artery, fetal aorta, middle cerebral artery and uterine arteries were recorded. Fetuses were assigned to one of the following groups according to the final recording prior to delivery: group 1, normal S/D ratios in the examined vessels; group 2, abnormal S/D ratio in the umbilical artery or fetal aorta with normal uterine artery studies; group 3, abnormal Doppler studies in all examined vessels; and group 4, absent end-diastolic velocity in the umbilical artery or fetal aorta and abnormal S/D ratio in the uterine arteries. NRBC counts showed a stepwise increase from group 1 to group 4. Multivariate analysis revealed that Doppler results of the umbilical artery, fetal aorta and uterine arteries were independent determinants of NRBC counts. Increasing abnormalities in fetal blood flow as detected by Doppler studies were associated with increasing NRBC counts.

Several studies have evaluated the association between NRBC counts and perinatal outcome. Minior et al.[32] studied 73 consecutive growth-restricted neonates (i.e. birth weight below the 10th centile for gestational age) on whom a complete blood count had been obtained during the first day of life. All infants who had any confounding variables (i.e. maternal diabetes or hemoglobinopathy, multiple gestation, or chromosomal or congenital anomalies) were excluded. The authors described a significant association between elevated NRBC counts and adverse short-term neonatal outcome (such as neonatal intensive care admission and duration of stay, respiratory distress and intubation, thrombocy-topenia, hyperbilirubinemia, intraventricular hemorrhage and neonatal death). In addition, elevated NRBC counts were significantly associated with Cesarean delivery for non-reassuring fetal status. A stepwise regression analysis established that NRBC counts were superior to gestational age at delivery or birth weight in the prediction of neonatal intraven-tricular hemorrhage, neonatal respiratory distress and neonatal death. The authors concluded that an elevated NRBC count independently predicted adverse perinatal outcome in growth-restricted fetuses.

In a subsequent study, Minior *et al.*[33] evaluated 237 neonates who were admitted to the neonatal intensive care unit. Birth weights of 43 neonates (18%) were below the 10th centile for gestational age and these were considered SGA. Perinatal outcomes were evaluated prospectively. Small-for-gestational-age neonates with high NRBC counts had significantly lower umbilical artery pH and were more likely to require mechanical ventilation or blood pressure support agents. Subgroup analysis demonstrated that SGA neonates with elevated NRBC counts had significantly more adverse outcomes than did SGA neonates with normal NRBC counts. The authors suggested that an elevated NRBC count distinguished the fetus with growth restriction from the small but otherwise healthy fetus[33].

Neurodevelopment

In 1995, Phelan *et al.*[34] compared umbilical cord NRBC data from 46 neurologically impaired term neonates with NRBC counts of 83 healthy term neonates. The purpose of their study was to identify a possible relationship between the presence of NRBCs, hypoxic-ischemic encephalopathy and long-term neo-natal neurological impairment. The authors showed that the neurologically impaired neonates exhibited a significantly higher number of NRBCs per 100 WBCs (34.5 ± 68 vs. 3.4 ± 3.0, respectively; $p < 0.00001$). The non-reactive-impaired neonates exhibited the highest mean NRBC count and the longest

clearance times. The authors concluded that NRBC data appeared to aid in the identification of the presence of fetal asphyxia and might assist in the timing of fetal neurological injury[34].

In a subsequent study, Phelan *et al.*[35] attempted to establish the role of NRBC and lymphocyte counts in fetal neurological injury. One hundred and one term infants with hypoxic–ischemic encephalopathy and perma-nent neurological handicap were divided into two groups: infants with preadmission injury as manifested by a non-acceleratory FHR pattern from admission to delivery, and infants with acute injury, as determined by a normal FHR pattern upon admission, which was subse-quently followed by a sudden prolonged FHR deceleration. The NRBC count was elevated and the elevation lasted longer in infants with preadmission injury. Again, the authors con-cluded that NRBC counts could effectively be used to time the onset of neurological injury[35].

Early-onset neonatal seizures are commonly considered an initial sign of neurological injury. Blackwell *et al.*[36] studied the relationship between NRBC counts and early-onset neonatal seizures, and showed that NRBC counts were significantly higher in infants who seized within the first 72 h of life. Buonocore *et al.*[37] suggested that an elevated NRBC count at birth not only reflected a fetal response to perinatal hypoxia, but also was a reliable index of perinatal brain damage. Elevated NRBC counts were found in neonates with abnormal cerebral artery Doppler studies at the age of 48–72 h, infants with hypoxic–ischemic encephalopathy at 6 months of age, and in 3-year old children who demonstrated abnormal developmental status.

Pregnancy complications

It has been documented that neonatal NRBC counts are elevated in pregnancies complicated by active and passive maternal cigarette smoking[38,39], gestational diabetes[40], prematurity with histological chorioamnionitis[41], ABO incompatibility[42], meconium aspiration syn-drome[43] and prolonged pregnancy[44] (Table 1).

Table 1 *Nucleated red blood cell (NRBC) counts in different types of pregnancy complications*

Study variable	Condition present	Condition absent	p Value
Smoking			
active[38]	0.5, 0–5*	0.0005, 0–0.6	0.02
passive[39]	0.36, 0–5.1*	0.24, 0–17.3	
Gestational diabetes[40]			
large for GA	0.56, 0–1.8*	0.0005, 0–0.6	< 0.001
appropriate for GA	0.13, 0–0.65*	0.0005, 0–0.6	< 0.001
Chorioamnionitis[41]	3.17, 1.04**	2.71, 1.27	0.005
ABS incompatibility[42]	13.2 ± 13.2***	8.3 ± 12.8	0.006
MAS[43]	0.007, 0–0.013*	0.003, 0–0.014	< 0.02
Prolonged pregnancy[44]	6.5, 0–24****	3.7, 0–14	< 0.05

GA, gestational age; MAS, meconium aspiration syndrome
*Absolute NRBCs × 10^9/l; median, range
**$NRBC^{log}$; mean, standard deviation
***NRBCs/100 WBCs; mean, standard deviation
****NRBCs/100 WBCs; median, range

Placental NRBC

Several authors have shown that NRBCs can be identified upon microscopic examination of the placenta. However, there is disagreement as to the implications of their presence. Whereas some believe that their occurrence in term fetuses is distinctly abnormal, others accept a ratio of 1 : 1.5 NRBCs to WBCs in fetal placental blood vessels as a normal finding[45]. There are no known standards for the normal range of intraplacental NRBC counts in preterm fetuses.

In 1994, Maier *et al.*[46] studied placentas from 300 high-risk newborns. Morphological placental abnormalities such as fetal vasculopathy and meconium phagocytosis were significantly correlated with umbilical vein EPO concentration $(r = 0.34)$. Furthermore, these EPO levels highly correlated with intraplacental NRBC counts $(r = 0.74)$. These findings are consistent with placental pathology resulting in fetal hypoxia and subsequent elevation of fetal EPO. In turn, the elevated EPO causes erythropoiesis and elevated NRBCs in both placental and peripheral vessels[46].

In 1997, Salafia *et al.*[47] studied 125 preterm singleton births delivered at 22–32 weeks' gestation. There were 92 cases of spontaneous prematurity (i.e. premature rupture of membranes and preterm labor with intact membranes) and 33 cases of pre-eclampsia. NRBC counts were obtained twice (within 3 h of life and again at 48 h of life). Neonates whose placenta demonstrated chronic marked uteroplacental vascular pathology exhibited stable, high levels of NRBC counts. However, neonates whose placenta showed acute inflammation revealed a rapid decline in NRBC counts. The authors hypothesized that this response reflects the differences in the mediators of NRBC release. The effects of acute inflammation on the release of NRBCs would be mediated by acute-phase cytokines (such as interleukin-6, which has short-term effects on bone marrow release of mature and immature myeloid and erythroid elements). In contrast, chronic uteroplacental vascular lesions probably result in elevated NRBC counts via the release of EPO[47].

SUMMARY

Recent studies have clearly demonstrated that intrauterine hypoxia results in a significant increase in the number of NRBCs in the fetal circulation. In addition, elevated umbilical cord NRBC counts have been suggested as predictors of short- and long-term adverse neonatal outcomes.

References

1. Miller DR, Baehner RL. *Blood Diseases of Infancy and Childhood*, 7th edn. St Louis, MO: Mosby, 1995:39–40
2. Green DW, Mimouni F. Nucleated erythrocytes in healthy infants and in infants of diabetic mothers. *J Pediatr* 1990;116:129–31
3. Kawamura T, Toyabe S, Moroda T, *et al.* Neonatal granulopoiesis is a postpartum event which is seen in the liver as well as in the blood. *Hepatology* 1997;26:1567–72
4. Sills RH, Hadley RAR. The significance of nucleated red blood cells in the peripheral blood of children. *Am J Pediatr Hematol Oncol* 1983;5:173–7
5. Geissler, Japha A. Beitrag zu den Anamieen junger Kinder. *Jahrbluch Linderheilk* 1901;56:627–47
6. Lippman HS. A morphologic and quantitative study of the blood corpuscles in the newborn period. *Am J Dis Child* 1924;27:473
7. Anderson GW. Studies on the nucleated red cell count in the chorionic capillaries and the cord blood of various ages of pregnancy. *Am J Obstet Gynecol* 1941;42:1–14
8. Fox H. The incidence and significance of nucleated erythrocytes in the fetal vessels of the mature human placenta. *J Obstet Gynaecol Br Commonw* 1967;74:40–3
9. Dorros G, Kleiner GJ, Romney SL. Fetal leukocyte pattern in premature rupture of amniotic membranes and in normal and abnormal labor. *Am J Obstet Gynecol* 1969;105:1269–73
10. Merenstein GB, Blackmon LR, Kushner J. Nucleated red-cells in the newborn. *Lancet* 1970;13:1293–4
11. Maier RF, Bohme K, Dudenhausen JW, Obladen M. Cord blood erythropoietin in relation to different markers of fetal hypoxia. *Obstet Gynecol* 1993;81:575–80
12. Ostlund E, Lindholm H, Hemsen A, Fried G. Fetal erythropoietin and endothelin-1: relation to hypoxia and intrauterine growth retardation. *Acta Obstet Gynecol Scand* 2000;79:276–82
13. Georgieff MK, Schmidt RL, Mills MM, Radmer WJ, Widness JA. Fetal iron and cytochrome c status after intrauterine hypoxemia and erythropoietin administration. *Am J Physiol* 1992;262:485–91
14. D'Souza SW, Black P, MacFarlane T, Jennison RF, Richards B. Haematologic values in cord blood in relation to fetal hypoxia. *Br J Obstet Gynecol* 1981;88:129–32
15. Snijders RJM, Abbas A, Melby O, Ireland RM, Nicolaides KH. Fetal plasma erythropoietin concentration in severe growth retardation. *Am J Obstet Gynecol* 1993;168:615–19
16. Zanjani ED, Gordon AS. Erythropoietin production and utilizing in fetal goats and sheep. *Isr J Med Sci* 1971;7:850–6
17. Widness JA, Garcia JF, Clemons GK, *et al.* Temporal response of immunoreactive erythropoietin to acute hypoxemia in the sheep fetus. *Pediatr Res* 1983;17:144A
18. Schooley JC, Mahlmann LJ. Erythopoietin production in the anephric rat. I. Relationship between nephrectomy, time of hypoxic exposure, and erythropoietin production. *Blood* 1972;39:31–9
19. Erslev AJ. Renal biogenesis of erythropoietin. *Am J Med* 1975;58:25–30
20. Widness JA, Teramo KA, Clemons GK, *et al.* Correlation of the interpretation of fetal heart rate records with cord plasma erythropoietin levels. *Br J Obstet Gynaecol* 1985;92:326–32
21. Altshuler G, Hyder SR. Nucleated erythrocytes. In Pitkin RM, Scott JR, eds. *Clinical Obstetrics and Gynecology*. Philadelphia: Lippincott-Raven, 1996:553–6
22. Benirschke K. Placenta pathology questions to the perinatologist. *J Perinatol* 1994;14:371–5
23. Donaldson C, Armitage WJ, Laundy V, *et al.* Impact of obstetric factors on cord blood donation for transplantation. *Br J Haematol* 1999;106:128–32
24. Lim FTH, Scherjon SA, van Bechhoven JM, *et al.* Association of stress during delivery with increased numbers of nucleated cells and hematopoietic progenitor cells in umbilical cord blood. *Am J Obstet Gynecol* 2000;183:1144–51
25. Hanon-Lundberg KM, Kirby RS, Gandhi S, Broekhuizen FF. Nucleated red blood cells in cord blood of singleton term neonates. *Am J Obstet Gynecol* 1997;176:1149–56
26. Hanon-Lundberg KM, Kirby RS. Nucleated red blood cells as a marker of acidemia in term neonates. *Am J Obstet Gynecol* 1999;181:196–201
27. Blackwell SC, Refuerzo JS, Hassan SS, Wolfe HM, Berry SM, Sorokin Y. Nucleated red blood cell counts in term neonates with umbilical artery pH ≤ 7.00. *Am J Perinatol* 2001;18:93–8
28. Soothill PW, Nicolaides KH, Campbell S. Prenatal asphyxia, hyperlacticemia, and erythroblastosis in growth retarded fetuses. *Br Med J (Clin Res Ed)* 1987;294:1051–3
29. Bernstein PS, Minior VK, Divon MY. Nucleated red blood cell counts in small for gestational age fetuses with abnormal umbilical artery Doppler studies. *Am J Obstet Gynecol* 1997;177:1079–84

30. Baschat AA, Gembruch U, Reiss I, Gortner L, Harman CR, Weiner CP. Neonatal nucleated red blood cell counts in growth-restricted fetuses: relationship to arterial and venous Doppler studies. *Am J Obstet Gynecol* 1999;181:190–5
31. Axt-Fliedner R, Ertan K, Hendrik HJ, Schmidt W. Neonatal nucleated red blood cell counts: relationship to abnormal fetoplacental circulation detected by Doppler studies. *J Ultrasound Med* 2001;20:189–90
32. Minior VK, Bernstein PS, Divon MY. Nucleated red blood cells in growth restricted fetuses: association with short-term neonatal outcome. *Fetal Diagn Ther* 2000;15:165–9
33. Minior VK, Shatzkin E, Divon MY. Nucleated red blood cell count in the differentiation of fetuses with pathologic growth restriction from healthy small-for-gestational-age fetuses. *Am J Obstet Gynecol* 2000;182:1107–9
34. Phelan JP, Ahn MO, Korst LM, Martin GI. Nucleated red blood cells: a marker for fetal asphyxia? *Am J Obstet Gynecol* 1995;173:1380–4
35. Phelan JP, Korst LM, Ahn MO, Martin GI. Neonatal nucleated red blood cell and lymphocyte counts in fetal brain injury. *Obstet Gynecol* 1998; 91:485–9
36. Blackwell SC, Refuerzo JS, Honor MW, *et al.* The relationship between nucleated red blood cell counts and early-onset neonatal seizures. *Am J Obstet Gynecol* 2000;182:1452–7
37. Buonocore G, Perrone S, Gioia D, *et al.* Nucleated red blood cell count at birth as an index of perinatal brain damage. *Am J Obstet Gynecol* 1999; 181:1500–5
38. Yeruchimovich M, Dollberg S, Green DW, Mimouni FB. Nucleated red blood cells in infants of smoking mothers. *Obstet Gynecol* 1999;93:403–6
39. Dollberg S, Fainaru O, Mimouni FB, Shenhav M, Lessing JB, Kuperminc M. Effect of passive smoking in pregnancy on neonatal nucleated red blood cells. *Pediatrics* 2000;106:E34
40. Yeruchimovich M, Mimouni FB, Green DW, Dollberg S. Nucleated red blood cells in healthy infants of women with gestational diabetes. *Obstet Gynecol* 2000;95:84–6
41. Leikin E, Garry D, Visintainer P, Verma U, Tejani N. Correlation of neonatal nucleated red blood cell counts in preterm infants with histologic chorioamnionitis. *Am J Obstet Gynecol* 1997;177: 27–30
42. Hanlon-Lundberg KH, Kirby RS. Association of ABO incompatibility with elevation of nucleated red blood cell counts in term neonates. *Am J Obstet Gynecol* 2000;183:1532–6
43. Dollberg S, Livny S, Mordecheyev N, Mimouni FB. Nucleated red blood cells in meconium aspiration syndrome. *Obstet Gynecol* 2001;97:593–6
44. Axt R, Ertan K, Hendrik J, Wrobel M, Mink D, Schmidt W. Nucleated red blood cells in cord blood of singleton term and post-term neonates. *J Perinat Med* 1999;27:276–81
45. Altshuler G. Pathology of the placenta. In Gilbert-Barness E, ed. *Potter's Pathology of the Fetus and Infant,* vol 1. St Louis, MO: Mosby, 1997:254–5
46. Maier RF, Gunther A, Vogel M, Dudenhausen JW, Obladen M. Umbilical venous erythropoietin and umbilical artery pH in relation to morphologic placental abnormalities. *Obstet Gynecol* 1994;84: 81–7
47. Salafia CM, Ghidini A, Pezzullo JC, Rosenkrantz TS. Patterns of change in early neonatal nucleated erythrocyte counts in preterm deliveries. *J Soc Gynecol Invest* 1997;4:178–82

Perinatal medicine in the information age

26

I. E. Zador, S. C. Blackwell, R. J. Sokol and M. I. Evans

INTRODUCTION

It is not unusual for authors writing a chapter for an 'updated' edition of a book just to revise and freshen up the older chapter. In trying to do exactly that with the chapter we wrote for the previous version of this book, we quickly realized how out of date the material presented had become in just a few years. This not only prompted us completely to rewrite this chapter but also allowed us to co-author this chapter with one of our junior faculty (S.B.) reflecting ideas from the information-age generation. As the 'digital decade' is knocking on the door of perinatal medicine, more and more fetomaternal health-care providers are encountering the information age in their practice. To reflect on these new realities this chapter focuses on a few selected innovative areas of computer technology that we felt might be of interest. We choose to elaborate along the lines of our research interest, which involves the design, development and implementation of a web-based perinatal electronic medical record (EMR). Currently, across the entire health-care industry the EMR represents a 'work in progress' as academic and commercial enterprises are diligently developing the EMR concept. Among many challenges, one that particularly stands out is the US government-mandated Health Insurance Portability and Accountability Act (HIPAA). HIPAA gives patients greater access to their own medical records and more control over how their personal health information is used. It also addresses the obligations of health-care providers and health plans to protect health information. By law, health plans, health-care clearinghouses and health-care providers who conduct certain financial and administrative

transactions electronically have until April 2003 to comply. The enormous task that lies ahead is to develop an EMR that can function across many diverse computer platforms, medical specialties, languages and governmental regulations, and at the same time keep pace with the rapidly evolving technologies. In this brief chapter we address EMR issues as they relate to areas of perinatal patient care, including issues related to information management in fetal ultrasound imaging.

TOWARDS A PERINATAL ELECTRONIC MEDICAL RECORD

Computerized perinatal database systems have been integral parts of clinical and research programs at academic obstetrics/gynecology departments since the 1970s[1]. These relational databases optimally link all obstetric data with both short- and long-term neonatal outcomes. They are episodic and longitudinal databases designed to enhance clinical care and expedite epidemiological research[2]. In particular, the ability to develop large perinatal datasets has facilitated the study of infrequent, but critically important, pregnancy complications[3,4].

Since 1985, at Wayne State University/Hutzel Hospital we have been using POPRAS forms for perinatal risk assessment[5]. Demographic and antenatal data are recorded at prenatal care sites and then sent to Hutzel Hospital for direct entry by trained technicians who batch-enter data after checks for completeness and internal consistency. The perinatal database is used to generate summaries of antepartum, intrapartum and neonatal findings, ultrasound reports and service statistics. It supports immediate availability of ultrasound reports and other key clinical information at multiple sites where care is provided. It has captured extensive obstetric and neonatal outcome data for over 100 000 consecutive births. Currently, the perinatal database is relational *and* in the Microsoft Access format; data in this format are easily converted into formats required by many different statistical programs including SPSS, SAS and Epistat. Thus, the data are accessible to faculty and fellows for research purposes.

Because of the significant manpower costs associated with this type of 'off-line' data entry, the feasibility of financially supporting a team of specific perinatal data entry personnel is a limiting factor for many departments. Even with database systems where patient information is inputted directly into a computerized medical record by physicians, nurses or other health-care team members (e.g. ultrasound technicians) the initial and maintenance hardware and network costs may also be prohibitive. For these reasons, there is much interest and enthusiasm in the development and application of an electronic medical record (EMR) that can run over the Internet.

There are several potential advantages and disadvantages to this approach (Table 1). First, if the perinatal EMR is maintained through an application service provider (ASP), there are limited computer and network infrastructure costs. As long as there is access to high-speed Internet connections, which are available at relatively low costs at most health-care sites, standard desktop computers can readily be used. Since the EMR application is administrated and maintained over the Internet at the server level, there is a low burden on the local client computer, which further decreases the departmental burden on in-house information technology support. The second advantage is immediate and widespread access to data from different health-care sites. Although a patient may have antenatal encounters at her prenatal care clinic or an off-site outside ultrasound unit, these data may be inputted into the same database that ultimately contains all in-patient data, thus providing potentially more seamless integration of antenatal out-patient and in-patient data. Furthermore, if the same EMR is used within a medical center, but at different hospitals, there is the potential for more uniform data collection, more consistent data definition and subsequently improved clinical care. This may be increased even more if disease-specific clinical pathways are part of the EMR. Of course, such technology is useful in support of a quality assurance program.

There are currently few entirely web-based perinatal database systems in clinical use. Concern over the stability and reliability of Internet access coupled with unknown security risks are major reasons for this hesitation. Although high-speed Internet access is relatively easy and inexpensive to obtain, the unknown risk of system downtime due to virus or denial of service attacks still plagues potential users. Furthermore, security and privacy of sensitive patient data is another issue. The potential for unauthorized remote access to patient information such as genetic testing or HIV test results by 'hackers' is surely a concern. Despite use of security measures, such as username and password protection, role-based security, IP address restriction and data

Table 1 *Potential advantages and disadvantages of an Internet-based perinatal database*

Advantages	Disadvantages
Limited computer and network costs	Unknown future down time of Internet
Immediate and widespread access	Security of system or data from 'hackers', denial of service attacks, or viruses
More standardized collection of data across health-care system	Unknown effect of future governmental regulations
Lower in-house IT costs	

encryption, administrators and risk managers remain wary. Soon-to-be released governmental guidelines for the electronic transmission of patient information are a further potential burden that affects initiation of an Internet-based system, because of the fear of an inability to be compliant with these regulations and the potential punitive action from the government[6].

In summary, regardless of the manner in which data are collected as part of a perinatal database, a good system must have three basic features. It must link information from all obstetric encounters; antepartum and delivery information must be linked to all other clinical information, such as data from prenatal ultrasound, antenatal testing and genetic testing. Second, obstetric conditions and outcomes must be actively linked to neonatal data; failure to link maternal and infant data threatens the utility of having a perinatal database. Finally, data must be able to be retrieved from the database, not merely collected, to be useful for research and vital statistics reporting.

EMERGING TRENDS FOR INFORMATION MANAGEMENT IN FETAL ULTRASOUND; THE DICOM STANDARD

The past decade witnessed astonishing improvements in fetal ultrasound imaging. The focus was and remains on improvements of image quality as demonstrated by the emergence of harmonic tissue imaging, color Doppler and most recently 3- and 4-dimensional ultrasound. However, despite major strides made in the image quality, the business of ultrasound information management is lagging. Ultrasound data acquisition, image archiving and reporting are still in a state of flux. There is, however, a strong indication that this will gradually change, possibly very rapidly. This transformation is being accelerated by the finalization and implementation of standards for ultrasound reporting and image archiving. The long-awaited full implementation of the digital imaging in medicine standard (DICOM) and the recent addition of DICOM structured reporting (DICOM SR) will significantly

enhance our ability for uniform and consistent ultrasound information management and integration into EMR.

WHAT IS DICOM?

DICOM is an acronym for Digital Imaging and Communications in Medicine. In 1985, the American College of Radiology and National Electrical Manufacturers Association published a standard, which addressed the issue of vendor-independent data transfers for digital medical images. Such connectivity is important to cost-effectiveness in health care. DICOM users can provide ultrasound services within facilities and across geographic regions, gain maximum benefit from existing resources, and keep costs down through compatibility of new equipment and systems. For example, computer workstations, ultrasound scanners, laser printers and host computers and mainframes made by multiple vendors and located at one site or many sites can 'talk to one another' by means of DICOM across an 'open-system' network.

The DICOM standard has become a catalyst for change in the medical imaging community and has created exciting opportunities for all of those involved by shaping the future of how images are used in our specialty. The goals of DICOM are to achieve compatibility and to improve the efficiency of workflow between imaging systems and other information systems in health-care environments worldwide. Despite the recent upheavals in the ultrasound industry related to mergers and acquisitions, all major diagnostic imaging vendors have incorporated the DICOM standard into their products. The majority of the professional societies throughout the world have supported and participated in the enactment of the standard as well. DICOM is used or will soon be used by virtually every medical profession that utilizes images within the health-care industry.

In summary, DICOM is a standard for the communication of medical images and associated information. DICOM relies on explicit and detailed models of how the patients, images, reports, etc. involved in ultrasound operations are described and how they are related.

DICOM divides much of the specification into parts. This was done so that parts can be expanded without having to republish the whole standard. The current version of DICOM 3.0 consists of nine parts. For example, part 1 of DICOM is the document that provides an overview of the rest of the standard. It provides a description of the design principles, defines many of the terms used and gives a brief description of all the other parts. For a detailed description of all the nine parts, we refer the reader to an excellent DICOM review[7].

DICOM STANDARD REPORTING (DICOM SR)

DICOM is now expanding into an area of structured documents. In particular, it is within the scope of DICOM to develop standards for documents that incorporate references to images and associated data. The recently released DICOM Structured Reporting (SR) supplement does just that. This recent addition to the DICOM standard is being actively developed for areas of radiology and cardiology and we can expect to see some applications in our specialty soon. As noted above, DICOM is the preferred standard for exchanging medical images and new ultrasound hardware manufactured during the past 3 years includes DICOM as a standard part of the equipment. However, one of the major drawbacks that limit DICOM adoption into fetal medicine is the limited amount of patient demographic and clinical information that can be exchanged with images. Because clinical findings and reports were not part of the DICOM standard, DICOM SR created an international standard for the exchange of non-image data among the vendors of ultrasound equipment. DICOM SR addresses the need for a mechanism and process for interchanging non-image information, including findings and reports in a structured or coded form. For example, there could be an anomaly on a fetal ultrasound image, along with an electronic annotation on the image. DICOM SR provides developers and manufacturers with the data-encoding mechanism to describe that region of interest, including the circle or annotation, and associate it with the corresponding images. DICOM SR's ability to standardize information to be exchanged opens a variety of opportunities in the fetal imaging laboratory. These include the ability to incorporate information from the ultrasound and cytogenetic laboratory into a comprehensive prenatal genetic report, or to export measurements from a fetal examination into a database or report electronically. DICOM SR enables the ultrasound hardware to transmit information in a standardized fashion and therefore will become an integral part of our effort to provide full integration of patient data into an EMR.

DICOM AS AN INTERNATIONAL STANDARD

In the USA, interest in ultrasound imaging and the general interest in electronic medical records has fostered the development of a group that has representation from all of the medical informatics standards bodies and professional groups. This group is the Healthcare Informatics Standards Planning Panel (HISPP), sponsored by the American National Standards Institute (ANSI). ANSI is the US representative to the International Standards Organization (ISO) and is the formal conduit for information exchange with CEN, the body that has responsibility for all medical informatics standards in Europe. The ISO also provides official communication with the Japanese standards organizations. As standards develop, co-ordination through ANSI HISPP and its international counterparts is vital if the end products are to be compatible. A look at the international nature of the imaging equipment business should serve to illustrate the importance of standards considerations that go beyond national boundaries.

PICTURE ARCHIVING AND COMMUNICATIONS SYSTEMS (PACS) IN FETAL IMAGING

In the past several years picture archiving and communications systems (PACS) technology gained wide acceptance, especially among the larger and financially well-to-do radiology imaging groups[8]. Fetal imaging, on the other hand, with its hands-on nature of the examination, is unlike that of any other image-acquisition modality. Fetal imaging is complex; it deals with organ systems and it has a unique need for color images when examination of fetal heart and Doppler studies are performed. Fetal imaging examination typically begins with a screening examination performed by a sonographer, followed by a directed, more limited examination by a fetomaternal specialist. Therefore, ultrasound images obtained by the sonographer must be of superb quality, inclusive of all areas of interest and readily comparable to previous studies. In clinical practice, however, the reliance on static images in the interpretation of fetal studies is minimal. Fetal studies are most commonly documented on videotape and supplemented by numerous static images outputted into low-cost thermal printers. The limited need for static digital image storage combined with the high cost of PACS systems has hampered the proliferation of digital storage in fetal ultrasound imaging. This is not to say that there is no need for digital storage once a cost-effective solution becomes available. With DICOM becoming a standard part of the ultrasound hardware and the wide availability of low-cost software packages (around $1000) designed to store and display DICOM images, we might anticipate a proliferation of low-cost PACS systems in fetal imaging.

CONCLUSION

Health care trails all other industries in its acceptance of electronic methods for information management. According to the October 2001 report from the American Medical Association, less than 5% of US physicians use electronic record systems; the majority relies on antiquated, paper-based methods[9,10]. The proportion of maternal medicine subspecialists using electronic medical records is probably even less. Nonetheless, new regulations from the US Department of Health and Human Services could finally force the health-care providers to enter the digital age. None of the upcoming regulations prohibits the use of paper records, but they require health-care organizations to document and manage so much information that paper-based offices will probably find themselves unable to comply.

Streamlining administrative functions through the use of information technology, including more efficient input and access of information, will significantly increase operational efficiency and the ability of practices to meet changing industry demands with greater ease. A major shift in physicians' attitudes will also play a significant role in the adoption of EMRs. A new generation of tech-savvy physicians, who will begin to play a more informed decision-making role in how information technology is utilized, is emerging.

The intrinsic benefits of EMRs can alleviate physician frustrations with paper-based methods, including concerns with legibility, inability to access records remotely, inefficiency and an inability to look at patient trends. In addition, EMRs reduce the high costs most practices incur related to the use of paper records, including transcription and storage.

It is estimated that data capture and particularly transcription for paper-based record keeping costs the health-care industry approximately $15 billion annually. Over time, as a result of the implementation of an EMR system, practices can reduce or eliminate transcription, storage and transportation costs, as well as costs for clerical support, professional liability, insurance premiums and supplies.

The value of the non-tangible benefits of an EMR is clear, but until real financial gain (or a neutral monetary impact, but improved documentation and adherence to best practices) is proven, the decision to implement an EMR as a component of practice management may be still in the distant future.

We hope that the outline of the embryonic research presented in this chapter provides some guide for the future of the EMR in perinatal medicine. Perhaps, in several years when our younger colleagues are asked to rewrite this chapter, EMR will not be of much interest, because more exciting technological innovations will be looming on the horizon.

References

1. Rosen MG, Sokol RJ, Chik L. Use of computers in the labor and delivery suite: an overview. *Am J Obstet Gynecol* 1978;132:589–94

2. Chik L, Sokol J, Kooi R, Pillay S, Hirsch J, Zador I. A perinatal database management system. *Meth Inf Med* 1981;3:133–41

3. Smith RS, Bottoms SF. Ultrasonographic prediction of neonatal survival in extremely low-birth-weight infants. *Am J Obstet Gynecol* 1993;169:490–3

4. Sorokin Y, Blackwell SC, Reinke T, Kazzi N, Berman S, Bryant D. Demographic and intrapartum characteristics of term pregnancies with early-onset neonatal seizures. *J Perinatol* 2001;21: 90–2

5. Sokol RS, Chik L. Perinatal computing. An overview. *Acta Obstet Gynecol Scand (Suppl)* 1982; 109:7–10

6. The buzz on HIPAA. How HIPAA will affect the electronic transmission of health information. *Health Devices* 2000;12:472–6

7. Clunie DA. DICOM Structured reporting. A web based publication; *Pixel Med Publishing* http://www.pixelmed.com/srbook.html

8. Reed G, Smith EM. Planning for a multi-imaging center picture archiving and communications system. *J Digit Imaging* 2001;14(2 suppl 1):9–11

9. AMA Policies related to computer-based patient records and electronic medical records. http://www.ama-assn.org/ama/pub/category/2906.html

10. Mikulich VJ, Liu YC, Steinfeldt J, Schriger DL. Implementation of clinical guidelines through an electronic medical record: physician usage, satisfaction and assessment. *Int J Med Inf* 2001;63: 169–78

Low-molecular-weight heparin in perinatal medicine

27

D. Blickstein and I. Blickstein

INTRODUCTION

Anticoagulation is prescribed in almost all medical and surgical disciplines. It is primarily indicated for treating deep vein thrombosis (DVT) and pulmonary embolism (PE), or for thromboprophylaxis against a wide range of thromboembolic events. Thromboprophylaxis is used in two groups of patients. The first comprises patients at constant risk of thromboembolism such as those with prosthetic heart valves, recurrent thromboembolism or with atrial fibrillation. The second group comprises patients who are at increased risk of thrombosis for a limited duration, such as the postoperative period or during pregnancy and the puerperium.

In recent years, inherited and acquired conditions, termed thrombophilia, were recognized as underlying the increased risk of thromboembolic phenomena during pregnancy and the puerperium[1]. In addition to DVT and PE, thrombophilia was also associated with vascular pathologies in the uteroplacental unit leading to adverse pregnancy outcome[1-3] and a wider range of indications for anticoagulation during pregnancy and the puerperium.

In the past, clinicians had to choose between two forms of anticoagulants: the oral derivatives of warfarin and heparin. Following the seminal study of Hall *et al.*[4], who extensively reviewed numerous reports on adverse fetal and neonatal outcomes related to warfarin anticoagulation, the manufacturers have contraindicated their use during pregnancy. Warfarin is currently restricted to specific indications when other anticoagulants are judged to be inadequate, such as thromboprophylaxis in patients with prosthetic heart valves[5]. Treatment with heparin, although safe for the fetus, is associated with maternal side-effects and needs close monitoring.

During the past two decades a third preparation – low-molecular-weight heparin (LMWH) – has been added to the arsenal of anticoagulants. This chapter reviews the current use of LMWH in perinatal medicine.

WHAT IS LMWH?

Heparin is a heterogeneous substance consisting of glycosaminoglycans of various molecular weights ranging from 3 to 30 kD. The anticoagulant effect of heparin requires a plasma co-factor – antithrombin III (ATIII). Heparin binds to ATIII, producing a conformational change that converts antithrombin from a slow progressive thrombin inhibitor to a very rapid inhibitor of thrombin and factor Xa. LMWH is derived from heparin by chemical or enzymatic depolymerization, producing fragments of approximately one-third the size of heparin. It appears that these fragments of heparin bind to ATIII and inactivate mainly factor Xa, and have less ability to inactivate thrombin, because the small fragments cannot bind simultaneously to both thrombin and ATIII[6].

Many forms of LMWH are available. A short list of the various LMWH preparations approved for use in the USA, Canada and Europe is shown in Table 1. The preparations differ by their pharmacokinetic and anticoagulant properties, and may not be clinically interchangeable. The duration of activity of LMWHs is measured by the $t_{1/2}$ anti-Xa, given in hours. The longer the $t_{1/2}$ anti-Xa the longer the duration of action. Hence, $t_{1/2}$ anti-Xa indirectly influences dosing with the particular preparation. The affinity of the product is represented by the anti-Xa to anti-IIa ratio. The higher the ratio the better the inactivation by the product of factor Xa.

There are several advantages and disadvantages of LMWH compared to unfractionated heparin. LMWH is usually given by the subcutaneous route and rarely intravenously, whereas heparin is given via both routes. Heparin binds to circulatory and cellular proteins and therefore its bioavailability and half-life are significantly less than that of LMWH. Monitoring the level of anti-Xa during treatment with LMWHs is rarely indicated, whereas checking the partial thromboplastin time (PTT) is obligatory during treatment with unfractionated heparin. By contrast to unfractionated heparin, there is a predictable dose–response relationship with LMWH, which translates to weight-adjusted dosing without laboratory monitoring. Thus, despite the fact that LMWHs are more costly than unfractionated heparin, savings of hospital costs

and monitoring counterbalance this expense. It should be remembered that LMWHs are by all means heparins with potential heparin-related side-effects and cross-sensitivity. Patients with known sensitivity to heparin should therefore not receive LMWHs. Complications such as hemorrhagic events, osteoporosis and heparin-induced thrombocytopenia (HIT) do occur with LMWHs, although the latter complication occurs with a much lower frequency (0.1% versus 2–3%). Altogether, LMWHs are as effective and safe as are unfractionated heparins, and are more convenient for the patient. Table 2 summarizes the differences between the two products.

Heparin and LMWHs do not cross the placental barrier and their effect during pregnancy is purely maternal[8]. It should be stressed that not all LMWHs are approved for use during pregnancy, and one should consult with the local health authority concerning the available LMWH.

The various regimens of unfractionated heparin and LMWH are summarized in Table 3.

Table 1 *Characteristics of some common LMWH preparations. Adapted from reference 7*

Generic name	Brand name	$t_{1/2}$ anti-Xa (h)	Anti-Xa to anti-IIa ratio
Nadroparin	Fraxiparin	3.74 ± 0.68	3.2
Enoxaparin	Clexane	3.95 ± 0.65–4.37 ± 0.47	2.7
Dalteparin	Fragmin	2.81 ± 0.84	2
Tinzaparin	Innohep	2.97 ± 1.01	1.9
Reviparin	Clivarin	3.3 ± 1.0	3.5

Table 2 *Comparison between heparin and LMWH*

	Heparin	LMWH
Molecular weight (kD)	5–30	3–10
Anti-Xa to anti-IIa ratio	1 : 1	2–4 : 1
Administration	IV or SC	SC or IV (rare)
Monitoring	needed (PTT)	seldom needed (anti-Xa)
Bioavailability (%)	30	90
Cost (drug)	low	high
Cost (monitoring)	high	low
Complications		
hemorrhagic events	+ +	+
thrombocytopenia (HIT)	+	very rare
osteoporosis	+	rare
drug allergy	+	+

Table 3 *Regimens of unfractionated heparin and LMWH*

Regimen	Dosage
Minidose unfractionated heparin	SC, 5000 U q 12 h
Moderate-dose unfractionated heparin	SC, q 12 h, anti-Xa-adjusted dose
Adjusted-dose unfractionated heparin	SC, q 12 h, PTT-adjusted dose
Prophylactic LMWH	SC, dalteparin 5000 U q 24 h
	SC, enoxaparin 40 mg q 24 h
Adjusted-dose LMWH	weight-adjusted full treatment doses (i.e. enoxaparin 1 mg/kg, q 12 h)
Postpartum anticoagulants	warfarin with a target INR of 2–3

LMWH IN THE TREATMENT OF ACUTE VENOUS THROMBOEMBOLISM

The risk of venous thromboembolism (VTE) in pregnancy is approximately six times greater than in the non-pregnant state[9]. PE occurs in about one sixth of the patients with untreated DVT and is the most common cause of maternal mortality[9].

Guidelines regarding the management of VTE during pregnancy are regularly updated. In the early 1990s, it was suggested that LMWH be used for acute DVT and PE instead of full heparinization. Recently, the *6th American College of Chest Physicians (ACCP) Consensus Conference on Antithrombotic Therapy* (2001) suggested that LMWHs were as effective and safe as unfractionated heparin for the treatment of acute DVT. The current recommendations for the treatment of VTE during pregnancy are either (a) weight-adjusted dose LMWH throughout pregnancy, or (b) intravenous heparin for at least 5 days followed by PTT-adjusted dose of heparin for the remaining pregnancy. Postpartum anticoagulation therapy should be administered for at least 6 weeks.

THROMBOPROPHYLAXIS WITH LMWH

The overall risk of DVT during pregnancy (0.05–1.8%) is higher in women with a previous event of DVT, with a recurrence rate of 1 : 71 cases[9]. Currently, five groups of pregnant patients at increased risk of VTE have been identified:

(1) *VTE associated with a transient risk factor* (i.e. with bed-rest, oral contraception, etc.). These patients should be closely observed during pregnancy and receive postpartum anticoagulants.

(2) *Single episode of idiopathic VTE*. For these patients there are several options: (a) close observation, (b) mini- to moderate-dose unfractionated heparin or (c) prophylactic LMWH. In any case, all patients should receive postpartum anticoagulants.

(3) *Single episode of idiopathic VTE and thrombophilia*. The same recommendations as in group 2. Because of the higher risk for VTE, it is suggested to be more active and to administer thromboprophylaxis in patients with ATIII deficiency.

(4) *No prior VTE and thrombophilia*. For these patients there are several options: (a) close observation, (b) minidose unfractionated heparin or (c) prophylactic LMWH. In any case, all patients should receive postpartum anticoagulants. Again, thromboprophylaxis should be strongly considered in patients with ATIII deficiency.

(5) *Multiple episodes of VTE and/or long-term anticoagulation*. For these patients there are several options: (a) PTT-adjusted dose of unfractionated heparin, (b) prophylactic LMWH or (c) weight-adjusted LMWH. These patients should receive long-term anticoagulation postpartum.

In summary, if prophylactic treatment is considered, it should be tailored according to the risk group. Both heparin and LMWH are options, but it appears that LMWH will largely replace unfractionated heparins[10].

LMWH AND ADVERSE PREGNANCY OUTCOME

An efficient uteroplacental unit associated with optimal fetal growth and development may be compromised by states related to maternal thrombophilia. Studies published in the past few years have shown that inherited thrombophilias are not only associated with increased risk of VTE during pregnancy and the puerperium, but also with an increased risk of vascular pathologies in the uteroplacental unit leading to adverse pregnancy outcome, such as first- and second-trimester miscarriages, intrauterine growth restriction (IUGR), intrauterine fetal death, placental abruption and pre-eclampsia[1,11].

Critical reading of the literature reveals two nuances on these aspects. On the one hand are the data of the European Prospective Cohort On Thrombophilia (EPCOT) study, which show a certain contribution of thrombophilia to adverse perinatal outcome[12]. On the other hand, there are numerous series that show a definitive role of thrombophilia in the pathogenesis of several adverse pregnancy outcomes[13]. Currently, there are two main controversies. The first relates to the validity of the evidence associating thrombophilia and gestational thromboembolic phenomena, and the second relates to the appropriate selection of patients and the timing of prophylactic anti-thrombotic therapy to prevent pregnancy loss and associated pregnancy complications[14]. These conflicting views are expected to be clarified in the near future when the results of several ongoing multicenter prospective studies will be published. Current data on treatment for women with inherited thrombophilia and pregnancy loss are mostly uncontrolled and include small series of patients treated mostly with LMWH. In addition, the optimal dosage of LMWH to prevent thrombophilia-associated adverse pregnancy outcome is yet unknown and is currently under prospective randomized trials[15].

The *2001 ACCP Consensus Conference on Antithrombotic Therapy* recommends evaluation for inherited thrombophilia as well as for the acquired antiphospholipid antibody (APLA) syndrome in women with recurrent pregnancy loss, prior severe pre-eclampsia, IUGR, placental abruption, or otherwise unexplained fetal demise. Management of pregnant patients is then subgrouped into five categories[10]:

(1) *Pregnant patients with APLA and previous pregnancy complications*. Treatment should consist of low-dose aspirin plus either of the following options: (a) mini- to moderate-dose unfractionated heparin; or (b) prophylactic LMWH.

(2) *Homozygous women for MTHFR*. These should be treated with folic acid before pregnancy or as soon as pregnancy is confirmed.

(3) *Women with thrombophilia and previous adverse pregnancy outcome*. One should consider low-dose aspirin plus either (a) minidose heparin; or (b) prophylactic LMWH. These patients should receive postpartum anticoagulants.

(4) *Women with APLA syndrome and history of VTE*. Long-term anticoagulation (warfarin) should be switched to either adjusted-dose unfractionated or LMW heparins throughout pregnancy and resumption of the long-term anticoagulant postpartum.

(5) *Women with APLA syndrome but without history of VTE or pregnancy loss*. Four approaches have been suggested: (a) surveillance only; (b) mindose heparin; (c) prophylactic LMWH; or (d) low-dose aspirin.

PERIPARTUM LMWH

Treatment during pregnancy can cause persistent peripartum anticoagulation that may complicate delivery. No significant difference in hemorrhagic complications was observed between LMWHs, mainly enoxaparin and dalteparin, and unfractionated heparins. Although bleeding complications appear to be very uncommon with LMWH, it was suggested to discontinue therapy 24 h prior to invasive procedures or before induction of labor[16].

The relation between LMWH and regional (epidural or spinal) anesthesia raised many concerns. These concerns explain why labor induction or Cesarean birth should be a planned elective procedure in women receiving LMWHs at the end of pregnancy.

The incidence of neurological complications resulting from hemorrhage associated with neural block is estimated to be less than 1 : 150 000 epidurals and less than 1 : 220 000 spinal blocks, and obviously traumatic needle or catheter placement may increase the risk of a spinal hematoma. Because the anti-Xa level does not predict the risk of bleeding, this test is not helpful in the management of laboring patients.

To reduce the risk of anesthesia-related hematoma, regional blockade should start at least 12 h after the last prophylactic LMWH dose and longer (24 h) if the patient receives a weight-adjusted dose of LMWH. When continuous epidural analgesia is performed, LMWH can be restarted 2 h after catheter removal.

DEALING WITH COMPLICATIONS

As mentioned above, bleeding is a rare complication in patients receiving LMWH, and should be even rarer when planned peripartum management is carried out. However, when bleeding occurs in a patient receiving LMWH, the antidote is protamine sulfate, as it is with unfractionated heparin. One should remember that protamine sulfate incompletely neutralizes the anti-Xa activity of LMWH, probably because it does not bind to very-low-molecular-weight components[17].

Heparin-induced thrombocytopenia is a rare complication of LMWHs. Nevertheless, a platelet count is recommended every 4 days during the first month, and monthly thereafter. Patients with the APLA syndrome are more prone to develop HIT. When a pregnant woman who requires continued anticoagulation develops HIT, one should switch to the heparinoid danaparoid sodium (Orgaran®)[16]. This effective agent, with an anti-Xa to anti-IIa ratio of 20, has limited cross-reactivity with LMWH and was safely used during pregnancy.

Data on heparin-induced osteoporosis are derived from menopausal women and are of limited application to the pregnant state. The prospective evaluation of bone density in 16 women receiving a dose of 40 mg daily of enoxaparin sodium showed no significant change in the mean bone density measurement from baseline to 6 weeks postpartum[18]. It is nonetheless advisable to prescribe supplemental calcium for malnourished patients or when weight-adjusted LMWH is administered throughout pregnancy.

Owing to the cross-sensitivity of the LMWHs, a heparin-induced skin reaction cannot usually be treated by substitution of one preparation for another, but as with HIT, one should change to the heparinoid danaparoid sodium.

SUMMARY

LMWHs are effective anticoagulants that are gradually replacing unfractionated heparins for various indications in perinatal medicine. Compared with unfractionated heparin, LMWHs have longer plasma bioavailability, lower incidence of serious side-effects, and a more predictable dose–response without laboratory monitoring. LMWHs are significantly more convenient to the patients and are considered safe for the fetus. In addition to the treatment and prevention of VTE events during pregnancy and the puerperium, LMWHs are at present prescribed for the prevention of recurrent pregnancy complications. Despite the safety of LMWHs, a planned induction of labor or elective abdominal birth is advisable in order to minimize bleeding and regional analgesia-related complications.

References

1. Blickstein D, Blickstein I. Fetal consequences of maternal inherited hypercoagulable states (thrombophilia). In Chervenak FA, Kurjak A, eds. *Fetal Medicine: The Clinical Care of the Fetus as a Patient*. Carnforth, UK: Parthenon Publishing, 1999:288–93

2. Mousa HA, Alfirevic Z. Thrombophilia and adverse pregnancy outcome. *Croat Med J* 2001; 42:135–45

3. Brenner B. Inherited thrombophilia and pregnancy loss. *Thromb Haemost* 1999;82:634–40

4. Hall JG, Pauli RM, Wilson KM. Maternal and fetal sequelae of anticoagulation during pregnancy. *Am J Med* 1980;68:122–40

5. Chan WS, Anand SS, Ginsberg JS. Anticoagulation of pregnant women with mechanical heart valves. *Arch Intern Med* 2000;160:191–6

6. Hirsh J, Warkentin TE, Shaughnessy SG, *et al.* Heparin and low molecular weight heparin. *Chest* 2001;119:64S–94S

7. Samama MM, Gerotziafas GT. Comparative pharmacokinetics of LMWHs. *Semin Thromb Hemost* 2000;26:31–8

8. Fejgin MD, Lourwood DL. Low molecular weight heparins and their use in obstetrics and gynecology. *Obstet Gynecol Surv* 1994;49:424–31

9. Eldor A. Thrombophilia, thrombosis and pregnancy. *Thromb Haemost* 2001;86:104–11

10. Ginsberg JS, Greer I, Hirsh J. Use of antithrombotic agents during pregnancy. *Chest* 2001;119:122S–131S

11. Brenner B. Inherited thrombophilia and pregnancy loss. *Thromb Haemost* 1999;82:634–40

12. Prestoneon FE, Rosendaal FR, Walker ID, *et al.* Increased fetal loss in women with heritable thrombophilia. *Lancet* 1996;348:913–16

13. Kupferminc MJ, Eldor A, Steinman N, *et al.* Increased frequency of genetic thrombophilia in women with complications of pregnancy. *N Engl J Med* 1999;340:9–13

14. Blickstein D. Thrombophilia in obstetrics and gynecology. In Ben-Refael Z, Shoham Z, eds. *The Second World Congress on Controversies in Obstetrics, Gynecology and Infertility*. Bologna, Italy: Monduzzi Editore, 2001:105–9

15. Brenner B. Pregnancy and thrombophilia: are they related? Can the complications be prevented? In Ben-Refael Z, Shoham Z, eds. *The Second World Congress on Controversies in Obstetrics, Gynecology and Infertility*. Bologna, Italy: Monduzzi Editore, 2001: 119–24

16. Gris JC. Risks and benefits of low molecular weight heparins in obstetrics and gynecology. In Ben-Refael Z, Shoham Z, eds. *The Second World Congress on Controversies in Obstetrics, Gynecology and Infertility*. Bologna, Italy: Monduzzi Editore, 2001:125–8

17. Hirsh J, Levine MN. Low molecular weight heparin. *Blood* 1992;79:1–17

18. Casele HL. Prospective evaluation of bone density in pregnant women receiving the low molecular weight heparin enoxaparin sodium. *J Matern Fetal Med* 2000;9:122–5

Breast cancer and pregnancy   28

E. Mathieu, P. Merviel, E. Barranger, J. M. Antoine and S. Uzan

The association of breast cancer with pregnancy is rare. It is defined as the onset of breast cancer during pregnancy or during the year following delivery.

Since Wolkman's initial description of carcinomatous mastitis of pregnancy, the prognosis of these tumors has remained poor, mainly because of the patients' young age. The management of breast cancer associated with pregnancy is delicate and must be ensured by a multidisciplinary team of gynecologists, obstetricians and oncologists.

We will consider two different situations:

(1) Diagnosis of breast cancer during the course of a pregnancy or shortly after pregnancy;
(2) Pregnancy occurring after breast cancer.

Although the literature is currently rich in publications concerning these problems, they are essentially limited series or isolated cases and never randomized trials.

BREAST CANCER DURING PREGNANCY OR SHORTLY AFTER PREGNANCY

Epidemiology

Between 0.2 and 3.8% of all cases of breast cancer are associated with pregnancy[1]. The rate is 8% in women under 45 and 18% in women under 30. Breast cancer occurs during the course of one to three per 10 000 pregnancies, with a total of about 250 to 300 cases annually in France[2].

In a French multicenter study published in 1994[3], 60% of 178 cases of breast cancer associated with pregnancy occurred during the pregnancy (respectively, 37%, 33% and 30% during the first, second and third trimesters),

while the remaining 40% occurred during the first 6 months postpartum.

Mean age at onset ranges from 31.5 to 35 years[3] but is tending to increase, owing to the increasing number of late pregnancies, and especially to the increase in medically assisted reproduction.

Pathophysiology

Many authors consider that women who have a term pregnancy at a young age have a degree of protection against the risk of breast cancer, owing to the associated maturation of the mammary glands and the protective effect of progesterone. Conversely, pregnancy occurring later in life favors the growth of cells already transformed by menstrual estrogen secretion[4].

Several explanations have been forwarded for the occurrence and aggressiveness of pregnancy-associated breast cancer (PABC):

(1) A vascular theory, in which the arterio-venous and lymphatic hypervascularization occurring in pregnancy contributes to the higher proportion of patients who have node metastases or generalized cancer during pregnancy than outside pregnancy[5].
(2) An immunological theory, based on the immune tolerance induced by pregnancy. This is held to explain the lack of immune reactivity to neoplastic proliferation and the frequency of metastatic forms at diagnosis[6].
(3) A hormonal theory, in which prolactin is considered to be responsible for the poor prognosis of breast tumors diagnosed during the third trimester of pregnancy[7].

Histopathology

The histological types are the same as those occurring outside pregnancy[8]. The most frequent PABC are infiltrating ductal forms (78%), as in non-pregnant women under 40. Lobular forms represent 9% and medullary forms 4%[9].

The frequency of inflammatory tumors is increased in pregnancy, to 14.3% according to Tretli et al.[10] and to 25–28% according to Juret and Dargent[2]. However, it is difficult to evaluate the precise inflammatory nature of these tumors, owing to the edema and breast congestion of pregnancy; the latter probably explains why the frequency of forms is overestimated. Inflammatory tumors with overlying inflammation represent 33% of PABC cases, while carcinomatous mastitis represents 7.5%[3]. Pathologically, these tumors are characterized by their frequent multifocal nature, involvement of the nipple and dermis, neoplastic emboli of the dermal lymphatics and frequent axillary, supraclavicular or internal mammary node involvement.

The histoprognostic stage in the Scarff, Bloom and Richardson (SBR) classification is also higher. In a review of 200 cases of PABC, 8% were SBR1, 39% SBR2 and 53% SBR3[11].

Radioimmunohistochemical assay of hormone receptors is hindered by receptor saturation due to the high circulating hormone levels during pregnancy, but it can be performed.

Node invasion is more frequent, affecting 47% of patients according to Rosemond and Maier[12], and 89% according to Ribeiro and Palmer[13]. Petrek reported axillary node invasion in 61% of patients with PABC, compared to only 28% of control non-pregnant women[9]. Similarly, metastatic progression is more frequent, with rates ranging from 11 to 32%[3]. Distant metastases occur mainly in the liver, lungs and bone (as observed outside pregnancy), and sometimes in the placenta. Potter and Schoeneman[14] found placental metastases in patients with inflammatory PABC, although with no apparent impact on the outcome of pregnancy. Fetal metastases have never been described. The last authors recommended routine pathological examination of the placenta, as did Dunn in 1999[15].

Diagnosis

All breast abnormalities can and must be investigated during pregnancy. The diagnostic work-up is the same as in non-pregnant women, being based on clinical, radiological (mammography and especially sonography) and histological findings[16–18]. Breast cancer must be sought particularly before medically assisted reproduction, after age 38 or even 35, according to the team[19,20].

The breasts must be examined routinely in early pregnancy. The malignancy is often more advanced at diagnosis than outside pregnancy, with an interval between onset and diagnosis of 5 to 15 months according to the series[10]. According to Giacalone et al.[3], only 58% of these tumors measure 5 cm or less at diagnosis (stage T0: 0%; stage T1: 28.3%; stage T2: 43.2%), compared to 85% in non-pregnant women. The size of the lesion is frequently overestimated, with a mean clinical size of 47 mm, but a mean pathological size of only 30.9 mm. In the French study[3], 84.5% of women had single tumors, 8.5% had two distinct tumors and 7% had multifocal cancer.

Mammography (with uterine protection) is perfectly feasible during pregnancy, the delivered dose (10–50 mRad) being well below the toxic threshold (150 mRad before 12 weeks of amenorrhea, 1500 mRad thereafter)[21,22]. The results are sometimes difficult to interpret (40% false-negative rate), owing to breast congestion[23]. The main value of mammography is thus to reveal microcalcifications. Note that a normal mammogram does not rule out breast cancer.

Sonographic examination of the breasts is particularly valuable in this setting, and can also be used to guide needle biopsy. Fine-needle aspiration cytology is only meaningful if positive, as is the case outside pregnancy. It has poor positive-predictive value in this context, owing to the lobular hyperplasia frequently associated with pregnancy. Cytological examination of a discharge can contribute to the diagnosis. Histological examination (Tru-Cut biopsy under local anesthesia) is the key to diagnosis, with a sensitivity and specificity of 94%.

The extension work-up must comprise a chest radiograph and sonography of the liver; scintigraphy, skeletal radiography and computed tomography must only be done after delivery[24]. Tumor marker values (CA 15-3 and ACE) are difficult to interpret during pregnancy[25].

Prognosis

Maternal prognosis

The prognostic factors in PABC are the same as those in non-pregnant women, with one or two minor exceptions:

(1) Diagnostic delay is pejorative: the initial disease is more likely to be advanced (24% of Pev forms, versus 4% outside pregnancy) and metastatic (11% versus 2.5%)[3].

(2) The woman's age seems to have more influence on survival than does onset during pregnancy or the postpartum period. These cases of breast cancer occurring in young women are characterized by the high frequency of forms with poorer prognosis (T2–3, SBR II and III, BRCA1 or 2 mutations)[26].

Overall, the vital prognosis of women with pregnancy-associated breast cancer is poor. Giacalone et al.[3], in a series of 178 cases, found a lower survival probability in pregnant versus non-pregnant women, both at 3 years (57% versus 74%) and at 5 years (43% versus 64%). Overall survival is therefore reduced by about 10–15%, although these differences seem to dwindle in the longer term[24]. According to Gemignani and Moore, the poor prognosis is due to the young age of these patients. Stage for stage, pregnancy does not modify the prognosis[27,28].

Fetal prognosis

This is determined by two main risks, namely prematurity (usually iatrogenic)[29] and low birth weight. The latter is partly due to the increased risk of prematurity, but may also be favored by the mother's altered general state and by possible placental metastases[30]. In a retrospective study of 119 pregnancies associated with breast cancer, Zemlikis et al. reported miscarriage in 10.1% of cases, therapeutic abortion in 18.4% and live births in 71.5%. Cesarean section was used for 26% of deliveries, in order to allow treatment of breast cancer to be started more rapidly in 82% of cases[31].

Therapeutic management

A balance must be struck between treating the mother as rapidly as possible and respecting the fetus.

Therapeutic abortion is not routinely warranted, as it does not, in itself, have any positive impact on maternal outcome. In 1996 and 2000, therapeutic abortion was considered unhelpful by Espié and Cuvier[32,33]. Indeed, breast cancer can be treated during pregnancy. However, the mother's choice between termination and treatment while pregnant will depend on the prognosis, which must be clearly discussed with her. The main prognostic factors (apart from the prognosis factors of the tumor itself: tumor stage, node (N) involvement, SBR, receptors, flow cytometry, Cer2b2) are the term of pregnancy at diagnosis, parity and the patient's decision on whether to continue or terminate her pregnancy.

Treatment principles are the following:

(1) Surgery is generally possible, although it is more hemorrhagic owing to local congestion and hypervascularization[29], especially close to term. Treatment can be conservative if radiotherapy can be administered rapidly, but the best treatment is often mastectomy. In 1998, among a series of 22 patients with stage T1 or T2 breast cancer, Kuerer[34] used conservative treatment in nine cases and mastectomy

in 13, and found no significant survival difference between the two groups.

(2) Anesthesia must be administered with the usual precautions during pregnancy, including fetal monitoring.

(3) Radiotherapy must be avoided during the period of organogenesis and should be reserved, if possible, for the postpartum period. Indeed, even when administered after day 42 of pregnancy, radiotherapy has been implicated in cases of neurological abnormalities, intrauterine growth retardation, fetal death *in utero*, chromosomal mutations in offspring and postnatal leukemia[25].

(4) Chemotherapy can be started during the fourth month, as there are teratogenic and mutagenic risks during the first trimester (miscarriage, and organ, gonadal and skeletal damage). It must be continued until term, but delivery should be avoided during the 3 weeks following the last course. In a study of 164 women who received chemotherapy during pregnancy, Murray *et al*. reported finding birth defects in 11.5% of neonates exposed in the first trimester, while the risk appeared to be nil after exposure in the second and third trimesters[35]. Similarly, after reviewing the literature, Bernik *et al*.[36] in 1998 and Berry *et al*.[37] in 1999 concluded that chemotherapy could be used from the fourth month of pregnancy. Giacalone's 1999 study[38] focused on 20 women who received chemotherapy while pregnant. Mean gestational age during the first course was 26 weeks, and delivery occurred at a mean term of 34.7 weeks. Two patients received chemotherapy during the first trimester, and miscarriage and intrauterine death occurred during the second trimester. There were five complications of prematurity (transient respiratory distress syndrome) and three complications of chemotherapy (anemia, leukopenia and IUGR). The 16 children with long-term follow-up (mean 42.3 months) developed normally. Thus, 95% of pregnancies exposed to chemotherapy gave rise to live births, with little morbidity. However, follow-up data are currently inadequate, and women must be warned that many uncertainties remain.

The study by Berry *et al*.[37] concerned 24 women receiving chemotherapy for breast cancer during pregnancy. These patients, who had primary cancer or recurrences, received four chemotherapy cycles, from the second quarter, including fluorouracil, doxorubicin and cyclophosphamide, with no antenatal complications. The Apgar score, birth weight and neonatal course were normal. The authors concluded that breast cancer could be treated with chemotherapy from the beginning of the fourth month of pregnancy, without major complications for childbirth or neonatal stage, despite the absence of prospective and randomized trials. One case of fetal cardiac toxicity of doxorubicin was described but not confirmed[39]. Cyclophosphamide, vinca-alkaloids, antracyclines, epirubicin and Navelbine can be used during pregnancy. The doxorubicin and FEC should be preferred[40]. There are no data on neoadjuvant chemotherapy during pregnancy.

(5) Hormone therapy must not be used during pregnancy, because it has no proven efficacy and may be teratogenic[41]. However, Isaacs *et al*.[42] reported a recent case of tamoxifen treatment for metastatic breast cancer during pregnancy, without adverse effects. Most authors consider that this treatment should only be envisaged in the postpartum period, possibly in combination with chemical castration (according to hormone receptor status).

(6) Maternal breast-feeding is contraindicated, especially during chemotherapy.

(7) Antenatal counselling is crucial to inform the couple of the risks of the various options. Thorough fetal and obstetric monitoring is necessary, with clinical, biological and sonographic examinations at relatively short intervals. Some authors recommend routine amniocentesis before starting chemotherapy. If

the chemotherapy regimen is potentially cardiotoxic, fetal echocardiography should be done in a specialized unit. Maternal monitoring should focus on gastrointestinal, infectious and hematological complications; in particular, there is a danger of aplasia and clotting disorders close to term.

Certain risks should be anticipated in the newborn, such as neutropenia, respiratory distress, gastroenteritis and septicemia, especially if the fetus has been exposed to chemotherapy less than 3 weeks before birth. These children require long-term follow-up to detect gonadal, endocrine (thyroid and adrenal), oncological and hematological disorders.

The choice of treatment thus depends on the individual patient. It must be made by a multidisciplinary team and explained to the patient first. The following therapeutic indications may be proposed[25]:

(1) When the diagnosis is made during the first trimester, therapeutic abortion should be offered, but the mother's decision is final. If the tumor is progressive or metastatic at diagnosis, therapeutic abortion is strongly recommended[25]; treatment of the cancer can be started immediately afterwards. If the woman decides to continue with her pregnancy, treatment during the first trimester is surgical (including mastectomy), complementary treatment being postponed until the second trimester, if possible.

(2) During the second trimester, surgery is feasible and delivery should be induced as soon as the fetus is viable. Complementary treatment can be started postpartum. If neoadjuvant chemotherapy is indicated immediately, it can be started during the fourth month of pregnancy. Note that the last course must be scheduled at least 3 weeks before the likely date of delivery. Surgery is then performed in the immediate postpartum. When breast cancer is diagnosed during the third trimester, delivery is usually induced before starting treatment.

Routine physical examination of the breasts in early pregnancy, followed, if there is the slightest doubt, by sonography and biopsy, will reduce the diagnostic delay and hasten treatment of the mother. The poor prognosis of breast cancer associated with pregnancy is due more to the frequency of inflammatory and metastatic forms, and to these women's young age, than to the pregnancy itself.

PREGNANCY AFTER BREAST CANCER

A growing number of women are choosing to have children after being treated for breast cancer. Indeed, 10% of all new cases of breast cancer diagnosed in France (more than 25 000 cases) involve women under 40 years of age. Of young women treated for breast cancer 7% become pregnant, less than 2 years after treatment in 72% of cases[43]. Three questions arise in this setting:

(1) Fertility after breast cancer treatment;
(2) The influence of pregnancy on the prognosis of breast cancer;
(3) The optimal moment to conceive after breast cancer treatment.

Effects of adjuvant treatments for breast cancer on ovarian function and fertility

Many of these young and potentially fertile women wish to know the effects of adjuvant treatment on their fertility and the potential impact of a future pregnancy on their prognosis. Medical adjuvant treatments such as chemotherapy, tamoxifen and gonadotropin releasing hormone (GnRH) analog are increasingly prescribed and can transiently or permanently affect fertility.

Cyclophosphamide and alkylating agents are the leading cause of amenorrhea and ovarian insufficiency. They are linked not only to age, but also to the dose and duration of treatment[44]. In 1999, Lower et al.[45] reported the occurrence of amenorrhea in a third of women receiving chemotherapy for breast cancer among a population of 109 nonmenopausal women; menopause occurred within 1 year after chemotherapy in 45% of cases. Menstrual abnormalities are more frequent after age 35 years ($p < 0.005$), but 28% of women under 35 develop persistent disorders.

The fertility rate after chemotherapy has been estimated at approximately 8% before age 40 and 11% before age 35[25].

Influence of a new pregnancy on the prognosis of previously treated breast cancer

A number of arguments point to a negative impact of pregnancy on the prognosis of breast cancer. In a population of 126 non-menopausal women treated with neoadjuvant chemotherapy for breast cancer, Poikonen et al.[46] observed a beneficial influence ($p = 0.02$) of chemotherapy-induced amenorrhea and irregular menses on the 5-year disease-free survival rate among young patients with receptor-positive tumors.

The individual prognosis of women with previously treated breast cancer will, of course, influence their decision to start a pregnancy. However, even for women with good-prognosis breast cancer, questions remain as to the role of estrogen in the growth acceleration and activation of micro-metastases, and the role of the hormones of pregnancy in tumor recurrence. Despite these data, it seems that pregnancy occurring after treatment of good-prognosis breast cancer does not worsen the outcome. In contrast, poor-prognosis cancer tends to contraindicate pregnancy, if only for 'familial' reasons.

Published retrospective studies generally show acceptable survival rates when pregnancy occurs after treatment of breast cancer; for example, in 1989, Clark and Chua[43] reported a 5-year survival rate of 78% ($n = 136$).

Retrospective case–control studies mostly show similar survival rates among women with a history of breast cancer of a given stage, regardless of subsequent pregnancies. In 1999, Velentgas et al.[47] compared 53 women who became pregnant after breast cancer with similar women who did not become pregnant, on the basis of the stage at diagnosis and

relapse-free survival. Sixty-eight per cent of the pregnant women had at least one live birth. Miscarriage occurred in 24% of cases (versus 18% in a comparable population with no history of breast cancer). The relative risk of death among women who become pregnant after breast cancer was 0.8 (0.3–2.3) after adjustment for age. These results do not therefore suggest that pregnancy after breast cancer has a negative effect on survival.

The prognostic influence of pregnancy 5 years after breast cancer ($n = 50$) was studied by Von Schoultz et al.[48] in a population of 2119 women under age 50 with operable breast cancer treated in Sweden between 1971 and 1988. The authors found no detrimental effect of pregnancy on the outcome of breast cancer. After adjustment for age and node status, the relative risk of death among pregnant women after breast cancer, compared to non-pregnant women, was 0.48 ($p = 0.14$; median survival 7 years), suggesting the possibility of a reduction in the risk of distant metastasis.

A study[49] based on the Danish breast cancer register between 1977 and 1997 examined the relative risk of death among women who became pregnant after breast cancer and women who did not. Among a total of 5725 women under age 45, 173 became pregnant after being treated for breast cancer. Patients who took their pregnancy to term after breast cancer treatment had a non-significant reduction in the risk of death (relative risk 0.55 (95% CI 0.28–1.06), $p = 0.08$) compared with those who did not, after adjustment for age at diagnosis, disease stage and reproductive history before diagnosis of cancer.

Recently, 94 patients who became pregnant after diagnosis of early-stage breast cancer were identified in institutions participating in International Breast Cancer Study Group (IBCSG) studies. A comparison group of 188 was obtained by randomly selecting, from the IBCSG database, two patients matched for nodal status, tumor size, age and year of diagnosis, and who were free of relapse for at least as long as the time between breast cancer diagnosis and completion of pregnancy for each pregnant patient. The study of 5- and

10-year survival percentages indicated that subsequent pregnancy does not adversely affect the prognosis of early-stage breast cancer[50].

Thus, terminating a pregnancy that occurs after breast cancer does not appear to improve the subsequent prognosis.

Optimal time to start a pregnancy after breast cancer therapy

Pregnancy after breast cancer must not be considered as a negative event for prognosis. For women with good-prognosis tumors (carcinoma *in situ*; T1, SBR I, Rh positive, N negative carcinoma) the optimal 'minimal' interval between the end of cancer treatment and conception is 1 year[51].

For women with breast cancer of other stages, local recurrence rate is maximum after 2 years in N negative patients, and after 4 years in N positive patients[52,53]. Clark's study[43] of 136 patients showed that 72% of pregnancies occurred a mean of 2 years after the end of treatment for breast cancer. Women who conceived within 6 months of the end of treatment had a poorer prognosis than those who conceived between 6 and 24 months later, with 5-year survival rates of, respectively, 54 and 78%. The survival rate was 100% among women who waited 5 years or more to conceive. The optimal interval is thus probably 5 years for these women, and always after the end of tamoxifen treatment.

Pregnancies occurring after breast cancer do not carry particular risks. They require more intensive monitoring, but the risk of complications, especially birth defects, does not appear to be increased. Breast-feeding should be avoided, however. These pregnancies must be planned:

(1) Effective contraception must be used until pregnancy (if authorized).
(2) Before authorizing pregnancy, it is preferable to have a multidisciplinary team examine the patient's entire file, focusing on initial prognostic factors.

CONCLUSION

The care of pregnant breast cancer patients is a challenging clinical situation that, historically, has sought to strike a balance between maternal and fetal outcome. For women in this situation, the emotions surrounding pregnancy can be overshadowed by those aroused by the diagnosis of breast cancer and its subsequent treatment. The risk to the unborn child plays a major role in the decision process. Overall, the prognosis of patients with pregnancy-associated breast cancer is worse because a large proportion of patients have more advanced disease at diagnosis. However, stage for stage, the prognosis is similar.

References

1. Kitchen P, McLeman D. Breast cancer and pregnancy. *Med J Aust* 1987;147:337–9
2. Dargent D. *Cancer du sein et grossesse*. Traité d'obstétrique: pathologie médico-chirurgicale de la grossesse. Paris: Masson, 1985:210–20
3. Giacalone PL, Bonnier P, Laffargue F, Dilhuydy MH, Piana L. Cancer du sein pendant la grossesse. Etude multicentrique à propos de 178 cas. Presented at *XVIèmes Journées Nationales de la Société Française de Sénologie et de Pathologie Mammaire*. Dijon, 1994
4. Cappelaere P. Cancer du sein et grossesse. In *Cours Supérieur Francophone de Cancérologie: Le Cancer du Sein*. Paris: ICI Pharma éditeur, 1992
5. King RM, Welch JS, Martin JK, Coulan CB. Carcinoma of the breast associated with pregnancy. *Surg Gynecol Obstet* 1985;160:228–32
6. Barnavon Y, Wallack M. Management of the pregnant patient with carcinoma of the breast. *Surg Gynecol Obstet* 1990;171:347–52
7. Haagensen C. The treatment of breast carcinoma occurring during pregnancy or lactation. In

Diseases of the Breast. London: Saunders, 1971

8. Slavin JL, Billson VR, Ostor AG. Nodular breast lesions during pregnancy and lactation. *Histopathology* 1993;22:481–5

9. Petrek J, Dukoff R, Rogatko A. Prognosis of pregnancy associated breast cancer. *Cancer* 1991; 67:869–72

10. Tretli S, Kvalheim G, Thoresen S, Host H. Survival of breast cancer patients diagnosed during pregnancy or lactation. *Br J Cancer* 1988;58:382–4

11. Dargent D, Mayer M, Lansac J, Carret JL. Cancer du sein et grossesse: à propos de 96 cas. *J Gynecol Obstet Biol Reprod (Paris)* 1976;5:783–804

12. Rosemond G, Maier W. The complication of pregnancy on breast cancer? In *Breast Cancer Management. Early and Late*. London: Heinemann, 1971:227–35

13. Ribeiro GG, Palmer MK. Breast carcinoma associated with pregnancy: a clinician's dilemma. *Br J Med* 1977;2:1524–7

14. Potter J, Schoeneman M. Metastasis of maternal cancer to the placenta and fetus. *Cancer* 1970; 25:380–8

15. Dunn JS. Breast carcinoma metastatic to the placenta. *Obstet Gynecol* 1999;10(6):747–51

16. Uzan S, Gaudet R. Cancers du sein: épidémiologie, anatomie pathologique, dépistagre, diagnostic, évolution, principes du traitement. *La revue du Praticien* 1998;48:787–96

17. Barrat J, Marpeau L, Demuynck B. Cancer du sein et grossesse. *Rev Fr Gynecol Obstet* 1993;88: 544–9

18. Sorosky JL, Scott-Conner CEH. Breast disease complicating pregnancy. *Obstet Gynecol Clin North Am* 1998;25(2):353–63

19. Venn A, Watson L, Bruinsma F, Giles G, Healy D. Risk of cancer after use of fertility drugs with *in-vitro* fertilisation. *Lancet* 1999;354(9190):1573–4

20. Rossing MA, Daling JR. Complexity of surveillance for cancer risk associated with *in-vitro* fertilisation. *Lancet* 1999;354(9190):1586–90

21. Gorins A, Lenhardt F, Espié M. Cancer du sein et grossesse: épidémiologie, diagnostic, pronostic. *Contracept Fertil Sex* 1996;24:153–6

22. Samuels TH, Liu FF, Yaffe M, Haider M. Gestational breast cancer. *Can Assoc Radiol J* 1998; 49(3):172–80

23. Donegan W. Breast cancer with pregnancy. In Ariel IM, Cahan AC, eds. *Treatment of Precancerous Lesions and Early Breast Cancer*. Baltimore: Williams and Wilkins, 1993:214–22

24. Querleu D, Crepin G, Verhaeghe M, Laurent LC, Demaille LC, Lesoin A, Evain P. Cancer du sein et grossesse: quelle attitude adopter en 1985? In Masson, ?, ed. *VII Journées de la Société Française de Sénologie et de Pathologie Mammaire*. Paris, 1985: 285–92

25. Merviel P, Salat-Baroux J, Uzan S. Cancer du sein et grossesse. *Bull Cancer* 1996;83(4):266–75

26. Bonnier P. Le jeune âge est-il un facteur pronostic des cancers du sein? In *Pathologie du Sein de la Femme Jeune*. 1994:209–26

27. Moore HC, Foster RS. Breast cancer and pregnancy. *Semin Oncol* 2000;27(6):646–53

28. Gemignani ML, Petrek JA. Breast cancer during pregnancy: diagnostic and therapeutics dilemmas. *Adv Surg* 2000;34:273–86

29. Mignot L. Grossesse et cancer du sein. In Espie M, Gorins A, eds. *Le Sein*. Paris: Eska éd, 1995: 528–33

30. Cappelaere P, Querleu D, Demaille A. Influence de la grossesse sur l'évolution et le pronostic du cancer. In *Médecine Perinatale*. Paris: Arnette éd, 1986:129–38

31. Zemlikis D, Lishner M, Degendorfer P, Panzarella T, Burke B, Sutcliffe FB, Koren G. Maternal and fetal outcome after breast cancer in pregnancy. *Am J Gynecol Obstet* 1992;166:781–7

32. Espié M, Cuvier C. Traitement du cancer du sein pendant la grossesse. *Contracept Fertil Sex* 1996; 24(11):805–10

33. Cuvier C, Espié M. Traitement du cancer du sein pendant la grossesse. *Oncologie* 2000;2(5):276–82

34. Kuerer HM, Cunningham JD, Bleiweiss IJ, Doucette JT, Divino CM, Brower ST, Tartter PI. Conservative surgery for breast carcinoma associated with pregnancy. *Breast J* 1998;4(3):171–6

35. Murray CL, Reicher JA, Anderson J, Twiggs LB. Multimodal cancer therapy for breast cancer in the first trimester of pregnancy. *J Am Med Assoc* 1984;252:2607–8

36. Bernik SF, Bernik TR, Whooley BP, Wallack MK. Carcinoma of the breast during pregnancy: a review and update on treatment options. *Surg Oncol* 1998;7(1,2):47–9

37. Berry DL, Theriault RL, Holmes FA, Parisi VM, Booser DJ, Singletary SE, Buzdar AU, Hortobagyi GN. Management of breast cancer during pregnancy using a standardized protocol. *J Clin Oncol* 1999;17(3):855–61

38. Giacalone PL, Laffargue F, Benos P. Chemotherapy for breast carcinoma during pregnancy: a French National Survey. *Cancer* 1999;86(11):2266–72

39. Meyer-Wittkopf M, Barth H, Emons G, Schmidt S. Fetal cardiac effects of doxorubicin therapy for carcinoma of the breast during pregnancy: case report and review of the literature. *Ultrasound Obstet Gynecol* 2001;18(1):62–6

40. Williams S, Schilsky R. Antineoplastic drugs administration during pregnancy. *Semin Oncol* 2000;27(6):618–22

41. Halaviki-Clarke L, Cho E, Onojafe I, Liao DJ, Clarke R. Maternal exposure to Tamoxifen during pregnancy increases carcinogen-induced

mammary tumourigenesis among female rat offspring. *Clin Cancer Res* 2000;6(1):305–8

42. Isaacs RJ, Hunter W, Clark K. Tamoxifen as systemic treatment of advanced breast cancer during pregnancy – case report and literature review. *Gynecol Oncol* 2001;80(3):405–8

43. Clark RM, Chua T. Breast cancer and pregnancy: the ultimate challenge. *Clin Oncol (R Coll Radiol)* 1989;1(1):11–18

44. Reichman BS, Green KB. Breast cancer in young women: effect of chemotherapy on ovarian function, fertility and birth defects. *J Natl Cancer Inst Monogr* 1994;16:125–9

45. Lower EE, Blau R, Gazder P, Tummala RJ. The risk of premature menopause induced by chemotherapy for early breast cancer. *Women's Health Gend Based Med* 1999;8(7):949–54

46. Poikonen P, Saarto T, Elomaa I, Joensuu H, Blomqvist C. Prognostic effect of amenorrhea and elevated serum gonadotropin levels induced by adjuvant chemotherapy in premenopausal node-positive breast cancer patients. *Eur J Cancer* 2000;36(1):43–8

47. Velentgas P, Daling JR, Malone KE, Weiss NS, Williams MA, Self SG, Mueller BA. Pregnancy after breast carcinoma: outcomes and influence on mortality. *Cancer* 1999;85(11):2424–32

48. Von Schoultz E, Johansson H, Wilking N. Influence of prior and subsequent pregnancy on breast cancer prognosis. *J Clin Oncol* 1995;13: 430–4

49. Kroman N, Jensen MB, Melby M. Should women be advised against pregnancy after breast-cancer treatment? *Lancet* 1997;350:319–322

50. Gelber S, Coates AS, Goldhirsch A, Castiglione-Gertsch M, Marini G, Lindtner J, Edelmann DZ, Gudgeon A, Harvey V, Gelber RD. Effect of pregnancy on overall survival after the diagnosis of early-stage breast cancer. *J Clin Oncol* 2001; 19(6):1671–5

51. Serin D, Escoute M. Cancer du sein et grossesse. In Namer M, ed. *Cancer du Sein: Compte-Rendu du Cours Supérieur Francophone de Cancérologie.* Springer, 2001

52. Hery M. Facteurs pronostiques des cancers du sein sans envahissement ganglionnairepN0. Histoire naturelle des cancers du sein N–. Evolution des facteurs pronostiques en fonction du temps. *Oncologie* 2000;2(5):255–60

53. Kerbrat P. Cancer du sein N+. Analyse des récidives locales chez 2970 patientes traitées dans 6 études prospectives. In *Le Sein Inflammatoire Malin. Les Récidives Loco-régionales.* Toulouse: Arnette, 2000:129–68

Substance abuse during pregnancy 29

L. S. Voto and A. J. Siufi

INTRODUCTION

The issue of substance abuse in pregnancy continues to be a major health concern. This review focuses on two aspects of its untoward fetal effects:

(1) The toxic fetal effects;
(2) The neonatal withdrawal syndrome.

It is of the utmost importance to make all updated information available to the obstetrician and neonatologist to allow them to recognize and manage these entities. The purpose of this paper was to analyze and comment on the information in the literature and add our experience on clinical presentation, differential diagnosis, therapeutic options and perinatal results associated with intrauterine drug exposure.

FREQUENCY AT THE DALMACIO VELEZ SARSFIELD HOSPITAL, BUENOS AIRES, ARGENTINA

No conclusive statistical studies on drug addiction in pregnancy are available for Argentina. However, the Pregnant Adolescents Office at the Dalmacio Vélez Sársfield Hospital, Buenos Aires, Argentina, has determined the frequency of this condition among its population. Most patients attending this office come from the Buenos Aires quarter called Ciudadela and especially from Fuerte Apache, one the lowest socioeconomic zones in Buenos Aires. In 1998 we performed a cross-sectional study by means of a questionnaire and found out that half of our pregnant population had taken some kind of illicit drug on at least one occasion during pregnancy, although less than 1% of them reported habitual substance abuse.

Several publications[1,2] have reported that the incidence of intrauterine exposed newborns ranges from 3 to 50% depending on the study target population. The largest urban areas tend to show increasing rates.

During the year 2000 the Dalmacio Vélez Sársfield Hospital recorded 1900 deliveries. Of these, 1050 patients underwent an ELISA radioimmunoassay for HIV, rendering 14 reactive tests. Four of these HIV-positive patients kept attending our hospital and underwent preventive treatment to avoid vertical transmission. Therefore, HIV screening allowed for the detection of 1.4% of infected patients. It is mandatory that developing countries adopt routine screening methods to prevent vertical HIV transmission. Prenatal detection of substance abuse should be routinely screened as well, as most of the neonates born to such patients, either intoxicated or in withdrawal, are admitted to the NICU without a diagnosis and treated for other pathologies.

DIAGNOSIS

Maternal substance abuse should be disclosed during pregnancy and recorded in the clinical history of the patient, regardless of the magnitude of the addiction, to establish the degree of fetal involvement and to reduce this risk factor through modification of maternal behavior.

What are the risk factors?

The following risk factors may be identified:

(1) Family conflict situations and, consequently, the untoward effects of the home

environment have negative influences on the child.

(2) Unmarried pregnant adolescents display a four times higher incidence of illicit drug abuse, excluding marijuana[3].

(3) Home violence is strongly related to substance abuse. An individual shows a five-fold and three-fold incidence of substance abuse in cases when he or she has been raped or physically assaulted, respectively[4]. The incidence of severe depression and suicidal attempts is greater in this population than the general mean[5,6].

(4) Argentina also holds an association between the tattoo culture and drug addiction.

How do we diagnose?

The clinical history based on information provided by the patient herself has traditionally been used to establish the prevalence and frequency of substance abuse. However, this method is subject to deceit and minimization.

Urine toxicological screening during prenatal visits has become a possibility to detect substance abuse, although its high cost ($60 for each determination) is a drawback in developing countries like Argentina. Moreover, fraud is also possible if the patient stops substance abuse a few days before urine tests are scheduled. Besides, this screening provides information about drug addiction but not about abuse patterns, mental condition or physical alterations resulting from it. Although cocaine is rapidly metabolized and disappears from human serum within a few hours of consumption, its metabolites benzoylecgonine and methylestherecgonine are excreted in the urine for prolonged periods of time and reach higher concentrations in urine than in serum. Radioimmunoassay is the most sensitive method and may detect urinary benzoylecgonine concentrations of 2–20 ng/ml even 4–5 days after cocaine abuse. False-negative results may be caused by an undetectable concentration of benzoylecgonine or, in the case of enzymatic methods, by alterations in urinary concentration or pH. False-positive results are rare because of the lack of cross-reactivity with other drugs or therapeutic agents. Most drug screening procedures show high sensitivity but low specificity; therefore, a positive urine test should be confirmed with a more sensitive and specific method. These confirmatory methods are gas chromatography, with or without mass spectrophotometry, and high-performance liquid chromatography; these show both high sensitivity and high specificity but are technically more complex and time-consuming. The timing of the last cocaine ingestion may be calculated through the relationship among the benzoylecgonine, methylestherecgonine and cocaine dosages.

Identification of drug-exposed newborns

Urinary tests Drug metabolite detection in neonatal urine may fail, depending on the time elapsed since the last maternal drug usage or on the moment of urinary collection. For instance, a test may render a negative result if the mother stopped using drugs a few days before delivery or if the urine sample was not obtained immediately after birth.

Hair tests These tests display some technical difficulties both in the procedure and in the collection of neonatal samples.

Meconium tests As in adults, the fetal liver metabolizes drugs into hydrosoluble derivatives excreted in the bile and urine. In the fetus, drug metabolites accumulate in the meconium either by biliary defecation or through the presence of metabolites in the amniotic fluid, or both. The fetus rarely defecates *in utero*; therefore, fetal waste products accumulate throughout gestation. These factors may explain why drug metabolite concentrations and recovery are higher in meconium than in neonatal urine, which is in fact excreted *in utero*. The fact that meconium analysis is easy and rapid, highly sensitive and specific, turns it into the test of choice to detect intrauterine drug exposure. Meconium is easily collected directly from the diaper. The test may be positive even 2–3 days after birth. Cocaine was the drug most commonly detected in meconium tests, followed by opiates. Radioimmunoassay for the detection of opiates also detects morphine and heroin, but not methadone. Therefore, any medication containing codeine and used significantly during pregnancy may be detected as an opiate in the meconium test. The analgesics used during labor, such as meperidine, do not cross-react with the opiate radioimmunoassay, except when administered at very elevated concentrations.

The spectrum of fetal effects caused by these drugs may be compared with an iceberg: the top represents the effects easily identifiable through the information reported by the mother or the neonatal clinical manifestations. Beneath there is a considerable group of exposed neonates apparently normal at birth and whose mothers deny substance abuse. These neonates may be detected only by using a high degree of suspicion based on maternal characteristics, meconium screening in the neonatal period or specially designed questionnaires.

Screening through questionnaires designed specifically to detect substance abuse This has proved to be more sensitive than urinary tests and to have a lower rate of false-negative results. The Substance Abuse Subtle Screening Inventory (SASSI)[7] and the Michigan Alcohol Screening Test (MAST), among others, validate this statement. SASSI used a psychology-based questionnaire with 78 items to identify individuals with addictions, including alcohol and other drugs. It allows for the identification of people who either have had an addiction or are prone to it. The urinary test, instead, only identifies recent drug abuse. The SASSI questionnaire is usually completed in 10–15 min and has reported an 89–97% accuracy rate and a 5–10% miss rate[7–10]. Further analysis showed that this questionnaire could predict a substance use disorder in adults in about 95% of the cases compared with a trained clinician prediction. According to a

personal communication by Miller in 1994, the false-negative and false-positive rates detected were 9% and 6%, respectively. The questionnaire is generally self-administered, but can be read to individuals with minimal reading skills by trained office staff. An automated scoring and reporting service provided by Professional Alternatives Inc., Toledo, Ohio, corroborated the accuracy of this screening tool, designed objectively to differentiate addicted from non-addicted women[8]. The questionnaire asks about alcohol and drug use and its consequences, and is divided into two sets: six 'subtle' scales, and two 'face valid' scales. The subtle scales are not intended to measure substance abuse but to make the measure 'fake-proof' or 'lie-proof', and are presented before the second set to avoid respondent defensiveness. The 'face valid' set is composed of two scales developed by the Indiana Division of Addiction Services: the Risk Prediction Scale for Alcohol and the Risk Prediction Scale for Drugs. This screening tool was implemented in our Vélez Sársfield Hospital patients and detected a 4% rate of patients with a substance abuse disorder versus a 0.7% rate of women who spontaneously reported their addiction.

FETAL TOXICITY

Fetal toxicity manifestations are: intrauterine growth restriction; congenital anomalies; fetal demise; placental abruption; and preterm birth.

Intrauterine growth restriction

The association between cigarette smoking and intrauterine growth restriction (IUGR) has been thoroughly studied. In fact, smoking in pregnancy is strongly linked to decreased birth weight: smokers compared with non-smokers are likely to deliver infants with a mean birth weight of about 187 g less. This effect is directly related to the number of cigarettes smoked, and is greater in long-term smokers. We retrospectively analyzed 10 050 perinatal histories at the Vélez Sársfield

Hospital and detected 14.5% of smokers with a birth weight reduction of up to 200 g in their babies, compared with non-smokers. According to our findings presented at the *2001 Argentine Congress of Perinatology* held in Buenos Aires, Argentina, the difference detected was greater after term.

Fetal alcohol syndrome displays several features including IUGR either before or after birth. Moreover, low birth weight is the most reliable indicator of prenatal alcohol exposure.

Mothers who use cocaine during pregnancy show a 19% incidence of IUGR. Heroin abuse during gestation is also associated with significant IUGR and prematurity. Some obstetricians advocate the use of a methadone-administration protocol to replace morphine or heroin maternal addiction, thus avoiding withdrawal symptoms and allowing for a term gestation and larger and healthiest fetuses.

Congenital anomalies

Newborns of smokers compared with non-smokers are more often affected with anencephaly, congenital heart defects and orofacial clefts. Several studies have reported that cigarette smoking is associated with intrauterine death and sudden infant death, and all evidence indicates that prenatal nicotine exposure causes mild though quantifiable deficiencies in growth rate, intellectual development and behavior. These effects are allegedly mediated by carbon monoxide causing chronic tissue hypoxia, and by nicotine stimulating catecholamine release and producing utero-placental vasoconstriction. Passive smoking effects are additive. Despite all these reports, we have not found any significant association between smoking and congenital malformations in our hospital database.

Alcohol is a major teratogen. Alcohol consumption during pregnancy may produce a wide range of defects from spontaneous abortion to severe behavioral alterations and physical anomalies. The risk of spontaneous abortion is twice as high in pregnant women who drink more than three alcoholic beverages per day than in non-drinkers. The incidence of the fetal alcoholic syndrome, one of the main consequences of ethanol in pregnancy, is 2.2 per 1000 liveborns. This syndrome was first described by Jones *et al.* in 1973. It includes pre- and postnatal growth retardation, craniofacial anomalies (wide upper lip, broad nose, micrognathia, microphthalmia, short palpebral fissures, short nose), joint contractures, cardiovascular defects and central nervous system dysfunction such as microcephaly, diverse degrees of mental retardation and neurobehavioral alterations. It is the main known cause of mental retardation. Its incidence is higher than that of Down's syndrome and cerebral paralysis. The degree of mental retardation is related to the severity of dysmorphogenesis. Microcephaly is a frequent finding, probably as a consequence of the overall retardation in cerebral growth. Newborns often either die or present with growth deficiency. No conclusive data exist about the ethanol volume required to be ingested to produce this syndrome. It is generally accepted that the ingestion of up to 45 ml/day of alcohol does not affect the incidence of congenital anomalies.

Marijuana

About 14% of pregnant women are marijuana consumers. D-9 tetrahydrocannabinol crosses the placenta and therefore poses a threat of potential fetal damage. However, few studies in humans have found an increase in the risk of congenital anomalies.

Cocaine

Several fetal anomalies have been reported in women regularly using cocaine during pregnancy. These include central nervous system, urinary and genital anomalies, mainly related to fetal circulatory compromise. Skeletal defects and isolated atresias are also present in affected newborns. Follow-up during childhood revealed that these children showed a lower degree of interaction with other children and neurobehavioral alterations such as hypertonicity, tremors and a significant learning deficit until 4–5 years of age (Toxicology Department of the University of Buenos Aires, Argentina).

At the Vélez Sársfield Hospital we have identified three newborns possibly affected by maternal cocaine use, one with prune belly syndrome[11,12] and concomitant hypospadias, another one with holoprosencephaly and the third with neonatal seizures due to temporal ischemia diagnosed with nuclear magnetic resonance.

Prematurity and fetal demise

It is very difficult to establish conclusively the influence of drugs on these two variables. All the drugs mentioned above, especially cocaine and heroin, have been implicated in prematurity and fetal death. Of course, any substance abused during pregnancy may affect maternal and perinatal health. Substance abuse interferes with the adequate nutrition and rest necessary for an intact immunological system. Addicted women generally consume diverse substances that make it difficult to establish the origin of a certain effect. Moreover, deficient nutrition or rest, venereal infections and other variables associated with substance abuse may be the direct cause of the adverse effect studied and seriously confound scientific investigations. Therefore, the development of an intrauterine exposed child may be better evaluated with a multifactorial model including prenatal and postnatal factors and the relationship among these variables.

A multifactorial developmental model

Prenatal influences Some drugs indirectly affect the fetus, either impairing maternal nutrition, or producing vasoconstriction resulting in hypoxia and diminished maternal–fetal nutrient transfer. Prenatal exposure to psychoactive substances including alcohol produces a wide range of effects, the severity and type of which are difficult and sometimes impossible to control in clinical research. In the first place, it is important to determine the quantity, frequency and duration of substance abuse. Second, the different factors related to drug and alcohol consumption contribute either additionally or synergistically to the effects of the drug itself; for instance, prenatal exposure to cocaine and heroin may affect synergistically rather than additionally the severity of neonatal abstinence syndrome. Last, genetic factors, both maternal and fetal, play an important role in the occurrence of affected offspring; cholinesterase, the main enzyme metabolizing cocaine, for example, although reduced in most pregnant women, sometimes persists or increases, therefore regulating fetal exposure to cocaine.

Postnatal influences The prognosis for children prenatally exposed to narcotics seems to be partly based on family environment, especially as the child grows. The addicted mother's characteristics affect maternal–infant interaction and have an impact on infant neurobehavioral progress. Mothers who use drugs or undergo withdrawal symptoms tend to detach themselves from their infants and sometimes from the caretaking responsibilities for the infant. This combination between insecure mothers and unresponsive infants often results in pathological maternal–infant relationships.

Home violence is still another factor associated with substance abuse. Many drug-using women have been or are physical abuse victims. Children are often witnesses or victims of such violence. Among the multiple consequences on development and behavior, post-traumatic stress produces either of two opposite effects on the infant: the inability to control impulses, an attraction towards danger and a tendency to exhibitionism; or an emotional separation, lethargy and inhibition. The neurophysiological alterations typical of the post-traumatic syndrome resemble those of prenatal cocaine exposure. Prenatal cocaine exposure and subsequent violence deteriorate infant behavior and neurophysiological function synergistically.

Drug- and/or alcohol-addicted women often present with other psychopathological problems, especially depression. Maternal depression has been shown to elicit difficulties in maternal–infant interaction, psychosomatic symptoms in preschool age, lesions, learning disabilities and depression paired with attention deficits during school age. Although genetic factors may contribute to them, these problems are mostly a consequence of unrewarding interactive behavior and parenting.

In summary, the prognosis for an *in utero* drug-exposed child depends on the child's dynamic interaction with social environmental demands. The following example gives an overall view of the problem. A neonate born at 38 weeks' gestation from a cocaine-addicted mother with poor nutrition during pregnancy and minimal prenatal care, after 3 days of hospitalization, will show slight hypotonia, disturbed sleep patterns and unresponsiveness. The mother will feel frustrated, overwhelmed and depressed, and continue using cocaine to feel better. The child's impairment in the ability to respond to her stimuli will elicit her feelings of inadequacy, and deepen her depression and cocaine dependence. Her positive interactions with her child will be rare. The child will be unresponsive to external stimulation and seldom vocalize except when crying; the mother's feelings of depression and frustration and consequently her drug/alcohol addiction will increase. At 2 years of age, the child will show delayed language and cognitive development.

What is the cause of the child's deficits? Is it the biological vulnerability caused by poor maternal nutrition or prenatal cocaine exposure? Or is it maternal depression or an inadequate environmental stimulation? A multivariate developmental model takes into account all these factors, each one of which modifies and potentiates the rest; altogether they constitute a complex model inaccessible through any single risk factor.

NEONATAL WITHDRAWAL SYNDROME

Definition

The neonatal withdrawal syndrome is an evidence of physical dependence characterized by: central nervous system hyperirritability; gastrointestinal dysfunction; respiratory distress; and vague autonomic symptoms.

These symptoms are opposite to the effects of the drug of dependence; they are caused by drug withdrawal, which produces a central nervous system hyperarousal during re-adaptation to abstinence.

Clinical presentation

Neonatal clinical onset of withdrawal symptoms varies depending on the drug used, timing and quantity of last maternal ingestion, *in utero* exposure duration, maternal and fetoneonatal metabolism and excretion, drug half-life and other unidentifiable factors. Therefore, because methadone has a longer half-life than heroin, its withdrawal symptoms tend to appear later than heroin withdrawal symptoms. In both cases the newborn appears both physically and behaviorally normal at birth. Symptoms begin to appear during the first 24–48 h of life, although according to the drug of dependence they may not appear until day 5 or 10[3,5,6]. Ethanol abstinence elicits early symptoms, generally 3–12 h after birth[13,14]. If more than a week has elapsed since the last maternal ingestion, the incidence of neonatal abstinence is relatively low[15].

Narcotic withdrawal, including methadone, appears frequently within 48–72 h of birth[14,16], but its appearance may be delayed by up to 4 weeks[17]. Sub-acute narcotic withdrawal symptoms may last over 6 months[18].

Abstinence of sedatives and hypnotic drugs is difficult to diagnose because it usually appears several days after birth. Barbiturate withdrawal symptoms appear at a mean of 4–7 days after delivery with a wide range of 1–14 days[19,20]. Similarly, other sedatives and hypnotics have been reported to display a late onset of symptoms: 12 days for diazepam[21] and 21 for chlordiazepoxide[22].

Non-opiate abstinence rarely requires pharmacological treatment. It is mostly characterized by neurological irritability.

Most cases of opiate abstinence (55–94%) require pharmacological treatment and present with a more complex syndrome characterized by: neurological irritability (reduction of sleep between feedings, myoclonic jerks, tremors, irritability, increase in spontaneous movements, acute cry, increased muscular tone, hyperactive tendinous reflexes, increased Moro reflex, seizures and yawning), gastrointestinal dysfunction (poor feeding, constant and unco-ordinated sucking, vomiting, diarrhea, dehydration and poor weight gain); respiratory distress (costal retraction, tachipnea and moaning) and autonomic signs (dribbling, nasal flaring, fever, marble skin, unstable thermoregulation and frequent sneezing). All these symptoms have been described by Loretta Finnegan[23].

Most studies show that methadone, used to replace morphine or heroin in an attempt to achieve better perinatal results, when administered at high doses late in pregnancy, is associated with higher neonatal concentrations and increased abstinence symptoms[24–27]. A study of 21 neonates of methadone-dependent women[26] revealed that higher maternal dosages were associated with abrupt reductions in neonatal plasma concentrations and more severe abstinence symptoms. Many obstetricians have reduced the maternal methadone dose to < 20 mg/kg after several studies[28–30] demonstrated that at lower doses methadone produces a lower incidence and severity of neonatal withdrawal syndrome. Some authors refuse to use methadone at all during late pregnancy[31]. Others[31,32] still use increasing methadone doses during late pregnancy. Cocaine withdrawal syndrome may be mediated by dopamine, serotonin or both. Thus, dopamine agonists such as amantadine, desipramine and bromocriptine, and serotonin antagonists such as triptophane, have all been used in adults undergoing cocaine abstinence[33]. However, no publication has quantified cocaine abstinence syndrome in neonates.

Many studies have assessed the behavior and neurological signs of cocaine-exposed infants through scoring systems primarily designed to evaluate opiate abstinence. Either cocaine or its metabolites have been detected in neonatal urine as long as 7 days after birth[34]. Abnormal neurological signs have been more frequently observed in intrauterine exposed newborns 2 or 3 days after delivery. Cocaine intoxication and abstinence show similar symptoms. Neonates exposed *in utero* to stimulating drugs (amphetamines, cocaine or both) have proved to be less symptomatic than those exposed to opiates[35,36], and newborns exposed to a combination of stimulant and narcotic drugs had an abstinence score similar to the score of those exposed only to opiates[37]. In an open study using an opiate score, all drug-exposed newborns, including those exposed only to cocaine, showed a higher abstinence score than non-exposed infants. Based on this score, 6%, 14% and 35% of neonates exposed to cocaine only, heroin only or cocaine plus heroin, respectively, qualified to receive treatment[38]. Finnegan *et al.*[23] have suggested that a separate score to evaluate cocaine exposure would certainly be more appropriate.

We frequently find in our maternal–fetal departments patients who have never been interrogated regarding substance abuse, or restless babies showing intense and prolonged crying, increased muscular tone, tremors, etc. without any detectable cause. The neonatal withdrawal syndrome should be included among the differential diagnosis in routine perinatal history recording. As we have already seen, the signs and symptoms of this syndrome are non-specific and may mimic sepsis, neurological compromise, or gastrointestinal or metabolic disorders.

Non-pharmacological treatment

Nurses will use diverse interventions to provide the baby with comfort and support. They will dress the baby to avoid heat loss and compensate for the energy expended by the increased muscular activity and central nervous system hyperirritability. For the same reason, they will try to reduce environmental sensory stimulation. They will provide frequent small feedings to optimize caloric intake and gastro-intestinal tolerance. However, this measure should not be applied whenever neonatal gastrointestinal tolerance is adequate and weight loss is minimal, as it implies greater stimulation and manipulation. A hypercaloric formula will be used to avoid excessive weight loss and diarrhea. The following parameters will be carefully observed: sleeping habits, body temperature stability, weight gain or loss and vital sign variations.

Pharmacological treatment

Loretta Finnegan[23] developed a score for objective measurement of withdrawal symptoms and to establish follow-up guidelines. In this score each withdrawal symptom is rated according to its significance. The score helps to determine the severity of the symptoms, to achieve an objective assessment, to establish the onset of pharmacological therapy and to evaluate clinical response to treatment. Its use is indicated in cases of: positive maternal toxicological screening, maternal history of drug abuse or high suspicion index through screening questionnaires, or positive neonatal toxicological screening (urine, meconium and maternal milk).

Indications for pharmacological treatment

Indications are seizures, severe feeding problems, diarrhea and vomiting, sleeplessness and fever > 39°C in the absence of infection. Scoring starts as a routine procedure: babies below 32 weeks' gestation will not display the usual withdrawal symptoms; the abstinence syndrome score will therefore be applied to all infants over 32 weeks' gestation and to selected neonates born prematurely before 32 weeks, every 4 h during the first 48 h of life.

Treatment will be instituted on the basis of the score's daily mean (Finnegan's score >8–10) and worsening of the score (increasing scores or score >8–10).

The score obtained should be an element for treatment decision-making, rather than a direct guide to dose usage, as for blood glucose values in diabetic patients. If the score approaches 7, recording should be continued every 4 h until two figures rate <2 to discard late exacerbation.

Treatment should be discontinued when two successive recordings are <2.

Drugs most frequently used in the treatment of neonatal withdrawal syndrome

These are morphine, phenobarbital, opium tincture, diazepam, clonidine, methadone, chlorpromazine and paregoric.

Morphine sulfate is the treatment of choice in cases of withdrawal syndrome due to opiate addiction. However, when addiction is detected early in pregnancy, it is convenient to replace self-administered morphine with a methadone decreasing dose protocol with informed consent. This will allow the baby to be born healthier, with greater birth weight and gestational age.

Morphine sulfate

Parenteral morphine is contraindicated in neonates, owing to the toxicity of its components: sodium bisulfite producing anaphylactic reaction, tachypnea, pruritus and rash, and phenol producing hyperbilirubinemia. It is available in tablets containing 2, 4 and 0.4 mg/ml of morphine sulfate. It is administered similarly to opium tincture.

Its advantages are: oral administration, inhibition of bowel motility, mild sedation improving sucking effectiveness, increase in nutrient consumption and effective treatment for seizures secondary to withdrawal.

Its disadvantages are: requirement of large doses and a long abstinence period.

Methadone

Little information is available in the literature regarding methadone for the neonatal withdrawal syndrome. The initial dose used is

0.05–0.1 mg/kg every 6 h. Unresponsiveness requires successive increases of 0.05 mg until the abstinence signs decrease. The effective dose should then be administered every 12–24 h. It is discontinued by lowering the effective dose by 0.05 mg/kg per day. Once discontinued the concentration in the neonate decreases slowly, owing to the long half-life of methadone (15–40 h). Oral methadone contains 8% alcohol.

Phenobarbital

Phenobarbital is the treatment of choice for non-opiate withdrawal syndrome. An initial dose of 16 mg/kg is used eliciting a blood level of 20 µg/ml. Maintenance dose is 2–8 mg/kg per day. After the neonate symptoms have stabilized, the maintenance dose is reduced by 10–20% daily.

Its advantage is a reduction in irritability and insomnia. It is the drug of choice for non-narcotic withdrawal syndrome.

Its disadvantages are: little or no effect on gastrointestinal symptoms, long half-life and development of tolerance, ineffectiveness in the treatment of seizures secondary to the neonatal withdrawal syndrome, toxic levels very near therapeutic doses, damage to the sucking reflex.

Clonidine

It is administered at an initial dose of 0.5–1 µg/kg in one oral take. Maintenance dose is 3–5 µg/kg per day divided every 6 h.

Its benefits are: shorter treatment period and absence of adverse effects. It is the therapy of choice in adult alcohol abstinence syndrome.

The only refractory symptom seems to be insomnia, although few publications have been devoted to its effects in neonatology.

CONCLUSION

The complex issue of substance abuse is a major topic of concern affecting all ages, racial and ethnic groups and socioeconomic classes. When a child is conceived and becomes the victim of such context, the most severe end of a continuum of physical, psychic, social and cultural consequences manifests in the offspring. If medicine's ultimate aim is prevention, this is no doubt a great opportunity for perinatologists to detect addictions during gestation and implement not only medical but also psychosocial measures to bring the reproductive-age woman and her partner back to a renewed conscience of health, and rescue the baby from illness.

References

1. American Academy of Pediatrics Committee on Drugs. Policy Statement: Neonatal drug withdrawal (RE9746). *Pediatrics* 1998;101:1079–88
2. Khalsa JH, Gfroerer J. Epidemiology and health consequences of drug abuse among pregnant women. *Semin Perinatol* 1991;15:265–70
3. Mensch B, Kandel DB. Drug use as a risk factor for premarital teen pregnancy and abortion in a national sample of young white women. *Demography* 1992;29:409–29
4. Berenson AB, San Miguel VV, Wilkinson GS. Violence and its relationship to substance abuse in adolescent pregnancy. *J Adolesc Health* 1992;13:470–4
5. Bayatpour M, Wells RR, Holford S. Physical and sexual abuse as predictors of substance use and suicide among pregnant teenagers. *J Adolesc Health* 1991;13:128–32
6. Steer RA, Stholl TO, Heidiger ML, Fisher RL. Self reported depression and negative pregnancy outcomes. *J Clin Epidemiol* 1992;45:1093–9
7. Horrigan TJ, Piazza NJ, Weinstein L. The Substance Abuse Subtle Screening Inventory is more cost effective and has better selectivity than urine toxicology for the detection of substance abuse in pregnancy. *J Perinatol* 1996;16:526–30

8. Miller G. *The Substance Abuse Subtle Screening Inventory Manual*. Bloomington, Indiana: Addiction Research & Consultation, 1985

9. Cooper SE, Robinson DAG. Use of Substance Abuse Subtle Screening Inventory with a college population. *J Am Public Health* 1987;36:180–4

10. Craeger C. SASSI test breaks through denial. *Professional Counselor* 1965;4

11. Bingol *et al*. Prune belly syndrome associated with maternal cocaine abuse. *Am J Hum Gen* 1986;39:A51

12. Chasnoff *et al*. Cocaine use in pregnancy. *N Engl J Med* 1985;313:666

13. Pierog S, Chandavasu O, Wexler I. Withdrawal symptoms in infants with the fetal alcohol syndrome. *J Pediatr* 1977;90:630–3

14. Nichols MM. Acute alcohol withdrawal syndrome in a newborn. *Am J Dis Child* 1967;113:714–15

15. Steg N. Narcotic withdrawal reactions in the newborn. *Am J Dis Child* 1957;94:286–8

16. Zelson C, Rubio E, Wasserman E. Neonatal narcotic addiction: 10 year observation. *Pediatrics* 1971;48:178–89

17. Kandall SR, Gartner LM. Late presentation of drug withdrawal symptoms in newborns. *Am J Dis Child* 1974;127:58–61

18. Desmond MM, Wilson GS. Neonatal abstinence syndrome: recognition and diagnosis. *Addict Dis* 1975;2:113–21

19. Bleyer WA, Marshall RE. Barbiturate withdrawal syndrome in a passively addicted infant. *J Am Med Assoc* 1972;221:185–6

20. Desmond MM, Schwanecke RP, Wilson GS, Yasunaga S, Burgdorff I. Maternal barbiturate utilization and neonatal withdrawal symptomatology. *J Pediatr* 1972;80:190–7

21. Rementeria JL, Bhatt K. Withdrawal symptoms in neonates from intrauterine exposure to diazepam. *J Pediatr* 1977;90:123–6

22. Athinarayanan P, Pierog SH, Nigam SK, Glass L. Chlordiazepoxide withdrawal in the neonate. *Am J Obstet Gynecol* 1976;124:212–13

23. Finnegan L, Kaltenbach K, Weiner S, Haney B. Neonatal cocaine exposure: assessment of risk scale. *Pediatr Res* 1990;27:10A

24. Harper RG, Solish G, Feingold E, Gersten-Woolf NB, Sokal MM. Maternal ingested methadone, body fluid methadone, and the neonatal withdrawal syndrome. *Am J Obstet Gynecol* 1977;129:417–24

25. Doberczak TM, Kandall SR, Wilets I. Neonatal opiate abstinence syndrome in term and preterm infants. *J Pediatr* 1991;118:933–7

26. Doberczak TM, Kandall SR, Friedmann P. Relationships between maternal methadone dosage, maternal–neonatal methadone levels, and neonatal withdrawal. *Obstet Gynecol* 1993;81:936–40

27. Rosen TS, Pippenger CE. Disposition of methadone and its relationship to severity of withdrawal in the newborn. *Addict Dis* 1975;2:169–78

28. Madden JD, Chappel JN, Zuspan F, Gumpel J, Mejia A, Davis R. Observation and treatment of neonatal narcotic withdrawal. *Am J Obstet Gynecol* 1977;127:199–201

29. Ostrea EM, Chavez CJ, Strauss ME. A study of factors that influence the severity of neonatal narcotic withdrawal. *J Pediatr* 1976;88:642–5

30. Strauss ME, Andresko M, Stryker JC, Wardell JN. Relationship of neonatal withdrawal to maternal methadone dose. *Am J Drug Alcohol Abuse* 1976;3:339–45

31. Sutton LR, Hinderliter SA. Diazepam abuse in pregnant women on methadone maintenance: implications for the neonate. *Clin Pediatr (Phila)* 1990;29:108–11

32. Kreek MJ, Schecter A, Gutjahr CL, *et al*. Analyses of methadone and other drugs in maternal and neonatal body fluids: use in evaluation of symptoms in a neonate of mother maintained on methadone. *Am J Drug Alcohol Abuse* 1974;1:409–19

33. Giannini AJ, Baumgartel P, DiMarzio LR. Bromocriptine therapy in cocaine withdrawal. *J Clin Pharmacol* 1987;27:267–70

34. Chasnoff IJ, Bussey ME, Savich R, Stack CM. Perinatal cerebral infarction and maternal cocaine use. *J Pediatr* 1986;108:456–9

35. Oro AS, Dixon SD. Perinatal cocaine and methamphetamine exposure: maternal and neonatal correlates. *J Pediatr* 1987;111:571–8

36. Dixon SD, Bejar R. Echoencephalographic findings in neonates associated with maternal cocaine and methamphetamine use: incidence and clinical correlates. *J Pediatr* 1989;115:770–8

37. Ryan L, Ehrlich S, Finnegan L. Cocaine abuse in pregnancy: effects on the fetus and newborn. *Neurotoxicol Teratol* 1987;9:295–9

38. Fulroth R, Phillips B, Durand DJ. Perinatal outcome of infants exposed to cocaine and/or heroin *in utero*. *Am J Dis Child* 1989;143:905–10

The dilemma of toxoplasmosis

30

M. Mahran

Toxoplasmosis is a common infection, which infects animals and humans; it has been around for thousands of years. One area of great concern is toxoplasmosis in pregnancy. The parasite may pass from mother to baby. Recently, it has also been recognized that some infected babies may develop eye problems many years later.

HISTORY AND BACKGROUND

The first convincing evidence of congenitally acquired toxoplasmosis in man was demonstrated in 1939 by Wolf Cowen and Paige. This led to a worldwide intensification of research on toxoplasmosis. *Toxoplasmosa gondii* was described as early as 1908.

More than 10 000 papers and almost 100 monographs have been published on toxoplasmosis in man and animals, and today many of the questions related to the biology and medical importance of *T. gondii* have been clarified. There are still a number of unsolved problems.

T. gondii has a worldwide distribution and is one of the most prevalent parasites among mammals and birds. The whole life cycle can, however, be completed only in the intestine of the cat (and other species of Felidae). Only these animals excrete the oocytes that become infective after a period of maturation that lasts for a few days. Under favorable conditions oocytes remain viable for many months. All other animals and birds, as well as man, may be infected by *T. gondii*, but once ingested the parasite multiplies only asexually by endogenesis, forming pseudocysts and cysts, and will not be excreted.

Sources of infection to man include cats, pigs, cattle, goats, poultry and horses.

Animals susceptible to toxoplasmosis infection include: dogs, exotic animals such as lion, giraffe, zebra, squirrel, rhesus monkeys, opossum and spotted hyena; and birds such as canaries, finches, siskins and linnets.

Women who are infected before pregnancy are immune and the organism will not be transmitted to the fetus, except in rare circumstances when the mother is severely immunocompromised and reactivation occurs.

CLINICAL PICTURE

The infection is usually asymptomatic in the mother, but can be devastating for the fetus. If the infection is acquired early in pregnancy, abortion may result. Damage to the fetus can occur if infection occurs at any stage of the pregnancy, but is more likely when infection takes place in the first trimester. Congenital toxoplasmosis may be recognized at birth. The classic tetrad of signs that may be found in any combination are:

(1) Hydrocephalus (or microcephaly);
(2) Chorioretinitis;
(3) Cerebral calcifications;
(4) Convulsion (in fully developed cases).

Infants often die within a few months. The majority of infected infants, however, will appear clinically normal at birth; stigmata of the infection appear within a few months, or do not become apparent for many years. Affected children may also present with mental retardation, spasticity, jaundice, fever hepatosplenomegaly, lymphadenopathy, diarrhea, strabismus cataract, pneumonitis, rash, hyperthermia and ambrosial bleeding.

CONFIRMATION OF DIAGNOSIS

Diagnosis can be confirmed by the following:

(1) Cordocentesis: to avoid unnecessary termination of uninfected fetuses, facilities for fetal blood sampling would be required to establish whether fetal infection has occurred. Cordocentesis:
   (a) Can be undertaken only after 18 weeks;
   (b) Carries a risk of fetal loss;
   (c) Can be done only in a few centers.
(2) Amniocentesis: isolation of parasites can be carried out only in special centers and may take 45 days.
(3) Polymerase chain reaction (PCR): to detect *Toxoplasma* DNA.

SIZE OF THE PROBLEM IN EGYPT

Considering that the incidence of acute *Toxoplasma* infection in pregnant women is about two per thousand and we have 1.8 million deliveries a year, the number of maternal *Toxoplasma* infections, in Egypt, is about 3600 each year. As many surveys proved that transplacental transmission occurs in nearly 50% of cases, the number of fetal *Toxoplasma* infections would be about 1800 cases per year. The chronological distribution of these fetal infections is as follows: 15% occur in the first trimester; 30% occur in the second trimester; and 55% occur in the third trimester.

TEN COMMON QUESTIONS ASKED BY PATIENTS

Does cat ownership contribute to the risk of toxoplasmosis?

Recent studies published in *The Journal of the American Medical Association* (1996) have tried to answer this question. Cat ownership or exposure does not appear to be a risk factor for seroconversion even in HIV-infected patients. In fact, if the published results were taken too literally, the possession of a cat would be interpreted as protective. This conclusion suggests that other risk factors may be much more important in producing infection in adults.

Why is toxoplasmosis serious?

Infection is serious, not because of the effect on the pregnant woman, but because of the effect on the fetus. The mother may not even have any complaints or have only a mild illness. The effects on the fetus, especially early in the pregnancy, can be disastrous resulting in a seriously handicapped baby who might require much individual care.

I have been told that I am susceptible to *Toxoplasma* infection. What should I do?

Patients who are susceptible should avoid sources of infection. They should not be cleaning cat litter trays. Hands should be washed after gardening or playing in the sand-pit and root vegetables should be washed before consumption. Meat should be well-cooked and milk should be pasteurized.

Will treatment remove all risk?

Treatment during pregnancy is likely to reduce significantly the risk of a baby being infected. However, some babies have already been infected before treatment is started and these babies may be born affected.

What happens when my baby is born?

At birth the baby is carefully examined for evidence of *Toxoplasma* infection. Blood is also tested. The majority of babies will appear normal. If there is any evidence of infection, the baby will be tested again and should be given treatment. This will often continue for 1 year. It is hoped that such treatment will reduce the number of patients that develop eye problems in later life.

Should I have been treated when I had toxoplasmosis diagnosed 2 years ago?

In the non-pregnant individual, treatment is not necessary in the vast majority of cases. Infection before conception is usually not a risk for that pregnancy. For a few patients, doctors may decide that drug treatment is necessary.

Why is it so difficult to interpret the blood results?

The reason is that there are a vast number of tests, and each test has particular difficulties of interpretation. Most local laboratories use only one test. Thus it is necessary to refer difficult cases to reference laboratories.

If I have an infected baby, does this mean that all of my future children will be infected?

The only pregnancy that is usually affected is the one in which the mother had the first *Toxoplasma* infection. Yet, as it can take some time for the infection to settle, it is recommended that a woman who is well waits 6 months before she becomes pregnant again.

If my baby is normal at birth will it develop any illness later in life?

Long-term follow-up studies of apparently normal infected babies suggest that many will develop symptoms, especially eye problems, later in life. It may be up to 18 years later. Therefore it is very important that babies are tested at birth to determine if they are infected. If they are infected, babies should be treated even if they appear normal.

Is *Toxoplasma* a cause of repeated abortion?

Toxoplasma is definitely not a cause of repeated abortion. *Toxoplasma* gives a long-acting solid immunity, except in the single situation when it is undermined by HIV infection. A woman who is exposed to *Toxoplasma* infection before becoming pregnant has no problems. She does not need any treatment. In spite of this solid scientific fact, confirmed by leading authorities, *Toxoplasma* is still being accused of causing habitual abortion. Thousands of women are receiving chemotherapy and antibiotics unnecessarily and even exposing the fetuses to teratogenic risk associated with some medicines.

There is no doubt that public education is extremely necessary to inform people about the facts of this disease, its obstetric complications and prophylaxis.

Bibliography

Ashburn D. History and general epidemiology. In Darrel O, Yen H, Joss AWL, eds. *Human Toxoplasmosis*. 1992

Wallon M, Liou C, Garner P, Peyron F. Congenital toxoplasmosis: systematic review of evidence of efficacy of treatment in pregnancy. *Br Med J* 1999:318

Evans R. Life cycle and animal infection. In Darrel O, Yen H, Joss AWL, eds. *Human Toxoplasmosis*. 1992

Royal College of Obstetricians and Gynaecologists. Prenatal screening for toxoplasmosis in the UK: report of a multidisciplinary working group. London: RCOG, 1992

Hall SM. Congenital toxoplasmosis. *Br Med J* 1992:305

Should we be using repeated doses of antenatal corticosteroids? 31

J. P. Newnham, T. J. M. Moss, I. Nitsos, D. Sloboda and J. Challis

INTRODUCTION

Despite a multitude of research studies and interventions in recent years, the incidence of preterm birth is not decreasing. Neonatal morbidity, however, has been reduced and survival is now expected at very early gestational ages. One of the reasons for the improved outcomes is the use of antenatal corticosteroids to promote fetal maturation.

The discovery that corticosteroids can 'mature' fetal lungs prior to preterm birth was made in the late 1960s by Professor GC (Mont) Liggins[1,2]. Using the sheep model he found that cortisol is a central component in maturation of the fetal lungs in late gestation and that pharmacological administration to the pregnant ewe will improve pulmonary function after preterm birth. In 1972, Liggins and Howie reported the results of a randomized controlled trial confirming that antenatal administration of betamethasone reduces the incidence of respiratory distress syndrome, intraventricular hemorrhage and death in the newborn period[3]. Since that time at least 16 more randomized controlled trials have been published, confirming the original observations[4]. These trials, however, were all based on the use of a single course of corticosteroid, typically consisting of two or four injections given to the pregnant woman intramuscularly over a 48-h period. In recent years, use of repeated injections has become common, given in the hope that more will be better[5,6]. This chapter reviews evidence suggesting that the effectiveness and safety of this practice needs to be evaluated further by appropriate studies.

NORMAL PHYSIOLOGY

The fetus grows and develops in an environment characterized by very low levels of cortisol[7]. Through most of gestation, the fetal hypothalamic–pituitary–adrenal (HPA) axis produces very little cortisol and the placenta contains an enzyme system to protect the fetus from the mother's cortisol. This enzyme is called 11-betahydroxysteroid dehydrogenase 2 (11-βHSD2) and converts active cortisol from the mother to inactive cortisone. In later gestation, the fetal HPA axis becomes activated resulting in an increase in circulating cortisol. The result is three-fold (Figure 1). First is the maturation of the lungs and virtually all other organs. Second is the inhibition of growth presumably to enable redirection of energy stores for the purpose of preparing for extrauterine life. Third is the initiation of the cascade of events that lead to parturition. These actions of cortisol are consistent with known effects at later times of life, with inhibition of growth being a central feature.

PHARMACOLOGY OF CORTICOSTEROIDS

Cortisol and the other glucocorticoids are powerful regulators of cell differentiation and maturation. Many of the physiological effects of these hormones can be produced by therapeutic administration of corticosteroids that are their synthetic counterparts. In the original study reported by Liggins and Howie[3], betamethasone was the agent chosen, but dexamethasone has similar effects. These drugs have actions similar to cortisol but are not

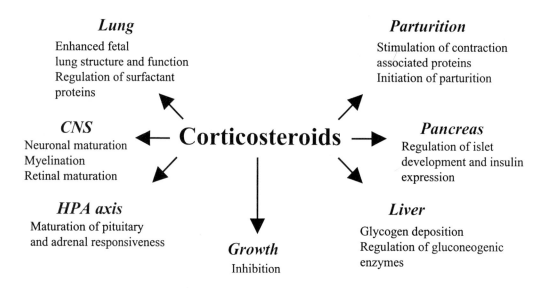

Figure 1 *The physiology of corticosteroids in normal fetal development*

inactivated by 11-βHSD2 and can thus cross the placenta and exert effects on the fetus. The agents are given intramuscularly to the pregnant woman and have a slow release resulting in betamethasone levels having a half-life of approximately 6 h in the mother, and 12 h in the fetus[8]. A single dose of hydrocortisone does not have a measurable effect on lung function[9,10]. Drugs such as prednisolone are ineffective because they have poor transplacental passage[9,11], and thus do not alter fetal lung development in pregnancies in which the mother uses corticosteroids for conditions such as asthma.

Repeated courses of corticosteroids have found their way into clinical practice because the duration of benefit from a single course is unknown. In the original study reported by Liggins and Howie[3], a protocol was chosen based on a single course of two injections 24 h apart. The evidence that this protocol is optimum is lacking and there has been little research investigating this vital question. Indeed, it remains unknown whether a second injection is of any further benefit. In our sheep studies, a single injection has been found to produce profound improvements in newborn lung function, with no change in effect between 2 and 7 days after treatment[12].

EFFECTS ON FETAL ORGAN SYSTEMS

Lungs

The improvement in postnatal lung function following a single course of antenatal corticosteroids amounts to a 50% decrease in the incidence and severity of respiratory distress syndrome[4]. In the sheep model, we have observed that a single maternal or fetal intramuscular injection of betamethasone, in a dose of 0.5 mg/kg maternal weight or estimated fetal weight respectively, doubles functional volume of the preterm lung in a 48-h period[10,13]. The result is demonstrable by increased compliance and reduced requirements for artificial ventilation. From a mechanistic perspective, the effect results from both increased surfactant production and anatomical changes[14]. Morphologically, the pulmonary effects of antenatal betamethasone are to make the alveoli fewer and larger, with thinner walls. The lifelong consequences of these alterations in alveolar development are unknown.

In humans, repeated doses of corticosteroids are given in the hope the therapy will further improve postnatal lung function. There is, however, no evidence from clinical studies to date that this hope is fulfilled, although our sheep studies do provide some support. When betamethasone is given to the pregnant ewe at weekly intervals on four occasions before elective preterm birth, postnatal lung function when compared with controls is sequentially improved with a 150% increase in compliance and a four-fold increase in volume[15].

Growth

Single-course therapy in humans has been shown in randomized controlled trials to have no measurable effect on birth weight[4]. This lack of an effect has been perplexing because of the well-known effects of cortisol in inhibiting growth, and it is presumed the duration of exposure is too short to exert an action. In our sheep model (Figure 2), maternal injections of betamethasone produced consistent effects on growth with a reduction in birth weight of 15% after a single dose and 27% after three or four doses[15]. The effect on growth is still demonstrable if the pregnancy continues to term[16].

If, however, the betamethasone injections are given intramuscularly to the fetus by ultrasound guidance, rather than to the mother, then the effects on growth are different[16,17]. Fetal treatments, either single or repeated, do not restrict growth, at least to the extent that is measurable with sample sizes typical in this field of research. The lack of an effect on growth is accompanied by improvements in postnatal lung function similar to those seen after maternal treatments[16], and circulating levels of betamethasone in the fetus are at least as high after fetal injection as in the fetal circulation after maternal injection[18]. How, then, can the differential effect of route of administration on fetal growth be explained? It is possible the observation points to a placental effect of maternal treatment on fetal growth, which may or may not also occur in humans. Alternatively, the finding may reflect differences in pharmacokinetics with different routes of treatment. Experiments to answer these two questions are in progress in our laboratory.

The findings from these sheep-based studies raise the possibility that corticosteroid injections could be given to the fetus rather than to the mother if clinical studies were to show that repeated maternal doses carry unacceptable effects. Such an approach may have several advantages, including a lower overall dose of drug administered to the combined maternal–fetal unit and a reduction in effect on maternal glucose tolerance in cases of diabetes. There are, however, compelling reasons why it would be premature to use this approach at the current time. As yet, there is no firm evidence in humans of harm resulting from repeated

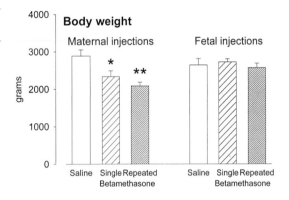

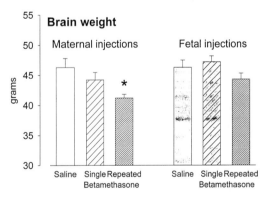

Figure 2 *Body and brain weights in sheep at 125 days' gestation (term is 150 days) following single or repeated betamethasone injections to the mother or fetus starting at 104 days' gestation and continued weekly until delivery[17]. Repeated maternal intramuscular betamethasone injections significantly reduced body and brain weights. Single injections at 104 days to the mother significantly reduced body weight. There were no significant effects observed after direct injections to the fetus. *$p < 0.05$, **$p < 0.001$*

doses to the mother. Further, the procedure of fetal injection would inevitably carry risks of exacerbation of preterm labor and introduction of infection. If the fetal approach is to be explored in clinical practice in coming years, the procedure must be restricted to randomized controlled trials of rigorous design and with the power to uncover potential risks as well as benefits.

Central nervous system

It has been known for many years from animal studies that corticosteroids have actions on the developing brain. The randomized controlled trials of single-course therapy in humans have shown no apparent effects on postnatal performance up to 20 years of age[19–23], but we do not have information on the effects of repeated doses on intellect or behavior.

Our sheep studies have provided evidence that antenatal corticosteroids may have many actions on the fetal brain that could be manifest as altered function in later life. Betamethasone treatments to the mother have been shown to reduce weights of the whole brain, cerebrum, cerebellum and brain stem[24]. The reductions in weight and volume persist to term gestation. Electron microscopy has also indicated significant effects on myelination. The first region to be studied was the optic nerve, chosen because it represents an isolated central nervous system tract that is actively myelinating at the time that corticosteroids are typically given[25]. Both single and repeated betamethasone treatments inhibited myelination within the optic nerves. Myelination was similarly inhibited in the corpus callosum[26]. The mechanism underpinning these observations is likely to be mediated by oligodendrocytes that are known to ensheath the axons with myelin and are regulated by corticosteroids. Myelin is crucial in the process by which the axons can rapidly transmit signals, and inhibition of myelination can be expected to alter the complex system of neuronal wiring that is active in late gestation. Our studies have also shown effects of antenatal corticosteroids on other components of the developing brain. Within the corpus callosum, repeated treatments to the pregnant ewe resulted in significant reductions in both astrocyte and capillary tight junction formation[27]. Astrocytes play many roles including neurotransmitter processing, maintenance of the myelin sheath and formation of the blood–brain barrier.

We are not able to predict the postnatal consequences, if any, of these observations. Nor are we certain at this time whether the effects shown in our sheep model occur in humans. We do know, however, that in rhesus monkeys corticosteroids affect the developing brain by retarding differentiation and maturation of pyramidal hippocampal neurons and granule cells in the dentate gyrus[28], indicating that at least in one primate species antenatal corticosteroids affect brain development.

Some of the consequences for fetal brain development of fetal rather than maternal injection have been studied. Repeated fetal injections with corticosteroids did not significantly affect brain growth[17] or optic nerve myelination[29], but comparable studies of astrocyte function and the blood–brain barrier have yet to be performed.

The eye

There are no data from human studies of the effects of repeated doses of antenatal corticosteroids on development of the eye. The second phase of retinal cell generation occurs at a time in gestation when treatment with these drugs begins. In our sheep model, we have observed that repeated doses of maternally administered corticosteroids result in thinner measures of the ventral periphery and area centralis of the retina[30]. At term gestation, total eye size was also significantly reduced when compared to saline-treated controls. These findings indicate a need to include assessments of vision in the follow-up of children in randomized controlled trials of repeated antenatal corticosteroid treatments.

Direct fetal injection with corticosteroids also has effects in delaying the processes of retinal maturation However, there are in addition changes resulting from the process of performing the injections themselves[29]. We know that introduction of a needle into fetal sheep under ultrasound guidance does not have significant effects on circulating fetal catecholamine levels[31], but further research is needed to explore other possible consequences.

Hypothalamic–pituitary–adrenal (HPA) axis

Under normal conditions cortisol maintains negative feedback to the hypothalamus to regulate release of corticotropin releasing hormone (CRH) and arginine vasopressin (AVP) and thus its own circulating levels. Further, in humans, cortisol positively feeds forward to stimulate production of placental CRH. Pharmacological administration of corticosteroids at early times in gestation has the potential to re-set thresholds for these loops. Experiments in sheep have shown that cortisol levels normally rise during the first 40 min after preterm birth and this rise was attenuated by prior treatment with either single or repeated doses of antenatal corticosteroids to the pregnant mother[15]. Cord blood cortisol levels at term were similar in corticosteroid-treated lambs and controls but adrenocorticotropin (ACTH) levels were increased[32]. This alteration in ACTH levels was not accompanied by any differences in mRNA encoding key pituitary and hypothalamic neuropeptides when examined by *in situ* hybridization. Postnatal studies of sheep that had been exposed to single and repeated antenatal corticosteroids before birth have provided evidence of long-standing alterations in the developing HPA axis. Postnatal intravenous infusion of CRH and AVP, given for the purpose of evaluating pituitary and adrenal function, revealed an altered responsiveness at 1 year of age in animals exposed before birth to maternal administration of corticosteroids[33]. Further, these effects were dependent on dose and route of administration. One single dose of antenatal maternal corticosteroid resulted in hypersecretion of cortisol to CRH and AVP challenge at 1 year of postnatal age. This observation suggests that

adrenal development in these animals was compromised, in a way that altered postnatal responsiveness. In animals that had received direct fetal intramuscular corticosteroids in late gestation, however, the ACTH response to CRH and AVP was attenuated, suggesting altered pituitary development. Experiments to determine the effects of dose and route of corticosteroid administration on the developing pituitary and adrenal are in progress in our laboratory.

Glucose tolerance and insulin resistance

Corticosteroid treatment in adult life is known to predispose to diabetes, but the implications for the fetus of antenatal administration are unknown. None of the randomized controlled trials of single-course treatment in humans has included follow-up with the capacity to address this issue. Using the sheep model, we have studied the relationships between corticosteroid exposure before birth, fetal growth restriction and postnatal glucose metabolism[34]. Single or repeated betamethasone injections were given to either the ewe or the fetus, and the lambs were then left to deliver spontaneously at term gestation. Studies were performed at 3, 6 and 12 months of age. The fetal growth restriction that results from repeated maternal betamethasone treatments was observed to persist to 3 months of age, but by 6 months their weights had exhibited catch-up. Birth weights and postnatal growth after fetal betamethasone injections were similar to those of controls. The lower weights in the repeated maternal betamethasone animals were accompanied by reduced blood pressures, a finding consistent with observations from other animal models of growth restriction. Glucose responses to an intravenous glucose challenge were similar in all groups, but an increased insulin response was observed in those that had been exposed to antenatal betamethasone regardless of number or route of treatments. These findings indicate that altered glucose metabolism in later life results from antenatal betamethasone exposure independent of any effect on prenatal growth.

RANDOMIZED CONTROLLED TRIALS OF REPEATED DOSES

The wealth of information from animal studies and the supporting data from human cohort studies provide a compelling case for randomized controlled trials of repeated antenatal corticosteroid treatments in clinical practice. Indeed, it is surprising that the research community over the past two decades has reported so many trials of single-course treatment with little attention to the effectiveness and safety of repeated treatments. Several randomized trials of repeated treatments are now under way in the USA, Australia, Canada and United Kingdom[35]. It will, however, be several years before the final results of these trials are available and firm conclusions can be drawn. In the meantime should we be prescribing repeated courses? To address this issue, the National Institutes of Health (http://odp.od.nih.gov/consensus/cons/112/112_statement.htm) hosted a Consensus Development Conference in August 2000. The group recommended on the basis of existing evidence that single-course treatment should continue for all pregnant women between 24 and 34 weeks' gestation who are at risk of preterm delivery within 7 days. Repeated courses, however, should not be used routinely and be reserved for patients enrolled in randomized controlled trials.

The results from the ongoing animal studies and human cohorts provide invaluable information to assist in the design of the randomized trials, and the extent of postnatal follow-up. There is a clear need for children in these trials to have thorough assessment through child and adult life. Particular attention will be warranted for all aspects of central nervous system development including behavior and vision, and the possibility of a lifelong predisposition to insulin resistance and diabetes.

The evolving story of the use of antenatal corticosteroids to enhance fetal maturation before preterm birth highlights the benefits of co-ordinated research programs spanning the spectrum from laboratory benches to animal studies and human trials. Preterm birth remains one of the great unsolved challenges in medicine. Improved methods of promoting fetal maturation promise to reduce further mortality and morbidity for the many children who will suffer from this complication of pregnancy.

References

1. Liggins G. Premature parturition after infusion of corticotrophin or cortisol into foetal lambs. *J Endocrinol* 1968;42:323–9
2. Liggins GC. Premature delivery of foetal lambs infused with glucocorticoids. *J Endocrinol* 1969;45:515–23
3. Liggins G, Howie R. A controlled trial of antepartum glucocorticoid treatment for prevention of the respiratory distress syndrome in premature infants. *Pediatrics* 1972;50:515–25
4. Crowley PA. Antenatal corticosteroid therapy: a meta-analysis of the randomized trials, 1972 to 1994. *Am J Obstet Gynecol* 1995;173:322–35
5. Brocklehurst P, Gates S, McKenzie-McHarg K, Alfirevic Z, Chamberlain G. Are we prescribing multiple courses of antenatal corticosteroids? A survey of practice in the UK. *Br J Obstet Gynaecol* 1999;106:977–9
6. Quinlivan JA, Evans SF, Dunlop SA, Beazley LD, Newnham JP. Use of corticosteroids by Australian obstetricians – a survey of clinical practice. *Aus NZ J Obstet Gynaecol* 1998;38:1–7
7. Challis JRG, Cox DB, Sloboda DM. Regulation of corticosteroids in the fetus: control of birth and influence on adult disease. *Semin Neonatol* 1999;4:96–7
8. Ballard PL, Granberg P, Ballard RA. Glucocorticoid levels in maternal and cord serum after prenatal betamethasone therapy to prevent respiratory distress syndrome. *J Clin Invest* 1975;56:1548–54
9. Schmidt PL, Sims ME, Strassner HT, Paul RH, Mueller E, McCart D. Effect of antepartum glucocorticoid administration upon neonatal respiratory distress syndrome and perinatal infection. *Am J Obstet Gynecol* 1984;148:178–86
10. Jobe AH, Polk D, Ikegami M, *et al.* Lung responses to ultrasound-guided fetal treatments with corticosteroids in preterm lambs. *J Appl Physiol* 1993;75:2099–105

11. Block MF, Kling OR, Crosby WM. Antenatal glucocorticoid therapy for the prevention of respiratory distress syndrome in the premature infant. *Obstet Gynecol* 1977;52:186–90

12. Ikegami M, Polk DH, Jobe AH, *et al*. Effect of interval from fetal corticosteriod treatment to delivery on postnatal lung function of preterm lambs. *J Appl Physiol* 1996;80:591–7

13. Ikegami M, Polk DH, Jobe AH, *et al*. Postnatal lung function in lambs after fetal hormone treatment. Effects of gestational age. *Am J Respir Crit Care Med* 1995;152:1256–61

14. Willet KE, Jobe AH, Ikegami M, Newnham J, Brennan S, Sly PD. Antenatal endotoxin and glucocorticoid effects on lung morphometry in preterm lambs. *Pediatr Res* 2000;48:782–8

15. Ikegami M, Jobe AH, Newnham J, Polk DH, Willet KE, Sly P. Repetitive prenatal gluco-corticoids improve lung function and decrease growth in preterm lambs. *Am J Respir Crit Care Med* 1997;156:178–84

16. Jobe AH, Newnham J, Willet K, Sly P, Ikegami M. Fetal versus maternal and gestational age effects of repetitive antenatal glucocorticoids. *Pediatrics* 1998;102:1116–25

17. Newnham JP, Evans SF, Godfrey M, Huang W, Ikegami M, Jobe A. Maternal, but not fetal, administration of corticosteroids restricts fetal growth. *J Maternal-Fetal Med* 1999;8:81–7

18. Berry LM, Polk DH, Ikegami M, Jobe AH, Padbury JF, Ervin MG. Preterm newborn lamb renal and cardiovascular responses after fetal or maternal antenatal betamethasone. *Am J Physiol* 1997;272:R1972–9

19. MacArthur B, Howie R, Dezoete J, Elkins J. Cognitive and psychosocial development of 4-year-old children whose mothers were treated antenatally with betamethasone. *Pediatrics* 1981; 68:638–43

20. MacArthur B, Howie R, Dezoete J, Elkins J. School progress and cognitive development of 6-year-old children whose mothers were treated antenatally with betamethasone. *Pediatrics* 1982; 70:99–105

21. Smolders-de Haas H, Neuvel J, Schmand B, Treffers P, Koppe J, Hoeks J. Physical develop-ment and medical history of children who were treated antenatally with corticosteroids to prevent respiratory distress syndrome: a 10- to 12-year follow-up. *Pediatrics* 1990;86:65–70

22. Schmand B, Neuvel J, Smolders-de Haas H, Hoeks J, Treffers P, Koppe J. Psychological development of children who were treated ante-natally with corticosteroids to prevent respiratory distress syndrome. *Pediatrics* 1990;86:58–64

23. Dessens AB, Haas HS, Koppe JG. Twenty-year follow-up of antenatal corticosteroid treatment. *Pediatrics* 2000;105:E77

24. Huang WL, Beazley LD, Quinlivan JA, Evans SF, Newnham JP, Dunlop SA. Effect of corticosteroids on brain growth in fetal sheep. *Obstet Gynecol* 1999;94:213–18

25. Dunlop SA, Archer MA, Quinlivan JA, Beazley LD, Newnham JP. Repeated prenatal cortico-steroids delay myelination in the ovine central nervous system. *J Maternal-Fetal Med* 1997;6:309–13

26. Huang W, Harper C, Evans S, Newnham J, Dunlop S. Repeated prenatal corticosteroid administration delays myelination of the corpus callosum in fetal sheep. *Int J Dev Neurosci* 2001; 19:415–25

27. Huang WL, Harper CG, Evans SF, Newnham JP, Dunlop SA. Repeated prenatal corticosteroid administration delays astrocyte and capillary tight junction maturation in fetal sheep. *Int J Dev Neurosci* 2001;19:487–93

28. Uno H, Lohmiller L, Thieme C, *et al*. Brain damage induced by prenatal exposure to dexamethasone in fetal rhesus macaques. I. Hippocampus. *Dev Brain Res* 1990;53:157–67

29. Quinlivan J, Beazley L, Braekevelt C, Evans S, Newnham J, Dunlop S. Repeated ultrasound guided fetal injections of corticosteroid alter nervous system maturation in the ovine fetus. *J Perinat Med* 2001;29:112–27

30. Quinlivan J, Beazley LD, Evans SF, Newnham JP, Dunlop SA. Retinal maturation is delayed by repeated, but not single, maternal injections of betamethasone in sheep. *Eye* 2000;14:93–8

31. Newnham JP, Polk DH, Kelly RW, Padbury JF, Evans SF, Ikegami M. Catecholamine response to ultrasonographically guided percutaneous blood sampling in fetal sheep. *Am J Obstet Gynecol* 1994; 171:460–5

32. Sloboda D, Newnham J, Challis J. Effects of repeated maternal betamethasone administration on growth and hypothalamic–pituitary–adrenal function of the ovine fetus at term. *J Endocrinol* 2000;165:79–91

33. Sloboda DM, Moss TJ, Gurrin LC, Newnham JP, Challis JRG. The effect of prenatal betamethasone administration on postnatal ovine hypothalamic–pituitary–adrenal function. *J Endocrinol* 2002; in press

34. Moss TJ, Sloboda DM, Gurrin LC, Harding R, Challis JRG, Newnham JP. Programming effects in sheep of prenatal growth restriction and glu-cocorticoid exposure. *Am J Physiol Reg Integrative Comparative Physiol* 2001;281:R960–70

35. Spencer C, Neales K. Antenatal corticosteroids to prevent neonatal respiratory distress syndrome. We do not know whether repeated doses are better than a single dose. *Br Med J* 2000;320: 325–6

Fetal macrosomia: prediction, timing and mode of delivery

32

C. Yabes-Almirante

DEFINITION

Fetal macrosomia is defined as a birth weight greater than 4500 g (9 lbs 15 oz)[1,2]. Actually, it is a misnomer, because the birth weight is known only with certainty after delivery. It implies excessive growth beyond the cut-off figure regardless of gestational age. One author[3] advanced this more appropriate definition of macrosomia as the birth weight below which no birth complications such as shoulder dystocia should occur.

RISK FACTORS FOR MACROSOMIA

It would be prudent to review the process of fetal growth to be able to understand the occurrence of fetal macrosomia. The fetus grows *in utero* at different rates[4]. From conception to 20 weeks' gestational age, growth is constant and growth parameters are similar throughout the world, across the spectrum of environmental conditions[5]. After 20 weeks, growth is steady until 34 to 37 weeks, when the maximum growth occurs[6]. During this period, the fetus increases in weight by more than 200 g a week. There is a sharp decline to 150 g a week after the 37the week, then to 100 g at the 40th week; after the 40th week growth may be down to zero. Figure 1 depicts the fetal growth rate at different ages of gestation as plotted by Brenner *et al.* for the USA in 1976[6].

In the latter half of the third trimester, true differences in fetal growth begin to appear. These are caused by limitations of the fetal supply line, maternal age, parity, socioeconomic status, race, maternal height, heart volume, smoking, prolonged gestation, maternal obesity, diabetes[4] and fetal sex[7]. This will explain why the average birth weight of one region's population differs from the birth weight of another region's population. The maternal factors as stated previously can explain variation in birth weight. However, this is true only in 50% of cases[8]. Paternal factors according to the same study have no significant effect on the birth weight[8].

Fetal overgrowth occurs at this stage of pregnancy and some investigators relate this to decompensation in protein turnover, level of lipids and amino acids and hormones, such as leptin, and growth factors[8].

Maternal diabetes is the strongest risk factor for fetal macrosomia. The incidence is doubled[9] and in other maternal conditions with derangement of carbohydrate metabolism the incidence of macrosomia is likewise increased,

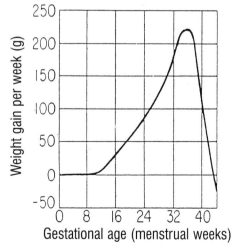

Figure 1 *Average fetal weight gain per week during pregnancy. Maximum growth is observed from about 34 to 37 weeks with a sharp decline thereafter. The post-date infant is often lighter than its term counterpart. (Reprinted with permission from reference 6)*

as shown in Table 1[9-16]. Preconception control of blood sugar in diabetic woman has an influence on the incidence of macrosomia. A study was performed in 50 women who attended a preconception diabetic clinic and who later became pregnant[17]. The glycosylated hemoglobin levels were compared between those with macrosomia and those without. The average HbA_{IC} in mothers with macrosomia was 6.8 ± 0.68 and those without macrosomia 6.3 ± 0.7 ($p < 0.05$). This implies that better metabolic control during the preconception period will lessen the risk of macrosomia.

It goes without saying that very good glycemic control in diabetic women will lessen the incidence of macrosomia. A study was done on 55 type 1 diabetic first pregnancies[10]. The incidence of macrosomia was 53.7% despite very good glycemic control. The only difference was higher fetal insulin, C peptide and leptin levels in macrosomic infants compared to non-macrosomic babies. This variability of fetal growth response to mild hyperglycemia led the authors to suggest identifying other factors involved in the modulation of fetal growth.

The risk of macrosomia is 20% in undiagnosed gestational diabetes mellitus[18]. The level of maternal glycemia in non-diabetics is associated with increased newborn birth weights[18]. These data support the relationship between maternal glucose level and increased birth weight of the newborn which is contrary to the findings of a more recent study[10]. There is a 32% risk of macrosomia[9] if two or three of these factors are present together: prolonged gestation, obesity and multiparity. On the other hand, 34% of macrosomic infants are born to mothers without any risk factors[9]. These facts have to be considered when fetal macrosomia is suspected.

Is a prior delivery to a macrosomic baby a risk factor? Yes, the chance of delivering another baby weighing more than 4500 g is 5–10%[15].

The pre-pregnancy body mass index (BMI) is a variable predictive of macrosomia separate from the blood glucose levels, as shown in a study of 94 women with GDM[19]. The BMI of women with macrosomic infants was 32.2 compared to those without macrosomic babies (28.2 kg/m^2).

The fasting maternal triglyceride level of more than 259 mg/dl was identified as a risk factor[16] and this was confirmed in a study of 146 Japanese women who had a positive diabetes screen but a normal OGTT.

Table 1 *Maternal factors; percentage risk of fetal macrosomia for each factor and authors of studies*

Maternal risk factors	Risk of fetal macrosomia	Authors
Maternal diabetes	double	Boyd 1983[9]
Type 1 diabetes	53.7%	Lepercq 2001[10]
GDM		
Untreated	20%	Adams 1998[11]
BS control 5.3 mmol	8.8%	Hod 1998[12]
Borderline	6%	Naylor 1996[13]
Normal OGTT	2%	Naylor 1996[13]
>42 wks AOG	2.5%	Ventura 2000[14]
Any 2 or 3 are present	32.0%	Boyd 1983[9]
Obesity		
Weight gain >15 kg		
Multiparity		
Previous macrosomic baby	5–10%	Okun 1997[15]
Triglycerides >259 mg/dl	OR 11.6 (1–122) $p = 0.04$	Kitajima 2001[16]
No risk	34%	Boyd 1983[9]

Hypertriglyceridemia was correlated with macrosomia (OR 11.6; 95% CI 1–122; $p = 0.04$).

Table 1 shows the maternal factors and the percentage of risk of having a macrosomic baby for each factor. Maternal diabetes gives the highest risk at a range of 53.7% to double the rate. Gestational diabetes mellitus if untreated has a 20% chance of macrosomia. Thirty-four per cent of macrosomic babies may not be related to any risk factors at all.

Genetic (parental height and stature), racial and ethnic factors interact with environmental factors during pregnancy to influence birth weight.

DIAGNOSIS

The medical literature confirms the difficulty of predicting fetal macrosomia, because the three major strategies used have substantial limitations. The strategies are: clinical risk factors; clinical estimation; and ultrasonography. A more accurate prediction may result by combining the three strategies.

Clinical risk factors

A high index of suspicion should be raised in the following conditions: maternal diabetes, maternal impaired glucose tolerance, obesity and excessive weight gain, previous macrosomic baby, prolonged gestation, parental stature, multiparity, male fetus, need for labor augmentation, prolonged second stage, maternal ethnicity and maternal age less than 17 years. The percentages of risk are documented in Table 1.

Clinician estimation

Clinician estimation of fetal weight by abdominal palpation and fundal height measurement are well documented to have a 300-g (11.6-oz) error[8,15]. This is due to the variance of volume of amniotic fluid, maternal body habitus and configuration of the uterus that complicates estimation.

Clinical fetal estimation was compared by several authors to that of the ultrasound estimation using different formulas[20–22], including that of the cheek-to-cheek diameter (CCD), upper arm or thigh subcutaneous tissue measurement, and ratio of thigh subcutaneous tissue to femur length[21]. The accuracy of the estimate compared to the actual birth weight in both the clinical and ultrasonography estimate is similar, prompting one author[22] to recommend that physicians continue to use clinical method to estimate fetal weight, multiparous women providing their own estimates.

Ultrasonography estimate

Ultrasound allows direct measurement of the fetus before delivery. Birth weight is estimated from the different measurements (BPD, FL, FAC) of the body parts of the fetus using a computer-generated formula. The formula is derived after regression analysis of the different measurements, which are inputted into the computer. Usually the subjects are normal pregnant women; obese woman or mothers with GDM are excluded. When this formula is used to estimate the weight of the fetus of the GDM mother, the accuracy will be low. The formula derived from one population may not be accurate in estimating the birth weight of another population.

This is the reason why a separate formula for estimating fetal weight for our population was made in 1989[23]; the mean birth weight of our population is 3000 g. Validation of the formula had $r = 0.996$ and a mean error of 69.71 g. When the formula was used to estimate the weight of suspected macrosomic babies, the accuracy was low and most often there was an underestimation[24]. A new formula was generated using the BPD, FL and FAC ultrasound measurements done within 5 days of babies suspected of weighing 3500 g and above. This improved the estimation of the birth weight to a mean error of 207 g[24]. Sokol and co-investigators[25] used a similar strategy to improve estimation of macrosomic babies.

Several researchers validated the formulas proposed by different authors in estimating the weight of macrosomic infants[26–29]. All 31 formulas[26] had poor accuracy for prediction of macrosomia. The number of large errors of prediction for all formulas was greatest in fetuses that were below the 10th centile or above the 90th centile[28].

The imprecise prenatal diagnosis of fetal macrosomia by ultrasound biometry of the BPD, FL and FAC have led to other studies, such as the measurement of soft tissue thickness[21,30], but results are inconsistent. MRI[31,32] and 3D ultrasound studies show some improvement in accuracy. The limitation is the cost, so MRI is recommended only in clinical situations where an accurate weight estimate is essential. MRI has also been used to measure the fetal shoulder, the bisacromial diameter (BAD)[33].

Volume measurement of the fetal arm and thigh by 3D ultrasound was studied by several investigators either alone or together with 2D biometry. The formula generated for estimating birth weight has a mean error ranging from 25.8 g to 38.6 g to 121.8 g and the absolute per cent error from 5.1% to 6.1%[32,34,35]. One researcher found that the most accurate estimation for macrosomic fetuses had an absolute per cent error of 8.8%[36].

Another study[37] was performed in 50 term pregnant women generating a formula that included the arm (AV) and thigh volume (TV) as well as the BPD, FL and FAC. The mean error was 81 g in estimating the fetal weight of the average-sized baby and the macrosomic fetus. The formula is shown below:

$$EFW (kg) = -4.42 + 0.07(TV) - 0.183(AV) - 0.17(BPD) + 0.005(AC) + 1.32(FL)$$

Table 2 shows the comparison of the three studies that performed fetal estimation of weight using 2D and 3D ultrasound measurement[37-39]. It shows that adding volume measurements to the 2D measurements improves the accuracy.

SHOULDER DYSTOCIA

Shoulder dystocia is the most feared complication of fetal macrosomia. It is a rare occurrence, with an incidence of 0.15–11% of vaginal deliveries[40-44]. Table 3[42-46] shows the frequency of shoulder dystocia and macrosomia as

Table 2 Studies showing the comparison of 2D versus 3D ultrasound measurement in the estimation of fetal weight, by mean error or percentage error

Authors	Mean error	% error
Brinkley et al. 1984[38]		
2D	73 g	—
3D	69.8 g	—
Lee et al. 1997[39]		
2D	—	−0.6% ± 8.8%
3D	—	−0.03% ± 6.1%
Almirante 2001[37]		
2D	207 g	3.72 ± 0.05
3D	81 g	2.77 ± 0.09

studied by different authors using vaginal births[43-45] and term infants[41,42,46] as subjects.

The incidence of macrosomia ranges from a low of 0.8% to a high of 13% and the incidence of shoulder dystocia ranges from a low of 0.13% to a high of 11%. The incidence of 12% is in the study on macrosomic infants. With 4750 g as a cut-off, shoulder dystocia is increased to seven times in the non-diabetic women and with non-assisted delivery, while this increases to 34% or ten times in the diabetic women and with assisted delivery (see Table 3). This is a good reason for fetal macrosomia in diabetics and non-diabetics to be considered separately by most studies and the ICD-10[2]. There is asymmetry in fetal growth among infants of diabetic mothers – a disproportionate growth of the fetal chest and shoulders compared with the fetal head[19] – making them more prone to shoulder dystocia.

Other than the studies mentioned in Table 3, there are other authors who give different statistical data on shoulder dystocia and brachial plexus injury. Twenty-six per cent to 58% of shoulder dystocia and 24% to 44% of brachial plexus injuries occur in babies weighing less than 4000 g[47,48]. Most studies, however, show that beyond 4500 g the risk of shoulder dystocia is increased, with rates from 9.2% to 24%[41,47,49,50]. The risk of brachial plexus injury increased with increasing birth weight, 3% for weight above 4500 g and 6.7% for weight above 5000 g[41,42]. The rates of shoulder dystocia are further doubled or trebled in

Table 3 *Incidence by different authors of macrosomia (mac) and shoulder dystocia by vaginal birth and among term infants*

Population	Macrosomia		Shoulder dystocia		Authors
	Number	%	Number	%	
16 416 deliveries	133	0.8	mac 3	3	Gonen *et al.* 2000[44]
			no mac 14	0.1	
63 761 infants no diabetes			80	0.13	Bryant *et al.* 1999[42]
			< 5000	3	
			> 5000	6.7	
175 886 vaginal births			6238	3	Nesbitt *et al.* 1998[43]
no diabetes			< 4750 g	14.3	
not assisted delivery			> 4750 g	21.1	
diabetes			< 4750 g	27.3	
assisted delivery			> 4750 g	34.8	
66 086 term infants	8815	13	97	11	Gregory *et al.* 1998[41]
14 157 vaginal deliveries			21	0.15	Martinetti *et al.* 2000[45]
505 macrosomic infants	504		60	12	Wojtasinska *et al.* 2000[46]

diabetic pregnancies: 19.5% to 50% in birth weights above 4500 g[47].

Vacuum- and forceps-assisted births[45] in both diabetic and non-diabetic mothers have an increased incidence of 35% to 45% of shoulder dystocia. This is seen in Figure 2[43]. This figure shows that, with increasing birth weight, the incidence of shoulder dystocia increases in an almost linear fashion until the birth weight of 4250 g, when the increase of shoulder dystocia in diabetics almost doubles. Assisted deliveries, whether in diabetics or non-diabetics, are associated with a higher incidence of shoulder dystocia than non-assisted deliveries.

PREVENTION

Can macrosomia be prevented?

Some authors claim that (a) tight glycemic control and elective early delivery and (b) insulin therapy for fetal overgrowth at 28 weeks' gestation in diabetic mothers could reduce macrosomia; a reduction from 17.9% to 8.8%[12] in the first instance and from 71.43% to 33.33% in the second instance. The association between pre-pregnancy weight and excessive maternal weight gain during pregnancy brought out advocates of optimal weight before attempting pregnancy and limitation of weight gain to 15 kg[51], especially in those with a positive glucose screen.

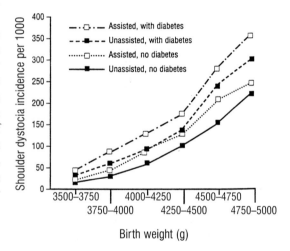

Figure 2 *Frequency of shoulder dystocia for increasing birth weight by maternal diabetes status and method of vaginal delivery – spontaneous or assisted. (Reprinted with permission from reference 43)*

Can shoulder dystocia be predicted?

Studies show[41,43,52] that macrosomia is the most important factor associated with shoulder dystocia. Diagnosis is difficult despite knowledge of risk factors and despite the advent of new technologies.

What is the recurrence rate of shoulder dystocia in subsequent deliveries? Two studies available have a wide range of recurrence rates from 1.25% to 13.8%[53].

A proposal for determining which fetal ultrasonographic parameter can best predict the neonatal BAD was made[33], and this was identified as the fetal chest circumference; however, correlation with actual measurement at birth was not very high ($r = 0.67$; $p = 0.003$).

Shoulder dystocia remains unpredictable and occurs even in infants with normal birth weight. Therefore, it may not be preventable.

MANAGEMENT OF SUSPECTED FETAL MACROSOMIA

From a study of 16 416 deliveries[44], only 45% of cases of fetal macrosomia will be confirmed from the 100% suspected; 84% will be undiagnosed, of which 10% will undergo emergency Cesarean section and 74% will deliver vaginally. The incidence of macrosomia is 0.8%. There is a 3% rate of brachial plexus injury among macrosomic infants. Eighty-six per cent of the confirmed macrosomic infants had a predelivery estimation of fetal weight and only 18.3% were correctly identified.

The proposed management of suspected fetal macrosomia should be viewed in the context of the above statistical data. Only 18.3% of macrosomic babies were correctly identified. Once diagnosis is made, will the labor be induced at 38 weeks or will an expectant delivery until 42 weeks be chosen? Cochrane Review found that labor induction did not reduce Cesarean section rate (OR 0.85; 95% CI 0.50–1.46) or instrumental delivery (OR 0.98; 95% CI 0.46–1.98). There was evidence of a trend to lower clavicular fracture and brachial plexus injury, but this needs confirmation by larger studies. Early induction of labor is not recommended.

Elective Cesarean section

Elective Cesarean section was proposed to prevent birth trauma for suspected macrosomic babies. However, evidence[42] shows that, to prevent a single case of permanent injury, 155–588 Cesarean deliveries will have to be performed in suspected macrosomic infants without diabetic complications. The authors did not take into account the sensitivity of ultrasound diagnosis to arrive at the figure. Another study[54], considering the inaccuracy of ultrasound diagnosis, calculated that more than 1000 Cesarean deliveries would be required to prevent one permanent injury, at a cost of millions of dollars for each injury avoided. Therefore, elective Cesarean section for suspect macrosomia in non-diabetics is not advocated.

For mothers with diabetes, elective Cesarean section for an estimated weight of 4500 g will need 443 Cesarean deliveries to prevent one permanent brachial plexus injury[55], so elective Cesarean section for estimated 4500-g babies is also not recommended. However, for babies estimated to weigh more than 4500 g, an elective Cesarean section would be considered, because of the increased risk of shoulder dystocia, as shown by Nesbitt et al.[43].

Since complications such as shoulder dystocia, brachial plexus injury or Erb–Duchenie paralysis cannot be predicted by estimated birth weight alone, the patient's obstetric history, progress during labor and adequacy of the pelvis should be taken into consideration before any intervention such as a Cesarean section. As shown in Figure 2, assisted deliveries increase the risk of shoulder dystocia, so instead of carrying out a mid-forceps delivery for prolonged second stage, a Cesarean section would be a better option. For infants weighing more than 4500 g a required mid-forceps delivery has a 50% chance of shoulder dystocia[43], more data to support doing a Cesarean section instead of a mid-forceps extraction.

With increasing awareness of the inprecision and unpredictability of the diagnosis of fetal macrosomia, hopefully more investigators will look for methods to improve diagnosis using newer technology. Decisions on mode and timing of delivery of these high-risk infants will then be more standardized and the multidisciplinary team of health professionals will be alerted earlier, so that they are ready to receive these babies.

References

1. The American College of Obstetricians and Gynecologists. Fetal macrosomia. ACOG Practice Bulletin 22. *2001 Compendium of Selected Publications* 2001:929–39

2. International Statistical Classification of Diseases and Related Health Problems Tenth Revision (ICD-10) PO8. Disorders related to long gestation and high birth weight. Geneva: WHO 1992:173

3. Zamorski MA, Biggs WS. Management of suspected fetal macrosomia. *Am Fam Physician* 2001;Jan15: 1–5

4. Lin CC, Evans MI. Normal fetal growth. In Lin CC, Evans MI, eds. *Intrauterine Growth Retardation: Patho-physiology and Clinical Management*. New York: McGraw-Hill, 1984:39

5. Grunewald P. Growth of the human fetus, normal growth and its variation. *Am J Obstet Gynecol* 1966; 94:1112

6. Brenner WE, Edelman DA, Hendricks CH. A standard of fetal growth for the United States of America. *Am J Obstet Gynecol* 1976;126:555

7. Wollschlaeger K, Nieder J, Koppe I, *et al*. A study of fetal macrosomia. *Arch Gynecol Obstet* 1999;263: 51–5

8. Lepercq J, Timsit J, Harguel-de Mouzon S. Etiopathology of fetal macrosomia. *J Gynecol Obstet Biol Reprod* 2000;29(Suppl):6–12

9. Boyd ME, Usher RH, Mclean FH. Fetal macrosomia: prediction, risks, proposed management. *Obstet Gynecol* 1983;61:715–22

10. Lepercq J, Taufin P, Dubois-Laforque D, *et al*. Heterogeneity of fetal growth in type 1 diabetic pregnancy. *Diabetes Metab* 2001;27:339–44

11. Adams KM, Li H, Nielson RL, *et al*. Sequelae of unrecognized gestational diabetes. *Am J Obstet Gynecol* 1998;178:1321–32

12. Hod M, Bar J, Peded Y. Antepartum management protocol. Timing and mode of delivery in gestational diabetes. *Diabetes Care* 1998;21:B113–17

13. Naylor CD, Sermer M, Chen E, *et al*. Cesarean delivery in relation to birth weight and gestational glucose tolerance; pathophysiology or practice style? Toronto Trihospital Gestational Diabetes Investigators. *J Am Med Assoc* 1996;275:1165–70

14. Ventura SJ, Martin JA, Curtin SC, *et al*. Births: final data for 1998. *Natl Vital Stat Rep* 2000;48: 1–100

15. Okun N, Verma, Mitchell BF, *et al*. Relative importance of maternal constitutional factors and glucose intolerance of pregnancy in the development of newborn macrosomia. *J Matern Fetal Med* 1997;6:285–90

16. Kitajima M, Oka S, Yasuhi I, *et al*. Maternal serum triglyceride at 24–32 weeks gestation and new-born weight in nondiabetic women with positive diabetic screens. *Obstet Gynecol* 2001;97: 776–80

17. Delgado Del Rey M, Herranz L, Martin Vaquero P, *et al*. Role of glycosylated hemoglobin of preconception stage in diabetic pregnancy outcome. *Med Clin (Barc)* 2001;117:45–8

18. Verma A, Mitchell BF, Demianczuk N, *et al*. Relationship between plasma glucose levels in glucose intolerant women and newborn macrosomia. *J Matern Fetal Med* 1997;6:187–93

19. McFarland MB, Trylovich CG. Langero. Anthropometric differences in macrosomic infants of diabetic and non diabetic mothers. *J Maternal Fetal Med* 1998;7:292–5

20. Sherman DJ, Arieli S, Tovbin J, *et al*. A comparison of clinical and ultrasonic estimation of fetal weight. *Obstet Gynecol* 1998;91:212–17

21. Chauhan SP, West DJ, Scardo JA, *et al*. Antepartum detection of macrosomic fetus; clinical versus sonographic, including soft tissue measurements. *Obstet Gynecol* 2000;95:639–42

22. O'Reilly-Green C, Divon M. Sonographic and clinical methods in the diagnosis of macrosomia. *Clin Obstet Gynecol* 2000;43:309–20

23. Almirante CY. Assessment of fetal growth by ultrasonic measurement in Filipinos. Master of Science Thesis, University of Zagreb, 1990

24. Teh N, Almirante CY. Sonographic estimation of fetal weight using the standard formula for the general population versus using a corrected factor for LGA fetuses at or near term. *9th Annual Convention Fetus as a Patient*, Book of Abstracts:28

25. Sokol RJ, Chik L, Dombrowski MP, Zador IE. Correctly identifying the macrosomic fetus: improving ultrasonography based prediction. *Am J Obstet Gynecol* 2000;182:1489–95

26. Combs CA, Rosenn B, Miodovnik K, *et al*. Sonographic EFW and macrosomia: is there an optimum formula to predict diabetic fetal macrosomia? *J Matern Fetal Med* 2000;9:55–61

27. Alsulyman OM, Ouzounlan JG, Kjos SL. The accuracy of intrapartum, ultrasonographic fetal weight estimation in diabetic pregnancies. *Am J Obstet Gynecol* 1997;177:503–6

28. Simon NV, Levisky JS, Shearer DM, *et al*. Influence of fetal growth patterns on sonographic estimation of fetal weight. *J Clin Ultrasound* 1987;13:367–83

29. Chauhan SP, Hendrix MW, Magarin EF, *et al*. Limitations of clinical and sonographic estimates of birth weight: experience with 1034 parturients. *Obstet Gynecol* 1998;91:72–7

30. Santolaya-Furgas J, Meyer WJ, Ganthier DW. Intrapartum fetal subcutaneous tissue/femur

length ratio: an ultrasonographic clue to fetal macrosomia. *Am J Obstet Gynecol* 1994;171:1072–5

31. Tukeva TA, Salim H, Poutanen VP. Fetal shoulder measurements by fast and ultra fast MRI techniques. *J Magn Reson Imaging* 2001;13:938–42

32. Schild RL, Fimmers R, Hansmann M. Fetal weight estimation by three-dimensional ultrasound. *Ultrasound Obstet Gynecol* 2000;16:445–52

33. Winn HN, Holcomb W, Shunneway JB, *et al.* The neonatal bisacromial diameter: a prenatal sonographic evaluation. *J Perinat Med* 1997;25:486–7

34. Liang RI, Chang FM, Yao BL, *et al.* Predicting birth weight by fetal upper-arm volume with use of three-dimensional ultrasonography. *Am J Obstet Gynecol* 1997;177:632–8

35. Song TB, Moore TR, Lee JI, *et al.* Fetal weight prediction by thigh volume measurement with three-dimensional ultrasonography. *Obstet Gynecol* 2000;96:157–61

36. Favre R, Bader AM, Nisand G. Prospective study on fetal weight estimation using limb circumferences obtained by three dimensional ultrasound. *Ultrasound Obstet Gynecol* 1995;6:140–4

37. Almirante CY. Estimation of fetal weight by 3D vs 2D ultrasound. *XVII International Society Fetus as a Patient Congress.* Book of Abstracts 2001:20

38. Brinkley JF, McCallum WD, Muramatsu SK, *et al.* Fetal weight estimation from lengths and volumes found by three-dimensional ultrasound measurement. *J Ultrasound Med* 1984;3:163–8

39. Lee W, Comstock CH, Kirk JS, *et al.* Birth weight prediction by three-dimensional ultrasonographic volume of the fetal thigh and abdomen. *J Ultrasound Med* 1997;10:779–805

40. Nocon JJ, McKenzie DR, Thomas IJ, *et al.* Shoulder dystocia an analysis of risks and obstetric maneuvers. *Am J Obstet Gynecol* 1993;168:1732–9

41. Gregory KD, Henry OA, Ramicone E, *et al.* Maternal and infant complications in high and normal weight infants by method of delivery. *Obstet Gynecol* 1998;92:507–13

42. Bryant DR, Leonardi MR, Landwehr JB, *et al.* Limited usefulness of fetal weight in predicting neonatal brachial plexus injury. *Am J Obstet Gynecol* 1999;179:686–9

43. Nesbitt TS, Gilbert WM, Herrchen B. Shoulder dystocia and associated risk factors with macrosomic infants born in California. *Am J Obstet Gynecol* 1998;179:476–80

44. Gonen R, Bader D, Ajami M. Effects of a policy of elective cesarean delivery in cases of suspected fetal macrosomia on the incidence of brachial plexus injury and the rate of cesarean delivery. *Am J Obstet Gynecol* 2000;183:1296–300

45. Martinetti E, Zanini A, Caghosis PM, *et al.* Risk factors and neonatal outcome on shoulder dystocia. *Minerva Ginecol* 2000;52:63–8

46. Wojtasinska M, Belfrage P, Gjessing L. Large fetus – a retrospective study [abstract]. *Tidsskr Nor Laegeform* 2000;120:1848–50

47. Acker DB, Sachs BP, Friedman EA. Risk factors for shoulder dystocia in the average-weight infant. *Obstet Gynecol* 1986;67:614–18

48. Sacks DA, Chen W, Irion O, *et al.* Estimating fetal weight in the management of macrosomia. *Obstet Gynecol Surv* 2000;55:229–39

49. Berard J, Dufour P, Vinatier D, *et al.* Fetal macrosomia, risk factors and outcome. A study of the outcome concerning 100 cases > 4500 g. *Eur J Obstet Gynecol Reprod Biol* 1998;77:51–9

50. Hill DJ, Petrik J, Arany E. Growth factors and the regulation of fetal growth. *Diabetes Care* 1998;21(Suppl 2):B60–9

51. Zhu F, Tao G, Shi K. Prospective study on the correlation factors of fetal macrosomia [abstract]. *Human Yi Ke Da Xue Bao* 1988;23:59–61

52. Lewis DF, Edwards MS, Asrat T, *et al.* Can shoulder dystocia be predicted? Preconceptive and prenatal factors. *J Reprod Med* 1998;43:654–8

53. Lewis DF, Raymond RC, Perkins MB, *et al.* Recurrence rate of shoulder dystocia. *Am J Obstet Gynecol* 1995;172:1369–71

54. Rouse DJ, Owen J. Prophylactic cesarean delivery for fetal macrosomia diagnosed by means of ultrasonography – a Faustian bargain? *Am J Obstet Gynecol* 1999;181:323–8

55. Lipocomb KR, Gregory K, Shaw K. The outcome of macrosomic infants weighing at least 4500 g: Los Angeles Country and University of Southern California Experiences. *Obstet Gynecol* 1995;85:558–64

Clinical dimensions of pre-eclampsia 33

E. V. Cosmi, F. Pierucci, G. Madonna Terracina, R. La Torre, L. Maranghi, E. Cosmi and M. M. Anceschi

INTRODUCTION

Hypertensive disorders of pregnancy are the leading cause of maternal and perinatal mortality, and morbidity in developing and developed countries. Their incidence varies according to the population studied and the criteria used for the diagnosis. As a general rule, hypertension in pregnancy is classified as follows:

(1) Chronic hypertension;
(2) Pre-eclampsia–eclampsia;
(3) Pre-eclampsia superimposed upon chronic hypertension;
(4) Transient hypertension.

Chronic hypertension is diagnosed if there is persistent elevation of blood pressure of at least 140 mmHg over 90 mmHg on two occasions, more than 6 h apart before 20 weeks' gestation, or a hypertension that occurs for the first time during pregnancy, but persists over 42 days postpartum. Pre-eclampsia–eclampsia (PE) is a disorder of pregnancy that accounts for 70% of hypertensive disorders in pregnancy, and its diagnosis is determined by increased arterial pressure, proteinuria and edema. Transient hypertension can be defined as elevated blood pressure during pregnancy after 20 weeks' gestation without proteinuria or edema; blood pressure returns to normal values within 12 weeks postpartum.

The etiology of PE is still unknown. Delivering the baby is the only definite treatment. PE is a disease unique to pregnancy that complicates from 5% to 7% of low-risk pregnancies and as many as 25% of high-risk pregnancies. PE classically includes a triad of clinical signs and symptoms: hypertension, proteinuria and pathological edema, e.g. glottis, central nervous system (CNS). Thus far, efforts to elucidate the causative factor or factors involved in the development of this disease have yielded a variety of biochemical and hemodynamic markers associated with the disease, but none of these markers has been shown to antedate the clinical manifestation by a significant interval. The benefits of acute pharmacological control of severe hypertension prior to and/or post-delivery are generally accepted.

The prerequisite for the development of PE is the presence of the placenta. More than 50 years ago, Ernest W. Page[1] suggested that the characteristic feature of the pre-eclamptic placenta was its exposure to decreased perfusion secondary to abnormal placentation. Normal pregnancies are characterized by endovascular invasion by the fetal trophoblast of maternal spiral arteries (Figures 1 and 2), with enlargement of their luminal diameter and disappearance of smooth muscle from the vessel wall. These changes provide a large-bore, low-resistance circuit for perfusion characteristic of the intervillous space. However, in cases of PE the maternal vessels become less compliant because the smooth muscle layer remains intact or proliferates thereby increasing vascular resistance, which leads to a generalized vasoconstriction that affects practically every organ system (Figure 3). Normally during early pregnancy, placentation takes place in a relatively hypoxic environment which, however, permits appropriate embryonic development. Intervillous blood flow increases at around 10–12 weeks' gestation and results in exposure of the trophoblast to increased oxygen tension (PO_2). Prior to this, low PO_2 seems to prevent trophoblast differentiation towards an invasive phenotype. In mammalian systems, the effects of oxygen tension are mediated by hypoxia

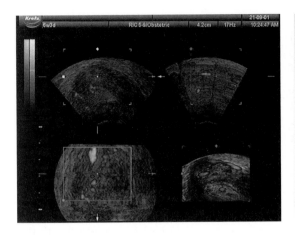

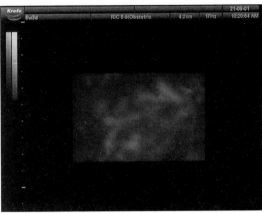

Figure 1 *Three-dimensional reconstruction of trophoblastic erosion of endometrial capillaries at 6 weeks' gestation (see Color Plate U)*

Figure 2 *Angio four-dimensional reconstruction of trophoblastic erosion of endometrial capillaries (the same case as in Figure 1) (see Color Plate V)*

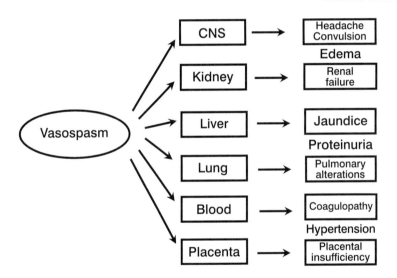

Figure 3 *Pathophysiological consequences of generalized vasoconstriction in pre-eclampsia–eclampsia. CNS, central nervous system*

inducible factor-1 (HIF-1). The ontogeny of HIF-1 α-subunit expression during the first trimester of gestation parallels that of transforming growth factor-β_3 (TGF-β_3), an inhibitor of early trophoblast differentiation. Expression of both molecules is high in early pregnancy and falls at around 10 weeks' gestation, when intervillous space PO_2 levels are believed to increase. TGF-β_3 expression is increased in pre-eclamptic placentae when compared to age-matched controls. Inhibition of TGF-β_3 by

antisense oligonucleotides or antibodies restores the invasive capability to the trophoblast cells in pre-eclamptic explants[2]. It has been speculated that if PO_2 fails to increase, or the trophoblast does not detect this increase, HIF-1α and TGF-β expression remains high, resulting in shallow trophoblast invasion, thus predisposing the pregnant woman to PE.

Other conditions can decrease placental blood supply and increase the risk of PE. Pre-existing maternal conditions that are associated

305

with microvascular diseases, such as hypertension or diabetes, or that are thrombophilic, such as anticardiolipin antibody syndrome, or obstetric conditions that increase placental mass, such as hydatidiform moles or twin pregnancies, increase the risk of PE[3]. However, the disease requires more than lowered placental perfusion. Perfusion can be further compromised by activation of the coagulation cascade, particularly platelets, with attendant microthrombi formation. Additionally, plasma volume is decreased by loss of fluid from the intravascular space, further compromising organ blood flow. The maternal factors that can predispose to the disorder are genetic, immunological, environmental and behavioral. In the presence of these factors, placental derangements can lead to the multisystemic maternal disease characterized by endothelial dysfunction, which is the final common pathway in the pathophysiology of PE.

GENETIC FACTORS

Some data suggest that genetic factors play a major role in development of PE. Genetic involvement is very difficult to evaluate, because PE occurs only in pregnant women. Moreover, there is a fetal genetic contribution that can be evaluated only after birth.

Most of the family data suggest that the maternal genotype is responsible for susceptibility, with little fetal contribution[4]. Nevertheless, there is a striking lack of concordance between monozygous twins. An Australian study[5] that has investigated maternal vs. fetal genetic causes of PE by assessing concordance between twins has not found concordant female twin pairs.

The impact of paternal factors is proved by the loss of protective effect of multiparity with the change of the partner. Lie et al.[6], using data based on the Norwegian population, have found that men who fathered a pre-eclamptic pregnancy were nearly twice as likely to father a pre-eclamptic pregnancy in different women (odds ratio (OR) 1.8; 95% confidence interval (CI) 1.2–2.6), regardless of whether or not they were previously affected by PE. Robillard et al.[7] have suggested the use of the term 'primipaternity' instead of 'primigravidity' to describe the epidemiological standard of PE. Further support for a fetal contribution is indirectly suggested by data showing that a prolonged cohabitation[8], with a long sperm exposure before pregnancy, is a protective factor from the development of PE. Graves[9] has proposed that PE may be due to mutation of a paternally imprinted (i.e. genetically 'silenced'), maternally active gene which must be expressed by the fetus in order to establish a normal placenta in the first pregnancy.

Several studies converge on the view that PE is under multifactorial control. Broughton-Pipkin[10] has suggested a cluster of polymorphisms which, in conjunction with environmental factors, predispose to the development of this condition. Several genes have been investigated on the basis of their hypothetical pathophysiological effects. Chromosomal exclusion mapping suggested a role for a gene(s) on chromosome 1, 3, 9, 18 or 4. Human leukocyte antigen (HLA) system has been widely investigated, but linkage studies have ruled out any direct influence of HLA genes (HLA-DRβ and HLA-G) on the development of the disease[11,12]. A polymorphism in the angiotensin-converting enzyme (ACE) gene, associated with essential hypertension in the non-pregnant population, was investigated in African-American women, but this study failed to demonstrate any association of the ACE gene with PE[13]. Two candidate genes, concerned with clotting, lie on chromosome 1: factor V Leiden and methylenetetrahydrofolate reductase (MTHFR) genes. In a recent study, thrombophilic mutations were found in 67% of women with severe PE[14]. The gene mutation of factor V makes it resistant to activated protein C, which is present in about 20% of women with PE; factor V mutation was found in 8.9% of former pre-eclamptic women as compared with 4.2% in controls[15]. The MTHFR gene C677T polymorphism is associated with reduced MTHFR activity and hyperhomocysteinemia[16]. The latter is a common finding in pre-eclamptic patients. Lachmeijer et al.[17] have found a significant excess of the TT genotype (homozygosity for C677T mutation) in women with PE with mild hyperhomocys-teinemia (values > 75th centile) with respect to women with PE without hyperhomocys-teinemia. However, they did not find any mutation in excess in women with PE with strictly defined hyperhomocysteinemia (values > 97.5th centile) relative to controls. Two other studies have reported excess homozygosity for TT in women with PE[18,19].

Gene mutations may predispose towards PE, but they do not seem to be a prerequisite. Several other genes have been investigated, such as superoxide dismutase gene, nitric oxide synthase gene and tumor necrosis factor T2 mutation, but the results are inconclusive. A very promising candidate in PE seems to be the angiotensinogen gene, which lies on chromo-some 1. The frequency of the variant T235 was found significantly increased in pre-eclamptic women in association with a raised plasma angiotensinogen concentration[20]. Nevertheless, a study in the UK failed to demonstrate any increased frequency of the T235 variant in pre-eclamptic women when compared to controls[21].

In conclusion, it is most likely that genetic factors are involved in development of PE, although it is not possible to identify exactly the maternal, paternal and fetal contribution to the disease and the gene(s) involved.

IMMUNE MALADAPTATION

The hypothesis of an abnormal maternal immune response to the trophoblast is largely based on epidemiological studies. The concept of 'primipaternity' as a risk factor for PE may be related to an altered immune response of the mother to antigens on the trophoblast. Moreover, a spontaneous abortion or blood transfusion is associated with a lower risk of PE in a subsequent pregnancy[22,23]. A long sperm exposure is a protective factor[24], and women using barrier methods of contraception have twice the likelihood of developing PE[25,26]. Finally, the incidence of PE after donor insem-ination was higher than expected[27]. In addition to epidemiological studies, there are numerous reports of immunological phenomena in PE. These include antibodies against endothelial

cells, increased circulating immune complexes, complement activation, enhanced activity of cytokines and the same pathological findings in acute atherosis and allograft rejection. The majority of studies do not report modifications in the concentration of IgG, IgM, IgA and IgD levels in pre-eclamptic pregnancies with respect to normal pregnancies.

Syncytiotrophoblasts are devoid of classical class I and II HLA. This prevents recognition by maternal T-lymphocytes, but leaves these cells susceptible to their attack by natural killer cells. Nevertheless, invading cytotrophoblasts, which are the cells in contact with maternal tissues, express the relatively non-polymorphic class I molecule HLA-G, which protects them from recognition by natural killer cells[28–30]. HLA-G on invasive cytotrophoblasts has a pivotal role in escaping maternal immune sur-veillance, and trophoblast invasion may be dependent on appropriate cytokines produced by uterine large granular lymphocytes and other decidual cells in response to HLA-G expression[31,32]. Attenuated HLA-G expression in pre-eclamptic placentae was reported in several studies[33,34], but it has not yet been elucidated whether this finding is related to an aberrant trophoblast differentiation or a structural gene mutation.

The prime candidates as mediators between immune maladaptation and endothelial activa-tion are the cytokines. In PE there are increased levels of tumor necrosis factor (TNFα-), interleukin (IL)-1, IL-2 and IL-6, and the source of cytokines may be decidual leukocytes. Increased IL-6 and IL-1 receptor antagonist levels in PE correlate with high concentrations of these adhesion molecules[35]. Hamai et al. reported that abnormal cytokine production in women destined to have PE is already present in the first trimester, and these findings are concordant with an altered maternal–fetal immunological adaptation[36,37].

Normal pregnancy is characterized by acti-vated neutrophils, and neutrophil activation is further increased in PE. Complement factors can activate neutrophils; markers for comple-ment activation are increased in PE and correlate with elevated IL-6 and elastase levels[38-40]. Mellembakken *et al.*[41] reported neutrophil activation in PE, shown by systemic increases in myeloperoxidase, but they could not detect systemic complement activation.

Redman *et al.*[42] suggested that the endothelial dysfunction observed in PE is part of a more generalized intravascular inflammatory reaction involving intravascular leukocytes, as well as the clotting and complement systems. They suppose that PE rises when a universal maternal intravascular inflammatory response to pregnancy decompensates in particular cases, which may occur because either the stimulus or the maternal response is too strong. Faas *et al.*[43,44] suggest that in the instance in which the zygote is not able perfectly to regulate the inflammatory response at the implantation site, but can still implant, the inflammatory response may impair implantation[45,46]. In these cases, implantation will be defective and the inflammatory response will not be down-regulated. At this point, since the woman is pregnant, a mild pro-inflammatory stimulus (induced by implantation) may induce a persistent generalized inflammatory response[47]. This inflammatory response may ultimately lead to the signs of PE and will not stop, unless pregnancy is terminated.

ENDOTHELIAL CELL DYSFUNCTION

Many observations point to a central role of the endothelial cells in the pathogenesis of PE. There is morphological evidence of endothelial cell injury in the kidney and in the placental bed and adjacent uterine vessels. Moreover, functional derangements or biochemical evidence of damaged endothelial cells have been described in pre-eclamptic women. These morphological and functional changes of the endothelial cells can be held directly responsible for triggering the clinical syndrome of PE and include arterial vasospasm in every organ system, increased thrombocyte aggregation and capillary permeability leading to hypertension, proteinuria, edema and, often, to hemolysis, elevated liver enzymes, low platelet count (HELLP) syndrome[48,49] (Figure 4).

It is an attractive hypothesis that pre-eclamptic women have a circulating factor, the so-called 'factor X', that is the 'missing link' between ischemic placenta and endothelial damage[50]. A current hypothesis identifies oxygen free radicals and lipoperoxides as the link between reduced placental perfusion and endothelial dysfunction. One of the primary sources of oxidative stress is reduced organ perfusion with subsequent return to normal oxygenation. The enzyme xanthine oxidase/dehydrogenase is increased in response to hypoxia and it is preferentially functioning as the oxidase form to produce uric acid and a superoxide radical[51]. With restitution of oxygen delivery, there is an abundant production of this radical. Adaptive mechanisms appear to prevent the formation of reactive oxygen species in normal pregnant women. In pre-eclamptic women, increased xanthine oxidase/dehydrogenase and increased oxidase activity in the invasive cytotrophoblast have been observed[52]. Reactive oxygen species are quite labile; however, there are stable products of lipid oxidation, such as malondialdehyde (MDA) or oxidized-low-density lipoprotein (ox-LDL), that may act as circulating factors responsible for endothelial damage. MDA is increased in the blood of pre-eclamptic women[53,54]. We have reported an enhanced susceptibility of LDL to copper-induced oxidization[55] in PE; we also observed a positive correlation between plasmatic uric acid levels and susceptibility of LDL to oxidization (unpublished data). Antibodies against oxidative epitopes on LDL are apparently increased in women with established PE[56,57]. Poranen *et al.*[58] have reported a higher placental lipid peroxidation and a lower placental superoxide dismutase and glucose-6-phosphate dehydrogenase activity in PE as compared to normal pregnancy. Placentae from women with PE contain more lipid peroxides and MDA than normal placentae; moreover, the content of antioxidative agents is reduced in pre-eclamptic placentae[59].

Recently, Regan *et al.*[60] did not find a significant difference in urinary 8,12-iso-iPF2α-VI (a chemically stable, free radical catalyzed product) levels between pre-eclamptic and

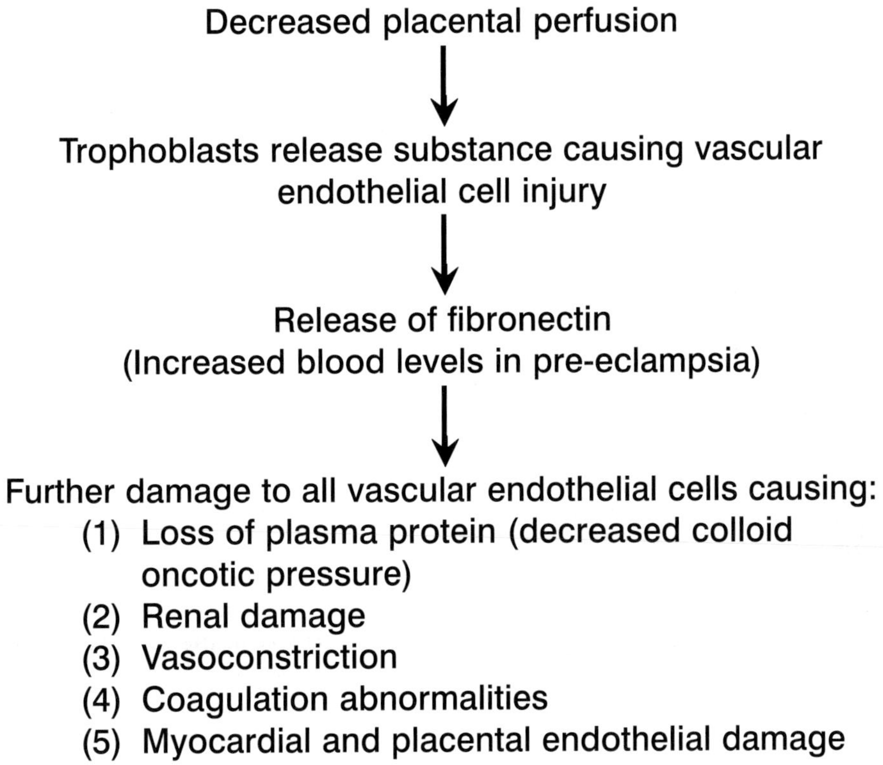

Decreased placental perfusion

↓

Trophoblasts release substance causing vascular
endothelial cell injury

↓

Release of fibronectin
(Increased blood levels in pre-eclampsia)

↓

Further damage to all vascular endothelial cells causing:
    (1) Loss of plasma protein (decreased colloid
        oncotic pressure)
    (2) Renal damage
    (3) Vasoconstriction
    (4) Coagulation abnormalities
    (5) Myocardial and placental endothelial damage

Figure 4 *Multisystem effects of decreased placental perfusion*

normal women, before or at diagnosis of PE. These data raise the question of the importance of oxidative stress for the development of the disease. The evaluation of the role of oxidative stress in the pathogenesis of PE is difficult, because almost every study has been performed after clinical signs of PE. The results are consistent with the hypothesis that enhanced systemic oxidative stress is a late phenomenon, but a localized oxidative stress in the decidual-placental tissues may be present long before the clinical manifestations of PE.

The endothelium releases several endothelium-derived factors that are involved in (1) the maintenance of vascular tone, (2) the preservation of normal endothelial permeability and (3) the inhibition of leukocyte adhesion and migration, platelet activation and smooth muscle cell proliferation. With activation or injury, endothelial cells lose these functions and produce procoagulants, vasoconstrictors (e.g. endothelin) and mitogens,

causing increased capillary permeability, vasospasm and platelet aggregation.

Increased vascular resistance is the main feature of PE. The findings of increased uterine artery resistance index and more frequent notching of the uterine artery Doppler velocimetry profile can be observed in the second trimester, representing a powerful predisposing factor for intrauterine growth retardation (IUGR) and PE (Figure 5).

Angiotensin II sensitivity is markedly increased in pre-eclamptic women, already before the clinical manifestation of the disease[61,62]. This feature can be explained by reduced production in damaged endothelial cells of vasodilating prostaglandins, particularly PGI_2. PGI_2 is the main cyclo-oxygenase product of endothelial cells, and it is a potent vasodilator and inhibitor of platelet aggregation. Thromboxane A_2 (TXA_2), the principal cyclo-oxygenase product of arachidonic acid in platelets, has the opposite effect on vascular tone and platelet function. The imbalance between TXA_2 and PGI_2 may explain many clinical features of PE, but it is uncertain if it is the major pathogenetic mechanism for the development of the disease[63–65]. Other possible agents involved are depicted in Figure 6.

PE is associated with impairment of endothelial-dependent relaxation in maternal arteries, while endothelial-independent relax-

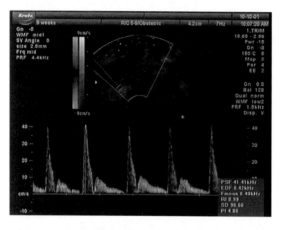

Figure 5 *Three-dimensional color Doppler of right uterine artery coupled with protodiastolic notch in a pregnant woman at 9 weeks' gestation, age 38 years, gravida 1, para 0. Note the high resistance index (RI) (0.99) (see Color Plate W)*

ation is normal. Nitric oxide (NO) is the endothelial-derived relaxing factor; it is a simple radical gas with a short half-life, and *in vivo* its activity is dependent on both NO synthesis and NO degradation. NO is synthesized from the amino acid L-arginine by nitric oxide synthase (NOS). Three isoforms of NOS have been identified: an endothelial (eNOS), a neuronal and a macrophage (inducible) type[66]. Endothelial NOS is activated by shear stress[67] or stimulation of G1-protein receptors (e.g. by acetylcholine or serotonin)[68]. NO degradation occurs mainly by its reaction with oxyhemoglobin in erythrocytes or by reacting with superoxide, leading to the formation of peroxynitrite, a highly cytotoxic agent[69]. Several studies have reported data supporting the role of increased NO activity as a prime contributor to systemic vasodilatation in normal pregnancies[70,71]. The exact role of NO in PE is not clear. Serum levels of NO metabolites have been reported to be reduced, increased or unchanged[72–75]. Recently, Shaamash *et al.*[76] observed an increase in serum NO production in normal pregnancies and significantly higher total nitrite and nitrate levels in the maternal sera of the pre-eclamptic and eclamptic women

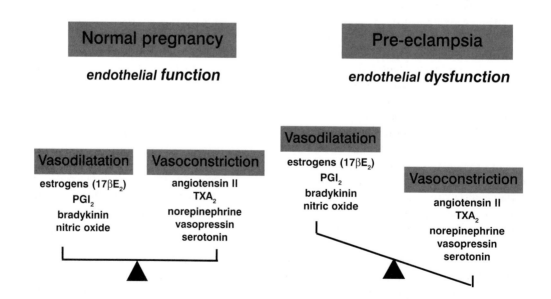

Figure 6 *Imbalance between vasodilators and vasoconstrictors in pre-eclampsia vs. normal pregnancy. $17\beta E_2$, 17β-estradiol; PGI_2, prostaglandin I_2; TXA_2, thromboxane A_2*

compared with those of normal pregnant women. The high levels of NO in PE may represent a compensatory/protective mechanism to maintain blood flow and limit platelet aggregation in the fetal–maternal circulation. Lopez-Jaramillo[77] has observed higher levels of nitrate and lower levels of cyclic guanosine monophosphate (GMP) in pre-eclamptic women with respect to normal pregnancy. The contradiction of the results between the production of NO, evaluated by the nitrate levels, and the action of NO, evaluated by the cGMP levels, could be related to a higher inactivation of NO in PE. Free radical superoxide inactivates NO, and these findings may provide a relationship between oxidative stress and NO function in PE.

Maternal plasma levels of the vasoactive peptide endothelin-1 (ET-1) are increased in PE when compared with normal pregnancy. Endothelins are the most potent vasoconstrictors yet identified. The increased production is a reflection of extensive endothelial damage[78–81].

Fibronectin is produced by fibroblasts, endothelial cells and platelets and is a marker of endothelial damage. Fibronectin levels are higher in pre-eclamptic women before the clinical manifestation of the disease, showing an early involvement of endothelial cells, before the hypertension is clearly manifested[82–85]. The endothelial involvement in the pathogenesis of PE is supported also by the evidence of increased levels of factor VIII-related antigen (von Willebrand factor), thrombomodulin, growth factor activity and disturbance of the tissue plasminogen activator (tPA)/plasminogen activator inhibitor (PAI) balance[86–92].

Adrenomedullin is a novel peptide with a potent vasodilatory action; the plasma levels of adrenomedullin are increased during normal pregnancy and it may contribute to the low placental vascular resistance[93,94]. Although fetoplacental adrenomedullin levels are reported to increase in PE, maternal plasma levels may be elevated, decreased or they may resemble those in normal pregnancy[95–98]. Increased levels of adrenomedullin in PE may represent a compensatory mechanism to hypoxia, but the role of this peptide in the pathogenesis of the disease has to be further investigated.

ORGAN SYSTEMS INVOLVEMENT

Hemodynamic changes

Hemodynamic changes occurring in pre-eclamptic pregnancies should be considered in the context of the hemodynamic adaptations that occur in normal pregnancy[99]. Maternal cardiovascular adaptation to pregnancy involves enormous changes. Cardiac output increases in early pregnancy, initially as a result of an increased heart rate, soon followed by an increased stroke volume. Cardiac output continues to increase until mid-pregnancy and remains stable afterward, with a possible small decline in the last weeks of pregnancy. Blood pressure decreases in early pregnancy, reaching a minimum in mid-pregnancy. Consequently, peripheral vascular resistance is reduced throughout pregnancy. Plasma volume increases in normal pregnancy by about 40%. There are two essentially theoretical models of the hemodynamic characteristics of PE:

(1) Reduced plasma volume, vasoconstriction and hypoperfusion of placenta and kidneys;
(2) Elevated cardiac output and compensatory vasodilatation.

The reduction in plasma volume is due to distribution of extracellular fluid to the interstitial space as a result of an increase of both vascular resistance and capillary permeability.

The vasospasm in PE is a greater response to normal concentrations of endogenous pressors; women with PE have higher sensitivity to all endogenous pressors thus far tested. They are sensitive to vasopressin[100] which can elicit marked blood pressure elevation, seizures and oliguria in some patients. Sensitivity to epinephrine and norepinephrine is also increased[101], but the most striking difference is seen in the sensitivity of the pre-eclamptic woman to angiotensin II. Pre-eclamptic women are much more sensitive to angiotensin II than normal pregnant and non-pregnant women. It would be expected that the cardiac output in pre-eclamptic women would fall in response to a decreased pre-load, related to vasospasm. This has been reported by some investigators, but most studies indicate that cardiac output is normal or slightly reduced in PE[102]. The high cardiac output, observed by other groups[103], may be the result of treatment (e.g. hydralazine) rather than a pathophysiological finding.

Coagulation system

The coagulation system is intimately involved in the pathogenesis of PE. There is substantial evidence of increased platelet activation and circulating levels of factors stored within platelets, reflecting platelet activation. Several studies have demonstrated increased levels of the platelet granule protein β-thromboglobulin in women with PE as compared with normal pregnant controls; thromboxane production is increased whereas antithrombin III is decreased in women with PE, compared with normal pregnant controls[104]. PE is associated with thrombocytopenia; its mechanism is yet to be fully elucidated, but there is evidence to implicate an immune mechanism.

Low platelets associated with hemolysis and elevated liver enzymes that characterize the HELLP syndrome have been recognized in PE for at least 100 years[105]. The diagnostic criteria include all three of the following laboratory findings: hemolysis (characteristic peripheral blood smear and serum lactate dehydrogenase levels > 600 IU), serum aspartate aminotransferase levels > 70 IU and platelet count < 100 000/μl[106]. A disseminated intravascular coagulation (DIC) occurred in 15% of women with HELLP syndrome and it is suggested that a subclinical DIC is present in all women with this syndrome[107]. The pathogenesis of HELLP syndrome remains an enigma; it has been speculated that this syndrome represents the severe end of the spectrum of liver involvement in this condition, possibly resulting from increasing vasospasm. The appearance of the HELLP syndrome is extremely variable because it may develop in the absence of significant proteinuria and hypertension.

Studies of coagulation factors have shown that PE accentuates a state of hypercoagulability already present in normal pregnancy[108]. There is an early rise in factor VIII-related antigen : coagulation activity ratio which correlates with the severity of the disease and the level of hyperuricemia[109]. Levels of fibrinopeptide A have been reported to be elevated or unchanged in normal pregnancy but increased in women with PE[110].

Antithrombin III, protein C and protein S levels are essentially unchanged in normal pregnancy, but are decreased in the majority of women with PE[111].

Liver dysfunctions

The liver dysfunctions complicating PE are uncertain. Abnormal liver function tests have been reported to occur in 20–30% of pregnancies complicated by PE[112]. They are speculated to reflect liver dysfunction occurring as a result of vasoconstriction of the hepatic vascular bed. Possibly the most worrying complications in PE are hepatic infarction and rupture. Infarction is thought to result from intense hepatic vasospasm. Hepatic rupture is a fortunately rare, but frequently fatal, complication; the pathogenesis is thought to involve liver necrosis, hypervascularity and vessel rupture, leading to subcapsular hematoma or hemoperitoneum[113].

Renal function

Renal function deteriorates in PE in two stages:

(1) Impairment of tubular function, reflected by a reduction in uric acid clearance and development of hyperuricemia;
(2) Impairment of glomerular filtration and development of proteinuria of intermediated selectivity.

Proteinuria reflects the involvement of the renal glomerulus in PE; there is a selective loss of intermediated weight proteins such as albumin, transferrin and γ-globulin. This in turn leads to a decrease in the amount of circulating plasma proteins and a fall in plasma oncotic pressure contributing to the tendency to generalized edema in PE. Edema has been found in 35% of normotensive pregnancies, and only a generalized edema that involves the body and face after 12 h of bed rest should be considered clearly abnormal. Particularly, edema of the glottis poses a big challenge to the anesthesiologist.

Cerebral sequelae

The principal and clinically most relevant cerebral sequelae of PE are eclamptic convulsions[114]. There are two essential models to explain the pathogenesis of eclamptic seizures:

(1) Eclampsia is a result of focal cerebral vasospasm and hypoperfusion;
(2) Hypertension results in a breakthrough in cerebral autoregulation with forced overdistension of intracranial arteries, resulting in endothelial injury. This is hypothesized to lead to extravasation of fluid across the disrupted endothelium into the interstitial spaces, resulting in cerebral edema.

In summary, evidence suggests that the most likely explanation of eclampsia is the intense vasoconstriction that leads to abnormal electrical activity and thus triggers seizures. Cerebral vasodilatation reported by some investigators is likely to reflect vasodilatation in response to treatment.

CONCLUSION

Pre-eclampsia–eclampsia (PE) affects virtually all organ systems, e.g. cardiovascular, liver and renal systems, CNS, the placenta and the coagulatory system.

The majority of research supports the hypothesis that the endothelial cell dysfunction is the final common pathway, directly responsible for triggering the clinical syndrome. However, the etiology of the disease is still unknown. Probably there is no single cause for PE, but different factors could be contributory. Immunological maladaptation has been suggested to play a role in defective placentation and endothelial damage. The putative misalliance of fetal trophoblast with maternal tissue in the uteroplacental vascular bed may give rise to an increase in cytokines that induce oxidative stress. Genetic predisposition and maternal vascular pathology could be modulating factors in this process.

There is a consistent overlap between observations in PE and normal pregnancy, and PE could be not a separate, distinct abnormality of pregnancy, but rather could represent an extension of pregnancy-induced changes. Most women with PE feel fine and pregnancy outcome is often uneventful. Thus, there is a pressing need for definition of biophysical/biochemical aspects, including molecular biology, of PE that are suited for the prediction of poor maternal or perinatal outcome. Regarding the pathophysiology of PE, there is a general consensus that recognizes a generalized vasoconstriction in almost every organ system, including the uteroplacental–fetal circulation, and that under these circumstances there should be instituted the proper management of the disease. Finally, one should be aware that the so-called normal brachial artery blood pressure does not exclude an already compromised uteroplacental–fetal circulation.

References

1. Page EW. The relation between hydatid moles, relative ischemia of the gravid uterus, and the placental origin of eclampsia. *Am J Obstet Gynecol* 1939;37:291–3
2. Caniggia I, Winter J, Lye SJ, Post M. Oxygen and placental development during the first trimester: implications for the pathophysiology of pre-eclampsia. *Placenta* 2000;21:S25–30
3. Roberts JM, Cooper DW. Pathogenesis and genetics of pre-eclampsia. *Lancet* 2001;357:53–6
4. Cooper DW, Brennecke SP, Wilton AN. Genetics of pre-eclampsia. *Hypertens Preg* 1993;12:1–23

5. Treloar SA, Cooper DW, Brennecke SP, Grehan MM, Martin NG. An Australian twin study of the genetic basis of pre-eclampsia and eclampsia. *Am J Obstet Gynecol* 2001;184: 374–81

6. Lie RT, Rasmussen S, Brunborg H, Gjessing HK, Lie-Nelsen E, Irgens LM. Fetal and maternal contributions to risk of pre-eclampsia. *Br Med J* 1998;316:1343–7

7. Robillard PY, Dekker GA, Hulsey TC. Revisiting the epidemiological standard of pre-eclampsia: primigravidity or primipaternity. *Eur J Obstet Gynecol Reprod Biol* 1999;84:37–41

8. Robillard PY, Hulsey TC, Perianin J, Janky E, Miri EH, Papiernik E. Association of pregnancy-induced hypertension with duration of sexual cohabitation before conception. *Lancet* 1994; 344:973–5

9. Graves JA. Genomic imprinting, development and disease – is pre-eclampsia caused by a maternally imprinted gene? *Reprod Fertil Dev* 1998;10:23–9

10. Broughton-Pipkin F. What is the place of genetics in the pathogenesis of pre-eclampsia? *Biol Neonate* 1999;76:325–30

11. Hayward C, Livingstone J, Holloway S, Liston WA, Brock DJ. An exclusion map for pre-eclampsia: assuming autosomal recessive inheritance. *Am J Hum Genet* 1992;50:749–57

12. Humphrey KE, Harrison GA, Cooper DW, Wilton AN, Brennecke SP, Trudinger BJ. HLA-G deletion polymorphism and pre-eclampsia–eclampsia. *Br J Obstet Gynaecol* 1995;102:707–10

13. Tamura T, Johanning GL, Goldenberg RL, Johnston KE, DuBard MB. Effect of angiotensin converting enzyme gene polymorphism on pregnancy outcome, enzyme activity and zinc concentration. *Obstet Gynecol* 1996;88:497–502

14. Kupferminc MJ, Faith G, Many A, Gordon D, Eldor A, Lessing JB. Severe pre-eclampsia and high frequency of genetic thrombophilic mutations. *Obstet Gynecol* 2000;96:45–9

15. Dizon-Towson DS, Nelson LM, Easton K, Ward K. The factor V Leiden mutation may dispose women to severe pre-eclampsia. *Am J Obstet Gynecol* 1996;175:902–5

16. Lockwood CJ. Inherited thrombophilias in pregnant patients. *Prenat Neonat Med* 2001;6:3–14

17. Lachmeijer AM, Arngrimsson R, Bastiaans EJ, Pals G, ten Kate LP, de Vries JI, Kostense PJ, Aarnoudse JG, Dekker GA. Mutations in the gene for methylenetetrahydrofolate reductase, homocysteine levels, and vitamin status in women with a history of pre-eclampsia. *Am J Obstet Gynecol* 2001;184:394–402

18. Shoda S, Arimani T, Hamada H, Yamada N, Hamaguchi H, Kubo T. Methylenetetrahydrofolate reductase polymorphism and pre-eclampsia. *J Med Genet* 1997;34:525–6

19. Kupferminc MJ, Eldor A, Steinman N, Many A, Bar-Am A, Jaffa A, Fait G, Lessing JB. Increased frequency of genetic thrombophilia in women with complications of pregnancy. *N Engl Med J* 1999;340:9–13

20. Kobashi G. A case-control study of pregnancy-induced hypertension with a genetic predisposition: association of a molecular variant of angiotensinogen in Japanese women. *Hokkaido J Med Sci* 1995;102:489–90

21. Morgan L, Baker PN, Broughton Pipkin F, Kalsheker N. Maternal and fetal angiotensinogen gene allele sharing in pre-eclampsia. *Br J Obstet Gynaecol* 1999;106:244–51

22. Strickland DM, Guzick DS, Cox K, Gant NF, Rosenfeld CR. The relationship between abortion in the first pregnancy and development of pregnancy-induced hypertension in the subsequent pregnancy. *Am J Obstet Gynecol* 1986; 154:146–8

23. Feeney JG, Tovey LA, Scott JS. Influence of previous blood-transfusion on incidence of pre-eclampsia. *Lancet* 1977;1:874–5

24. Trupin LS, Simon LP, Eskenazi B. Change in paternity: a risk factor for pre-eclampsia in multiparas. *Epidemiology* 1996;7:240–4

25. Robillard PY, Hulsey TC, Perianin J, Yanky E, Miri EH, Papiernik E. Association of pregnancy-induced hypertension with duration of sexual cohabitation before conception. *Lancet* 1994; 344:973–5

26. Klonoff Cohen HS, Savitz DA, Cefalo RC, McCann MF. An epidemiologic study of contraception and pre-eclampsia. *J Am Med Assoc* 1989; 262:3143–7

27. Serhal PF, Craft I. Immune basis for pre-eclampsia: evidence from oocyte recipients. *Lancet* 1987;2:744

28. Mowbray J, Jalali R, Chaouat G, Clark DA, Underwood J, Allen WR, Mathias S. Maternal response to paternal trophoblast antigens. *Am J Reprod Biol* 1997;37:421–6

29. Loke YWK, King A. Immunology of human placental implantation: clinical implications of our current understanding. *Mol Med Today* 1997; 3:153–9

30. Shorter SC, Starkey PM, Ferrey BL, Clover LM, Sargent PL, Redman CW. Antigenic heterogeneity of human cytotrophoblast and evidence for the transient expression of MHC class I antigens distinct from HLA-G. *Placenta* 1993;14: 571–82

31. Clark DA. Cytokines, deciduas, and early pregnancy. *Oxf Rev Reprod Biol* 1993;15:83–110

32. Rouas-Freiss N, Marchal RE, Kirszenbaum M, Dausset J, Carosella ED. The alpha-1 domain of HLA-G2 inhibits cytotoxicity induced by natural killer cells: is HLA-G the public ligand for

natural killer cell inhibitory receptors. *Proc Natl Acad Sci USA* 1997;94:5249–54

33. Hara N, Fujji T, Yamashita T, Kozuma S, Okai T, Taketani Y. Altered expression of human leukocyte antigen G (HLA-G) on extravillous trophoblasts in preeclampsia: immunohisto-logical demonstration with anti-HLA-G specific antibody '87G' and anticytokeratin antibody 'CAM.2'. *Am J Reprod Immunol* 1996;36:349–58

34. Faas MM, Schuiling GA, Baller JFW, Visscher CA, Bakker WW. A new animal model for human pre-eclampsia: ultra-low-dose endotoxin infusion in pregnant rats. *Am J Obstet Gynecol* 1994;171:158–64

35. Krauss T, Kuhn W, Lakoma C, Augustin HG. Circulating endothelial adhesion molecules as diagnostic markers for the early identification of pregnant women at risk for development of pre-eclampsia. *Am J Obstet Gynecol* 1997;177:443–9

36. Hamai Y, Fujii T, Yamashita T, Kozuma S, Okai T, Taketani Y. Pathogenetic implication of interleukin 2 expressed in pre-eclamptic decid-ual tissue. A possible mechanism of deranged vasculature of the placenta associated with pre-eclampsia. *Am J Reprod Biol* 1997;38:83–8

37. Hamai Y, Fujii T, Yamashita T, Nishina H, Kozuma S, Mikami Y, Taketani Y. Evidence for an elevation in serum interleukin 2 and tumor necrosis factor-α levels before the clinical manifestations of pre-eclampsia. *Am J Reprod Biol* 1997;38:89–93

38. Haeger M, Unander M, Andersson B, Tarkowski A, Arnestad JP, Bengtsson A. Increased release of tumor necrosis factor-alpha and interleukin 6 in women with the syndrome of hemolysis, elevated liver enzymes, and low platelet count. *Acta Obstet Gynecol Scand* 1996;75:695–701

39. Rebelo I, Carvalho-Guerra F, Pereira-Leite L, Quintanilha A. Comparative study of lactoferrin and other blood markers of inflammatory stress between pre-eclamptic and normal pregnancies. *Eur J Obstet Gynecol Reprod Biol* 1996;64:167–73

40. Prieto JA, Panyutich AV, Heine RP. Neutrophil activation in pre-eclampsia. Are defences and lactoferrin elevated in pre-eclamptic patients. *J Reprod Med* 1997;42:29–32

41. Mellembakken JR, Hogasen K, Mollines JE, Hack E, Abyholm T, Videm V. Increased systemic activation of neutrophils but not complement in pre-eclampsia. *Obstet Gynecol* 2001;97:371–4

42. Redman WG, Sacks GP, Sargent IL. Pre-eclampsia: an excessive maternal inflammatory response to pregnancy. *Am J Obstet Gynecol* 1999;180:499–506

43. Faas MM, Schuiling GA. Pre-eclampsia and the inflammatory response. *Eur J Obstet Gynecol Reprod Biol* 2001;95:213–17

44. Faas MM, Schuiling GA, Bakker WW. Low dose endotoxin infusion: a new model. Reply. *Am J Obstet Gynecol* 1995;172:1634–5

45. Tuohy JF, James DK. Pre-eclampsia and trisomy 13. *Br J Obstet Gynaecol* 1992;99:434–9

46. Boyd PA, Lindenbaum RH, Redman C. Pre-eclampsia and trisomy 13: a possible association. *Lancet* 1987;2(8556):425–7

47. Ros HS, Lichtenstein P, Lipworth L, Cnattingius S. Genetic effects on the liability of developing pre-eclampsia and gestational hypertension. *Am J Med Genet* 2000;91:256–60

48. Gaber LW, Spargo BH, Lindheimer ND. Renal pathology in pre-eclampsia. *Baillieres Clin Obstet Gynaecol* 1994;8:443–68

49. Shankling DR, Sibai BM. Ultrastructural aspects of pre-eclampsia. I. Placental bed and uterine boundary vessels. *Am J Obstet Gynecol* 1989;161:735–41

50. Van Beek E, Peeters LH. Pathogenesis of pre-eclampsia: a comprehensive model. *Obstet Gynecol Surv* 1998;53:233–9

51. Hamer I, Wattiaux R, Wattiaux-DeConick S. Deleterious effects of xanthine oxidase on rat liver endothelial cells after ischemia/reperfusion. *Biochim Biophys Acta* 1995;1269:145–52

52. Many A, Hubel C, Fischer SJ, Roberts JM, Zhou Y. Invasive cytotrophoblast manifest evidence of oxidative stress in pre-eclampsia. *Am J Pathol* 2000;156:321–31

53. Hegberts J. Circulating markers of oxidative stress are raised in normal pregnancy and pre-eclampsia. *Br J Obstet Gynaecol* 1999;106:751

54. Yanik FF, Amanvernetz R, Yanik A, Celik C, Kokcu A. Pre-eclampsia associated with increased lipid peroxidation and decreased serum vitamin E levels. *Int J Gynaecol Obstet* 1999;64:27–33

55. Pierucci F, Piazze Garnica JJ, Cosmi EV, Anceschi MM. Oxidability of low density lipoproteins in pregnancy-induced hypertension. *Br J Obstet Gynaecol* 1996;103:1159–61

56. Branch Ware D, Mitchell MD, Miller E, Palinsky W, Witzum JL. Pre-eclampsia and serum antibodies to oxidised low density lipoprotein. *Lancet* 1994;343:645–6

57. Uotila J, Solakivi T, Yaakkola O, Tuimala R, Lehtimaki T. Antibodies against copper oxidised and malondialdehyde-modified low density lipoproteins in pre-eclamptic pregnancies. *Br J Obstet Gynaecol* 1998;105:1113–17

58. Poranen AK, Ekblad U, Uotila P, Ahotupa M. Lipid peroxidation and antioxidants in normal and pre-eclamptic pregnancies. *Placenta* 1996;17:401–5

59. Walsh SW. Maternal-placental interactions of oxidative stress and antioxidants in pre-eclampsia. *Semin Reprod Endocrinol* 1998;116:93–104

60. Regan CL, Levine RJ, Baird DD, Ewell GM, Martz KL, Sibai BM, Rokach J, Lawson JA, FitzGerald GA. No evidence for lipid peroxidation in severe pre-eclampsia. *Am J Obstet Gynecol* 2001;185:72–8

61. AbdAlla S, Lother H, el Massiery A, Quitterer U. Increased AT 1 receptor heterodimers in pre-eclampsia mediate in enhanced angiotensin II responsiveness. *Nat Med* 2001;7:1003–9

62. Granger JP, Alexander BT, Llinas MT, Bennet WA, Khalil RA. Pathophysiology of hypertension during pre-eclampsia linking placental ischemia with endothelial dysfunction. *Hypertension* 2001; 38:718–22

63. Mills JL, DerSimonian R, Raymond E, Morrow JD, Roberts LJ II, Clements JD, Hauth JC, Catalano P, Sibai B, Curet LB, Levine RJ. Prostacyclin and thromboxane changes predating clinical onset of pre-eclampsia: a multicenter prospective study. *J Am Med Assoc* 1999;282:356–62

64. Ylikorkala O, Viinikka L. The role of prostaglandins in obstetrical disorders. *Baillieres Clin Obstet Gynaecol* 1992;6:809–27

65. Rowe J, Campbell S, Gallery ED. Plasma from pre-eclamptic women stimulates decidual endothelial cell growth and prostacyclin but not nitric oxide production: close correlation of prostacyclin and thromboxane production. *J Soc Gynecol Invest* 2001;8:32–8

66. Marletta MA. Nitric oxide synthase: aspects concerning structure and catalysis. *Cell* 1994;78: 927–30

67. Wieczorek KM, Brewer AS, Myatt L. Shear stress may stimulate release and action of nitric oxide in the human fetal-placental vasculature. *Am J Obstet Gynecol* 1995;173:708–13

68. Flavahan NA, Vanhoutte PM. Endothelial cell signalling and endothelial dysfunction. *Am J Hypertens* 1995;8(5.Pt2):285–415

69. Verhaar MC, Rabelink TJ. The endothelium: a gynecological and obstetric point of view. *Eur J Obstet Gynecol Reprod Biol* 2001;94:180–5

70. Conrad KP, Joff GM, Kruszyna H, Kruszyna R, Rochelle LG, Smith RP, Chavez JE, Mosher MD. Identification of increased nitric oxide synthesis during pregnancy in rats. *FASEB J* 1993;7:566–71

71. Curtis NE, Gude NM, King RG. Nitric oxide in normal human pregnancy and pre-eclampsia. *Hypertens Pregn* 1995;14:339–49

72. Morris NH, Eaton BM, Dekker JA. Nitric oxide, the endothelium, pregnancy and pre-eclampsia. *Br J Obstet Gynaecol* 1996;103:4–15

73. Di Iorio R, Marinoni E, Emiliani S, Villaccio B, Cosmi EV. Nitric oxide in pre-eclampsia: lack of evidence for decreased production. *Eur J Obstet Gynecol Reprod Biol* 1998;76:65–70

74. Davidge ST, Billiar TR, Roberts JM. Plasma nitrites and nitrates, stable end products of nitric oxide, are elevated in women with pre-eclampsia. *Hypertens Preg* 1994;13:344

75. Davidge ST, Stranko CP, Roberts JM. Urine but not plasma nitric oxide metabolites are decreased in women with pre-eclampsia. *Am J Obstet Gynecol* 1996;174:1008–13

76. Shaamash AH, Elsnosy ED, Makhlouf AM, Zakhari MM, Ibrahim OA, El-dien HM. Maternal and fetal serum nitric oxide (NO) concentrations in normal pregnancy, pre-eclampsia and eclampsia. *Int J Gynecol Obstet* 2000;68:207–14

77. Lopez-Jaramillo P. Calcium, nitric oxide, and pre-eclampsia. *Semin Perinatol* 2000;24:33–6

78. Schiff E, Ben-Baruch G, Peleg E, Rosenthal T, Alcalay M, Devir M, Mashiach S. Immunoreactive circulating endothelin-1 in normal and hypertensive pregnancies. *Am J Obstet Gynecol* 1992; 166:624–8

79. Parlberg KM, de Jong CL, van Geijn HP, van Kamp GJ, Heinen AG, Dekker GA. Vasoactive mediators in pregnancy-induced hypertensive disorders: a longitudinal study. *Am J Obstet Gynecol* 1998;179:1559–64

80. Saijo Y, Maeda K, Nakya Y, Kamada M, Mitani R, Endo S, Irahara M, Yamano S, Aono T. Altered sensitivity to a novel vasoconstrictor endothelin-1 (1-31) in myometrium and umbilical artery of women with severe pre-eclampsia. *Biochem Biophys Res Commun* 2001;286:964–7

81. Nishikawa S, Miyamoto A, Yamamoto H, Ohshika H, Kudo R. The relationship between serum nitrate and endothelin-1 concentrations in pre-eclampsia. *Life Sci* 2000;67:1447–54

82. Paarlberg KM, de Jong CL, van Geijn HP, van Kamp GJ, Heinen AG, Dekker GA. Total plasma fibronectin as a marker of pregnancy-induced hypertensive disorders: a longitudinal study. *Obstet Gynecol* 1998;91:383–8

83. Halligan A, Bonnar J, Sheppard B, Darling M, Walshe J. Haemostatic, fibrinolytic and endothelial variables in normal pregnancies and pre-eclampsia. *Br J Obstet Gynaecol* 1994;101:488–92

84. Yoshida A, Nakao S, Kobayashi M, Kobayashi H. Flow-mediated vasodilation and plasma fibronectin levels in pre-eclampsia. *Hypertension* 2001;36:400–4

85. Islami B, Shoukir Y, Dupont P, Campana A, Bischof P. Is cellular fibronectin a biological marker for pre-eclampsia? *Eur J Obstet Gynecol Reprod Biol* 2001;97:40–5

86. Heshe S, Silveira A, Hansten A, Blonbach M, Bremme K. Haemostatic, endothelial and lipoprotein parameters and blood pressure levels in women with a history of pre-eclampsia. *Thromb Haemost* 1999;81:538–42

87. Hayman R, Brochelsby J, Kenny L, Baker P. Pre-eclampsia: the endothelium, circulating factor(s)

and vascular endothelial growth factor. *J Soc Gynecol Invest* 1999;6:310

88. Boffa MC, Valsecchi L, Fausto A, Gozin D, Viganò D'Angelo F, Safa O, Castiglioni MT, Amiral J, D'Angelo A. Predictive value of plasma thrombomodulin in pre-eclampsia and gestational hypertension. *Thromb Haemost* 1998;79:1092–5

89. de Moerloose P, Mermillod N, Amiral J, Reber G. Thrombomodulin levels during normal pregnancy, at delivery and in the post partum: comparison with tissue-type plasminogen activator and plasminogen activator inhibitor-1. *Thromb Haemost* 1998;79:554–6

90. Nakabayashi M, Yamamoto S, Suzuki K. Analysis of thrombomodulin gene polymorphism in women with severe early-onset pre-eclampsia. *Semin Thromb Haemost* 1999;25:473–9

91. de Boer K, Lecander I, ten Cate JW, Borm JJ, Treffers PE. Placental-type plasminogen activator inhibitor in pre-eclampsia. *Am J Obstet Gynecol* 1998;158:518–22

92. Astedt B, Lidoff C, Lecander I. Significance of the plasminogen activator inhibitor of placental type (PAI-2) in pregnancy. *Semin Thromb Haemost* 1998;24:431–5

93. Lauria MR, Standley CA, Sorokin Y, Yejelian FD, Cotton DP. Adrenomedullin levels in normal and pre-eclamptic pregnancy at term. *J Soc Gynecol Invest* 1999;6:318–21

94. Jerat S, Morrish DW, Davidge ST, Kaufman S. Effect of adrenomedullin on placental arteries in normal and pre-eclamptic pregnancies. *Hypertension* 2001;37:227–31

95. Di Iorio R, Marinoni E, Letizia C, Alò P, Villaccio B, Cosmi EV. Adrenomedullin, a new vasoactive peptide is increased in pre-eclampsia. *Hypertension* 1998;32:758–63

96. Di Iorio R, Marinoni E, Cosmi EV. Adrenomedullin in pre-eclampsia. *Lancet* 1998;351:676–7

97. Hata T, Miyazaki K, Matzui K. Decreased circulating adrenomedullin in pre-eclampsia. *Lancet* 1997;350:1600

98. Kanenishi K, Kuwabara H, Ueno M, Sakamoto H, Hata T. Immunohistochemical adrenomedullin expression is decreased in the placenta from pregnancies with pre-eclampsia. *Pathol Int* 2000;50:536–40

99. Cosmi EV, Di Renzo GC. *Hypertension in Pregnancy*. Bologna: Monduzzi Publishers, 1992

100. Pascoal IF, Lindheimer MD, Nalbantian-Brandt C, Umans JG. Pre-eclampsia selectively impairs endothelium-dependent relaxation and leads to oscillatory activity in small omental arteries. *J Clin Invest* 1998;15:101(2):464–70

101. Kublickiene KR, Lindblom B, Kruger K, Nisell H. Pre-eclampsia: evidence for impaired shear stress-mediated nitric oxide release in uterine circulation. *Am J Obstet Gynecol* 2000;183:160–6

102. Sibai BM, Mabie WC. Hemodynamics of pre-eclampsia. *Clin Perinatol* 1991;18:727–47

103. Bosio PM, McKenna PJ, Conroy R, O'Herlihy C. Maternal central hemodynamics in hypertensive disorders of pregnancy. *Obstet Gynecol* 1999;94:978–84

104. Fitzgerald DJ, Rocki W, Murray R. Thromboxane A2 synthesis in pregnancy-induced hypertension. *Lancet* 1990;335:751–4

105. Weinstein L. Syndrome of haemolysis, elevated liver enzymes and low platelet count: a severe consequence of hypertension in pregnancy. *Am J Obstet Gynecol* 1982;142:159–67

106. Sibai BM. The HELLP syndrome: much ado about nothing? *Am J Obstet Gynecol* 1990;162:311–16

107. Audibert F, Friedman SA, Frangieh AY, Sibai BM. Clinical utility of strict diagnostic criteria for the HELLP syndrome. *Am J Obstet Gynecol* 1996;175:460–4

108. Perry KG Jr, Martin JN Jr. Abnormal hemostasis and coagulopathy in pre-eclampsia and eclampsia. *Clin Obstet Gynecol* 1992;35:338–50

109. Caron C, Goudemand J, Marey A, Beague D, Ducroux G, Drouvin F. Are haemostatic and fibrinolytic parameters predictors of pre-eclampsia in pregnancy-associated hypertension? *Thromb Haemost* 1991;66:410–14

110. Bellart J, Gilabert R, Angles A, Piera V, Miralles RM, Monasterio J, Cabero L. Tissue factor levels and high ratio of fibrinopeptide A:D-dimer as a measure of endothelial procoagulant disorder in pre-eclampsia. *Br J Obstet Gynaecol* 1999;106:594–7

111. Dekker GA, de Vries JI, Doelitzsch PM. Underlying disorders associated with severe early-onset pre-eclampsia. *Am J Obstet Gynecol* 1995;173:1042–8

112. Romero R, Vizoso J, Emamian M. Clinical significance of liver dysfunction in pregnancy-induced hypertension. *Am J Perinatol* 1988;5:146–51

113. Henny CP, Lim AE, Brummelkamp WH. A review of the importance of the multidisciplinary treatment following spontaneous rupture of the liver capsule during pregnancy. *Surg Gynecol Obstet* 1983;156:593–8

114. Douglas KA, Redman CW. Eclampsia in the United Kingdom. *Br J Obstet Gynaecol* 1994;309:1395–400

Pathophysiology of pre-eclampsia 34

P. Merviel, L. Carbillon, J.-C. Challier, M. Beaufils and S. Uzan

INTRODUCTION

Implantation of the human embryo leads to the invasion by the extraembryonic trophoblast of the endometrium and to the colonization of the uterine arteries. This phenomenon enables the embryo to be anchored in the uterine wall and thus makes possible the maintenance of the pregnancy and fetal growth via the placenta. For this semi-allogeneic graft to occur, the endometrium must first undergo structural and biochemical modifications, called 'decidualization'. The interactions between the embryo and various components of the decidua then lead to implantation in the strict sense of the term. Finally, the trophoblastic cells transform the uterine vascular system; this change, together with the action of vasomotor factors, will adequately nourish the fetal–placental unit[1].

Pre-eclampsia is characterized by hypertension (>140/90 mmHg) and proteinuria (>0.3 g/l). It is secondary to an anomaly of the invasion of the uterine spiral arteries by cytotrophoblast cells. The aim of this review is to reconsider the pathophysiology of pre-eclampsia.

AN ANOMALY OF THE EXTRAVILLOUS CYTOTROPHOBLASTIC INVASION OF THE UTERINE SPIRAL ARTERIES

The extravillous cytotrophoblast cells (EVCT) must invade the decidua before they modify the walls of the spiral arteries[2,3]. The trophoblast behaves like a 'pseudo-tumor' invading the endometrium, which tolerates it in a controlled way. Any anomaly between the factors promoting and those limiting this invasion may cause a pregnancy-related disease. Pre-eclampsia is one of these[4].

To invade the decidua, the trophoblast cells need both to recognize the different components of the membrane and of the extracellular matrix (integrins, cadherin) and to break them down (metalloproteases). To control this invasion, the endometrium modifies the composition of its extracellular matrix (ECM), secretes transforming growth factor (TGF)β and protease inhibitors (TIMP)[5]. Moreover, the decidua is colonized by immune-system cells (NK, lymphocytes and macrophages), which are responsible for the local production of cytokines that promote or inhibit the trophoblastic invasion.

The establishment of the uteroplacental vascular system begins with the invasion of the maternal decidua by the EVCT. Two successive and interdependent phenomena are necessary to accomplish the complete transformation of the uterine spiral arteries by the trophoblastic cells[6,7].

The first vascular invasion by the cytotrophoblast

During the first trimester (from 8 until 12 weeks, approximately), the EVCT sheathes the outer wall of the decidual capillaries and the intra-endometrial branches of the uterine spiral arteries, thereby creating a trophoblastic shell around these vessels. The trophoblast cells invade from the exterior towards the inner capillary walls, where they are organized in loose but interrelated clusters of trophoblastic shells. These intravascular plugs obstruct almost all of the decidual capillaries. The plugs are more of a filter than a barrier[8]. Nonetheless, the permeability of these plugs enables plasma, with some maternal red blood cells, to diffuse past them towards pools of blood that result from the vascular invasion and that are the future intervillous spaces[9].

Oxygen partial pressure

This anatomical phenomenon results in the increase of oxygen partial pressure (Po_2) upstream from these plugs and its decrease downstream from them. The increased Po_2 observed upstream diminishes lipid peroxidation in the endothelial cells of the intramyometrial spiral arteries, which in turn is translated into an increase in PGI_2 and a diminution of TXA_2 (and the consequent increase in the vasodilatation of these vessels). The increase in Po_2 also diminishes production of endothelin 1 (ET-1), which is vasoconstrictive. Downstream from these plugs, the reduced Po_2 works towards guaranteeing the best possible environment for the embryo's organogenesis. Inversely, the high pressure upstream from the plugs increases the release of NO by the endothelins of the myometrial spiral arteries and thus helps to increase local vasodilatation further[10]. Rodesch et al.[11] showed that placental Po_2 is lower than endometrial Po_2 during the first trimester, but between 8 and 12 weeks, Po_2 increases progressively. Moreover, because first-trimester embryos lack defense systems against oxygen free radicals, this low Po_2 level protects their tissues against the harmful effects of oxygen. Finally, embryos at this term have embryonic hemoglobin, which has a greater affinity for oxygen in low partial pressure conditions, such as those encountered in plasma.

Hemostasis in the vascular spaces

The existence of plugs in the endometrial capillaries should theoretically be accompanied by a stacking of maternal red blood cells upstream and the appearance of extensive thrombi. This is not observed in vivo, however, because of systems that regulate local hemostasis: thrombomodulin, tissue factor and plasminogen activator. These local factors work together to ensure that blood flows through the uterine spiral arteries and to prevent extravasation following the EVCT invasion. Thrombomodulin (TM) is secreted by the endothelial cells and activates protein C, which has a proteolytic activity and inhibits the

formation of blood clots. By its anticoagulant action, TM prevents the formation of intravascular thromboses. Tissue factor (TF) is a pro-coagulant factor located on the membranes of endometrial stromal cells (during the secretory phase) and of perivascular decidual cells. Stimulable by progesterone, it contributes to the perivascular endometrial hemostasis necessary after the EVCT vascular invasion (by synthesizing thrombin, which transforms fibrinogen into fibrin). At the same time, fibrinolysis in the decidua is inhibited by the activation of plasminogen activator inhibitor, type 1 (PAI-1) and the diminution of tPA and uPA (tissue-type and urokinase-type plasminogen activators). Some authors have hypothesized that arterial–venous shunts may exist upstream from the plugs, which might explain the diminution of maternal blood intake at the plugs and thus the absence of thrombi. This has never been shown clearly during pregnancy. Remember that the uterine spiral arteries are connected in parallel to the uterine radiate arteries and are not the final branches of the latter. Accordingly, supplemental blood reaching the placenta during pregnancy (in connection with the opening of the vascular space and the increase in the maternal heart rate) is distributed evenly throughout all the spiral arteries; the blood influx is thus moderated. In these conditions arterial–venous shunts do not seem strictly necessary.

Hemodynamic protection of the embryo

The plugs in the decidual capillaries provide hemodynamic protection for the embryo, by preventing strong vascular pressure in the blood lakes. The increased sinuosity of the spiral arteries at the beginning of pregnancy (which have a damping effect on maternal blood flow) and the extraembryonic celom also play a role in this protection. In cases of spontaneous abortions, it is frequently observed that, due to the absence of intravascular plugs, the mother's blood has flooded the intervillous lakes[12]. This leads to the cessation of the embryonic–placental circulation and the death of the embryo.

Early maternal–embryonic exchanges, followed by embryonic–maternal exchanges

At the beginning of pregnancy, the embryo evacuates its wastes towards the yolk sac. There is no embryonic circulation and the pressure in the villous capillaries is less than that in the blood lakes. The exchanges therefore occur solely towards the embryo from the mother (transfer of nutrients and oxygen). From 4 to 5 weeks, fetal heart activity begins and pressure in the villous capillaries increases, thereby enabling exchanges from the embryo to the mother. The plugs in the maternal vessels protect these embryonic–maternal exchanges, because a substantial increase in the blood lake pressure would interrupt them and cause a vascular collapse of the villous vessels (and lead the embryo to stop thriving).

The first trophoblastic invasion can be observed from 5 weeks in the intraendometrial arteries. Between 5 and 8 weeks, the plugs obstruct the vascular lumina almost completely and prevent the passage of maternal blood to the intervillous lakes; they then progressively disaggregate from week 8 through week 13.

The second vascular invasion by the cytotrophoblast

The second trophoblastic invasion of the intramyometrial spiral arteries thus occurs between 13 weeks and 18 weeks, at which time it is completed. Because these are continuous phenomena, an intramyometrial vascular invasion can sometimes be observed before 13 weeks[13].

Starting at 8 weeks and through 13 weeks, the trophoblastic shell surrounding the decidual spiral arteries becomes discontinuous, persisting only at the anchoring villi of the placenta. This induces the progressive release of the intravascular plugs. A portion of the trophoblastic cells from the plugs will move backwards to colonize the inner wall of the intramyometrial spiral arteries and then penetrate into the thickness of the vascular wall[14]. This intraparietal encroachment causes the endothelial cells and the smooth muscle cells of the tunica media and the internal elastic layer to disappear progressively[15]. The latter is replaced by a fibrin deposit that deprives the vessels of their contractility. The trophoblast cells progressively develop an endothelial phenotype because of the switch from E- to VE-cadherin and the acquisition of endothelial cell molecules such as VCAM-1 and PECAM-1[16]. Decreased resistance in the uterine arteries occurs and starts the continuous blood flow through the intervillous spaces that is necessary to fetal growth during the second and third trimesters. These anatomical and hemodynamic processes can be seen in a Doppler study by the disappearance of the uterine artery notch, by the increased diastolic flow through these arteries and by the blood flow that appears in the intervillous spaces. This progressive replacement of the collagen and elastin frame and the transformation of the intramyometrial spiral arteries is most often completed at 18 weeks, but sometimes requires several additional weeks (notches not infrequently disappear between the 22-week and 26-week Doppler ultrasound examinations). The defective development of the myometrial arterial network also plays a role in the persistence of the notches in preeclampsia. At the same time, the endothelial cells detach from the uterine veins and arteries, proliferate and migrate towards the internal face of the intervillous spaces, thus separating the fetal circulation from the maternal blood by a double cellular layer – trophoblastic and endothelial. During this period, the fetus acquires fetal hemoglobin (HbF) with oxygen-uptake capacities in line with its greater needs for growth.

Vasomotor factors

Pregnancy is associated with a diminution in blood pressure, a drop in systemic and uterine vascular resistance and a reduced response to various vasopressor (vasoconstrictive) agents. The uteroplacental vessels are subjected to various factors that regulate their vascular tone. Even before implantation, the sexual hormones regulate the balance in the uterus between vasoconstricting and vasodilating agents. During the follicular phase, NO secretion (together with 17β-estradiol) increases and then diminishes during the luteal phase. Similarly, ET-1 also diminishes during the follicular phase. Estradiol has an indirect vasodilating action (NO, ET-1 and prostaglandins) and inhibits vasoconstrictors, while progesterone functions as an estradiol antagonist. Nonetheless, progesterone alone or combined with estrogens inhibits the vasoconstrictive response to angiotensin II[17].

Schematically, uterine vascular tone is regulated principally by two opposing vasomotor systems: a vasoconstrictor system (endothelin/enkephalinase) and a vasodilator system (nitric oxide/guanylate cyclase). These agents are involved in the placental regulation of the vascular flow: they set up a local balance that enables adequate blood intake. Some diseases, such as the vascular complications of hypertension, may be due to the deregulation of these systems[18]. It is now generally agreed that endothelial cells, together with endocrine and nervous system factors, participate in regulating vasomotor tone[19,20]. They also ensure the continuous inhibition of platelet aggregation.

Case of pre-eclampsia

In pre-eclampsia, decidual resistance, more powerful than the trophoblastic invasion, prevents the EVCT from reaching the spiral arteries. Placentas of women with pre-eclampsia express lower levels of matrix metalloproteinase (MMP) 9, human lymphocyte antigen (HLA) G, hPL and α1β1 than those of women with normal pregnancies; the integrin α4β5 level is stable and that of α1β1 increases[21]. Moreover, neither does the switch from E-cadherin to VE-cadherin occur, nor are VCAM-1 and PECAM-1 produced[22]. These phenomena testify that these cytotrophoblasts have lost their capacity for deep invasion. Invasive EVCT dedifferentiates into syncytium (giant cells) that thereby lose their penetrating power; the increase in giant cells thus expresses

this initial impulse[23]. A related finding is the higher frequency of pre-eclampsia and intra-uterine growth restriction among nulliparas (75% of the cases); this may be associated with the fact that the arteries colonized in a first pregnancy can be invaded more easily during subsequent pregnancies. The role of the decidual NK cells may explain why a subsequent invasion is facilitated; they can be thought of as the endometrial memory of paternal antibodies. Pre-eclampsia was similar in nulliparas and in the multiparas who had changed partners (3.2 and 3%, respectively), but lower among multiparas with the same partner (1.9%). A similar finding is noted in pregnancies after oocyte donation, sperm donation or a long period of contraceptive use. Accordingly, we must consider pre-eclampsia as a disease of primipaternity rather than primigravidity[24].

In pre-eclampsia, the second trophoblastic invasion either does not occur or is incomplete, because of the lack of intravascular plugs. This is expressed by the persistence of uterine vasoconstriction. Blood intake into the intervillous spaces is diminished and fetal growth restriction ensues. The downstream consequence of this vasoconstriction is hypoxia, with an increase in lipid peroxidation[25,26] and in the TXA_2/PGI_2 ratio[27], both of which accentuate vasoconstriction and platelet aggregation. Thromboses and disseminated fibrin deposits are usually found in the placenta in this disease[28]. Moreover, downstream hypoxia increases ET-1 production and diminishes that of NO (also related to the reduction of the mechanical force of the artery wall).

Evidence of intravascular plugs is not found in pre-eclampsia. This absence explains why the Po_2 in the decidual spiral arteries is on the whole lower than that observed upstream from these plugs. This results in increased lipid peroxidation[29] and a decreased PGI_2/TXA_2 ratio, with vasoconstriction and platelet aggregation. This diminution of Po_2 also causes an increase in ET-1 and (in combination with the diminution of the mechanical forces on the vascular wall) a decrease in NO in the myometrial and decidual spiral arteries. The stimulant effect of ET-1 on the release of NO partly compensates for this NO decrease. Moreover, the absence of plugs (resulting in relative high pressure in the blood lakes) is responsible for the increase in the rate of spontaneous abortions and the fetal 'failure to thrive' observed in patients at risk of pre-eclampsia[30].

Pre-eclampsia is thus characterized by an increase in systemic vascular resistance and in vascular reactivity and by a change in the distribution of the pelvic blood flow that precedes the onset of hypertension[31]. All of these suggest a dysregulation in the normal vasomotor factors of pregnancy. During pre-eclampsia, the sympathetic system/normal pregnancy is activated[32]. Finally, chronic hypoxia, which results from a placentation defect, can induce the transcription of some genes[33], including those of ET-1 (vasoconstrictor), angiotensin conversion enzyme (hypertensive), plasminogen activator[34] (stimulating formation of active TGFβ, which inhibits the EVCT invasion) and cyclooxygenase-1 (COX-1, an enzyme involved in prostaglandin production).

THE INFLAMMATORY THEORY OF PRE-ECLAMPSIA

Pre-eclampsia is a disease characterized by a generalized dysfunction of the endothelial cell, linked to several factors: fatty acids, lipoproteins, lipid peroxide, tumor necrosis factor (TNFα), decay products of fibronectin and microvillous fragments of syncytiotrophoblastic cells. All these factors together result from a generalized intravascular inflammatory response present during pregnancy but exacerbated in pre-eclampsia[35]. During inflammation, leukocyte adhesion proteins in the vascular system increase, stimulated too early by thrombin and histamine and then in the hours that follow

by interleukin (IL-1) or TNFα. Vascular permeability then increases, together with extravasation, and cellular chemotaxis with phagocytosis.

During pre-eclampsia, granulocyte and monocyte activation occur together with the endothelial dysfunction; this increases the level of adhesion molecules (CD11b, CD64) or other factors (L-selectin and HLA-DR). These cells also cause an increase in TNFα, IL-6 and phospholipase A_2 (important inflammatory reaction mediators) and they produce and secrete oxygen free radicals. During pre-eclampsia, these radicals increase as does the expression of CD11b and CD64 (phagocytes), while L-selectin (granulocytes) and HLA-DR (monocytes) decrease. These disturbances also occur during normal pregnancies, but are significantly less important. Moreover, activated neutrophils produce some proteases, including elastase, which increase during pre-eclampsia. Elastase is associated with increased production of endothelins and factor VIII and plays a role in the endothelial alterations observed in this disease.

CONCLUSIONS

Pre-eclampsia is therefore a form of spontaneous abortion, incomplete because it involves only the vascular face of the implanted embryo. Along with the anomaly of the trophoblastic invasion of the uterine spiral arteries, we find local disruptions of vascular tone, of immunological balance and inflammatory status, sometimes associated with genetic predispositions. Pre-eclampsia, a disease defined in the second and third trimesters of pregnancy, is multifactorial from a pathophysiologic point of view, thus complicating its prediction and treatment as well as the efficacy of preventive measures against it.

References

1. Brosens I, Robertson WB, Dixon HG. The physiological response of the vessels of the placenta bed to normal pregnancy. *J Pathol Bact* 1967;93:569–79
2. Pijnenborg R. Establishment of uteroplacental circulation. *Reprod Nutr Dev* 1988;28:1581–6
3. Strickland S, Richards WG. Invasion of the trophoblast. *Cell* 1992;71:355–7
4. Zhou Y, Fisher SJ, Janatpour M, *et al*. Human cytotrophoblasts adopt a vascular phenotype as they differentiate: a strategy for successful endovascular invasion? *J Clin Invest* 1997;99:2139–51
5. Giudice LC, Saleh W. Growth factors in reproduction. *Trends Endocrinol Metab* 1995;6:60–9
6. Hustin J. Vascular physiology and pathophysiology of early pregnancy. In Bourne T, Jauniaux E, Jurkovic D, eds. *Transvaginal Colour Doppler*. Heidelberg: Springer-Verlag, 1995:47–56
7. Hustin J, Schaaps JP, Lambotte R. Anatomical studies of the utero-placental vascularization in the first trimester of pregnancy. *Trophoblast Res* 1988;3:49–60
8. Jaffe R, Jauniaux E, Hustin J. Maternal circulation in the first trimester human placenta – myth or reality? *Am J Obstet Gynecol* 1997;176:695–705
9. Meekins JW, Luckas MJM, Pijnenborg R, *et al*. Histological study of decidual spiral arteries and the presence of maternal erythrocytes in the intervillous space during the first trimester of normal human pregnancy. *Placenta* 1997;18:459–64
10. Nanaev A, Chwalisz K, Frank HG, *et al*. Physiological dilation of uteroplacental arteries in the guinea pig depends on nitric oxide synthase activity of extravillous trophoblast. *Cell Tissue Res* 1995;282:407–21
11. Rodesch F, Simon P, Donner C, *et al*. Oxygen measurements in the materno-trophoblastic border during early pregnancy. *Obstet Gynecol* 1992;80:283–5
12. Jaffe R, Dorgan A, Abramowicz JS. Color Doppler imaging of uteroplacental circulation in the first trimester: value in prediction pregnancy failure or complication. *Am J Roentgenol* 1995;164:1255–8
13. Jauniaux E, Jurkovic D, Campbell S. Current topic: *in vivo* investigation of the placental circulation by Doppler echography. *Placenta* 1995;16:323–31
14. Kam EPY, Gardner L, Loke YW, *et al*. The role of trophoblast in the physiological change in decidual spiral arteries. *Hum Reprod* 1999;14:2131–8
15. Lin S, Shimizu I, Suehara N, *et al*. Uterine artery Doppler velocimetry in relation to trophoblast migration into the myometrium of the placental bed. *Obstet Gynecol* 1995;85:760–5
16. Vicovac L, Aplin JD. Epithelial–mesenchymal transition during trophoblast differentiation. *Acta Anat* 1996;156:202–16
17. Myatt L. Current topic: control of vascular resistance in the human placenta. *Placenta* 1992;13:329–41
18. Seligman SP, Buyon JP, Clancy RM, *et al*. The role of nitric oxide in the pathogenesis of pre-eclampsia. *Am J Obstet Gynecol* 1994;171:944–8
19. Graf AH, Hutter W, Hacker GW, *et al*. Localization and distribution of vasoactive neuropeptides in the human placenta. *Placenta* 1996;17:413–21
20. Shepherd RW, Stanczyk FZ, Betha CL, *et al*. Fetal and maternal endocrine responses to reduced uteroplacental blood flow. *J Clin Endocrinol Metab* 1992;75:301–7
21. Merviel P, Challier JC, Carbillon L, *et al*. The role of integrins in human embryo implantation. *Fetal Diagn Ther* 2001;in press
22. Zhou Y, Damsky CH, Chiu K, *et al*. Pre-eclampsia is associated with abnormal expression of adhesion molecules by invasive cytotrophoblasts. *J Clin Invest* 1993;91:950–60
23. Genbacev O, Joslin R, Damsky CH, *et al*. Hypoxia alters early gestation human cytotrophoblast differentiation/invasion *in vitro* and models the placental defects that occur in pre-eclampsia. *J Clin Invest* 1996;97:540–50
24. Walsh SW. Pre-eclampsia: an imbalance in placental prostacyclin and thromboxane production. *Am J Obstet Gynecol* 1985;152:335–40
25. Maseki M, Nishigaki I, Hagihara M, *et al*. Lipid peroxide levels and lipid content of serum lipoprotein fractions of pregnant subjects with and without pre-eclampsia. *Clin Chim Acta* 1981;115:155–61
26. Nelson GH, Zuspan FP, Mulligan LT. Defects of lipid metabolism in toxemia of pregnancy. *Am J Obstet Gynecol* 1966;94:310–15
27. Fox H. Effect of hypoxia on trophoblast in organ culture: a morphologic and autographic study. *Am J Obstet Gynecol* 1970;107:1058–64
28. Tsukimori K, Maeda H, Shingu M, *et al*. The possible role of endothelial cells in hypertensive disorders during pregnancy. *Obstet Gynecol* 1992;80:229–33
29. Davidge ST, Hubel CA, Brayden RD, *et al*. Sera antioxidant activity in uncomplicated and pre-eclamptic pregnancies. *Obstet Gynecol* 1992;79:897–901

30. Jauniaux E, Watson AL, Hempstock J, *et al*. Onset of maternal arterial blood flow and placental oxidative stress. A possible factor in human early pregnancy failure. *Am J Pathol* 2000;157:2111–22

31. Oian P, Kjeldsen SE, Eide I, *et al*. Increased arterial catecholamines in pre-eclampsia. *Acta Obstet Gynecol Scand* 1986;65:613–17

32. Mochizuki M, Morikawa H, Yamasaki M, *et al*. Vascular reactivity in normal and abnormal gestation. *Am J Kidney Dis* 1991;17:139–43

33. Halliwell B. Free radicals, antioxidants, and human diseases: curiosity, cause or consequence? *Lancet* 1994;344:721–4

34. Estelles A, Gilabert J, Grancha S, *et al*. Abnormal expression of type 1 plasminogen activator inhibitor and tissue factor in severe pre-eclampsia. *Thromb Haemost* 1998;79:500–8

35. Redman CWG, Sacks GP, Sargent IL. Pre-eclampsia: an excessive maternal inflammatory response to pregnancy. *Am J Obstet Gynecol* 1999; 180:499–506

New therapeutic developments in brain-orientated intensive care in the term and preterm newborn

35

L. Cornette and M. I. Levene

INTRODUCTION

The developing brain is an extremely vulnerable organ and is subject to a wide range of insults that may alter its structure or function. Apart from congenital structural defects and inborn metabolic disorders, a variety of perinatal insults may affect brain function, i.e. hemorrhagic lesions (with or without post-hemorrhagic hydrocephalus), hypoxic/ischemic injury, infection and metabolic disorders (e.g. hyperbilirubinemia, hypoglycemia). The spectrum of long-term morbidity consists of cerebral palsy, seizure disorders, mental retardation, visual or hearing impairments, behavioral problems and learning disabilities.

Prevention and treatment strategies are complicated by the fact that each pattern of brain injury will vary with the severity and duration of the insult, as well as with the gestational age of the fetus or infant at the time of the insult. Indeed, the developing brain is intrinsically vulnerable. For instance, intraventricular hemorrhage (IVH) remains a major cause of morbidity and mortality in premature infants. At the present time, there is still insufficient evidence to recommend any specific treatment to prevent IVH; careful postnatal hemodynamic stabilization and ventilatory support remain most important. However, the increased use of imaging techniques such as magnetic resonance (MR) in neonatal intensive care[1] has provided us with promising new insights into hemorrhagic brain injury. For instance, optimization of MR acquisition techniques has recently led to the observation of punctate brain lesions, most likely representing areas of petechial hemorrhage,

which we are currently investigating for their clinical significance[2].

In addition, intense experimental animal work over the past decade has led to a considerably improved understanding of non-hemorrhagic brain injury, especially hypoxic/ischemic injury and central nervous system infection[3]. Hence, what follows is a concise overview of those pathophysiological mechanisms in both types of insult that may be amenable to neuroprotective intervention. We will distinguish between currently available therapies and more innovative strategies that may lead to future clinical applications.

PATHOPHYSIOLOGY

Hypoxic-ischemic encephalopathy

Hypoxic-ischemic encephalopathy (HIE) is an evolving process, which begins during the primary hypoxic-ischemic insult (primary injury) and extends into the recovery period (secondary injury)[4]. This dynamic concept is supported by the typical delay in onset of seizures and other signs of encephalopathy several hours following an insult[5], as well as in the delayed and sequential evolution of neuroimaging findings[6,7]. Typical patterns of vulnerability (e.g. putamen, thalamus and peri-Rolandic cortex) seem related to the intrinsic properties of neurons, rather than to a pattern of vascular supply or redistribution of cerebral blood flow[8].

Details of hypoxic-ischemic-reperfusion excitotoxicity have recently been discussed in excellent reviews[9,10]. In essence, when cerebral perfusion is too low to provide adequate cerebral oxygenation, a cascade of biochemical events is initiated. Depletion of oxygen during reduction in cerebral blood flow (CBF) initiates anaerobic metabolism (glycolysis). Reduction in oxidative phosphorylation results in depletion of adenosine triphosphate (ATP) and other high-energy reserves, but also accumulation of adenosine and hypoxanthine. Hence, failure of energy-dependent re-uptake pumps that normally move the excitatory neurotransmitter glutamate out of the synapse into glial cells leads to an overstimulation of the N-methyl-D-aspartate (NMDA)-type glutamate receptor. Cytotoxic edema is the result of lethal amounts of calcium and water influx into neurons through the NMDA channels. Calcium overload in turn leads to cell damage by activating proteases, lipases and endonucleases.

Reoxygenation of ischemic tissues during the recovery period is necessary to prevent additional damage to the neural tissue. However, adenosine and hypoxanthine are oxidized to xanthine and uric acid by xanthine oxidase. This produces damaging amounts of highly reactive superoxide radicals, converted by superoxide dismutase to hydrogen peroxide (secondary injury)[11,12]. Also, the weak free radical nitric oxide (NO) is produced through activation of NO synthase. NO disrupts mitochondrial function through both a direct membrane attack mechanism and indirect energy depletion. Mitochondrial disruption results in delayed neuronal death by either necrosis (passive process of cell swelling, and rupture of nuclear and cytoplasmatic membranes) or induction of apoptosis (active suicide program through caspase enzymes, see below).

Perinatal infection

Over the past decades, it was thought that periventricular leukomalacia in the preterm infant was caused by hypoperfusion of the boundary zones, i.e. the zone between the ventriculofugal and ventriculopetal arteries in the periventricular white matter. Since the demonstration that these 'arteries', in fact, reflect transcerebral venous structures[13], a rapidly expanding body of evidence currently provides support for a causal relationship between perinatal infection outside of the central nervous system and damage to the developing white matter through a range of inflammatory molecules[14,15]. Such an infection remote from the brain results in the production of inflammatory molecules that easily cross the (fetal) blood–brain barrier[16].

Pro-inflammatory cytokines such as interleukin (IL)-1β, IL-6 and tumor necrosis factor-α (TNF-α) enhance inflammation as they activate microglia/macrophages and stimulate production of adhesion molecules (see below) on endothelial and neutrophil surfaces. These cytokines are elevated in the amniotic fluid of women who give birth before term[17], in fetal blood obtained by cordocentesis in preterm infants suffering white matter damage[18], in traumatic head injury[19] and in hypoxic/ischemic conditions, facilitating the infiltration of leukocytes into reperfused tissue[20]. Whereas perinatal infection involves a more systemic inflammatory response, a local inflammatory response is involved in hypoxia-ischemia. However, the interaction between excitotoxicity and inflammation is complex. For example, IL-1β amplifies excitotoxic brain damage *in vivo*, whereas it ameliorates neuronal death *in vitro*[21]. IL-6 possesses both pro- and anti-inflammatory properties[22]. TNF-α protects embryonic rat hippocampal neuronal cultures against glutamate-induced cell death, but exacerbates glutamate-induced damage to fetal human neurons through blood–brain barrier disruption after hypoxia-ischemia[23].

Caspase enzymes play a key role in apoptosis during normal development, i.e. programmed cell death characterized by cytoplasmatic shrinkage, condensation of nuclear chromatin and DNA fragmentation. Caspase activity has also been observed in a variety of pathological conditions, including cerebral hypoxia-ischemia[24] and possibly also infection-induced inflammation[25]. A critical role for caspase-3 in response to excitotoxicity is suggested by a number of studies[26].

Finally, there is an important role of adhesion molecules, such as P-selectin and intercellular adhesion molecule-1 (ICAM-1). P-selectin and ICAM-1 are expressed on endothelial surfaces and thereby facilitate leukocyte adhesion. Again, levels of adhesion molecules are elevated in both infection and hypoxia-ischemia[27].

NEW THERAPEUTIC DEVELOPMENTS

Ongoing newborn brain injury can be interrupted through a careful selection from a whole arsenal of new neuroprotective strategies. Identification of newborns at high-risk for neurological morbidity needs to be extremely accurate, in view of the potential serious side-effects that are associated with more experimental interventions[28]. Therefore, selection of infants for early clinical interventions, which may be possible in the future, should take into account clinical information, biochemical parameters (e.g. brain-specific creatine kinase and protein S-100[29]), refined electrophysiological tests, and, if available, functional modalities such as diffusion-weighted MR imaging and, as recently reported in term infants suffering HIE, positron emission tomography[30]. It is also important to stress that any new strategy in perinatal brain care should supplement rather than replace standard brain-orientated approaches, facilitating an adequate perfusion and supply of nutrients to the brain (e.g. treatment of cerebral edema, convulsions, etc.). What follows is a concise overview of new neuroprotective strategies.

NEW STRATEGIES TESTED IN THE HUMAN NEWBORN

Cerebral hypothermia

Cerebral hypothermia has the potential to modify many of the likely causes of newborn brain injury, including the production of free radicals, excitotoxic amino acids and pro-inflammatory cytokines. Cerebral hypothermia also reduces metabolic rate, preserves tissue pH during impaired cerebral blood flow and inhibits events leading to apoptosis. By reducing and delaying several damaging processes, the technique may allow therapeutic agents to be neuroprotective at even longer intervals after the insult.

The cooling cap (circulation of cold water) together with overhead body heating is an effective method of selective brain cooling, minimizing adverse systemic effects[31]. Studies on adult animals have shown that lowering the brain temperature by as little as 3–4°C during global cerebral ischemia reduces neuronal cell damage dramatically[32]. Although brief hypothermia immediately after resuscitation has limited and inconsistent results, extended periods of mild to moderate cerebral cooling (from 24 to 72 h) attenuate brain damage and favorably affect the outcome in animals[33].

Hypothermia in the care of newborns and neonates is already well established during cardiothoracic open-heart surgery, neurosurgical procedures and acute head injury. Selective head cooling (72 h circulation of 10°C water through a coil of tubing wrapped around the head) in term infants after perinatal asphyxia is a safe and convenient method of quickly reducing brain temperature[34]. It should be instituted within several hours of birth, as delayed prolonged head cooling begun after the onset of post-asphyxial seizures is no longer neuroprotective[35]. The feasibility of moderate systemic hypothermia has recently been assessed in ten newborns at high risk of developing severe neonatal encephalopathy[36]. Hypothermia to a rectal temperature of 33–34°C was instituted within 6 h of birth. Electrolyte imbalances, increased blood viscosity and catecholamine mediated side-effects such as changes in blood pressure, glycemia, lactate levels, etc. were generally mild. However, in three out of the ten children, MR brain imaging revealed unusual patterns of injury which may be associated with hypothermia, i.e. transverse and straight sinus thrombosis, and extensive infarction. A recent study determined the neurodevelopmental outcome of infants with evidence of post-asphyxial encephalopathy, treated with head cooling and mild hypothermia[37]. The relatively wide range of outcomes indicated that its long-term efficacy is not proven in any clinical context. Further randomized, controlled studies through stringent multicenter trials are warranted to assess the efficacy and safety of prolonged systemic hypothermia after perinatal asphyxia.

Oxygen-free radical scavengers and inhibitors

Several free radical inhibitors have been examined in animal models. Desferrioxamine reduces free radicals in the newborn piglet brain by sequestrating iron, which is an important catalyst in the formation of free radicals, and reducing hydroxyl formation[38]. Lazeroids are 21-aminosteroids, able to scavenge peroxyl radicals in animal models of hypoxic-ischemic damage[39]. In newborn rats, the infarct volume could be reduced in a model of focal ischemia by application of allopurinol, i.e. a xanthine-oxidase inhibitor and free radical scavenger[40]. In a small randomized trial involving severely asphyxiated neonates, a beneficial effect of high-dose allopurinol (40 mg/kg) was recently observed on free radical status, post-asphyxial cerebral perfusion and electrical brain activity, without producing adverse effects[41].

FUTURE STRATEGIES IN BRAIN-ORIENTATED INTENSIVE CARE

The effectiveness and safety of a drug or brain protective procedure should have been successfully demonstrated in animal models before proceeding towards a clinical trial. Indeed, some of the target molecules exhibit fragile equilibria of biological activity, and hence, blocking their activity might also be harmful. Excellent reviews have been published on neuroprotective strategies that have shown promise in animal and adult studies[26]. We here summarize some strategies with the future potential of becoming a therapeutic strategy of neuroprotection in the newborn human brain.

Promoting endogenous protection

The preterm brain suffers increased vulnerability because of an immature blood–brain barrier, incomplete myelination and paucity of endogenous protectors[42]. Endogenous protector molecules or survival enhancers either promote oligodendrocyte differentiation and survival (oligotrophic function or protecting myelin formation) or enhance neuronal protection (neurotrophic function or suppressing programmed cell death mechanisms). These endogenously produced molecules and their receptors are induced following a range of insults, such as seizures, ischemia and hypoglycemia[26]. Several molecules are of interest for neuroprotection, such as insulin-like growth factors (IGFs), nerve growth factor (NGF), brain-derived neurotrophic factor (BDNF), neurotrophin-3 (NT-3), basic fibroblast growth factor (bFGF), platelet-derived growth factor (PDGF), ciliary neurotrophic factor (CNTF), transforming growth factor-β_1 (TGF-β_1), etc.[43]. In general, long-term *in vivo* survival of oligodendrocytes requires the concerted action of multiple extracellular signals[44]. In addition, several hormones, such as thyroid hormone[45] and corticosteroids[42] have an important but complex role in oligodendrocytic differentiation and neuronal growth.

IGF-I

In animals, IGF-I protects neuronal cells from calcium-mediated hypoglycemic damage and prevents apoptosis of cortical neurons following NMDA- and NO-mediated neurotoxicity[26]. It appears to be neuroprotective through two distinct derivatives, glycine-proline-glutamate and des-N-(1-3)-IGF-I[46]. IGF-I plays a crucial role in normal oligodendrocyte development and myelination and is currently under investigation for the promotion of remyelination in adults suffering from multiple sclerosis[47]. Since its production appears to be under the regulation of growth hormone (GH), it has been suggested that GH may exert neuroprotective effects similar to those shown by IGF-I[48]. IGF-I administration in animals is maximally effective when administered 2 h after an ischemic insult. However, the therapeutic window increases to 6 h when combining IGF-I administration with cerebral hypothermia, suggesting such a combination may offer real opportunity for future therapeutic intervention[46].

NGF

Negligible levels of NGF in the cerebrospinal fluid (CSF) of asphyxiated newborns may be a useful biochemical marker for early estimates of neuronal death and potentially adverse outcome[49]. Many of the neurotrophic factors cannot cross the blood–brain barrier and do not distribute properly after systemic administration. An elegant way to overcome this problem is to induce endogenous growth factor synthesis in affected brain regions by administering low molecular weight lipophilic drugs, such as β-adrenoceptor agonists[50]. Such increased responsiveness to NGF protection in rats is observed for higher gestational age[51].

VEGF and bFGF

These endogenous neuroprotective cytokines are capable of improving tissue resistance through neo-angiogenesis[52]. Future studies will focus on their possible benefits through exogenous enhancement.

IL-10

IL-10 is an anti-inflammatory cytokine that downregulates IL-1 and TNF-α. In animals, its systemic administration after middle cerebral artery occlusion significantly reduces infarct size[53]. IL-10 has also been studied extensively in infants suffering chronic lung disease, where it is present in the broncho-alveolar lavage fluid of term but not preterm infants[54]. Hence, it is to be tested whether IL-10 administration will reduce inflammation-related damage to the preterm white matter.

TGF-β$_1$

Administration of recombinant human TGF-β$_1$ reduces cortical infarction and neuronal loss in several brain regions[46]. Activin is a member of the TGF-β superfamily. It promotes the survival of neurons in culture and protects against toxicity[55].

Inflammatory response modifiers

Anti-inflammatory strategies may apply to both infectious and hypoxic/ischemic initiators of white matter damage[56]. Exogenous administration of inflammatory response modifiers is currently practised in adults with rheumatoid arthritis and in multiple sclerosis. Administration of these molecules aiming at neuroprotection is, however, still under study in animals; no reports are available on clinical trials in the newborn brain.

TNF-α antagonism

Increased permeability of the blood–brain barrier during hypoxia-ischemia can be attenuated by treatment with anti-TNF-α antibodies[57]. Intraventricular administration of anti-TNF-α antibodies, in a mouse model of middle cerebral artery occlusion, reduced both infarct volume and expression of ICAM-1[58]. Fetal blood sampling in patients with preterm labor and preterm premature rupture of the membranes indicated an increased availability of the soluble receptors of TNF-α compared to a control group. Administration of TNF-receptors, buffering the deleterious biological activity of TNF-α, may thus offer a neuroprotective strategy[59]. However, mortality increased with increasing doses of such receptors during a recent randomized trial in adults with septic shock, indicating TNF-α has benefits as well[60]. The use of anti-TNF-α antibodies in animal models of meningitis is controversial[61].

Cytokine-receptor blockers

The administration of the IL-1β receptor antagonist prevented preterm delivery in mice[62] and reduced brain injury in animal models of hypoxia-ischemia[63]. It has also been suggested that the IL-1β receptor antagonist acts through downregulation of ICAM-1 expression[64]. Etanercept, used in active rheumatoid arthritis and inflammatory bowel disease, is a fusion protein inhibiting the binding of TNF-α to its receptor[65]. Recently, its administration in a rat model of experimental brain injury has resulted in improved performance during a series of standardized motor tasks[19].

Caspase inhibition

In the developing rat brain, caspase inhibition interrupts programmed cell death and provides benefit over a prolonged therapeutic window after hypoxic-ischemic insults[66]. Caspase inhibition may also play a pivotal role in protecting oligodendrocytes during infection-induced inflammation[67].

Adhesion molecule antibodies

Using a rat model of hypoxia-ischemia, administration of anti-ICAM-1 antibodies[68] or anti-P-selectin antibodies results in a significant reduction of infarct size, polymorphonuclear leukocyte infiltration, brain edema and apoptosis[69]. However, whereas cellular adhesion molecule blockage reduces brain damage in experimental models, it may impair their physiological activity during further brain development and plasticity[70].

Excitotoxic cascade modifiers

In infants with asphyxia, CSF concentrations of excitatory amino acids, such as glutamate and aspartate, remain increased for some days[71]. Release of excitatory amino acids during and after cerebral ischemia in damaged brain regions can lead to epileptiform activity, which in turn can create an imbalance between CBF and cell metabolism, causing further brain damage.

Glutamate antagonists

Kynurenic acid has been shown to exert a strong neuroprotective effect against hypoxic-ischemic brain damage in adult[72] and neonatal animals[73]. NMDA-receptor antagonists, such as ketamine, cerestat, dizocilpine, dextromethorphan, MK-801 and phencyclidine, have been proven successful in animal studies, acting through a direct or indirect decrease of intracellular calcium accumulation[74]. Because of deleterious cardiovascular effects[75] and induction of apoptotic cell death in the immature brain[76], their use as neuroprotective agents in the neonate is currently not recommended. However, alternative pharmacological strategies are under way, modulating other sites of the NMDA–receptor complex.

NO-synthase inhibitors

Aminoguanidine is a relatively selective inhibitor of inducible NO synthase. When used in a neonatal ischemic rat model, the drug resulted in suppression of NO production after reperfusion and significant reduction of infarct size[77]. NO-synthase inhibition is a potential post-insult strategy and its usefulness could be extended when combined with cerebral hypothermia[78].

Miscellaneous

Sodium channel blockers

Voltage-dependent sodium channel blockers may have a role in the preservation of cerebral vascular reactivity and maintenance of normal CBF (autoregulation). Indeed, cerebral vasodilatation through vascular paralysis is a consistently observed phenomenon after prolonged asphyxia. In addition, sodium channel blockers can delay anoxic depolarization, attenuate extracellular accumulation of glutamate and reduce ATP depletion during ischemia[26]. However, these drugs seem neuroprotective only when given prior to a HIE insult in animal models[79].

Fructose-1,6-diphosphate

Fructose-1,6-diphosphate facilitates adaptive changes in membrane ionic permeability and enhances metabolic efficiency of cells during stress episodes via increased glycolysis, preventing generation of reactive oxygen intermediates and maintaining normal calcium homeostasis[80]. Its administration significantly reduced brain injury in a neonatal rat model of hypoxia-ischemia[81]. It is currently used in phase II clinical trials for improvement of heart recovery in bypass surgery. It may also become a new avenue in neuroprotection.

Creatine

Exogenous supplementation of creatine stabilizes ATP concentrations during anoxic conditions through raised phosphocreatine pools in neonatal mice[82]. Hence, creatine might also be neuroprotective in humans, by preventing hypoxic energy failure.

Not convincing strategies

Calcium channel blockers

Although reduction of intracellular calcium overload during hypoxic-ischemic injury is desirable, the use of calcium channel blockers does not convincingly prevent calcium toxicity. In animals, nimodipine did not result in a neuroprotective effect[83] and flunarizine yielded only partial protective effects[84]. Nicardipine has been tested in four severely asphyxiated infants, but hemodynamic management was severely impaired[85].

Magnesium sulfate

A number of pathophysiological mechanisms have been put forward to explain its neuroprotective effect in HIE, such as blockage of the NMDA receptor and voltage-dependent calcium channels, prevention of excitatory amino acids release, anticonvulsive action and reduced cell metabolism[71]. To date, research suggests that administration of magnesium sulfate can lower the incidence of cerebral palsy in immature neonates of less than 1500 g[86], and this is the subject of a number of ongoing randomized control trials. Human neonatal cortex, compared to older infants, has fewer NMDA receptors and a low potential of magnesium to block the receptors[87]. Accordingly, in a mouse model of excitotoxic neuronal death, magnesium offered protection only after the stage of brain development at which magnesium could block NMDA channels[88]. Obviously, such altered sensitivity suggests that therapeutic NMDA receptor block in newborns may require higher concentrations of magnesium sulfate than in older neonates. However, high doses of magnesium sulfate can cause potentially dangerous hypotension in asphyxiated infants[89]. A consistent therapeutic effect of magnesium still needs to be demonstrated in multicenter randomized, double-blind studies, but with the available evidence, it cannot be currently recommended for treatment of HIE.

Gangliosides

Monosialogangliosides are lipids that can be incorporated into neuronal cell membranes when administered systemically. However, their use in animal models resulted in only partial neuroprotective effects[90,91] and further research in this direction is not convincing.

CONCLUSION

Considerable progress has been made in understanding the pathophysiological mechanisms of neonatal brain damage. Various pathways are currently targeted as a potential means of inhibiting irreversible brain injury. A new arsenal of potential neuroprotective strategies have been evaluated in experimental models for their efficacy and long-term safety. The hope exists for their clinical implementation in the foreseeable future.

However, there seems to be a discrepancy between the promising results of animal experiments and a relatively weak body of evidence on clinical effectiveness in human newborns. Several reasons account for this discrepancy. First, our understanding of the complex pathophysiological processes defining onset, duration and severity of any cerebral insult is still incomplete. The question then arises whether we should consider the administration of protector molecules to all women likely to deliver a very preterm newborn, as brain damage may occur antenatally[92] and as responsiveness to endogenous protectors is higher for a younger gestational age[51]. Second, while the so-called therapeutic window can extend from several hours to a day or more in adults, this may not be the case in perinatal animals and presumably in human neonates, where the processes of neuronal necrosis and apoptosis may occur in a range of 2–6 h[93] Third, there may be inadequate brain penetration and/or dosage of the drug to block the targeted mechanism of damage. Fourth, measures of outcome may be insufficiently sensitive or efficient. Finally, there are many barriers to research in newborns, such as social and emotional factors that come with the unknown, leading parents to withhold from giving informed consent.

For all the above-mentioned reasons, we, as others[94], argue for further well-controlled, multicenter, randomized experimental trials of efficacy and safety of neuroprotective strategies in clinical neonatal settings. What we need is a more intense collaboration among basic (neuro)-scientists, clinicians and members of the pharmaceutical industry. The potential benefits for infants born in the future, their families and our whole society make this a high priority.

References

1. Barkovich AJ. Normal development of the neonatal and infant brain, skull and spine. In Barkovich AJ, ed. *Pediatric Neuroimaging*. Philadelphia: Lippincott Williams & Wilkins, 2000:13–69

2. Cornette L, Tanner SF, Ramenghi L, Miall L, Childs AM, Arthur RJ, Martinez D, Levene MI. Punctate lesions in the infant brain: MR imaging characteristics and clinical significance. *Arch Dis Child*;in press

3. de Haan HH, Gunn AJ, Gluckman PD. Experiments in perinatal brain injury: what have we learnt? *Prenat Neonat Med* 1996;1:16–25

4. Hope PL, Costello AM, Cady EB, Delpy DT, Tofts PS, Chu A, Hamilton PA, Reynolds EO, Wilkie DR. Cerebral energy metabolism studied with phosphorus NMR spectroscopy in normal and birth-asphyxiated infants. *Lancet* 1984;18:366–70

5. Johnston MV, Trescher WH, Taylor GA. Hypoxic and ischemic central nervous system disorders in infants and children. *Adv Pediatr* 1995;42:1–45

6. Barkovich AJ, Westmark K, Partridge C, Sola A, Ferriero DM. Perinatal asphyxia: MR findings in the first 10 days. *Am J Neuroradiol* 1995;16:427–38

7. Sie LT, van der Knapp MS, van Wezel-Meijler G, Taets van Amerongen AH, Lafeber HN, Valk J. Early MR features of hypoxic-ischemic brain injury in neonates with periventricular densities on sonograms. *Am J Neuroradiol* 2000;21:852–61

8. Johnston MV, Trescher WH, Ishida Q, Nakajima W. Neurobiology of hypoxic-ischemic injury in the developing brain. *Pediatr Res* 2001;49:735–41

9. Fellman V, Raivio KO. Reperfusion injury as the mechanism of brain damage after perinatal asphyxia. *Pediatr Res* 1997;41:599–606

10. du Plessis AJ, Johnston MV. Hypoxic-ischemic brain injury in the newborn. Cellular mechanisms and potential strategies for neuroprotection. *Clin Perinatol* 1997;24:627–54

11. Berger R, Garnier Y. Pathophysiology of perinatal brain damage. *Brain Res Rev* 1999;30:107–34

12. McCord JM. Oxygen-derived free radicals in post-ischemic tissue injury. *N Engl J Med* 1985;312:159–63

13. Moody DM, Bell MA, Challa VR. Features of the cerebral vascular pattern that predict vulnerability to perfusion or oxygenation deficiency: an anatomic study. *Am J Neuroradiol* 1990;11:431–9

14. Adinolfi M. Infectious diseases in pregnancy, cytokines and neurological impairment: an hypothesis. *Dev Med Child Neurol* 1993;35:549–53

15. Dammann O, Leviton A. Maternal intrauterine infection, cytokines, and brain damage in the preterm newborn. *Pediatr Res* 1997;42:1–8

16. Adinolfi M. The development of the human blood-CSF-brain barrier. *Dev Med Child Neurol* 1985;27:527–32

17. Yoon BH, Romero R, Jun JK, Park KH, Park JD, Ghezzi F, Kim BI. Amniotic fluid cytokines (interleukin-6, tumor necrosis factor-alpha, interleukin-1 beta, and interleukin-8) and the risk for the development of bronchopulmonary dysplasia. *Am J Obstet Gynecol* 1997;177:825–30

18. Yoon BH, Romero R, Yang SH, Jun JK, Kim IO, Choi JH, Syn HC. Interleukin-6 concentrations in umbilical cord plasma are elevated in neonates with white matter lesions associated with periventricular leukomalacia. *Am J Obstet Gynecol* 1996;174:1433–40

19. Knoblach SM, Fan L, Faden AI. Early neuronal expression of tumor necrosis factor-alpha after experimental brain injury contributes to neurological impairment. *J Neuroimmunol* 1999;95: 115–25

20. Bona E, Andersson AL, Blomgren K, Gilland E, Puka-Sundvall M, Gustafson K, Hagberg H. Chemokine and inflammatory cell response to hypoxia-ischemia in immature rats. *Pediatr Res* 1999;45:500–9

21. Loddick SA, Rothwell NJ. Commentary. Mechanisms of tumor necrosis factor alpha action on neurodegeneration: interactions with insulin-like growth factor-1. *Proc Natl Acad Sci USA* 1999; 96:9449–51

22. Martin-Ancel A, Garcia-Alix A, Pascual-Salcedo D, Cabanas F, Valcarce M, Quero J. Interleukin-6 in the cerebrospinal fluid after perinatal asphyxia is related to early and late neurological manifestations. *Pediatrics* 1997;100:789–94

23. Cheng B, Christakos S, Mattson MP. Tumor necrosis factors protect neurons against metabolic-excitotoxic insults and promote maintenance of calcium homeostasis. *Neuron* 1994;12:139–53

24. Nicholson DW, Thornberry NA. Caspases: killer proteases. *Trends Biochem Sci* 1997;22:299–306

25. Silverstein FS. Can inhibition of apoptosis rescue ischemic brain? *J Clin Invest* 1998;101:1809–10

26. Hagberg H, Blomgren K, Mallard C. Neuroprotection of the fetal and neonatal brain. In Levene MI, Chervenak FA, Whittle M, eds. *Fetal and Neonatal Neurology and Neurosurgery*. London: Churchill Livingstone, 2001

27. Silverstein FS, Barks JD, Hagan P, Liu XH, Ivacko J, Szaflarski J. Cytokines and perinatal brain injury. *Neurochem Int* 1997;30:375–83

28. Perlman JM. Markers of asphyxia and neonatal brain injury. *N Engl J Med* 1999;341:364–5

29. Nagdyman N, Kömen W, Ko HK, Müller C, Obladen M. Early biochemical indicators of hypoxic-ischemic encephalopathy after birth asphyxia. *Pediatr Res* 2001;49:502–6

30. Thorngren-Jerneck K, Ohlsson T, Sandell Q, Erlandsson K, Strand SE, Ryding E, Svenningsen NW. Cerebral glucose metabolism measured by positron emission tomography in term newborn infants with hypoxic ischemic encephalopathy. *Pediatr Res* 2001;49:495–501

31. Thoresen M, Simmonds M, Satas S, Tooley J, Silver IA. Effective selective head cooling during posthypoxic hypothermia in newborn piglets. *Pediatr Res* 2001;49:594–9

32. Wagner CL, Eicher DJ, Katikaneni LD, Barbosa E, Holden KR. The use of hypothermia: a role in the treatment of neonatal asphyxia? *Pediatr Neurol* 1999;21:429–43

33. Gunn AJ, Gunn TR, Gunning MI, Williams CE, Gluckman PD. Neuroprotection with prolonged head cooling started before postischemic seizures in fetal sheep. *Pediatrics* 1998;102:1098–106

34. Gunn AJ, Gluckman PD, Gunn TR. Selective head cooling in newborn infants after perinatal asphyxia: a safety study. *Pediatrics* 1998;102: 885–92

35. Gunn AJ, Bennet L, Gunning MI, Gluckman PD, Gunn TR. Cerebral hypothermia is not neuroprotective when started after postischemic seizures in fetal sheep. *Pediatr Res* 1999;46:274–80

36. Battin MR, Dezoete JA, Gunn TR, Gluckman PD, Gunn AJ. Neurodevelopmental outcome of infants treated with head cooling and mild hypothermia after perinatal asphyxia. *Pediatrics* 2001;107: 480–4

37. Azzopardi D, Robertson NJ, Cowan FM, Rutherford MA, Rampling M, Edwards AD. Pilot study of treatment with whole body hypothermia for neonatal encephalopathy. *Pediatrics* 2000;106: 684–94

38. Feng Y, LeBlanc MH, LeBlanc EB, Parker CC, Fratkin JD, Qian XB, Patel DM, Huang M, Smith EE, Vig PJ. Desmethyl trilazad improves neurologic function after hypoxic ischemic brain injury in piglets. *Crit Care Med* 2000;28:1431–8

39. Vannucci RC, Perlman JM. Interventions for perinatal hypoxic-ischaemic encephalopathy. *Pediatrics* 1997;100:1004–14

40. Palmer C, Vannucci RC, Towfighi J. Reduction of perintal hypoxic-ischemic brain damage with allopurinol. *Pediatr Res* 1990;27:332–6

41. Van Bel F, Shadid M, Moison RM, Dorrepaal CA, Fontijn J, Monteiro L, Van De Bor M, Berger HM. Effect of allopurinol on postasphyxial free radical formation, cerebral hemodynamics and electrical brain activity. *Pediatrics* 1998;101: 185–93

42. Dammann O, Leviton A. Brain damage in preterm new-borns: might enhancement of developmentally regulated endogenous protection open a door for prevention? *Pediatrics* 1999;104:541–50

43. Semkova I, Krieglstein J. Neuroprotection mediated via neurotrophic factors and induction of neurotrophic factors. *Brain Res Rev* 1999;30: 176–88

44. Barres BA, Schmid R, Sendtner M, Raff MC. Multiple extracellular signals are required for long-term oligodendrocyte survival. *Development* 1993;118:283–95

45. Pasquini JM, Adamo AM. Thyroid hormones and the central nervous system. *Dev Neurosci* 1994; 16:1–8

46. Gluckman PD, Pinal CS, Gunn AJ. Hypoxic-ischemic brain injury in the newborn: pathophysiology and potential strategies for intervention. *Semin Neonatol* 2001;6:109–20

47. McMorris FA, Mozell RL, Carson MJ, Shinar Y, Meyer RD, Marchetti N. Regulation of oligodendrocyte development and central nervous system myelination by insulin-like growth factors. *Ann NY Acad Sci* 1993;27:321–34

48. Gustafson K, Hagberg H, Bengtsson BA, Brantsing C, Isgaard J. Possible protective role of growth hormone in hypoxia-ischemia in neonatal rats. *Pediatr Res* 1999;45:318–23

49. Riikonen RS, Korhonen LT, Lindholm DB. Cerebrospinal nerve growth factor – a marker of asphyxia? *Pediatr Neurol* 1999;20:137–41

50. Culmsee C, Stumm RK, Schafer MK, Weihe E, Krieglstein J. Clenbuterol induces growth factor mRNA, activates astrocytes, and protects rat brain tissue against ischemic damage. *Eur J Pharmacol* 1999;379:33–45

51. Cheng Y, Gidday JM, Yan Q, Shah AR, Holtzman DM. Marked age-dependent neuroprotection by brain-derived neurotrophic factor against neonatal hypoxic-ischemic brain injury. *Ann Neurol* 1997; 41:521–9

52. Milner R, Anderson HJ, Rippon RF, McKay JS, Franklin RJ, Marchionni MA, Reynolds R, Ffrench-Constant C. Contrasting effects of mitogenic growth factors on oligodendrocyte precursor cell migration. *Glia* 1997;19:85–90

53. Spera PA, Ellison JA, Feuerstein GZ, Barone FC. IL-10 reduces rat brain injury following focal stroke. *Neurosci Lett* 1998;251:189–92

54. Jones CA, Cayabyab RG, Kwong KY, Stotts C, Wong B, Hamdan H, Minoo P, deLemos RA. Undetectable interleukin (IL)-10 and persistent IL-8 expression early in hyaline membrane disease: a possible developmental basis for the predisposition to chronic lung inflammation in preterm new-borns. *Pediatr Res* 1996;39: 966–75

55. Schubert D, Kimura H, LaCorbiere M, Vaughan J, Karr D, Fischer WH. Activin is a nerve cell survival molecule. *Nature* 1990;344:868–70

56. Dammann O, Leviton A. Brain damage in preterm new-borns: biological response modification as a strategy to reduce disabilities. *J Pediatr* 2000;136: 433–8

57. Yang GY, Gong C, Qin Z, Liu XH, Lorris Betz A. Tumor necrosis factor alpha expression produces increased blood-brain barrier permeability following temporary focal cerebral ischemia in mice. *Brain Res Mol Brain Res* 1999;69:135–43

58. Yang GY, Gong C, Qin Z, Ye W, Mao Y, Betz AL. Inhibition of TNFalpha attenuates infarct volume and ICAM-1 expression in ischemic mouse brain. *Neuroreport* 1998;22:2131–4

59. Romero R, Maymon E, Pacora P, Gomez R, Mazor M, Yoon BH, Berry SM. Further observations on the fetal inflammatory response syndrome: a potential homeostatic role for the soluble receptors of tumor necrosis factor alpha. *Am J Obstet Gynecol* 2000;183:1070–7

60. Fisher CJ Jr, Agosti JM, Opal SM, Lowry SF, Balk RA, Sadoff JC, Abraham E, Schein RM, Benjamin E. Treatment of septic shock with the tumor necrosis factor receptor: Fc fusion protein. The Soluble TNF Receptor Sepsis Study Group. *N Engl J Med* 1996;334:1697–702

61. Bogdan I, Leib SL, Bergeron M. Tumor necrosis factor-α contributes to apoptosis in hippocampal neurons during experimental group B Streptococcal meningitis. *J Infect Dis* 1997;176:693–7

62. Romero R, Tartakovsky B. The natural interleukin-1 receptor antagonist prevents interleukin-1-induced preterm delivery in mice. *Am J Obstet Gynecol* 1992;167:1041–5

63. Hagberg H, Gilland E, Bona E, Hanson LA, Hahin-Zoric M, Blennow M, Holst M, McRae A, Soder O. Enhanced expression of interleukin (IL)-1 and IL-6 messenger RNA and bioactive protein after hypoxia-ischemia in neonatal rats. *Pediatr Res* 1996;40:603–9

64. Yang GY, Mao Y, Zhou LF, Gong C, Ge HL, Betz AL. Expression of intercellular adhesion molecule 1 (ICAM-1) is reduced in permanent focal cerebral ischemic mouse brain using an adenoviral vector to induce overexpression of interleukin-1 receptor antagonist. *Brain Res Mol Brain Res* 1999;65: 143–50

65. Blam ME, Stein RB, Lichtenstein GR. Integrating anti-tumor necrosis factor therapy in inflammatory bowel disease: current and future perspectives. *Am J Gastroenterol* 2001;96:1977–97

66. Cheng Y, Deshmukh M, D'Costa A, Demaro JA, Gidday JM, Shah A, Sun Y, Jacquin MF, Johnson EM, Holtzman DM. Caspase inhibitor affords neuroprotecion with delayed administration in a rat model of neonatal hypoxic-ischaemic brain injury. *J Clin Invest* 1998;101:1992–9

67. Shibata M, Hisahara S, Hara H, Yamawaki T, Fukuuchi Y, Yuan J, Okano H, Miura M. Caspases determine the vulnerability of oligodendrocytes in the ischemic brain. *J Clin Invest* 2000;106:643–53

68. Kyrkanides S, Olschowka JA, Williams JP, Hansen JT, O'Banion MK. TNF alpha and IL-1 beta mediate intercellular adhesion molecule-1 induction via microglia-astrocyte interaction in CNS radiation injury. *J Neuroimmunol* 1999;95:95–106

69. Suzuki H, Hayashi T, Tojo SJ, Kitagawa H, Kimura K, Mizugaki M, Itoyama Y, Abe K. Anti-P-selectin antibody attenuates rat brain ischemic injury. *Neurosci Lett* 1999;265:163–6

70. Cotman CW, Hailer NP, Pfister KK, Soltesz I, Schachner M. Cell adhesion molecules in neural

plasticity and pathology: similar mechanisms, distinct organizations? *Prog Neurobiol* 1998;55: 659–69

71. Hagberg H, Thornberg E, Blennow M, Kjellmer I, Lagercrantz H, Thiringer K, Hamberger A, Sandberg M. Excitatory amino acids in the cerebrospinal fluid of asphyxiated infants: relationship to hypoxic-ischemic encephalopathy. *Acta Paediatr* 1993;82:925–9

72. Park CK, Nehls DG, Graham DI, Teasdale GM, McCulloch J. The glutamate antagonist MK-801 reduces focal ischemic brain damage in the rat. *Ann Neurol* 1988;24:543–51

73. Andine P, Lehmann A, Ellren K, Wennberg E, Kjellmer I, Nielsen T, Hagberg H. The excitatory amino acid antagonist kynurenic acid administered after hypoxic ischemia in neonatal rat offers neuroprotection. *Neurosci Lett* 1988;90:208–12

74. Hattori H, Morin AM, Schwartz PH, Fujikawa DG, Wasterlain CG. Posthypoxic treatment with MK-801 reduces hypoxic/ischemic damage in the neonatal rat. *Neurology* 1989;39:713–18

75. Hurstveit O, Maurset A, Oye I. Interaction of the chiral forms of ketamine with opioid, phencyclidine, and muscarinic receptors. *Pharmacol Toxicol* 1995;77:355–9

76. Ikonomidou C, Bosch F, Miksa M, *et al.* Blockade of NMDA receptors and apoptotic neurodegeneration in the developing brain. *Science* 1999;283:70–4

77. Tsuji M, Higuchi Y, Shirqishi K, Kume T, Akaike A, Hattori H. Protective effect of aminoguanidine on hypoxic-ischemic brain damage and temporal profile of brain nitric oxide in neonatal rat. *Pediatr Res* 2000;47:79–83

78. Johnston MV, Trescher WH, Ishida A, Nakajima W. Novel treatments after experimental brain injury. *Semin Neonatol* 2000;5:75–86

79. Levine V, Pourcyrous M, Bada HS, Parfenova H, Yang W, Korones SB, Leffler CW. Preservation of cerebrovascular tone and reactivity by sodium channel inhibition in experimental prolonged asphyxia in piglets. *Pediatr Res* 2000;47:376–80

80. Roig T, Bartrons R, Bermudez J. Exogenous fructose 1,6-bisphosphate reduces K+ permeability in isolated rat hepatocytes. *Am J Physiol* 1997;273: C473–8

81. Sola A, Berrios M, Sheldon RA, Ferriero DM, Gregory GA. Fructose-1,6-biphosphate after hypoxic ischemic injury is protective to neonatal rat brain. *Brain Res* 1996;741:294–9

82. Wilken B, Ramirez JM, Probst I, Richter DW, Hanefeld F. Anoxic ATP depletion in neonatal mice brainstem is prevented by creatine supple-

mentation. *Arch Dis Child Fetal Neonatal Ed* 2000;82:F224–7

83. LeBlanc MH, Vig V, Randhawa T, Smith EE, Parker CC, Brown EG. Use of polyethylene glycol-bound superoxide dismutase, polyethylene glycol-bound catalase, and nimodipine to prevent hypoxic ischemic injury to the brain of newborn pigs. *Crit Care Med* 1993;21:252–9

84. Berger R, Lehmann T, Karcher J, Garnier Y, Jensen A. Low dose flunarizine protects the fetal brain from ischemic injury in sheep. *Pediatr Res* 1998;44:277–82

85. Levene MI, Gibson NA, Fenton AC, Papathoma E, Barnett D. The use of a calcium-channel blocker, nicardipine, for severely asphyxiated newborn infants. *Dev Med Child Neurol* 1990;32:567–74

86. Nelson KB, Gretherm JK. Can magnesium sulfate reduce the risk of cerebral palsy in very low birth-weight infants? *Pediatrics* 1995;95:263–9

87. Chahal H, D'Souza SW, Barson AJ, Slater P. Modulation of magnesium of N-methyl-D-aspartate receptors in developing human brain. *Arch Dis Child Fetal Neonatal Ed* 1998;78:F116–20

88. Marret S, Gressens P, Gadisseux JF, Evrard P. Prevention by magnesium of excitotoxic neuronal death in the developing brain: an animal model for clinical intervention studies. *Dev Med Child Neurol* 1995;37:473–84

89. Whitelaw A. Systematic review of therapy after hypoxic-ischaemic brain injury in the perinatal period. *Semin Neonatol* 2000;5:33–40

90. Hadjiconstantinou M, Yates AJ, Neff NH. Hypoxia-induced neurotransmitter deficits in neonatal rats are partially corrected by exogenous GM1 ganglioside. *J Neurochem* 1990;55:864–9

91. Tan WK, Williams CE, Gunn AJ, Mallard EC, Gluckman PD. Pretreatment with monosialoganglioside GM1 protects the brain of fetal sheep against hypoxic/ischemic injury without causing systemic compromise. *Pediatr Res* 1993;34:18–22

92. de Vries LS, Eken P, Groenendaal F, Rademaker KJ, Hoogervorst B, Bruinse HW. Antenatal onset of haemorrhagic and/or ischaemic lesions in preterm infants: prevalence and associated obstetric variables. *Arch Dis Child Fetal Neonatal Ed* 1998;78:F51–6

93. Islam N, Aftabuddin M, Moriwaki A, Hori Y. Detection of DNA damage induced by apoptosis in the rat brain following incomplete ischemia. *Neurosci Lett* 1995;188:159–62

94. Lucey JF. Neuroprotection and perinatal brain care: the field of the future, currently going nowhere!? *Pediatrics* 1997;100:1030–1

Index